Textbook of Diagnostic and Therapeutic Procedures in Allergy

Editors

Pudupakkam K. Vedanthan

University of Colorado Anschutz Campus
Aurora, Colorado USA

Harold S. Nelson

National Jewish Health
Denver, Colorado, USA

Hugo P.S. Van Bever

National University, Singapore

Mandakolathur R. Murali

Massachusetts General Hospital
and
Harvard Medical School
Boston, Massachusetts, USA

CRC Press
Taylor & Francis Group
Boca Raton London New York

CRC Press is an imprint of the
Taylor & Francis Group, an **informa** business

A SCIENCE PUBLISHERS BOOK

Cover picture credit: Personal Collections of the following authors. From Left to Right Pictures:

1. Hibiscus flower: Dr. Saibal Moitra (saibal.moitra@gmail.com)
2. Alair Catheter Expanding basket: Dr. Ali Musani (ALI.MUSANI@cuanschutz.edu)
3. Nasal Polyp: Dr. Jerald Koepke (jwkmlk@gmail.com), Dr. William K. Dolen (BDOLEN@augusta.edu)
4. CT Sinuses: Dr. Mary Beth Cunnane (MaryBeth_Cunnane@meei.harvard.edu)

First edition published 2024
by CRC Press
2385 NW Executive Center Drive, Suite 320, Boca Raton FL 33431

and by CRC Press
4 Park Square, Milton Park, Abingdon, Oxon, OX14 4RN

© 2024 Pudupakkam K. Vedanthan, Harold S. Nelson, Hugo P.S. Van Bever and Mandakolathur R. Murali

CRC Press is an imprint of Taylor & Francis Group, LLC

Library of Congress Cataloging-in-Publication Data (applied for)

ISBN: 978-1-032-21653-9 (hbk)
ISBN: 978-1-032-21654-6 (pbk)
ISBN: 978-1-003-26942-7 (ebk)

DOI: 10.1201/9781003269427

Typeset in Times New Roman
by Radiant Productions

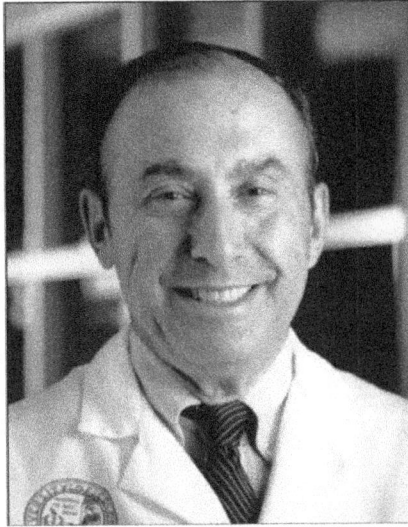

Late Dr. Henry Neumann Claman
December 13, 1930–September 3, 2016.
"A Renaissance Man"

Preface

National Jewish Health & University of Colorado, Denver, Colorado USA

It is my privilege to introduce the first edition of this novel and exciting textbook Diagnostic and Therapeutic Procedures in Allergy. This was a vision by the editors to provide a comprehensive yet practical reference, targeted at the clinician, for the commonly encountered procedures within the field of allergy and immunology. The textbook is truly unique since it provides a single source for both the commonly and uncommonly used tests within the field, while providing the advantages and limitations for the various tests. Additionally, for each test, rational, indications, precautions and interpretation are provided. The textbook is comprised of 15 chapters authored by an international faculty and laid out by clinical disease area, diagnostics in, asthma, food sensitivity, urticaria, allergic contact dermatitis, atopic dermatitis, drug sensitivity, immune deficiency, allergen immunotherapy, insect allergy, aerobiology, environmental control measures, biologics and concluding with controversial procedures in allergy. Another unique feature of this textbook is the amalgamation of eastern and western medicine through two chapter on the role of yoga and acupuncture. The reader will find the book not only illuminating but serve as an ongoing reference for their clinical practice. The textbook covers the breadth and depth of diagnostic testing while written by world renowned faculty with expertise in their respective areas of focus. I would like to thank the editors P.K. Vedanthan, H. Nelson, H Van Bever and M. Murali. I also want to thank the authors and co-authors for their tireless work in submitting overviews of the highest quality in a timely manner. Finally, I would like to acknowledge the publisher CRC Press (Taylor & Francis) for the guidance, and assistance in bringing to fruition a one-of-a-kind textbook.

Rohit Katial, MD, FAAAAI, FACAAI, FACP
Professor of Medicine
Associate Vice President of Education
Director, Center for Clinical Immunology

Irene J, and Dr. Abraham E. Goldminz,
Chair In Immunology and Respiratory Medicine
National Jewish Health & University of Colorado, Denver

International Asthma Services (www.saahns.org) (IAS)

International Asthma Services (IAS) under the chairmanship of Dr. Pudupakkam K. Vedanthan (Dr. PK) is proud to continue its global educational outreach. IAS is fortunate and thankful for the opportunity to present this unique 'textbook of diagnostic and therapeutic procedures in allergy'. The uniqueness of this textbook is that, it is the FIRST book of its kind and quality in the field of allergy.

IAS has been active in several developing nations with the main hub being in India. IAS has successfully partnered with major educational institutions and universities across the globe to initiate several training programs for physicians, physician assistants, and allergy technicians to cater to the burgeoning needs of the specialty especially in the developing world. IAS is highly indebted to dedicated faculty, advisory board of academicians as well as volunteers across the globe.

Contents

Chapter 1

Principles of Diagnostic Tests

Vijaya Knight[1] and *Mandakolathur R. Murali*[2],*

Introduction

The utility of diagnostic tests lies in their interpretation within a clinical context. To make effective use of diagnostic test results, the clinician should understand the terminology used to describe the performance of a diagnostic test and the application of test performance parameters to clinical diagnosis.

Evaluation of a diagnostic test's performance falls into three categories:

1) Preanalytical variables that have an impact on laboratory test results include characteristics such as the age of the subject, gender, body mass index and dietary factors, timing of blood samples and interference with assay characteristics.

2) Analytic test characteristics that describe the performance of the test within the laboratory environment.

3) Diagnostic test characteristics that describe the test performance in relevant clinical populations. The scope of this chapter is to describe briefly the analytical characteristics of a diagnostic test and, to discuss in more detail, the clinical performance characteristics of diagnostic tests and how to interpret laboratory data in the context of disease.

4) Understanding heterogeneity of clinical and laboratory data across patient populations.

Preanalytical Variables

a) *AGE*: The normal ranges for some laboratory tests depend on the "age" of the patient and are best seen in pediatric populations. Examples include the levels of some coagulation factors and serum immunoglobulins which do not reach adult levels for many months after birth.

b) *GENDER*: The normal range of hormones depends on "gender," exemplified by levels of testosterone and estradiol. Variations in levels of estrogen and progesterone during the various phases of the menstrual cycle have an impact on evaluating women with cyclical urticaria.

[1] Associate Professor, University of Colorado School of Medicine, Department of Pediatrics, Section of Allergy, and Immunology, Children's Hospital, Colorado, Translational and Diagnostic Immunology Laboratory, 13123 East 16th Avenue, Aurora, Colorado 80045.

[2] Director of Clinical Immunology laboratory, Departments of Medicine and Pathology, Massachusetts General Hospital, Assistant Professor of Medicine, Harvard University, Boston, Massachusetts 02114.

Email: vijaya.knight@childrenscolorado.org

* Corresponding author: murali50@aol.com

c) *BODY MASS INDEX (BMI)*: Alterations in BMI have an impact on the values of some laboratory results. The strongest associations with BMI were noted for alanine transaminase (ALT), apolipoprotein A1, high-density lipoprotein (HDL)-cholesterol, hemoglobin, C-reactive protein (CRP), cystatin C, triglycerides, urate and creatine kinase.

d) *DIET, FASTING and TIMING OF BLOOD SAMPLING*: Values of triglycerides, glucose, creatinine, C-peptide and insulin are significantly upregulated when blood is drawn after breakfast or lunch, whereas testosterone is downregulated. Parameters that decrease when sampled during the day include total bilirubin, brain natriuretic peptide (BNP), myoglobin, cortisol, thyroid stimulating hormone (TSH), prolactin and adrenocorticotropic hormone (ACTH).

e) *INTERFERING SUBSTANCES*: Many automated laboratory tests are spectrophotometric, and therefore depend on measurable alterations in the color of plasma or serum after a chemical reaction. Examples of interference include hemolysis either *in vivo* or during phlebotomy rendering plasma and serum a pink to red hue, elevated bilirubin that makes plasma or serum acquire shades of orange or green, and lipemia that makes plasma and serum milky. When results are outside the range these interfering parameters should be excluded.

A recently emerging interfering substance is noted in subjects taking large doses of vitamin B7 or biotin. Biotin is used in some immunoassays as it can be coupled to molecules or antibodies and amplified by its affinity bind avidin. This method is sometimes used to measure analytes, such as hormones [e.g., thyroxine (T4), triiodothyronine (T3), TSH, parathyroid hormone (PTH), cortisol, follicle-stimulating hormone (FSH) and (luteinizing hormone (LH)], vitamin D or troponin, which is a marker of cardiac muscle injury. Interference by biotin may cause a false decrease or increase in the measurement of these analytes. Counseling patients to avoid these mega doses of biotin prior to phlebotomy coupled with laboratory initiatives to ascertain limits of biotin interference in their assays and verify abnormal data against a reference method not using biotin complexes is recommended by the United States Food and Drug Administration (FDA). The effect of medications on laboratory tests is used to monitor the therapeutic efficacy of a drug, such as the measurement of the International Normalized Ratio (INR) in those on coumadin analogs. Also, drugs such as cyclosporin, rituximab and azathioprine can alter T and B cell numbers and function, including levels of immunoglobulins.

Analytical Test Characteristics

Prior to implementation for clinical use, diagnostic tests go through extensive evaluation for their performance and utility in both laboratory and clinical environments. These data are submitted to organizations such as the FDA in the United States, the Central Drugs Standard Control Organization (CDSCO) in India or for CE-marking approval through the European IVD Regulatory Process. For diagnostic tests that receive approval from these organizations, "analytical test characteristics" are established by the manufacturer of the diagnostic test and are verified before implementation by the clinical laboratory performing the test. Diagnostic tests that are developed by a single laboratory are termed "Laboratory Developed Tests" or LDTs. The analytical performance characteristics for LDTs are developed and validated by the specific laboratory performing the assay. The onus of ensuring accurate and reliable performance of diagnostic tests falls on diagnostic test developers, therefore comprehensive and well-designed experiments should be implemented during test evaluation to make sure that the diagnostic test meets the required standards of analytical performance. Reference documents such as those published by the Clinical Laboratories Standards Institute (CLSI; www.clsi.org) and the FDA (https://www.fda.gov/regulatory-information/search-fda-guidance-documents/bioanalytical-method-validation-guidance-industry) provide guidelines for diagnostic test development and validation and establishment of test performance parameters. These reference documents are used widely by clinical laboratories and diagnostics manufacturers. The analytic characteristics of a diagnostic test are described in Table 1.

Table 1. Analytical test characteristics.

Assay Characteristic	Description
Accuracy	Accuracy reflects the relationship between the number obtained by a test and a true result. It is the closeness of agreement of the test result to the true or expected value. May include comparative studies between the test under evaluation and a gold-standard established method.
Precision	Reproducibility of the test or the ability of the test to generate the same result on repeated analyses under the same conditions. Calculation of precision of a test includes intra-assay (within run) variation, inter-assay (between run) variation and inter-operator variation.
Sensitivity	The lowest concentration of the analyte can be reliably detected by the test.
Specificity	The ability to accurately measure the specific analyte to the exclusion of other analytes. This is also known as "interference testing" and often includes analysis of the effect of hemolysis or lipemia on accurate measurement of an analyte in clinical samples such as serum or plasma.
Linearity	The linear range across which the test performs reproducibly and accurately. The upper and lower limits of the linear range of a test define the "analytical measurement range" or AMR. Clinical results are considered accurate only when they fall within the AMR.
Reference Range	Range of values that are characteristic of a normal population. Reference ranges generally include at least 95% of the reference population tested during the validation of the diagnostic test. For certain analytes whose concentration or levels change with age (e.g., serum immunoglobulins), age-specific reference ranges are critical.

Diagnostic Test Characteristics

Clinical sensitivity, specificity, positive and negative predictive values and likelihood ratios describe diagnostic test performance (Shreffler and Huecker 2021). These terms describe the ability of the diagnostic test to distinguish between people with the disease and people who do not have the disease; in other words, the test's ability to improve the physician's confidence in ruling in or ruling out disease. These parameters are influenced by disease prevalence and pre-test odds of the presence of disease based on clinical symptoms and other investigations. For the physician to make the most effective use of diagnostic test information, a good understanding of the diagnostic test's performance characteristics and their limitations in the clinical environment is necessary. Without this knowledge, unnecessary testing may lead a physician down an irrelevant diagnostic path and may result in unnecessary and oftentimes, expensive, additional diagnostic tests and procedures or even treatment.

Clinical Sensitivity and Specificity

Clinical sensitivity and specificity are indicators of the accuracy of a diagnostic test in a population with or without diseases.

Clinical sensitivity is defined as the ability of a diagnostic test to correctly identify "true positives" or people who have the disease that the test is designed to detect. Sensitivity is therefore calculated as "true positives/true positives + false negatives" and includes the population that has the disease. Clinical specificity, on the other hand, is defined as the ability of the test to accurately identify people who do not have the disease, otherwise known as "true negatives." Specificity is calculated as "true negatives/true negatives + false positives" and includes the population that does not have the disease. The sensitivity and specificity of a test are calculated using a 2 × 2 table (Table 2).

An example below explains the calculation of sensitivity and specificity for a given test; in this case, a newly developed serological assay for the detection of antibodies to the Severe Acute Respiratory Syndrome Coronavirus 2 (SARS-CoV-2) virus (Test X). Assume that in a population of 1,000 people, 200 are confirmed to have COVID-19 by PCR detection of SARS-CoV-2. Test X, which uses a finger prick blood sample to detect SARS-CoV-2 antibodies, is an easy method

Table 2. Calculation of sensitivity and specificity of a diagnostic test.

		Disease	
		Present	Absent
Diagnostic Test Under Evaluation	Positive	A – True Positive (TP)	B – False Positive (FP)
	Negative	C – False Negative (FN)	D – True Negative (TN)
Sensitivity and Specificity		Sensitivity = (A/A+C) × 100	Specificity = (B/B+D) × 100
		All persons with the disease	All persons without the disease

Table 3. Calculation of sensitivity and specificity for Test X.

		PCR for SARS-CoV-2	
		Positive	Negative
Test X	Positive	195	160
	Negative	5	640
Sensitivity and Specificity		Sensitivity = 97.5%	Specificity = 80%
		All persons with the disease	All persons without the disease

to determine what percentage of the population has been previously infected with the virus. If it performs satisfactorily, it may be used as a serosurveillance tool. However, it is necessary to determine whether Test X will accurately detect all people who have been previously infected with SARS-CoV-2 as identified by the gold-standard PCR test. The performance of Test X is therefore evaluated in serum samples collected from individuals who were PCR positive for SARS-CoV-2 and those who were PCR negative. Sensitivity and specificity for this new serological test are calculated using a 2 × 2 table (Table 3).

Table 3 indicates that Test X is highly sensitive and detects most people who have been previously infected with SARS-CoV-2. However, Test X has relatively lower specificity and therefore results in 20% false positive results.

Tests with high sensitivity accurately identify people with the disease and therefore are useful for "ruling out" disease, as a negative test will reliably be obtained in people who "do not" have the disease. On the other hand, a test with high specificity is useful for "ruling in" disease as a positive test result will reliably identify people who "do" have the disease. A combination of sensitivity and specificity for any given test determines its reliability for ruling or ruling out disease. For instance, a test with a sensitivity of 100% and specificity of 67% will not miss people with the disease but because of low specificity, it will result in a significant number of false positives (people who test positive but do not have the disease). Similarly, a test with a sensitivity of 80% and specificity of 100% will correctly identify all people without the disease; however, because of relatively low sensitivity, it will also result in several false negatives (people who have the disease but test negative).

How do sensitivity and specificity affect the performance of a test in any given population? Taking the example of Test X, which is highly sensitive, we can be sure that a person who tests negative with this test has a very low probability of having been infected with SARS-CoV-2. However, because this test is only 80% specific, it also results in a significant number of false positives, which would lead to the assumption that the prevalence of SARS-CoV-2 infection is much higher in this population than it really is.

Positive and Negative Predictive Values

While the sensitivity and specificity of a given test provide information on the performance of the test, these parameters are independent of disease prevalence in any given population. The diagnostic test's ability to correctly identify persons with and without disease changes as disease prevalence changes. A test with high sensitivity and low specificity will perform differently in its ability to identify true positives and true negatives depending on the prevalence of disease in the population. The probability that any given test will correctly identify people who have the disease, and at the same time also identify people who do not have the disease is defined by the Positive Predictive Value (PPV) and Negative Predictive Value (NPV) of the test, respectively (https://www.westgard.com/predictive-value.htm).

PPV is defined as the proportion of people who test positive and have the disease. PPV is calculated as the number of people who test positive and have the disease/total number of people who test positive.

NPV is defined as the probability that a person who tests negative with the diagnostic test does not have the disease. NPV is calculated as the number of people who test negative and do not have disease/number of people who tested negative.

The calculation of PPV and NPV for any given test is illustrated in Table 4.

Taking the example of Test X for the detection of SARS-CoV-2 antibodies, the PPV and NPV can be calculated as illustrated in Table 5.

Although the test has high sensitivity, the relatively lower specificity of the test affects PPV. Thus, a positive test will correctly identify people previously infected with SARS-CoV-2 only 55% of the time. On the other hand, the high NPV of the test indicates that negative results correctly identify people who were not previously infected with SARS-CoV-2 99% of the time. Thus, based on the PPV and NPV of Test X, a negative result is much more reliable than a positive result.

NPV and PPV are influenced by disease prevalence. When disease prevalence is low, PPV decreases, and the number of false positives increases. Table 6 shows how the NPV and PPV of Test X change when the prevalence of SARS-CoV-2 infection in the population changes. Although the sensitivity and specificity of Test X remain unchanged, the ability of Test X to correctly identify infected and uninfected person changes as disease prevalence changes.

Figure 1 shows that as disease prevalence increases, the likelihood of a positive test result increases, therefore PPV increases. When disease prevalence is high, Test X will be positive in

Table 4. Calculation of PPV and NPV.

		Disease			
		Present	Absent	Predictive Value	
Diagnostic Test Under Evaluation	Positive	A – True Positive (TP)	B – False Positive (FP)	PPV = (A/A+B) × 100	All positive results (A+B)
	Negative	C – False Negative (FN)	D – True Negative (TN)	NPV = (D/C+D) × 100	All negative results (C+D)
Sensitivity and Specificity		Sensitivity = A/A+C	Specificity = B/B+D		
		All persons with disease (A+C)	All persons without disease (B+D)		

Table 5. PPV and NPV of Test X.

		PCR for SARS-CoV-2		
		Positive	Negative	Predictive Value
Test X	Positive	195	160	PPV = 0.55%
	Negative	5	640	NPV = 0.99%
Sensitivity and Specificity		Sensitivity = 97.5%	Specificity = 80%	
		All persons with the disease	All persons without the disease	

Table 6. Influence of disease prevalence on PPV and NPV of Test X.

Prevalence of SARS-CoV-2 Infection (%)	PPV (%)	NPV (%)
5	20	99
10	35	99
20	55	99
40	76	97
60	88	96
80	95	88

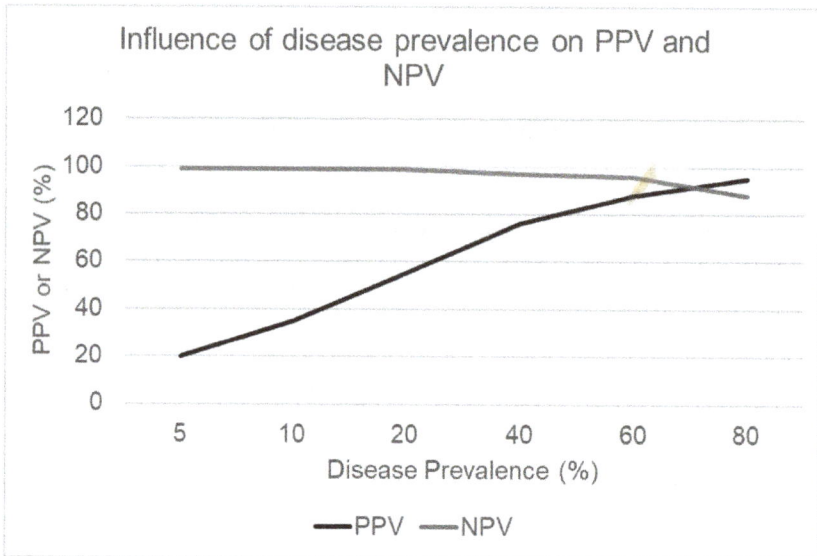

Figure 1. Comparison of the Effect of Disease Prevalence on PPV and NPV of Test X. Test X, developed for the detection of SARS-CoV-2 antibodies, has a sensitivity of 97.5% and a specificity of 80%. When disease prevalence changes from 5% to 80%, PPV also increases whereas NPV starts to decrease. PPV, Positive Predictive Value; NPV, Negative Predictive Value.

people who are infected and can be relied on to detect past SARS-CoV-2 infection. However, when disease prevalence is low, PPV is low and therefore leading to false positive results in people who do not have the disease, and Test X falsely overestimates disease prevalence.

Judicious use of diagnostic testing is therefore important. If the appropriate diagnostic test is used when the pre-test probability for the disease is high based on clinical findings or disease prevalence in a population, a positive test is more likely to be useful to confirm or refute a diagnosis than when tests are used indiscriminately. Antinuclear autoantibody (ANA) testing is an example of a diagnostic test that is frequently misused, resulting in unnecessary clinical follow-up and additional unnecessary testing of people with false positive results (Narain et al. 2004). A positive ANA in the absence of relevant clinical history or physical signs or symptoms has little clinical relevance, and when used indiscriminately will have a low PPV for autoimmune disease. However, ANAs are frequently positive in patients with autoimmune diseases such as systemic lupus erythematosus, Sjogren's syndrome and systemic sclerosis. When the pre-test probability for autoimmune disease is high (e.g., based on clinical findings), ANA is a useful, relatively low-cost, diagnostic tool with reasonably good PPV (Wei et al. 2020).

The use of prick skin tests or tests for specific IgE to food antigens, in the absence of a comprehensive clinical history, is another example of misguided practice in allergy. The PPV for the diagnosis of true food allergy, in this scenario, is very low and is inconsistent with principles of appropriate care. However, in a cohort of children with suspected anaphylaxis to peanuts, the PPV of skin tests are high and can guide the allergist to perform specific IgE to the components of peanut, such as Ara h2, Ara h3, Ara h5, Ara h6 and Ara 8, etc., to stratify for the risk of anaphylaxis from non-anaphylactic presentation such as hives. Sequential and pathogenesis-based testing forms the basis of oral immunotherapy to peanuts, ushering in an era of personalized and precision practice of allergy.

Screening and Confirmatory Tests

Screening tests, often employed to screen large populations for disease, should have high sensitivity to detect as many people with the disease as possible. These tests are often used to potentially detect underlying disease prior to symptom onset and therefore allow early intervention. Because screening tests are designed to maximize the detection of individuals with the disease, they may result in a not insignificant percentage of false positive results. Screening tests are followed by confirmatory tests, which are selected for high specificity, thus minimizing the number of false negatives.

The tuberculin skin test (Mantoux test) for evidence of exposure to *M. tuberculosis* is an example of a screening test. This test may yield false positive results in people who have received the BCG vaccine or who have been exposed to environmental non-tuberculous mycobacteria. Individuals who test positive undergo clinical follow-up that may include a chest X-ray, if necessary, to confirm a diagnosis of latent TB. While screening tests with high sensitivity are important to enable early and accurate detection of disease, they may cause harm if incorrectly implemented in populations that are not at risk for the disease, or if they are not followed up with confirmatory testing to confirm or refute a positive result. Some examples of screening and confirmatory tests are shown in Table 7.

Table 7. Examples of screening and confirmatory tests.

Disease	Screening Tests	Confirmatory Tests	References
Tuberculosis	Mantoux test	Chest X-ray, detection of *M. tuberculosis* by culture or PCR	Farhat et al. 2006; Sterling et al. 2020
Breast cancer	Mammography	Biopsy	Oeffinger et al. 2015
Prostate cancer	Prostate specific antigen	Prostate biopsy	Wolf et al. 2010
Celiac disease	Tissue transglutaminase (tTg) IgA, deamidated gliadin IgG and IgA	Small intestine biopsy	Maglione et al. 2016; Hadithi et al. 2007
Colorectal cancer	Fecal occult blood, colonoscopy	Biopsy	Lin et al. 2016
HIV	HIV-2 and HIV-2 antibody and HIV-1 p24 antigen immunoassay	HIV-1 and HIV-2 differentiation test; HIV-1 nucleic acid test	Hurt et al. 2017 (https://www.cdc.gov/hiv/pdf/guidelines_testing_recommendedlabtestingalgorithm.pdf)
Severe combined immunodeficiency	PCR analysis of T cell receptor excision circles (TREC)	Flow cytometry for lymphocyte subsets (percentage and absolute numbers)	Biggs et al. 2017
Systemic mastocytosis	Serum tryptase	Bone marrow biopsy for morphology of mast cells, CD2+ CD25+ cells; C-kit mutations	Valent et al. 2021

Receiver Operator Characteristics (ROC) Curve and Area Under the Curve (AUC)

Receiver Operator Characteristic (ROC) curve and Area Under the Curve (AUC) are used to measure the ability of a test to classify positive and negative results (Mandrekar 2010). A ROC curve is a probability curve that can be used to examine the sensitivity and specificity of a test at various numerical cut-points for positivity, and thereby choose optimal sensitivity and specificity for the diagnostic application. AUC or Area Under the Curve is a measure of how well positive and negative results are discriminated from each other. True Positive Rate (TPR or sensitivity) is plotted against False Positive Rate (FPR or 1-specificity) for all possible cut-off values that distinguish positive results from negative results to generate the ROC curve.

The ideal situation is where the cut-off value for a test separates true positives and true negatives with no overlap (Figure 2A). In this ideal situation, sensitivity and specificity are 100%, the ROC curve passes through the upper left corner of the graph (point 1, 0) and the AUC is 1. When the test cannot discriminate between true negatives and true positives, the ROC curve is close to a diagonal line connecting the origin and the upper right corner (point 1, 1), and the AUC is 0.5 (Figure 2C). Most tests fall between an AUC of 1 and 0.5, and the closer the AUC is to 1, the better the test's ability to distinguish between true positives and true negatives (Figure 2B).

By varying the cut-off point, the sensitivity of the test may increase or decrease, and correspondingly, specificity decreases or increases, as sensitivity and specificity are inversely related. Choosing the right cut-off point for a diagnostic is important; in some cases, such as a screening test where sensitivity is critical, it may be appropriate to lower the cut-off value to detect more positives. For a confirmatory test, higher specificity is important, and increasing the cut-off value may be appropriate. Thus, the ROC curve and AUC can be used to determine the most appropriate cut-off point to optimize sensitivity and specificity for a test. ROC curves and AUC can also be used to compare tests for their ability to accurately distinguish true positives and true negatives.

Likelihood Ratio (LR)

The sensitivity and specificity of a test can be combined into a single value, the Likelihood Ratio (LR) (Simel et al. 1991; Fierz and Bossuyt 2020). LRs are used to determine the diagnostic value of the test, taking into consideration the pre-test probability that the disease exists or the disease prevalence in a population.

Positive LR (LR+) is defined as the probability of a positive test in an individual with disease/the probability of a positive test in an individual without disease and is calculated as sensitivity/1-specificity. A positive LR of 1 or greater indicates that the diagnostic test is more likely to be positive in a person with the disease. Taking the example of Test X, whose sensitivity is 97.5% and specificity is 80%, the LR+ is 4.9, which means that a person with a positive test is 4.9 times more likely to have been previously infected with SARS-CoV-2.

Negative LR (LR–) is defined as the probability of a negative test in an individual with disease/the probability of a negative test in an individual with the disease and is calculated as 1-Sensitivity/Specificity. A negative LR of less than 1 indicates that a negative test is less likely to occur in a person with the disease. The lower the LR– value, the better the correlation of a negative test result with no disease.

LRs used in combination with pre-test probability for disease can greatly improve the post-test odds of disease detection. Pre-test probability can be defined in multiple ways; the disease prevalence in a population, the presence of certain clinical symptoms, findings on a physical examination that correlate with the disease, or radiological or other imaging findings.

Bayes theorem, named after Thomas Bayes, combines sensitivity, specificity and LRs of a test, with disease prevalence or pre-test probability of disease occurrence, to calculate the post-test

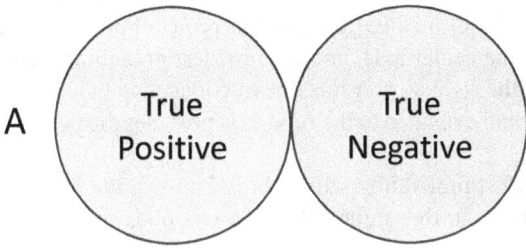

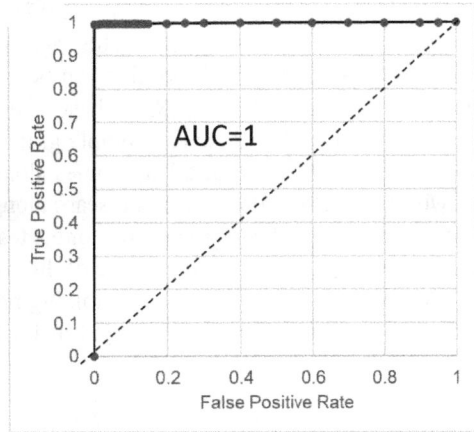

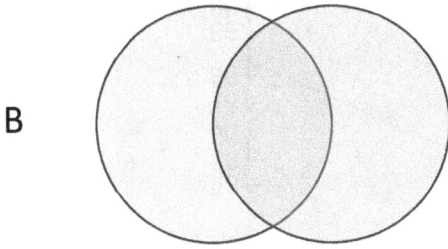

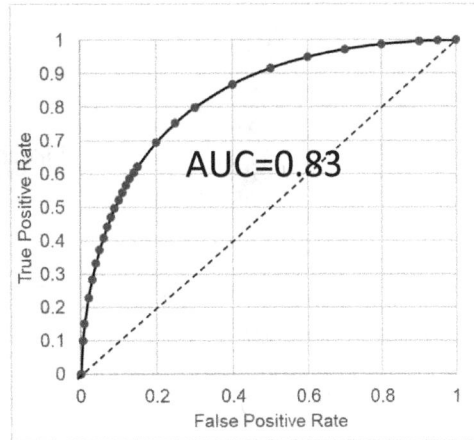

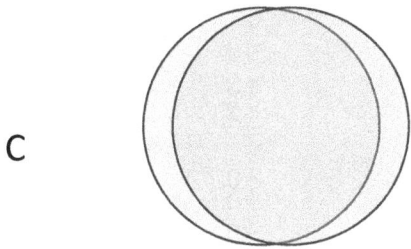

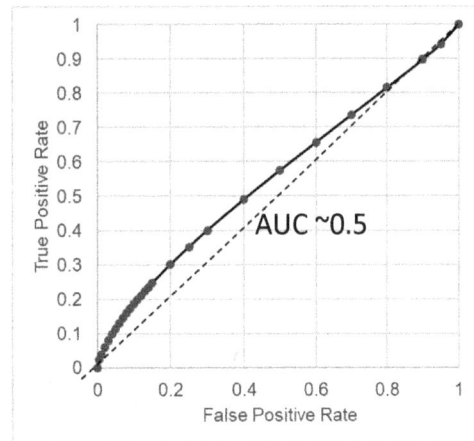

Figure 2. Comparison of ROC curves and AUC as Sensitivity and Specificity Change. (A) Test with 100% sensitivity and 100% specificity detects true positives and true negatives with no overlap; AUC is 1. (B) Test with 82% sensitivity and 83% specificity; AUC is 0.83. (C) Test with 57% sensitivity and 50% specificity; AUC is 0.52. ROC, Receiver Operator Characteristics; AUC or Area Under the Curve.

probability that disease exists (Johnson 2017). Bayes theorem can be simplified graphically using a tool known as Fagan's nomogram. The Fagan nomogram, developed by Dr. Terrence Fagan (Fagan 1975), is a visual graphical tool that can be used to combine pre-test probability for the presence of disease with the LR+ or LR– values of a diagnostic test intended to rule in or rule out said disease (Safari et al. 2016). This simple graphical tool includes the pre-test probability of disease on the left axis, the LR+ and LR– values along the center axis, and the post-test probability (also known as posterior probability) of disease along the right axis. A line drawn connecting the pre-test probability through the LR+ and LR– for the test and extended to the right axis provides the post-test probability of the presence or absence of disease.

An example of the utility of combining pre-test probability with LRs to improve the post-test odds of detecting disease is illustrated in Figure 3. In this figure, the post-test odds of a person

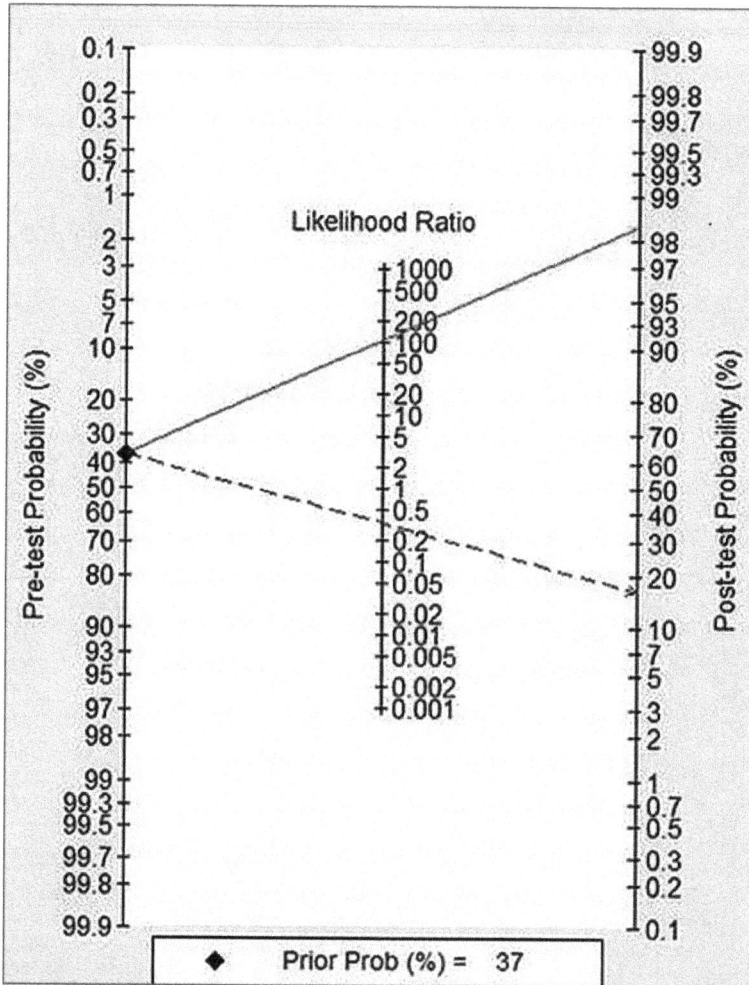

Figure 3. Application of Fagan's nomogram to Test X. Given disease prevalence at 20%, LR+ of 4.9 and LR– of 0.03, the post-test odds of a person testing positive for anti-SARS-CoV-2 antibodies having been infected with the virus is 55%, whereas the post-test odds of a person who tests negative having been infected with the virus is 0.07%. Therefore, a negative result with Test X is more reliable in ruling in disease than a positive result. LR or Likelihood Ratio. http://araw.mede.uic.edu/cgi-bin/testcalc.pl.

who tests positive for antibodies to SARS-CoV-2 having been previously infected with the virus is examined, using the diagnostic Test X characteristics of LR+ = 4.8 and LR− = 0.03 in a population where the prevalence of infection is 20%. Application of these data to Fagan's nomogram shows that a negative test is very likely to indicate no disease; post-test odds of infection are 0.7, whereas a positive test results in a 55% post-test probability for infection with SARS-CoV-2. Therefore, a positive test result, while increasing the post-test odds for SARS-CoV-2 infection, may still be falsely positive in 45% of people tested, whereas a negative test, will be negative in greater than 99% of uninfected people.

Applying Test Characteristics to the Diagnosis and Management of Allergy

Skin prick testing (SPT) and specific IgE analysis are widely used for the assessment of allergies. Inappropriate or indiscriminate use of these tests, particularly when assessing food allergy can have drastic consequences for patients, such as unnecessary avoidance of foods which can, in extreme cases, lead to malnourishment (Fleischer et al. 2011). The sensitivity and specificity of SPT and sIgE vary widely depending on the specific allergen and the patient population in which these test characteristics were determined. In general, both SPT and sIgE at the manufacturer's determined cut-off value of 0.35 kUA/L have reasonably good sensitivity (70% or higher, depending on the specific allergen), but poor specificity (as low as 21% for hazelnut allergen) (Ho et al. 2006; Soares-Weiser et al. 2014; Beyer et al. 2015). Thus, reliance on these test results alone for the diagnosis of allergy can result in a significant number of false positive results, leading to mislabeling patients as "allergic." A number of research groups have evaluated cut-off values for SPT and specific IgE, especially for food allergens, to increase the utility of these tests (reviewed in Foong et al. 2021; Foong and Santos 2021). By refining the cut-off values further, the patient population is better selected to include only those individuals who are more likely to have a clinical allergy. As reviewed by Foong et al. (Foong et al. 2021), diagnostic cut-offs with a 95% PPV were 7 kUA/L for egg, 15–34 kUA/L for peanut and 50 kUA/L for sesame, illustrating the challenges with using a blanket 0.35 kUA/L cut-off value for positivity, irrespective of the allergen. A 2020 update to the practice parameters for peanut allergy diagnosis (Greenhawt et al. 2020) illustrated the utility of likelihood ratios to improve the usefulness of SPT and sIgE testing. Making use of Fagan's nomograms, Greenhawt et al. showed that the post-test odds for a positive Ara h 2 sIgE result of 0.35 kUA/L increases significantly from 10% to 90% when the pre-test odds are 2% (e.g., general population) or 70% (e.g., selected based on clinical reactivity to peanut allergen), respectively (Greenhawt et al. 2020). These studies illustrate the need for the allergist to not only understand the performance characteristics of available laboratory tests but to also use them in the appropriate clinical context.

Understanding Heterogeneity of Clinical and Laboratory Data Across Patient Populations

a) *WATERFALL PLOTS*: The immune response to antigens (including tumors) is unique and personalized and is the outcome of immunogenetics and epigenetic factors. The heterogeneity has been captured in the display of clinical outcomes data to various therapeutic interventions in oncology as "waterfall plots." They provide a better understanding of the clinical outcome than just data depicting the means and standard deviation of the treatment and control groups. Waterfall plots are ideal for revealing how a net or mean value is arrived at in clinical studies. This is achieved by breaking down the cumulative effect of "positive" and "negative" contributions. It provides a panoramic view of the variability of data points in a study. Baseline parameters

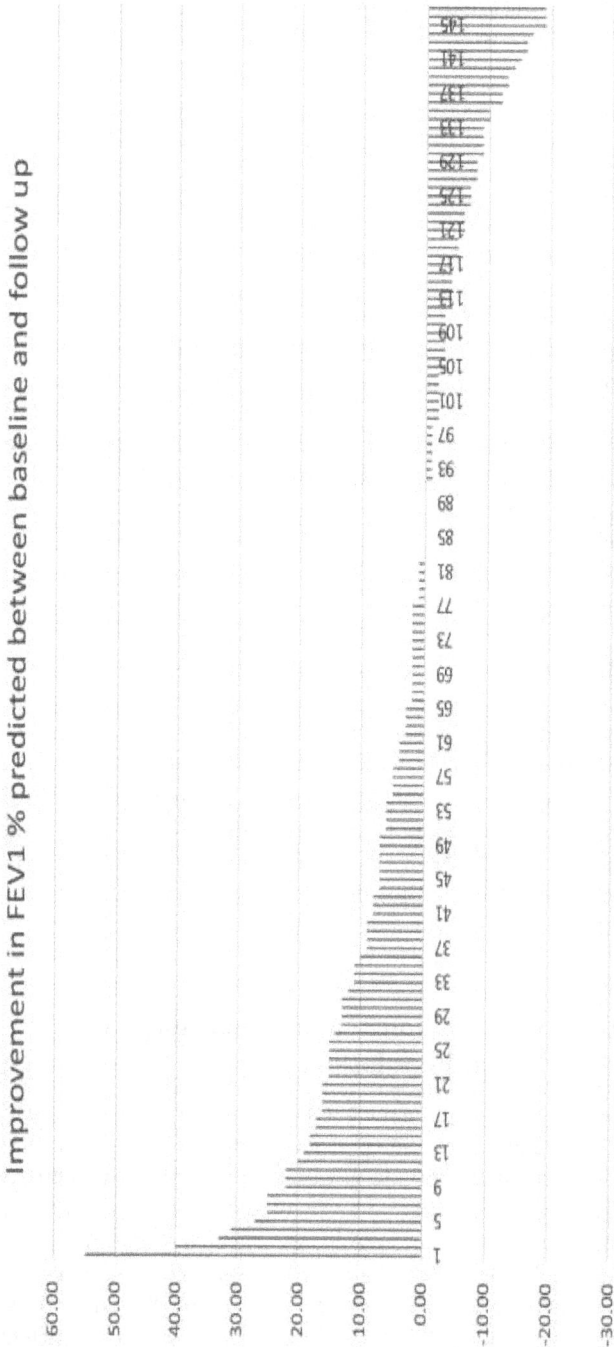

Figure 4. Waterfall Plot Depicting the Heterogeneity of the FEV1 Response in a Study on Asthma Control and Outcomes. Note that the majority had improvements in FEV1, a few had no alteration in FEV1 and a minority did show a decline in FEV1. The magnitude of the changes and heterogeneity in outcomes is more revealing than numbers for mean and standard deviation. FEV, Forced Expiratory Volume.

are depicted on the horizontal or X-axis, while vertical bars are drawn for each patient, either above or below the baseline. In studies of asthma the vertical axis Y may be used to depict the maximum % change from baseline for parameters, such as forced expiratory volume (FEV1), absolute eosinophil count, or decrease in oral corticosteroid (OCS) use. For FEV1, vertical bars above the baseline represent improvements in FEV1 with no change reflecting a null effect of the intervention and vertical bars below the baseline a deterioration in lung function. The latter suggests that the intervention did not modify the deterioration of lung function. Figure 4 is an example of changes in FEV1 plotted as an outcome of an intervention. The data are not presented randomly or in order of when a patient was enrolled into a study but are organized to provide a clear picture of the study subjects' response; from best to worst based on the parameter evaluated (Denton et al. 2020).

The individual bars, besides representing a single subject, can also be used to represent other salient patient characteristics, such as the effect of smoking on FEV1 of asthmatics by using a different color. Thus, a waterfall plot provides data about not only the primary outcome, such as FEV1 but also adds relevant information about the other risk factors (such as smoking or obesity) influencing the outcome.

b) *META-ANALYSIS*: Historical anecdotes, personal observations and hypothetical therapeutic modalities have been replaced by carefully planned, scientifically designed randomized controlled trials (RCT) in many fields and particularly in medicine ushering in an era of evidence-based medicine. This has resulted in many publications addressing the same question with each individual study reporting measurements that may have some error. A stringent statistical analysis that combines the result of these scientific studies is called "meta-analysis." Data derived from meta-analyses can identify patterns or trends among study results, endorsing some outcomes and identifying others that need further validation. This data is often presented in what is called a "Forest Plot" or as a "Blobbogram." In many of the clinical guidelines or practice parameters data is presented as a Forest plot and recommendations are made based on the quality of data used to derive the plot. Forest plots are commonly presented in two columns. The left-hand column lists chronologically the names of the RCT. The right-hand column is a plot of the measurement of effects (e.g., odds ratio) for each of the studies. The square is proportional to the weights used and the confidence interval is represented by horizontal lines. The summary measure also called pooled fixed effect is depicted by a diamond with the lateral points of the diamond, indicating the confidence intervals for the measurement. A solid vertical line representing no effect (null effect) for the outcome is also plotted. The net effect of the outcome derived from meta-analysis should fall on either side of the null effect line. In the example provided in Figure 5, it favors the combination of inhaled corticosteroids (ICS) plus systemic corticosteroids (SCS) over SCS alone in acute asthma (Kearns et al. 2020).

Conclusion

Diagnostic tests can be very useful tools to support clinical decisions and patient management. However, physicians should understand the limitations of diagnostic tests, their performance characteristics and the influence of pre-test probability on the value of diagnostic tests. A better understanding of integrating the clinical findings with judicious use of diagnostic tests greatly improves the utility of diagnostic tests in the management of all patients in general and particularly those with allergic and immunological diseases.

ICS + SCS vs SCS

Study	ICS + SCS n/N	SCS n/N	Odds Ratio (95%CI)	Odds ratio (95% CI)	Weight (%)
Silverman 2009	18/46	19/49		1.02 (0.44 to 2.32)	9.3
Upham 2011	56/91	55/88		0.96 (0.52 to 1.76)	17.4
Alangari 2014	75/458	82/448		0.87 (0.62 to 1.23)	53.4
Guttman 1997	8/30	12/30		0.5 (0.18 to 1.62)	5.3
Sung 1998	2/24	5/20		0.27 (0.05 to 1.60)	2.0
Starobin 2008	5/26	11/23		0.26 (0.07 to 0.93)	3.9
Razi 2017	12/50	29/50		0.23 (0.10 to 0.54)	8.6

Pooled Fixed Effect (95% CI) 0.73 (0.57 to 0.94)

Pooled Random Effect (95% CI) 0.61 (0.39 to 0.94)

Heterogeneity: Chi² = 13.5, DF = 6 (p = 0.04)
    I² (95%CI) = 55.5 (0.89 to 80.9)

Favours ICS/SCS   Favours SCS

0.1   0.5   1   2   10

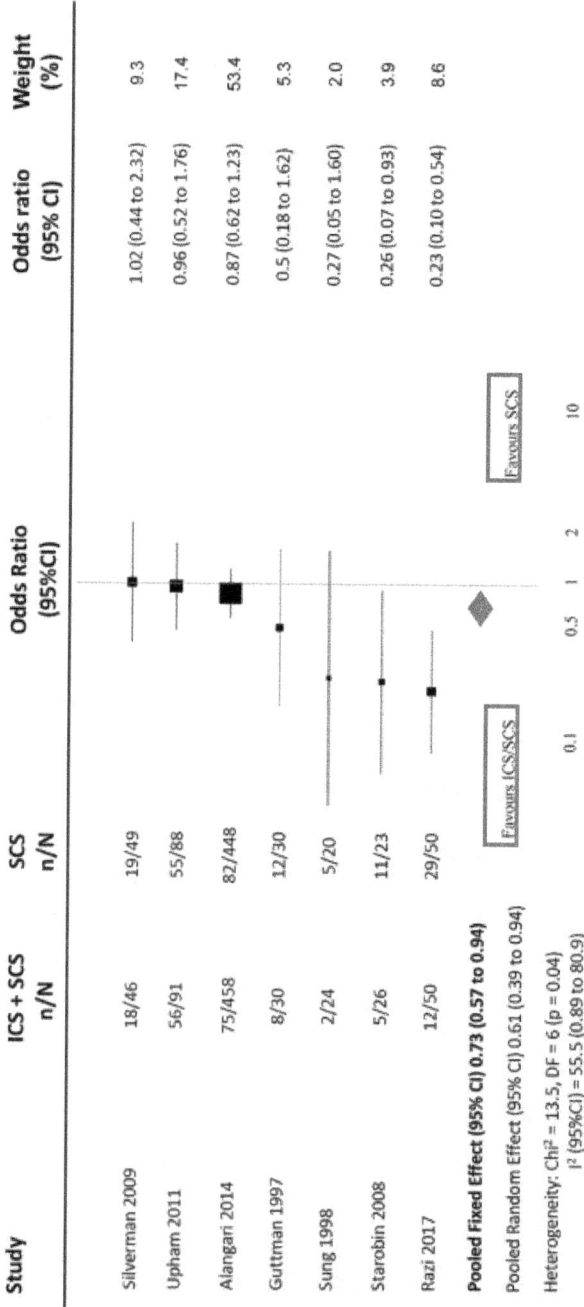

Kearns N, Ingrid M, Harper J, Beasley R and Weatherall M. Inhaled Corticosteroids in Acute Asthma: A Systemic Review and Meta analysis. J Allergy Clin Immunol Pract 2020;8:605-17

Figure 5. A Forest Data Plot of the Meta-Analyses. Outcome data derived from 7 studies addressing the value of adding ICS to SCS versus SCS alone in acute asthma favors the combination as a more effective regimen. A conclusion derived from meta-analysis is often used to develop treatment guidelines or practice parameters. ICS, Inhaled Corticosteroid; SCS, Systemic Corticosteroid.

Glossary of Abbreviations

ACTH – Adrenocorticotropic Hormone
ALT – Alanine Transaminase
ANA – Antinuclear Antibody
AUC – Area Under the Curve
BMI – Body Mass Index
BNP – Brain Natriuretic Peptide
CDSCO – Central Drugs Standard Control Organization
CLSI – Clinical Laboratory Standards Institute
CRP – C-Reactive Protein
FDA – Food and Drug Administration
FEV – Forced Expiratory Volume
FN – False Negative
FP – False Positive
FSH – Follicle Stimulating Hormone
HDL – High-Density Lipids
INR – International Normalized Ratio
kUA – Kilounit Allergen
LH – Luteinizing Hormone
LR – Likelihood Ratio
NPV – Negative Predictive Value
PPV – Positive Predictive Value
PTH – Parathyroid Hormone
RCT – Randomized Controlled Trials
ROC – Receiver Operator Characteristics
sIgE – Specific Immunoglobulin E
SPT – Skin Prick Test
TN – True Negative
TP – True Positive
TSH – Thyroid Stimulating Hormone

References

Beyer, K., Grabenhenrich, L., Hartl, M., Beder, A., Kalb, B., Ziegert, M. et al. 2015. Predictive values of component-specific IGE for the outcome of peanut and hazelnut food challenges in children. Allergy 70(1): 90–98.

Biggs, C. M., Haddad, E., Issekutz, T. B., Roifman, C. M. and Turvey, S. E. 2017. Newborn screening for severe combined immunodeficiency: A primer for clinicians. CMAJ 189(50): E1551–E1557.

Denton, E., Lee, J., Tay, T., Radhakrishna, N., Hore-Lacy, F., Mackay, A. et al. 2020. Systematic assessment for difficult and severe asthma improves outcomes and halves oral corticosteroid burden independent of monoclonal biologic use. J. Allergy Clin. Immunol. Pract. 8(5): 1616–1624.

Eng j. ROC analysis: Web-based calculator for ROC curves. Baltimore: Johns Hopkins University [updated 2014 March 19; cited 12.9.2021]. Available from: http://www.jrocfit.org.

Fagan, T. J. 1975. Letter: Nomogram for Bayes theorem. N Engl. J. Med. 293(5): 257.

Farhat, M., Greenaway, C., Pai, M. and Menzies, D. 2006. False-positive tuberculin skin tests: What is the absolute effect of BCG and non-tuberculous mycobacteria? Int. J. Tuberc. Lung Dis. 10(11): 1192–1204.

Fierz, W. and Bossuyt, X. 2020. Likelihood ratios as value proposition for diagnostic laboratory tests. J. Appl. Lab Med. 5(5): 1061–1069.

Fleischer, D. M., Bock, S. A., Spears, G. C., Wilson, C. G., Miyazawa, N. K., Gleason, M. C. et al. 2011. Oral food challenges in children with a diagnosis of food allergy. J. Pediatr. 158(4): 578–583 e571.

Foong, R. X., Dantzer, J. A., Wood, R. A. and Santos, A. F. 2021. Improving diagnostic accuracy in food allergy. J. Allergy Clin. Immunol. Pract. 9(1): 71–80.

Foong, R. X. and Santos, A. F. 2021. Biomarkers of diagnosis and resolution of food allergy. Pediatr Allergy Immunol. 32(2): 223–233.

Greenhawt, M., Shaker, M., Wang, J., Oppenheimer, J. J., Sicherer, S., Keet, C. et al. 2020. Peanut allergy diagnosis: A 2020 practice parameter update, systematic review, and grade analysis. J. Allergy Clin. Immunol. 146(6): 1302–1334.

Hadithi, M., von Blomberg, B. M., Crusius, J. B., Bloemena, E., Kostense, P. J., Meijer, J. W. et al. 2007. Accuracy of serologic tests and HLA-DQ typing for diagnosing celiac disease. Ann. Intern. Med. 147(5): 294–302.

Ho, M. H., Heine, R. G., Wong, W. and Hill, D. J. 2006. Diagnostic accuracy of skin prick testing in children with tree nut allergy. J. Allergy Clin. Immunol. 117(6): 1506–1508.

Hurt, C. B., Nelson, J. A. E., Hightow-Weidman, L. B. and Miller, W. C. 2017. Selecting an HIV test: A narrative review for clinicians and researchers. Sex Transm. Dis. 44(12): 739–746.

Johnson, K. M. 2017. Using Bayes' rule in diagnostic testing: A graphical explanation. Diagnosis (Berl) 4(3): 159–167.

Kearns, N., Maijers, I., Harper, J., Beasley, R. and Weatherall, M. 2020. Inhaled corticosteroids in acute asthma: A systemic review and meta-analysis. J. Allergy Clin. Immunol. Pract. 8(2): 605–617 e606.

Lin, J. S., Piper, M. A., Perdue, L. A., Rutter, C. M., Webber, E. M., O'Connor, E. et al. 2016. Screening for colorectal cancer: Updated evidence report and systematic review for the US preventive services task force. JAMA 315(23): 2576–2594.

Maglione, M. A., Okunogbe, A., Ewing, B. et al. 2016. Diagnosis of Celiac Disease [Internet]. Rockville (MD): Agency for Healthcare Research and Quality (US); 2016 Jan. (Comparative Effectiveness Reviews, No. 162.) Available from: https://www.ncbi.nlm.nih.gov/books/NBK344454/.

Mandrekar, J. N. 2010. Receiver operating characteristic curve in diagnostic test assessment. J. Thorac. Oncol. 5(9): 1315–1316.

Narain, S., Richards, H. B., Satoh, M., Sarmiento, M., Davidson, R., Shuster, J. et al. 2004. Diagnostic accuracy for lupus and other systemic autoimmune diseases in the community setting. Arch. Intern. Med. 164(22): 2435–2441.

Oeffinger, K. C., Fontham, E. T., Etzioni, R., Herzig, A., Michaelson, J. S., Shih, Y. C. et al. 2015. Breast cancer screening for women at average risk: 2015 guideline update from the American Cancer Society. JAMA 314(15): 1599–1614.

Safari, S., Baratloo, A., Elfil, M. and Negida, A. 2016. Evidence based emergency medicine; part 4: Pre-test and post-test probabilities and Fagan's nomogram. Emerg (Tehran) 4(1): 48–51.

Shreffler, J. and Huecker, M. R. 2021. Diagnostic testing accuracy: sensitivity, specificity, predictive values and likelihood ratios. [Updated 2021 Mar 3]. In: StatPearls [Internet]. Treasure Island (FL): StatPearls Publishing; 2022 Jan-. Available from: https://www.ncbi.nlm.nih.gov/books/NBK557491/.

Simel, D. L., Samsa, G. P. and Matchar, D. B. 1991. Likelihood ratios with confidence: Sample size estimation for diagnostic test studies. J. Clin. Epidemiol. 44(8): 763–770.

Sterling, T. R., Njie, G., Zenner, D., Cohn, D. L., Reves, R., Ahmed, A. et al. 2020. Guidelines for the treatment of latent tuberculosis infection: Recommendations from the National Tuberculosis Controllers Association and CDC, 2020. MMWR Recomm. Rep. 69(1): 1–11.

Soares-Weiser, K., Takwoingi, Y., Panesar, S. S., Muraro, A., Werfel, T., Hoffmann-Sommergruber, K. et al. 2014. The diagnosis of food allergy: A systematic review and meta-analysis. Allergy 69(1): 76–86.

Valent, P., Akin, C., Hartmann, K., Alvarez-Twose, I., Brockow, K., Hermine, O. et al. 2021. Updated diagnostic criteria and classification of mast cell disorders: A consensus proposal. Hemasphere 5(11): e646.

Wei, Q., Jiang, Y., Xie, J., Lv, Q., Xie, Y., Tu, L. et al. 2020. Analysis of antinuclear antibody titers and patterns by using HEP-2 and primate liver tissue substrate indirect immunofluorescence assay in patients with systemic autoimmune rheumatic diseases. J. Clin. Lab Anal. 34(12): e23546.

Wolf, A. M., Wender, R. C., Etzioni, R. B., Thompson, I. M., D'Amico, A. V., Volk, R. J. et al. 2010. American Cancer Society guideline for the early detection of prostate cancer: Update 2010. CA Cancer J. Clin. 60(2): 70–98.

Chapter 2

Routine Laboratory Tests

Vijaya Knight[1] and *Mandakolathur R. Murali*[2,*]

Introduction

Workup for atopy or allergic diseases typically includes evaluation of peripheral blood cells, serum levels of immunoglobulin E (IgE) and allergen-specific IgE (sIgE). In addition, measurement of serum tryptase may be of value when evaluating an anaphylactic reaction or when mast cell disorders are on the differential diagnosis. Analysis of markers of acute inflammation, including C-reactive protein and erythrocyte sedimentation rate, can be helpful when considering autoimmune or infectious etiologies in the differential diagnosis. This chapter describes the clinical utility of these routine diagnostic tests.

Complete Blood Count

The Complete Blood Count (CBC) is perhaps the most widely used laboratory test and has been refined and automated following decades of pioneering work (Verso 1964). The earliest known method for the analysis of blood cells was developed by Karl von Vierordt, a professor of theoretical medicine at the University of Tubingen in the mid-1800s. In addition to developing techniques to study blood flow and a prototype instrument for the measurement of blood pressure, Karl von Vierordt developed the first slide-based method for counting blood cells. In 1874, Louis-Charles Malassez, a French anatomist and histologist developed the first hemocytometer; Paul Erlich later developed methods to stain and differentiate the various peripheral blood leucocytes (Kay 2016) and Maxwell Wintrobe developed the Wintrobe hematocrit method in the early 1900s (Fred 2007). Automated blood counts became mainstream with the development of the Coulter counter that used electrical impedance to analyze and measure peripheral blood cells (Robinson 2013). The Coulter principle continues to form the basis of analytical measurements in modern hematology analyzers.

A CBC provides information on the relative percentages and absolute numbers (generally expressed per microliter (mcL) or liter (L) of blood) of red blood cells (RBCs), white blood cells (WBCs) and platelets, and includes hemoglobin concentration and various characteristics of RBCs (George-Gay and Parker 2003). When combined with a WBC differential, the percentages and

---
[1] Associate Professor, University of Colorado School of Medicine, Department of Pediatrics, Section of Allergy, and Immunology, Children's Hospital, Colorado, Translational and Diagnostic Immunology Laboratory, 13123 East 16th Avenue, Aurora, Colorado 80045.
[2] Director of Clinical Immunology laboratory, Departments of Medicine and Pathology, Massachusetts General Hospital, Assistant Professor of Medicine, Harvard University, Boston, Massachusetts 02114.
Email: vijaya.knight@childrenscolorado.org
* Corresponding author: murali50@aol.com

Table 1. Components of CBC with differential.

Parameter	Units	Description	Clinical Significance
WBC	Cells/L	Number of WBC per liter of blood	Low WBC counts: Bone marrow suppression due to infection, inherited bone marrow defects, autoimmune destruction of WBC and drug-induced bone marrow suppression. Elevated WBC counts: Response to infection or inflammation, immune dysregulation and malignancy
RBC	Cells/L	Number of RBC per liter of blood	Low RBC counts: Result in anemia and may be a consequence of blood loss, defective RBC production (e.g., iron deficiency, vitamin B12 or folic acid deficiency, PRCA, bone marrow failure and infections, such as Parvovirus B19), or increased destruction (autoimmune causes such as PNH, cold agglutinin disease; congenital hemolytic anemias, DIC, drug-induced hemolytic anemia, transfusion reactions, infections, such as malaria, mechanical trauma due to prosthetic heart valves). Elevated RBC counts (polycythemia): hypoxic conditions such as smoking or heart failure; malignancy such as PV.
Hemoglobin (Hb)	g/dL	Amount of hemoglobin expressed in grams per deciliter	Anemia: Hb is below the age-matched reference interval. Erythrocytosis: Elevated Hb count is an indirect reflection of increased RBC production, generally in response to low oxygen levels (e.g., smoking, living at a high altitude, COPD, lung or cardiac abnormalities, heart failure)
Hematocrit (Hct)	%	Also called "packed cell volume" or PCV. Hct is the ratio of the volume of RBCs to the total volume of blood	Low hematocrit: Associated with anemia (decreased RBC), nutritional deficiencies, and blood loss Elevated hematocrit: Associated with dehydration, conditions in which RBCs are increased, such as PV, lung or cardiac disorders leading to a hypoxic state
Mean Corpuscular Volume (MCV)	Femtoliters (fl) or cubic microns	Defines the size of red blood cells	Low MCV (< 80 fL): microcytic anemic commonly seen in iron deficiency, thalassemias and sideroblastic anemia Increased MCV (> 100 fL): macrocytic anemia, classified as megaloblastic anemia that occurs due to impaired DNA synthesis (e.g., folic acid and/or vitamin B12 deficiency, orotic aciduria) and non-megaloblastic anemia (e.g., chronic alcoholism, hypothyroidism, liver disease and primary bone marrow disease)
MCH (Mean Corpuscular Hemoglobin)	pg	Amount of hemoglobin per red blood cell	Low MCH: iron deficiency; thalassemias High MCH: vitamin B12 and/or folate deficiency

Parameter	Unit	Description	Clinical significance
MCHC (Mean Corpuscular Hemoglobin Concentration)	g/dL	Amount of hemoglobin per unit volume	Low MCHC (hypochromic): e.g., iron deficiency, poor absorption of iron and chronic blood loss. High MCHC (hyperchromic): e.g., hereditary spherocytosis, hemolytic anemias and hypersplenism
RDW (Red Cell Distribution Width)	%	Coefficient of RBC volume or RBC size variation	High RDW (variable sizes of RBCs): associated with nutritional deficiencies (iron, folate and vitamin B12), following blood loss. Low RDW: not associated with any specific hematological disorder
Platelets	Cells/L	Number of platelets per liter of blood	Thrombocytopenia (low platelet count): drug-induced, particularly following chemotherapy; hematological malignancies, autoimmunity and genetic causes. Thrombocytosis (high platelet count): primary or essential thrombocytosis, secondary to infection, inflammation or malignancies
Plateletcrit (PCT)	%	The volume occupied by platelets in blood	Genetics, age, race, alcohol consumption, physical activity can all modify PCT and MPV
MPV (Mean Platelet Volume)	Femtoliters (fl)	Calculated as the plateletcrit (PCT) by the total number of platelets	
% Segmented Neutrophils	%	Percentage of neutrophils with normal, segmented nucleus (typically 3–5 segments)	Neutropenia: drug-induced, following viral, bacterial, or parasitic infections, nutritional deficiencies, autoimmunity, bone marrow suppression, inherited defects in genes responsible for neutrophil development
Segmented Neutrophils (Absolute count) *	Cells/mcL	Calculated as (WBC count × % segmented neutrophils)/100	Neutrophilia: normal physiological variation, response to acute infection, inflammatory processes, such as rheumatoid arthritis, ulcerative colitis, chronic hepatitis, medications, neoplastic processes, genetic disorders (e.g., leukocyte adhesion defect 1 and LAD1) and corticosteroid therapy
Immature Neutrophils*	%	Percentage of immature forms (band forms, metamyelocytes, myelocytes or promyelocytes)	An increase in immature granulocytes may occur due to physiological stresses, such as pregnancy, infection, or inflammation; or following administration of G-CSF; or due to hematological malignancies
Immature Neutrophils (Absolute count)	Cells/mcL	Calculated as (WBC count × % immature granulocytes)/100	
% Lymphocytes	%	Percentage of lymphocytes	Lymphocytosis: infections such as CMV, infectious mononucleosis; drug hypersensitivity reactions, stress, LGL leukemia, CLL, early HIV-1 infection
Lymphocytes (Absolute count)	Cells/mcL	Calculated as (WBC count × %lymphocytes)/100	Lymphopenia: inherited defects in genes responsible for lymphocyte development, immunosuppressants, such as glucocorticoids, chemotherapy, malignancy and AIDS
% Monocytes	%	Percentage of monocytes	Monocytosis: malignancies, response to infections (e.g., infectious mononucleosis)
Monocytes (Absolute count)	Cells/mcL	Calculated as (WBC count × % monocytes)/100	

Table 1 contd. ...

...Table 1 contd.

Parameter	Units	Description	Clinical Significance
% Eosinophils	%	Percentage of eosinophils	Eosinophilia: allergic diseases, parasitic infections, drug reactions, neoplastic diseases such as acute eosinophilic leukemia, CML, systemic mastocytosis and hypereosinophilic syndromes
Eosinophils (Absolute count)	Cells/mcL	Calculated as (WBC count × % eosinophils)/100	
% Basophils	%	Percentage of basophils	Allergic reactions, neoplastic diseases, such as CML and acute myeloid leukemia
Basophils (Absolute count)	Cells/mcL	Calculated as (WBC count × % basophils)/100	

* The absolute neutrophil count (ANC) includes both mature and immature neutrophils.

absolute values of neutrophils, lymphocytes, monocytes, eosinophils and basophils are reported. CBC parameters including WBC differential are detailed in Table 1.

CBCs are performed using manual methods or automated instruments (hematology analyzers or hematology systems) (Chhabra 2018). While manual methods have the advantage of low cost and require little infrastructure, they are labor-intensive and have relatively low throughput. Automated methods offer the advantage of high throughput analysis but require significantly more investment. Most clinical laboratories now use automated analyzers for CBCs; however, unusual findings on an automated CBC require a manual review of a blood smear by a pathologist to identify and quantify unusual or abnormal cell types. The International Consensus Group for Hematology Review (Barnes et al. 2005) which included 17 laboratories from six countries published suggested consensus criteria and recommended actions for follow-up of abnormal findings following automated CBC analyses. These criteria include delta checks and delta limits (recognition of previous abnormal CBC findings and the extent to which results differ from each other), results exceeding or falling below instrument linearity, limits for the various CBC parameters and abnormal findings on the WBC differential (including immature or atypical granulocytes or lymphocytes, presence of blasts and other immature forms of neutrophils). The presence of atypical or immature cells typically triggers a manual slide review of the sample. Individual laboratories establish triggers for manual slide reviews according to their patient populations.

CBCs are routinely performed using ethylenediaminetetraacetic acid (EDTA) anticoagulated blood, which is collected via venipuncture. Blood must be thoroughly mixed with EDTA prior to analysis to avoid spurious results due to inadequate anti-coagulation, and preferably analyzed within 6–8 hours of collection for optimal results. However, individual laboratories perform validation studies to determine acceptable sample stability following venipuncture and may analyze samples up to 24–48 hours following collection.

CBCs can provide important information to support clinical findings; however, as with any laboratory tests, the results must be interpreted within the context of clinical findings (see Chapter 1, pre- and post-test probability). Peripheral blood parameters are influenced by circadian rhythms, age, sex and race, as well as by extrinsic environmental factors (Feriel et al. 2021). For instance, hemoglobin levels vary between males and females after puberty owing to increased testosterone production in males that supports increased RBC production, and blood loss due to menstruation in females that results in relatively lower hemoglobin levels. WBC counts vary with age as do the absolute counts of individual WBC populations; lymphocyte counts are highest in newborns and infants, and slowly decline and eventually stabilize in early adulthood. This contrasts with absolute neutrophil counts that are relatively low compared with lymphocytes in infancy and increase with age. CBC parameters must therefore be reported with appropriate age-matched reference intervals to be interpreted accurately. Race and ethnicity also influence CBC parameters; Enujung Lim et al. highlighted the challenges of developing race or ethnicity-specific reference intervals for a variety of laboratory tests, including the CBC (Lim et al. 2015). While the development of race-specific CBC reference intervals is much more challenging, the majority of clinical laboratories report CBCs with age-specific reference intervals.

Absolute Eosinophil Count (AEC)

Eosinophils make up approximately 0–6% of WBC. Normal peripheral blood contains approximately $0.05–0.5 \times 10^3$ eosinophils/mcL.

Eosinophils develop from CD34+IL5Rα+ progenitors, that in turn arise from common myeloid progenitor cells within the bone marrow (Blanchard and Rothenberg 2009). Mature eosinophils contain a variety of pre-formed granules including major basic protein-1 and -2 (MBP-1 and MBP-2), eosinophil cationic protein (ECP), eosinophil-derived neurotoxin (EDN) and eosinophil peroxidase (EPX) (Acharya and Ackerman 2014). A variety of pre-formed growth factors (GM-CSF), chemokines [Eotaxin, C-C Motif Chemokine Ligand 5 (CCL5)], and cytokines (IL-2,

Table 2. Causes of eosinophilia.

Cause	Description	References
Primary HES	Idiopathic: > 1,500 eosinophils/mcL for > six months. Lymphocytic variant: Associated with IL-5 producing aberrant T cells Myeloproliferative HES, may be associated with gene rearrangements in *PDGFRB, PDGFRA, FIP1L1* or *FGFR1* Episodic eosinophilia with angioedema	Dispenza and Bochner 2018
Allergic disorders	Seasonal allergy, allergic rhinitis, atopic dermatitis, asthma, EoE; generally associated with mild eosinophilia (< 1,500 eosinophils/mcL)	Jenerowicz et al. 2007; Nakagome and Nagata 2018; Chen et al. 2020
Infection	Parasites: Nematodes (e.g., Strongyloidiasis, ascariasis, trichinellosis, hookworm infestation), filariasis (tropical pulmonary eosinophilia), flukes (schistosomiasis, fasciolopsiasis) and protozoa (Isospora belli and Dientamoeba fragilis) Fungal infections (e.g., histoplasmosis, allergic bronchopulmonary aspergillosis (ABPA) and coccidiodomycosis) HIV, *M. tuberculosis* and non-tuberculous mycobacterial infections can be associated with eosinophilia	Chou and Serpa 2015; O'Connell and Nutman 2015; Prakash Babu et al. 2019
Drug hypersensitivity	DRESS (drug reaction with eosinophilia and systemic symptoms)/ examples of drugs causing DRESS: antibiotics (beta-lactam antibiotics, sulfamethoxazole, minocycline, dapsone, and vancomycin), anticonvulsants (phenobarbital and phenytoin), retroviral agents (raltegravir and abacavir). Blood eosinophils may not be elevated, and a normal AEC does not rule out DRESS.	De et al. 2018)
Neoplastic	Primary HES (*PDGFRB, PDGFRA, FIP1L1* or *FGFR1* gene rearrangements; these gene rearrangements result in increased tyrosinase activity leading to overproduction and over-activation of eosinophils), eosinophilic leukemia, chronic myeloid leukemia, systemic mastocytosis, T or B cell lymphoma, Sezary syndrome (cutaneous T cell lymphoma), solid tumors	Baer et al. 2018
Endocrine	Adrenal insufficiency and steroid-induced adrenal suppression	Beishuizen et al. 1999
Immunologic	Autoimmune: Inflammatory bowel disease, sarcoidosis, IgG4 disease, EGPA or Churg-Strauss Syndrome, connective tissue disorders Immunodeficiency: Omenn syndrome, HES due to STAT3 or DOCK8 pathogenic variants and WAS	Navabi and Upton 2016; Diny et al. 2017

IL-4, IL-5 and IL-13) are present within eosinophil granules. Eosinophil-specific granules may mediate pathological processes and in fact, tissue deposition of these granules is a frequent finding in eosinophil-associated disease (Tai et al. 1987; Tajima and Katagiri 1996). MBP-1, MBP-2 and EPX are toxic to certain cell types, including airway epithelial cells, cardiac muscle cells and endothelium, thereby contributing to respiratory dysfunction and organ damage in eosinophil-mediated diseases (Slungaard and Mahoney 1991; McBrien and Menzies-Gow 2017). Eosinophils produce reactive oxygen species (e.g., peroxides and superoxides) and inflammatory cytokines, present antigens to T cells and induce B cell proliferation and the production of IgE (Kita 2013). While these biological processes have a role in immune protection against parasitic infections, they also play a significant role in mediating allergic inflammation, making the eosinophil a central player in allergic disease.

The eosinophil is primarily a tissue-dwelling cell and is found in the gut, thymus, adipose tissue, uterus, and mammary glands in healthy individuals (Mishra et al. 1999). Detection of eosinophils in other organs and tissues is generally associated with the disease.

Analysis of eosinophils is a critical part of the laboratory workup when suspecting allergic disease and includes the percentage as well as the absolute count of eosinophils per mcL or L of blood. This information is obtained from a CBC with WBC differential or may be available separately as an "Absolute Eosinophil Count (AEC)" in some laboratories. The AEC can be easily calculated from the percentage of eosinophils obtained from the CBC and the total WBC count. The percentage of eosinophils on a CBC may not provide sufficient clinically actionable information because the AEC is dependent on the WBC count and the relative percentages of the other WBC populations.

An increase in AEC above the expected age-matched reference range is known as "Eosinophilia." Eosinophilia is defined as an AEC of > 500 cells/mcL and is classified into mild (500–1,500 eosinophils/mcL), moderate (1,500–5,000 cells/mcL) and severe (> 5,000 eosinophils/mcL). Eosinophilia may be driven by pathogenic gene variants (primary eosinophilia) or may be secondary to parasitic diseases, infection, autoimmunity, immunodeficiency, drug reactions or malignancy (secondary eosinophilia). Although the causes of eosinophilia are similar in adults and children, atopic dermatitis, asthma, eosinophilic esophagitis (EoE) and certain hematological malignancies are more common in children.

Hypereosinophilic syndrome (HES) encompasses a group of diseases that are defined by an AEC of > 1,500 cells/mcL for which no obvious cause has been defined, persistent eosinophilia for at least six months and evidence of organ damage (Dispenza and Bochner 2018). HES may be due to inherited genetic defects or myeloproliferative disorders. Damage to the skin, respiratory tract, heart, and central nervous system is most commonly seen in HES, although other organs may be involved as well.

The causes of eosinophilia are listed in Table 2.

Total and Specific Immunoglobulin E and Component Resolved Diagnostics

Immunoglobulin E (IgE) is the fifth of the five isotypes of immunoglobulins and was the last to be discovered. The presence of a "serum factor" causing allergy was proposed as early as 1919 (Ramirez 1919); however, it took several decades for this factor to be identified as IgE. IgE was discovered independently by two groups: Kimishige and Teruko Ishizaka in Denver (The United States) and Hans Bennich and S.G.O. Johansson in Uppsala (Sweden) (reviewed in Reference) (Johansson 2011). Since the discovery of IgE, much has been learned about its structure and function.

IgE is a 190 kDa monomer, composed of two identical heavy chains (epsilon; E) with four constant regions, and two light chains. IgE mediates its function by binding to its specific high and low-affinity receptors. The high-affinity IgE receptor (Fc-epsilon R1; FcεR1), the alpha chain of which binds to the constant region of IgE, is highly expressed on basophils, mast cells, eosinophils, peripheral blood dendritic cells, airway epithelial and smooth muscle cells, and intestinal epithelial cells (Campbell et al. 1998; Gounni et al. 2005; Kraft and Kinet 2007; Untersmayr et al. 2010). The low-affinity IgE receptor, also known as FcεRII or CD23, is expressed on a variety of immune and non-immune cells including T and B cells, antigen-presenting cells, and airway and gut epithelial cells (Conrad et al. 1994). FcεRII plays a significant role in the uptake of allergen-IgE complexes by antigen-presenting cells, thereby promoting the presentation of allergens to the immune system.

Although present in very low concentrations in plasma, IgE is a potent inducer of allergic responses. Free IgE has a half-life of two days, but when bound to its high-affinity receptor FcεR1, its half-life is extended to approximately two weeks (Normansell et al. 2014). IgE has an exceedingly high affinity for FcεR1; therefore, most FcεR1 binding sites are occupied by IgE and only a minute amount of allergen is required to result in cross-linking of FcεR1. Following cross-linking of FcεR1, mast cells and basophils degranulate and release pre-formed mediators of the allergic response (e.g., histamine, TNF-α and tryptase) and initiate synthesis of lipid mediators such as prostaglandins, leukotrienes and platelet-activating factor from membrane phospholipids. This IgE-mediated type 1 hypersensitivity response is responsible for typical features of allergy including sneezing, skin rash and/or watery eyes, and in severe cases can result in anaphylaxis.

Serum IgE is expressed in kU/L where one kU is equivalent to 2.44 ng/mL. Assays that measure total IgE are calibrated against the World Health Organization IgE reference standard, currently 11/234 which is the 3rd International Standard for serum IgE (Thorpe et al. 2014).

The concentration of IgE in peripheral circulation is age dependent. Serum IgE is very low at birth with cord blood samples having less than 4.8 ng/mL. Serum IgE levels increase thereafter, reaching maximal levels around 6–14 years of age in both sexes, and remaining steady at approximately 22–85 kU/L throughout adult life (Barbee et al. 1981; Gergen et al. 2009).

Increases in serum IgE occur in a variety of diseases including infectious diseases (parasitic infections, viral infections, such as with cytomegalovirus (CMV) or Epstein-Barr virus (EBV), mycobacterial infections, candidiasis, atopic diseases, inflammatory diseases (Kawasaki disease, eosinophilic granulomatosis with polyangiitis) or immunodeficiency (Hyper IgE syndrome, Omenn syndrome, Wiskott Aldrich syndrome, Immune dysregulation, Polyendocrinopathy, Enteropathy, X-linked (IPEX) syndrome) and malignancies (IgE myeloma and Hodgkin's lymphoma)). Low IgE levels, which are defined as less than 2.5 kU/mL, may be associated with decreases in other immunoglobulin classes, sinopulmonary infections, and autoimmunity (Smith et al. 1997). Isolated, clinically significant, decreases in serum IgE levels are rare.

Measurement of Serum IgE

The radioallergosorbent test (RAST), a solid phase sandwich immunoassay was developed in 1967 to detect allergen-specific IgE in serum samples (Wide et al. 1967). In brief, allergens are bound to a solid phase; in this case, a paper disk and incubated with serum. Allergen-specific IgE present in serum binds to the immobilized allergen and unbound IgE washes away. Bound, allergen-specific IgE is detected using radiolabeled anti-IgE. Radioactive counts are an indirect measure of the level of allergen-specific IgE, which is expressed in arbitrary units. Since the development of the first solid phase immunoassay for IgE, several new assays that use this principle have been developed. The paper disk has been replaced by other solid phase supports such as agarose, microcrystalline cellulose or polystyrene. Radiolabeled antibodies have been replaced by enzyme-conjugated antibodies whose substrates lead to a chemiluminescence or fluorescence readout. Specific IgE units have been standardized as well; serum levels of specific IgE are expressed in kU_A/L, where the "A" refers to "allergen-specific" and differentiates it from total IgE which is expressed as kU/L.

The US FDA-approved methods for total and specific IgE measurement include the ImmunoCAP system (Thermo Fisher Phadia), Immulite (Siemens), Hytec Automated System (Hycor), and Cobas (Roche Diagnostics). These automated methods have enabled high throughput testing for both total and specific IgE and have resulted in improved assay sensitivity, specificity, and reproducibility (Hamilton and Franklin Adkinson 2004).

Allergen-specific IgG may interfere with the detection of specific IgE due to competitive binding for limited antigen-binding sites. It is not uncommon for individuals to have IgG specific to a variety of allergens in circulation, and its presence may merely reflect exposure to the allergen in the absence of clinical consequences. Individuals on immunotherapy, however, can develop high levels of specific IgG, particularly IgG4, in response to therapy. These high titers, allergen-specific IgG antibodies may interfere with the detection of specific IgE, whose serum concentration is several orders of magnitude lower than IgG. To overcome this interference, specific IgE detection systems use solid phases, such as cellulose that provide a large surface area for allergen binding, thereby providing antigen binding sites in molar excess of potentially available allergen-specific antibodies.

Crude extracts of allergens are used as capture antigens for the measurement of allergen-specific IgE. However, because of the structural similarity between antigens (e.g., peanut and soybean allergens share antigenic features with birch pollen), the specificity of such allergen preparations can be low. Thus, a person with birch allergy may have elevated specific IgE to peanut or soybean. The American Academy of Allergy, Asthma, and Immunology (AAAAI) provides a useful reference table of pollens and cross-reacting food allergens (https://www.aaaai.org/tools-for-the-public/ conditions-library/allergies/oral-allergy-syndrome-(oas)).

The characterization of molecular components of individual allergens has led to "component resolved diagnostics" or CRD, particularly for food allergies (Tuano and Davis 2015). The ability to evaluate specific IgE to individual components of a food allergen has led to improved sensitivity and specificity of these assays. For instance, over 13 allergenic components have been defined in peanuts. Of these, specific IgE to the molecule Ara h 2 (a storage protein and peanut-specific marker) has been shown to be significantly associated with clinical allergy to peanuts (Hemmings et al. 2020). On the other hand, Ara h 8 is a PR-10 protein and is cross-reactive to tree pollen, especially birch, and is positive in oral allergy syndrome. Individuals who are positive for Ara h 2 have the potential for anaphylaxis and need to be evaluated for possible oral desensitization. Molecularly defined components are now available for a variety of allergens including peanut, egg, milk, wheat, soybean and a variety of tree nuts (Tuano and Davis 2015). The advantage of CRD is that these individual components of the allergen can either be purified from crude extracts or can be produced by recombinant protein technology, thereby allowing for a better definition of these allergenic proteins as well as their use in standardized assays.

Analysis of specific IgE, while a useful component of the laboratory workup for allergy, must be interpreted with caution and in the context of clinical history for allergy and relevant clinical findings. Particularly in the case of patients with very high total IgE levels (> 1,000 kU/L), false positive results for specific IgE to multiple allergens may be obtained (Merkel et al. 2015). In addition, a diagnosis of allergy, especially food allergy, cannot be made based on specific IgE measurements alone as there are no well-established clinically relevant cut-off values for food allergen-specific IgE (Greenhawt et al. 2020). Furthermore, the carbohydrate groups of IgE may bind to the lectins in foods, resulting in falsely elevated IgE values, that does not indicate specific food antigen binding to the Fab region of IgE (Shibasaki et al. 1992).

Serum Tryptase

Serum tryptase measurements form an important part of the laboratory workup in the field of allergy, particularly for the evaluation of mastocytosis, familial hypertryptasemia and anaphylaxis.

Tryptases are a subgroup of trypsin-family serine proteases and are one of the major products of mast cell degranulation (Payne and Kam 2004). Mast cells, which are tissue-resident granulocytes, play a key role in mediating allergic reactions. Mast cell degranulation can be triggered by cross-linking of allergen-specific IgE on the surface of mast cells as well as non-IgE-mediated mechanisms. The latter include physical stimuli, activation of neurokinin receptors, drugs acting via MRGPRX2 receptors as well as anaphylatoxins (C3a, C4a and C5a) derived from complement activation and T cell cytokines (Theoharides et al. 2019). This results in the release of pre-formed mediators like histamine, tryptase and heparin, as well as the subsequently synthesized lipid mediators like prostaglandins, platelet-activating factor and leukotrienes. In healthy individuals, tryptase is produced constitutively at basal levels. Although the biological function of tryptase has not been fully elucidated, tryptase may be involved in a variety of biological processes including airway homeostasis, gastrointestinal smooth muscle activity and contraction and relaxation of the vasculature [reviewed in (Hallgren and Pejler 2006)]. Tryptase may also play a role in mediating inflammation, chemotaxis, and fibroblast proliferation (Hallgren and Pejler 2006). These processes tend to be magnified in allergic reactions, thus suggesting a role for tryptase in the clinical presentation of IgE-mediated allergic diseases or mast cell disorders.

There are two main forms of tryptase, α-tryptase and β-tryptase, with approximately 90% sequence identity between the two. The α- and β-tryptase exist in mature (active) and immature (protryptase; inactive) forms within mast cells. Immature protryptase is spontaneously secreted by mast cells and constitutes most of what is measured in serum in healthy individuals. In the presence of heparin, protryptases are proteolyzed to their mature forms (α- and β-tryptase) and are present within mast cell secretory granules complexed with heparin proteoglycan (Sakai et al. 1996; Schwartz et al. 2003). These active, mature forms of tryptase are released when mast cells degranulate.

The genes encoding tryptase, *TPSAB1* and *TPSAB2* reside on the short arm of chromosome 16 (Le et al. 2019). *TPSAB1* is dimorphic and can give rise to either α or β tryptase, whereas *TPSAB2* codes for β-tryptase alone. Most individuals have four functional tryptase genes, which can generate phenotypes $\alpha\alpha$:$\beta\beta$, $\alpha\beta$:$\beta\beta$ or $\beta\beta$:$\beta\beta$. The diversity of tryptase genotypes is influenced by race and ethnicity (Trivedi et al. 2009); although individuals lacking the gene coding for α-tryptase have been identified (Soto et al. 2002), genetic deficiency of β-tryptase has thus far not been reported (Trivedi et al. 2009). These variations in genotype have an insignificant effect on serum tryptase levels; thus, despite the variation in genotype, all individuals with four tryptase coding genes have physiological levels of serum tryptase.

Hereditary α-tryptasemia (HaT) is an autosomal dominant condition in which there is an increase in the copy number of the *TPSAB1* gene (while gene duplication is found in the majority of individuals, three, four or even five gene copies have been reported) (Lyons et al. 2016; Sabato et al. 2018). In the UK, HaT occurs in approximately 5–8% of the general population (Robey et al. 2020). These individuals have increased production of a-tryptase and elevated baseline total tryptase levels, but normal mature tryptase levels.

Individuals with HaT can present with a variety of clinical symptoms including irritable bowel syndrome-like symptoms (abdominal pain; bloating) (Hamilton et al. 2021), skin flushing, itching or recurrent hives, joint hypermobility, changes in blood pressure or heart rate. More serious clinical presentations such as anaphylactic reactions, particularly to insect venom may occur (O'Connell and Lyons 2020). HaT is also associated with mastocytosis, a hematopoietic neoplasm in which clonal populations of mast cells infiltrate a variety of organs (Heybeli 2015).

Analysis of Serum Tryptase

Manual immunoassays such as ELISA can be used to measure serum tryptase levels; however, the automated fluorescent enzyme immunoassay (FEIA) developed by Thermofisher Phadia is much more widely used in clinical laboratories. This assay measures total tryptase, including all forms of α-tryptase and β-tryptase (ImmunoCAP™ Tryptase | Thermo Fisher Scientific). In this assay, anti-tryptase antibodies are immobilized on a cellulose sponge. Tryptase, present in serum samples, binds the anti-tryptase antibodies and is detected by an enzyme-conjugated anti-tryptase antibody followed by a developing agent. The enzyme-developing agent reaction results in fluorescence which is proportional to the amount of total tryptase in the sample.

Tryptase levels can be measured in both serum and plasma. Samples should be analyzed as soon as possible following collection, and preferably stored frozen if the analysis is delayed, thus avoiding degradation of tryptase.

Serum tryptase levels range from 1–11.4 ng/mL in healthy individuals. Values greater than 11.4 ng/mL are considered elevated; however, the patient's basal tryptase value must also be considered when evaluating an acute episode such as anaphylaxis. Tryptase levels that are greater than 1.2x baseline tryptase level + 2 ng during a symptomatic episode are indicative of mast cell activation, even if measured tryptase levels are within the normal range (Valent et al. 2012). Although the diagnosis of anaphylaxis is made clinically, tryptase levels measured within 30–120 minutes of a reaction can be helpful to differentiate anaphylaxis from clinical conditions (asthma exacerbation, panic attacks, C1-inhibitor deficiency, ACE-inhibitor induced angioedema, and vasovagal syncope) that present similarly.

Table 3. Elevated tryptase levels.

Condition	Description
Anaphylaxis	Correlates with the severity of anaphylaxis; does not distinguish between IgE mediated (e.g., insect venom allergy) and non-IgE mediated (e.g., reaction to NSAIDs) anaphylaxis; tryptase levels begin to rise within minutes of clinical symptoms of anaphylaxis and reach maximal levels within 30–90 minutes. In severe reactions, tryptase levels may remain elevated for a longer period
Systemic or Cutaneous Mastocytosis	Baseline total tryptase is generally > 20 ng/mL; activating mutations of *KIT*, cytopenias or other hematological malignancies may be present
Mast Cell Activation Syndrome (MCAS)	Characterized by episodes of symptoms related to mast cell activation, an elevated tryptase level
Hereditary α-Tryptasemia (HaT)	Elevated total tryptase, *TPSAB1* gene copy number analysis
Malignancy	Mast cell leukemia, chronic eosinophilic leukemia, acute and chronic myeloid leukemia, myelodysplastic syndrome, myeloproliferative syndromes, myelomastocytic leukemias. The source of tryptase is neoplastic mast cells or basophils

Abbreviations: IgE; Immunoglobulin E; NSAID; Non-Steroidal Anti-Inflammatory Drug.

Raised serum tryptase levels reflect mast cell degranulation and are not specific to IgE- or non-IgE-mediated reactions. Thus, an elevated tryptase level must be correlated with clinical and other significant laboratory findings. Conditions in which tryptase can be elevated are listed in Table 3.

Acute Phase Reactants: Erythrocyte Sedimentation Rate (ESR) and C-Reactive Protein (CRP)

Analysis of ESR and CRP are widely used in the laboratory work of a variety of clinical conditions. While these tests, when used in conjunction with clinical findings and in the context of other laboratory findings, can be very useful, it is important to note that these tests are not specific to any clinical condition.

Erythrocyte Sedimentation Rate: ESR is the rate at which RBCs settle in a sample of anticoagulated blood over a specific time interval (typically 60 minutes). This phenomenon was first observed in 1897 by Dr. Edmund Biernacki, who noted that the rate at which RBCs settled was related to the amount of fibrinogen in the blood (Grzybowski and Sak 2012). A method for measuring ESR was described by Drs. R. Fahraeus and A. Westergren in 1921, following which it became a laboratory tool for the evaluation of both acute and chronic diseases (Grzybowski and Sak 2012). The Westergren method for measurement of ESR rapidly became the laboratory standard and while automated and more rapid methods have replaced this original method, new technologies for the measurement of ESR are standardized against the Westergren reference method. The International Committee for Standardization in Hematology (ICSH) provides guidelines for the standardization of ESR measurement methods, using the Westergren method as a reference (Jou et al. 2011).

ESR measured by the Westergren method uses sodium citrate anticoagulated blood. Samples should preferably be analyzed within 2 hours or stored at 4°C if the analysis is delayed. The sample is transferred into a Westergren tube (a 2.5 mm bore tube that is graduated in mm from 0–200) and allowed to stand for 60 minutes. The column of settled RBCs is measured at the end of 60 min and ESR is reported in mm/hr.

Inaccurate ESR results may occur if the ESR tube is tilted, results are read before or after 60 minutes, the ratio of blood to anticoagulant is suboptimal, or bubbles are present in the tube.

While individual laboratories should validate reference ranges specific to their instruments or method of analysis, commonly accepted ESR reference ranges are 0–15 mm/hr for males, and 0–22 mm/hr for females (Bottiger and Svedberg 1967).

A variety of factors influence the ESR.

1. *Increased plasma proteins*: An increase in plasma proteins (e.g., immunoglobulins and/or acute phase proteins such as fibrinogen, CRP, haptoglobin, complement proteins, prothrombin, plasminogen and alpha-1 antitrypsin) due to an ongoing inflammatory process leads to clumping of RBCs, or rouleaux (stacks) formation, allowing them to settle at a more rapid rate. Additionally, RBCs are inherently negatively charged and repel each other, thus reducing clumping. Positively charged plasma proteins can neutralize the negative charge on the surface of RBCs, allowing them to clump, thereby increasing the ESR. Many of these inflammation-associated proteins increase in response to infection, malignancy, autoimmune processes or trauma; however, plasma proteins also increase during physiological changes such as pregnancy.

2. *RBC size*: Macrocytes settle rapidly leading to a falsely increased ESR. Conversely, microcytes settle less rapidly leading to relatively low ESR.

3. *Erythrocyte shape*: Spherocytes, as found in hereditary or autoimmune hemolytic anemia and sickle cells (sickle cell anemia) cannot aggregate, and therefore lead to a low ESR.

4. *Erythrocyte number*: A lower RBC count leads to an increased ESR whereas increased RBC counts as seen in polycythemic patients lead to a low ESR. Polycythemia decreases rouleaux formation and therefore artificially decreased ESR.

5. *Leukocytosis*: Increased WBC counts can impede the settling of RBCs, thereby decreasing the ESR.

6. *Physiological factors*: Females have a higher ESR than males. Pregnancy, menstruation and aging also increase ESR.

C-reactive Protein: C-reactive protein (CRP), first discovered by Tillet and Francis in 1930, is an acute phase, highly conserved, inflammatory protein that is synthesized by the liver. The name "C-Reactive Protein" or CRP is derived from the ability of the protein to react with the capsular (C)-polysaccharide of *Pneumococcus* (Black et al. 2004). CRP is produced chiefly by hepatocytes in response to increased levels of proinflammatory cytokines, interleukin-6 in particular. Plasma levels of CRP rise rapidly in response to infectious and immune stimuli and can result in a thousand-fold or greater increase within 24–72 hours. This rapid rise is generally accompanied by a rapid decrease in CRP levels with the resolution of the infectious or inflammatory process. Although CRP levels increase in acute or chronic inflammatory states, physiological factors such as age, sex and race can affect CRP levels. Mild to moderate increases in CRP occurs in association with metabolic dysfunction, such as obesity and insulin resistance.

CRP plays an important role in the clearance of pathogens and damaged or apoptotic cells, and activation of phagocytic cells and the complement cascade. While this protective or housekeeping function is beneficial, these very processes can turn pathological in the setting of an autoimmune or malignant process, or significant trauma, and can contribute to increased tissue damage.

CRP is typically measured in serum or plasma samples, collected by standard venipuncture. Immunoturbidimetry or nephelometry are commonly used, automated, techniques to measure CRP levels. Normal CRP levels are less than 10 mg/L. Values > 10 mg/L generally indicate clinically significant inflammation. High-sensitivity CRP (hsCRP) assays are capable of measuring very low concentrations of CRP, generally in the 3 to 10 mg/L range. These lower concentrations of CRP generally correlate with low-grade inflammation that may occur in a variety of metabolic stressors.

Clinical Utility of ESR and CRP

Both ESR and CRP are useful but non-specific laboratory tests and results must be interpreted with caution, considering a variety of factors, both physiological and pathological, that can affect the ESR. While an increased ESR or CRP may be indicative of an ongoing inflammatory process, it should be taken in the context of clinical and other relevant laboratory findings. For instance, CRP may be increased in DRESS Syndrome, which typically presents with fever, skin rash, lymphadenopathy and organ involvement, and is triggered by a severe adverse reaction to a variety of drugs including anticonvulsants and sulfonamide-containing antibiotics (Hubner et al. 2018). The occurrence of DRESS syndrome in patients who have an elevated CRP level and who are on antibiotics may result in a diagnostic dilemma because an infectious etiology may be suspected and treatment (withdrawal of the inciting drug) may be delayed.

Although increases in CRP and ESR tend to track together, discrepancies between the two do occur. Particularly in autoimmune diseases, such as rheumatoid arthritis, CRP and ESR are often elevated during an acute inflammatory episode. Laboratory findings in Systemic Lupus Erythematosus (SLE), however, can present an exception, while ESR is often elevated in SLE, CRP levels can be low (Gaitonde et al. 2008). Low CRP levels in SLE have been attributed to type 1 interferons which are highly elevated in SLE and inhibit the production of CRP in hepatocytes (Enocsson et al. 2009). Thus, elevated CRP in SLE patients may in fact be suggestive of acute infection, rather than inflammation driven by ongoing autoimmune processes.

CRP values tend to drop markedly following the initiation of treatment whereas ESR may take weeks to reach normal levels (Litao and Kamat 2014). ESR has therefore been proposed as a better monitoring tool for disease progression and response to therapy, particularly for chronic diseases such as rheumatoid arthritis, whereas CRP is likely to be more beneficial for the management of acute bacterial infections or acute inflammatory conditions.

Glossary of Abbreviations

ABPA – Allergic Bronchopulmonary Aspergillosis
ACE – Angiotensin Converting Enzyme
AEC – Absolute Eosinophil Count
AIDS – Acquired Immunodeficiency Syndrome
CBC – Complete Blood Count
CCL5 – C-C Motif Chemokine Ligand 5
CLL – Chronic Lymphocytic Leukemia
CML – Chronic Myeloid Leukemia
CMV – Cytomegalovirus
COPD – Chronic Obstructive Pulmonary Disease
CRD – Component Resolved Diagnostics
CRP – C-Reactive protein
DIC – Disseminated Intravascular Coagulation
dL – Deciliter
DOCK8 – Dedicator of Cytokinesis 8
DRESS – Drug Rash with Eosinophilia and Systemic Symptoms
EBV – Epstein-Barr Virus
ECP – Eosinophil Cationic Protein
EDN – eosinophil-Derived Neurotoxin
EDTA – Ethylenediaminetetraacetic Acid
EGPA – Eosinophilic Granulomatosis With Polyangiitis
EoE – Eosinophilic Esophagitis

EPX – Eosinophil Peroxidase
ESR – Erythrocyte Sedimentation Rate
FcεR1 – Fc-Epsilon Receptor 1
FDA – Food and Drug Administration
FEIA- Fluorescent Enzyme Immunoassay
FIP1L1 – Factor Interacting With PAPOLA And CPSF1
fL – Femtoliter
G-CSF – Granulocyte Colony Stimulating Factor
HaT – Hereditary Alpha Tryptasemia
Hb – Hemoglobin
HES – Hyper Eosinophilic Syndrome
HIV – Human Immunodeficiency Virus
IgE – Immunoglubulin E
IL-13 – Interleukin-13
IL-2 – Interleukin-2
IL-4 – Interleukin-4
IL-5 – Interleukin-5
IPEX – Immune Dysregulation, Polyendocrinopathy, Enteropathy, X-linked
kU – Kilo Unit
kUA – Kilo Unit Allergen
L – Liter
LAD – Leukocyte Adhesion Deficiency
LGL – Large Granular Lymphocyte
MBP – Major Basic Protein
MCH – Mean Corpuscular Hemoglobin
MCHC – Mean Corpuscular Hemoglobin Concentration
mcL – Microliter
MCV – Mean Corpuscular Volume
MPV – Mean Platelet Volume
NSAID – Non-Steroidal Anti-inflammatory Drug
PCT – Plateletcrit
PDGFRA – Platelet-Derived Growth Factor Receptor Alpha
PDGFRB – Platelet-Derived Growth Factor Receptor Beta
Pg – Picogram
PNH – Paroxsysmal Nocturnal Hematuria
PRCA – Pure Red Cell Aplasia
PV – Polycythemia Vera
RAST – Radioallergosorbent Test
RBC – Red Blood Cell
RDW – Red Cell Distribution Width
SIgE – Specific Immunoglobulin E
SLE – Systemic Lupus Erythematosus
STAT3 – Signal Transducer and Activator Of Transcription 3
TNFα – Tumor Necrosis Factor alpha
WAS – Wiskott Aldrich Syndrome
WBC – White Blood Cell

References

Acharya, K. R. and Ackerman, S. J. 2014. Eosinophil granule proteins: form and function. J. Biol. Chem. 289(25): 17406–17415.

Baer, C., Muehlbacher, V., Kern, W., Haferlach, C. and Haferlach, T. 2018. Molecular genetic characterization of myeloid/lymphoid neoplasms associated with eosinophilia and rearrangement of PDGFRA, PDGFRB, FGFR1 or PCM1-JAK2. Haematologica 103(8): e348–e350.

Barbee, R. A., Halonen, M., Lebowitz, M. and Burrows, B. 1981. Distribution of IgE in a community population sample: correlations with age, sex, and allergen skin test reactivity. J. Allergy Clin. Immunol. 68(2): 106–111.

Barnes, P. W., S. L. McFadden, S. J. Machin and E. Simson. 2005. The international consensus group for hematology review: suggested criteria for action following automated CBC and WBC differential analysis. Lab Hematol. 11(2): 83–90. doi: 10.1532/LH96.05019. PMID: 16024331.

Beishuizen, A., Vermes, I., Hylkema, B. S. and Haanen, C. 1999. Relative eosinophilia and functional adrenal insufficiency in critically ill patients. Lancet 353(9165): 1675–1676.

Black, S., Kushner, I. and Samols, D. 2004. C-reactive Protein. J. Biol. Chem. 279(47): 48487–48490.

Blanchard, C. and Rothenberg, M. E. 2009. Biology of the eosinophil. Adv. Immunol. 101: 81–121.

Bottiger, L. E. and Svedberg, C. A. 1967. Normal erythrocyte sedimentation rate and age. Br Med. J. 2(5544): 85–87.

Brightling, C. E., Chanez, P., Leigh, R., O'Byrne, P. M., Korn, S., She, D. et al. 2015. Efficacy and safety of tralokinumab in patients with severe uncontrolled asthma: a randomised, double-blind, placebo-controlled, phase 2b trial. Lancet Respir. Med. 3(9): 692–701.

Campbell, A. M., Vachier, I., Chanez, P., Vignola, A. M., Lebel, B., Kochan, J. et al. 1998. Expression of the high-affinity receptor for IgE on bronchial epithelial cells of asthmatics. Am. J. Respir. Cell Mol. Biol. 19(1): 92–97.

Castro, M., Wenzel, S. E., Bleecker, E. R., Pizzichini, E., Kuna, P., Busse, W. W. et al. 2014. Benralizumab, an anti-interleukin 5 receptor alpha monoclonal antibody, versus placebo for uncontrolled eosinophilic asthma: a phase 2b randomised dose-ranging study. Lancet Respir. Med. 2(11): 879–890.

Chen, Y., Yang, M., Deng, J., Wang, K., Shi, J. and Sun, Y. 2020. Elevated levels of activated and pathogenic eosinophils characterize moderate-severe house dust mite allergic rhinitis. J. Immunol. Res. 2020: 8085615.

Chhabra, G. 2018. Automated hematology analyzers: Recent trends and applications. J. Lab Physicians 10(1): 15–16.

Chou, A. and Serpa, J. A. 2015. Eosinophilia in patients infected with human immunodeficiency virus. Curr. HIV/AIDS Rep. 12(3): 313–316.

Conrad, D. H., Campbell, K. A., Bartlett, W. C., Squire, C. M. and Dierks, S. E. 1994. Structure and function of the low affinity IgE receptor. Adv. Exp. Med. Biol. 347: 17–30.

Corren, J., Weinstein, S., Janka, L., Zangrilli, J. and Garin, M. 2016. Phase 3 Study of Reslizumab in patients with poorly controlled asthma: effects across a broad range of eosinophil counts. Chest 150(4): 799–810.

De, A., Rajagopalan, M., Sarda, A., Das, S. and Biswas, P. 2018. Drug reaction with eosinophilia and systemic symptoms: an update and review of recent literature. Indian J. Dermatol. 63(1): 30–40.

Diny, N. L., Rose, N. R. and Cihakova, D. 2017. Eosinophils in autoimmune diseases. Front. Immunol. 8: 484.

Dispenza, M. C. and Bochner, B. S. 2018. Diagnosis and novel approaches to the treatment of hypereosinophilic syndromes. Curr. Hematol. Malig. Rep. 13(3): 191–201.

Enocsson, H., Sjowall, C., Skogh, T., Eloranta, M. L., Ronnblom, L. and Wettero, J. 2009. Interferon-alpha mediates suppression of C-reactive protein: explanation for muted C-reactive protein response in lupus flares? Arthritis Rheum 60(12): 3755–3760.

Feriel, J., Tchipeva, D. and Depasse, F. 2021. Effects of circadian variation, lifestyle and environment on hematological parameters: A narrative review. Int. J. Lab Hematol. 43(5): 917–926.

Fred, H. L. 2007. Maxwell Myer Wintrobe: new history and a new appreciation. Tex Heart Inst. J. 34(3): 328–335.

Gaitonde, S., Samols, D. and Kushner, I. 2008. C-reactive protein and systemic lupus erythematosus. Arthritis Rheum 59(12): 1814–1820.

George-Gay, B. and Parker, K. 2003. Understanding the complete blood count with differential. J. Perianesth Nurs 18(2): 96–114; quiz 115–117.

Gergen, P. J., Arbes, Jr., S. J., Calatroni, A., Mitchell, H. E. and Zeldin, D. C. 2009. Total IgE levels and asthma prevalence in the US population: results from the National Health and Nutrition Examination Survey 2005–2006. J. Allergy Clin. Immunol. 124(3): 447–453.

Gounni, A. S., Wellemans, V., Yang, J., Bellesort, F., Kassiri, K., Gangloff, S. et al. 2005. Human airway smooth muscle cells express the high affinity receptor for IgE (Fc epsilon RI): a critical role of Fc epsilon RI in human airway smooth muscle cell function. J. Immunol. 175(4): 2613–2621.

Greenhawt, M., Shaker, M., Wang, J., Oppenheimer, J. J., Sicherer, S., Keet, C. et al. 2020. Peanut allergy diagnosis: A 2020 practice parameter update, systematic review, and GRADE analysis. J. Allergy Clin. Immunol. 146(6): 1302–1334.

Grzybowski, A. and Sak, J. 2012. A short history of the discovery of the erythrocyte sedimentation rate. Int. J. Lab Hematol. 34(4): 442–444.

Hallgren, J. and Pejler, G. 2006. Biology of mast cell tryptase. An inflammatory mediator. FEBS J. 273(9): 1871–1895.

Hamilton, M. J., Zhao, M., Giannetti, M. P., Weller, E., Hufdhi, R., Novak, P. et al. 2021. Distinct small intestine mast cell histologic changes in patients with hereditary alpha-tryptasemia and mast cell activation syndrome. Am. J. Surg. Pathol. 45(7): 997–1004.

Hamilton, R. G. and Franklin Adkinson, Jr., N. 2004. *In vitro* assays for the diagnosis of IgE-mediated disorders. J. Allergy Clin. Immunol. 114(2): 213–225; quiz 226.

Hemmings, O., Du Toit, G., Radulovic, S., Lack, G. and Santos, A. F. 2020. Ara h 2 is the dominant peanut allergen despite similarities with Ara h 6. J. Allergy Clin. Immunol. 146(3): 621–630 e625.

Heybeli, C. 2015. Mast cells, mastocytosis, and related disorders. N Engl. J. Med. 373(19): 1885.

Hubner, S. T., Bertoli, R., Ratz Bravo, A. E., Schaueblin, M., Haschke, M., Scherer, K. et al. 2018. C-Reactive protein and procalcitonin in case reports of drug reaction with eosinophilia and systemic symptoms (DRESS) syndrome. Int. Arch Allergy Immunol. 176(1): 44–54.

Jenerowicz, D., Czarnecka-Operacz, M. and Silny, W. 2007. Peripheral blood eosinophilia in atopic dermatitis. Acta Dermatovenerol Alp Pannonica Adriat 16(2): 47–52.

Johansson, S. G. 2011. The History of IgE: From discovery to 2010. Curr. Allergy Asthma Rep. 11(2): 173–177.

Jou, J. M., Lewis, S. M., Briggs, C., Lee, S. H., De La Salle, B., McFadden, S. et al. 2011. ICSH review of the measurement of the erythrocyte sedimentation rate. Int. J. Lab Hematol. 33(2): 125–132.

Kay, A. B. 2016. Paul Ehrlich and the early history of granulocytes. Microbiol. Spectr. 4(4).

Kita, H. 2013. Eosinophils: multifunctional and distinctive properties. Int. Arch. Allergy Immunol. 161 Suppl 2: 3–9.

Kraft, S. and Kinet, J. P. 2007. New developments in FcepsilonRI regulation, function and inhibition. Nat. Rev. Immunol. 7(5): 365–378.

Le, Q. T., Lyons, J. J., Naranjo, A. N., Olivera, A., Lazarus, R. A., Metcalfe, D. D. et al. 2019. Impact of naturally forming human alpha/beta-tryptase heterotetramers in the pathogenesis of hereditary alpha-tryptasemia. J. Exp. Med. 216(10): 2348–2361.

Lim, E., Miyamura, J. and Chen, J. J. 2015. Racial/ethnic-specific reference intervals for common laboratory tests: a comparison among asians, blacks, hispanics, and white. Hawaii J. Med. Public Health 74(9): 302–310.

Litao, M. K. and Kamat, D. 2014. Erythrocyte sedimentation rate and C-reactive protein: how best to use them in clinical practice. Pediatr Ann. 43(10): 417–420.

Lyons, J. J., Yu, X., Hughes, J. D., Le, Q. T., Jamil, A., Bai, Y. et al. 2016. Elevated basal serum tryptase identifies a multisystem disorder associated with increased TPSAB1 copy number. Nat. Genet. 48(12): 1564–1569.

Massanari, M., Holgate, S. T., Busse, W. W., Jimenez, P., Kianifard, F. and Zeldin, R. 2010. Effect of omalizumab on peripheral blood eosinophilia in allergic asthma. Respir Med. 104(2): 188–196.

McBrien, C. N. and Menzies-Gow, A. 2017. The biology of eosinophils and their role in asthma. Front. Med. (Lausanne) 4: 93.

Merkel, P. A., O'Sullivan, M. D., Ridge, C. and Knight, V. 2015. Critique on the quantitative nature of IgE antibody measurements. J. Allergy Clin. Immunol. Pract. 3(6): 973–975.

Mishra, A., Hogan, S. P., Lee, J. J., Foster, P. S. and Rothenberg, M. E. 1999. Fundamental signals that regulate eosinophil homing to the gastrointestinal tract. J. Clin. Invest 103(12): 1719–1727.

Nakagome, K. and Nagata, M. 2018. Involvement and possible role of eosinophils in asthma exacerbation. Front Immunol. 9: 2220.

Navabi, B. and Upton, J. E. 2016. Primary immunodeficiencies associated with eosinophilia. Allergy Asthma Clin. Immunol. 12: 27.

Normansell, R., Walker, S., Milan, S. J., Walters, E. H. and Nair, P. 2014. Omalizumab for asthma in adults and children. Cochrane Database Syst. Rev. (1): CD003559.

O'Connell, E. M. and Nutman, T. B. 2015. Eosinophilia in infectious diseases. Immunol. Allergy Clin. North Am. 35(3): 493–522.

O'Connell, M. P. and Lyons, J. J. 2020. Hymenoptera venom-induced anaphylaxis and hereditary alpha-tryptasemia. Curr. Opin. Allergy Clin. Immunol. 20(5): 431–437.

Ortega, H. G., Liu, M. C., Pavord, I. D., Brusselle, G. G., FitzGerald, J. M., Chetta, A. et al. 2014. Mepolizumab treatment in patients with severe eosinophilic asthma. N Engl. J. Med. 371(13): 1198–1207.

Payne, V. and Kam, P. C. 2004. Mast cell tryptase: a review of its physiology and clinical significance. Anaesthesia 59(7): 695–703.

Prakash Babu, S., Narasimhan, P. B. and Babu, S. 2019. Eosinophil polymorphonuclear leukocytes in TB: What we know so far. Front. Immunol. 10: 2639.

Qu, S. Q., Qin, T. J., Xu, Z. F., Zhang, Y., Ai, X. F., Li, B. et al. 2016. Long-term outcomes of imatinib in patients with FIP1L1/PDGFRA associated chronic eosinophilic leukemia: experience of a single center in China. Oncotarget 7(22): 33229–33236.

Ramirez, M. 1919. Horse Asthma following blood transfusion: report of case. JAMA 73(13): 984–985.

Robey, R. C., Wilcock, A., Bonin, H., Beaman, G., Myers, B., Grattan, C. et al. 2020. Hereditary alpha-tryptasemia: UK prevalence and variability in disease expression. J. Allergy Clin. Immunol. Pract. 8(10): 3549–3556.

Robinson, J. P. 2013. Wallace H. Coulter: decades of invention and discovery. Cytometry A 83(5): 424–438.

Rothenberg, M. E., Wen, T., Greenberg, A., Alpan, O., Enav, B., Hirano, I. et al. 2015. Intravenous anti-IL-13 mAb QAX576 for the treatment of eosinophilic esophagitis. J. Allergy Clin. Immunol. 135(2): 500–507.

Sabato, V., Chovanec, J., Faber, M., Milner, J. D., Ebo, D. and Lyons, J. J. 2018. First identification of an inherited TPSAB1 quintuplication in a patient with clonal mast cell disease. J. Clin. Immunol. 38(4): 457–459.

Sakai, K., Ren, S. and Schwartz, L. B. 1996. A novel heparin-dependent processing pathway for human tryptase. Autocatalysis followed by activation with dipeptidyl peptidase I. J. Clin. Invest 97(4): 988–995.

Schwartz, L. B., Min, H. K., Ren, S., Xia, H. Z., Hu, J., Zhao, W. et al. 2003. Tryptase precursors are preferentially and spontaneously released, whereas mature tryptase is retained by HMC-1 cells, Mono-Mac-6 cells, and human skin-derived mast cells. J. Immunol. 170(11): 5667–5673.

Shibasaki, M., Sumazaki, R., Isoyama, S. and Takita, H. 1992. Interaction of lectins with human IgE: IgE-binding property and histamine-releasing activity of twelve plant lectins. Int. Arch. Allergy Immunol. 98(1): 18–25.

Simpson, E. L., Flohr, C., Eichenfield, L. F., Bieber, T., Sofen, H., Taieb, A. et al. 2018. Efficacy and safety of lebrikizumab (an anti-IL-13 monoclonal antibody) in adults with moderate-to-severe atopic dermatitis inadequately controlled by topical corticosteroids: A randomized, placebo-controlled phase II trial (TREBLE). J. Am. Acad. Dermatol. 78(5): 863–871 e811.

Slungaard, A. and Mahoney, Jr., J. R. 1991. Bromide-dependent toxicity of eosinophil peroxidase for endothelium and isolated working rat hearts: a model for eosinophilic endocarditis. J. Exp. Med. 173(1): 117–126.

Smith, J. K., Krishnaswamy, G. H., Dykes, R., Reynolds, S. and Berk, S. L. 1997. Clinical manifestations of IgE hypogammaglobulinemia. Ann. Allergy Asthma Immunol. 78(3): 313–318.

Soto, D., Malmsten, C., Blount, J. L., Muilenburg, D. J. and Caughey, G. H. 2002. Genetic deficiency of human mast cell alpha-tryptase. Clin. Exp. Allergy 32(7): 1000–1006.

Tai, P. C., Ackerman, S. J., Spry, C. J., Dunnette, S., Olsen, E. G. and Gleich, G. J. 1987. Deposits of eosinophil granule proteins in cardiac tissues of patients with eosinophilic endomyocardial disease. Lancet 1(8534): 643–647.

Tajima, K. and Katagiri, T. 1996. Deposits of eosinophil granule proteins in eosinophilic cholecystitis and eosinophilic colitis associated with hypereosinophilic syndrome. Dig. Dis. Sci. 41(2): 282–288.

Theoharides, T. C., Tsilioni, I. and Ren, H. 2019. Recent advances in our understanding of mast cell activation - or should it be mast cell mediator disorders? Expert Rev. Clin. Immunol. 15(6): 639–656.

Thorpe, S. J., Heath, A., Fox, B., Patel, D. and Egner, W. 2014. The 3rd International Standard for serum IgE: international collaborative study to evaluate a candidate preparation. Clin. Chem. Lab Med. 52(9): 1283–1289.

Trivedi, N. N., Tamraz, B., Chu, C., Kwok, P. Y. and Caughey, G. H. 2009. Human subjects are protected from mast cell tryptase deficiency despite frequent inheritance of loss-of-function mutations. J. Allergy Clin. Immunol. 124(5): 1099–1105 e1091–1094.

Tuano, K. S. and Davis, C. M. 2015. Utility of component-resolved diagnostics in food allergy. Curr. Allergy Asthma Rep. 15(6): 32.

Untersmayr, E., Bises, G., Starkl, P., Bevins, C. L., Scheiner, O., Boltz-Nitulescu, G. et al. 2010. The high affinity IgE receptor Fc epsilonRI is expressed by human intestinal epithelial cells. PLoS One 5(2): e9023.

Valent, P., Akin, C., Arock, M., Brockow, K., Butterfield, J. H., Carter, M. C. et al. 2012. Definitions, criteria and global classification of mast cell disorders with special reference to mast cell activation syndromes: a consensus proposal. Int. Arch. Allergy Immunol. 157(3): 215–225.

Verso, M. L. 1964. The evolution of blood-counting techniques. Med. Hist 8: 149–158.

Wenzel, S., Castro, M., Corren, J., Maspero, J., Wang, L., Zhang, B. et al. 2016. Dupilumab efficacy and safety in adults with uncontrolled persistent asthma despite use of medium-to-high-dose inhaled corticosteroids plus a long-acting beta2 agonist: a randomised double-blind placebo-controlled pivotal phase 2b dose-ranging trial. Lancet 388(10039): 31–44.

Wide, L., Bennich, H. and Johansson, S. G. 1967. Diagnosis of allergy by an *in-vitro* test for allergen antibodies. Lancet 2(7526): 1105–1107.

Chapter 3A

Diagnosis of Allergy and Asthma

Kwiat C., Nelson H. and *Hoyte F.* *

Introduction

In addition to a thorough history and physical exam, confirmatory diagnostic tests are crucial in the evaluation of environmental allergies and asthma. Obtaining diagnostic testing that is able to determine a patient's specific allergic sensitizations or objective measurement of lung function allows for better management and decreases long term morbidity/mortality from these conditions. The following chapter describes the most evidence based and widely used diagnostic tools for the diagnosis of allergy and asthma.

Allergy Skin Testing

Allergy skin prick testing (ASPT), in conjunction with a thorough clinical history, is the preferred diagnostic method for IgE-mediated reaction to environmental allergens. Comparative analyses have shown SPT to have the highest positive predictive value among available diagnostic tools for allergies. SPT is validated, safe, reliable, relatively inexpensive and easily performed in the outpatient setting. One advantage to SPT is that results are available to the clinician and patient immediately after the procedure.

Skin testing as a method of diagnosing allergic sensitization was first described in 1865 by Charles Blackley, who performed experiments during which he created abrasions in the skin and covered them with aqueous grass pollen on a piece of wet lint (Blackley 1873). The grass pollen was kept over the abraded skin with a piece of dry occlusive bandage for six hours. SPT became widely used in the 1970s after Pepys introduced a modified technique in which a hypodermic needle was passed through a drop of aqueous allergen placed on the skin. Instead of piercing the skin, the tip of the needle was used to gently lift the skin surface in an upward motion, lightly and superficially disrupting the skin (Hendrick et al. 1975). In this manner, cutaneous mast cells are effectively exposed to the allergen without skin puncture. This technique evolved into modern SPT which is routinely done today.

The mechanism of SPT involves provoking a localized hypersensitivity reaction on the skin by exposing cutaneous mast cells to aqueous solutions of allergens. The cutaneous mast cells of a patient sensitized to an aeroallergen have surface IgE receptors that crosslink and cause degranulation of its contents when exposed to enough aeroallergen locally (Bernstein et al. 2008). Upon degranulation, the mast cell releases its proinflammatory mediators which results in a raised wheal and erythema visible on the skin surface (Horsmanheimo et al. 1996). This reaction is then

---

National Jewish Health, Denver, Colorado USA.
* Corresponding author: hoyteF@njhealth.org

measured and compared against positive histamine and negative saline control. A positive reaction to SPT is evidence of sensitization but does not always correlate to the presence of a clinically relevant allergy. Evidence of sensitization through skin prick or serum testing alone is not sufficient for diagnosis without clinical history of reaction.

There are two general techniques of skin testing: prick/puncture and intradermal testing. The prick method is the most appropriate first step and is performed by applying small drops of aqueous solutions of allergens in either a 1:10 or 1:20 weight:volume extract solution on the skin of the back or the anterior surface of the forearms (Nelson et al. 1993). The droplets may be applied individually in a sequential manner or by using commercially available applicators that apply several different aeroallergens to individual areas of the skin at once, typically using lancets coated with the allergen. Droplets should be applied at a minimum of 2 cm apart to ensure accurate reading of the results (Nelson et al. 1993). Standardized panels for SPT generally consist of common regional aeroallergens (trees, grasses and weeds) as well as animal danders, dust mites, cockroaches and molds. Although many extracts are standardized, SPT can be customized for individual patients through puddle testing, whereby aqueous solutions are made from inhalants or foods mixed with saline and then applied to the skin.

After placement, measurements of both the wheal and erythema are taken, if present. The histamine control is measured approximately 10 minutes after placement and the rest are read approximately 15–20 minutes after placement (Adinoff et al. 1990). A result is considered positive if the wheal diameter measures 3 mm × 3 mm or more with negative saline control (Adinoff et al. 1990).

The accuracy of SPT can be affected by many factors, most notably the allergen extracts and application method/device used to perform the test. Allergen extracts are aqueous solutions made from naturally occurring allergen sources, such as individual animal hairs or dust mites, and can be standardized or non-standardized (Ansotegui et al. 2020). The potency of some standardized extracts in the United States is expressed as allergy units or Bioequivalent Allergy Units (BAUs), which is a measure of potency. Commercially available extracts that are not yet standardized are often labeled in Protein Nitrogen Units (PNU), which does not reflect potency (Dirksen et al. 1985). Aeroallergen extracts are more commonly standardized as opposed to food allergen extracts.

Several medications can also interfere with the results, most notably oral antihistamines, which should be held for at least 5 days prior to the examination to prevent false negative results (Dos Santos et al. 2009). Other medications that may cause false negative skin prick testing include tricyclic antidepressants, antipsychotics, methotrexate and omalizumab (Nolte and Stahl 1998; Isik et al. 2011). Skin prick testing is considered more sensitive than specific for allergic diseases and may result in false positive results. Although when combined with clinical history, the sensitivity and specificity of SPT for inhalant allergens is over 90% when standardized high-potency extracts are used during testing (Adinoff et al. 1990; Tschopp et al. 1998). In general, SPT for aeroallergens is more sensitive and specific for clinical allergies when compared to SPT for food allergies. For this reason, a convincing clinical history and a positive SPT are generally sufficient to establish a diagnosis of allergic rhinoconjunctivitis.

Skin testing for allergic sensitization can also be performed intradermally, a process in which 0.02–0.05 ml of an aqueous solution of allergen is injected underneath the dermis (Dolen 2001). A visible bleb of 2–3 mm is created on the skin, which is read 10–15 minutes after placement. Although a wide variety of concentrations of aeroallergen extracts are available for use, current practice parameters recommend a 100-to-1,000-fold dilution from the prick extract be used for intradermal skin testing (IDST) (Calabria and Hagan 2008). Interpretation of IDST results can be done in several ways, and there is a lack of evidence-based guidelines regarding which method is the most accurate. According to one survey of practicing allergists, over 80% use a threshold of wheal size 3 mm greater than the negative control as the definition of a positive test (Oppenheimer and Nelson 2006). IDST is used primarily for venom and drug allergy, and its use for aeroallergen tests remains controversial. In general, a thorough history, physical and SPT is sufficiently sensitive for a diagnosis of allergic rhinoconjunctivitis due to aeroallergens. Although there is evidence that IDST is more sensitive and more reproducible than SPT, it has also been shown to be significantly less specific and has a high false positive rate (Patel and Saltoun 2019). If a patient has negative skin prick testing for specific aeroallergens, performing IDST subsequently has a low positive predictive value for the detection of a clinically relevant allergy (Wood et al. 1999; Nelson et al. 2006). Therefore, SPT remains the preferred method of diagnosis of allergic sensitivity to aeroallergens.

Nasal Provocation Challenge

The Nasal Provocation Challenge (NPC) has been demonstrated to be an effective diagnostic tool for allergic and non-allergic rhinitis in research protocols but is not as widely used clinically in the United States. NPC is performed by directly placing an aqueous solution of allergen extract unilaterally to the nasal mucosa and subsequently assessing clinical parameters of hyperresponsiveness and allergic sensitization (Litvyakova and Baraniuk 2001). The allergen extract chosen can be one to which the patient has demonstrated sensitization on skin prick or serum-specific IgE testing. Alternatively, it can be an allergen to which a patient does not show sensitization on SPT or serum-specific IgE testing but is a likely culprit based on clinical history. The goal of the NPC is to reproduce the hypersensitivity response under supervised and controlled conditions.

An applicator device is placed into the wider nostril of the patient and delivers 50 to 100 microliters of test solution into the nose (Litvyakova and Baraniuk 2001). Ten minutes after delivery, clinical parameters of sensitization are evaluated using the total nasal symptom score (TNSS). The TNSS is a clinical calculator in which patients grade their symptoms of nasal congestion, rhinorrhea, sneezing, and nasal pruritus from 0–3 to measure symptom severity with 12 being the most severe score (Table 1) (Downie et al. 2004). Rhinoscopic examination with assessment of nasal airflow by anterior rhinomanometry is also performed both before and after the application of topical allergen solution to establish a baseline exam and determine clinical response (Litvyakova and Baraniuk 2001).

Using these methods, NPC uses both subjective and objective measurements to determine the clinical reaction. The NPC is considered positive if the score is over a certain threshold, typically greater than three. The NPC is also considered positive if anterior rhinomanometry reveals a greater than 40% decrease of nasal airflow after administration of aeroallergen, regardless of clinical symptom score (Litvyakova and Baraniuk 2001).

NPC has several practical applications that can aid in the diagnosis of allergic rhinitis in addition to skin prick testing and serum-specific IgE measurements. First, it can help clarify whether sensitization to a given aeroallergen is clinically relevant, as some patients may show sensitization to certain aeroallergens on skin prick testing, but not develop symptoms upon exposure in natural conditions (Kanthawatana et al. 1997). In patients demonstrating polysensitization to numerous aeroallergens on skin prick testing, NPC can aid in identifying the most provocative aeroallergens, which may greatly aid in writing immunotherapy prescriptions.

Furthermore, NPC can be used for definitive diagnosis when skin prick and serum-specific IgE testing are either both negative despite a convincing clinical history or their results are incongruent (Jang and Kim 2015). In addition, NPC has the advantage of targeting a patient's particular exposures,

Table 1. TNSS scoring assigned to each symptom to determine composite score.

Rating	Definition
0	Symptom is not present
1	Symptom is present, but not bothersome
2	Symptom is bothersome, but tolerable
3	Symptom is intolerable, interferes with daily life

aiding in the diagnosis of occupational rhinitis. In theory, NPC may also be used as a surrogate marker for airway hyperreactivity among patients for whom bronchial provocation testing may not be safe, as the mechanisms of hyperreactivity are similar in the upper and lower airway (Peebles and Hartert 1997; Canbaz et al. 2011). NPC should not be performed in patients who are pregnant, have a history of anaphylaxis to the aeroallergen under investigation, are experiencing acute viral or bacterial rhinosinusitis or are experiencing an acute exacerbation of the allergic disease.

Unfortunately, NPC has some disadvantages that have limited its use in clinical practice compared with skin prick and serum-specific IgE testing. First, there is a lack of a standardized testing protocol and clinical assessment, which makes the nasal symptom score a less accurate determination of test positivity (Jang and Kim 2015). Objective measurements, such as rhinoscopic exams with anterior rhinomanometry, are time-consuming, relatively invasive and more expensive to perform than standard skin prick testing. Furthermore, NPC is always performed in addition to skin prick and serum-specific IgE testing, which have relatively high specificity for allergic rhinitis themselves and are often sufficient for definitive diagnosis.

Peripheral Eosinophils

Eosinophils are a subtype of white blood cells that have been implicated in many disease states, including allergies and asthma. A normal eosinophil count on CBC with differential is generally between 0–500 cells per microliter, although the upper limit is variable depending on the source (Ramirez et al. 2018). The presence of peripheral eosinophilia, or a peripheral eosinophil count greater than the upper limit of normal, is a non-specific finding in some patients with allergic or atopic conditions. Allergic sensitization and CD4+ Th2 immune responses result in the activation and degranulation of mast cells and basophils, which are responsible for many of the symptoms of allergic diseases (Fulkerson and Rothenberg 2013). Mast cells, basophils and CD4+ Th2 also produce interleukin-5 (IL-5), a chemokine that promotes the propagation, proliferation and survival of eosinophils.

Eosinophils congregate in various tissues throughout the body where they can cause damage and inflammation by releasing contents of their granules, including major basic proteins, chemokines and growth factors (O'Sullivan and Bochner 2018). Eosinophils alone also promote the *de novo* production of many interleukins, including IL-4, which promotes the production of IgE. The clinical signs and symptoms of eosinophilia are dependent upon the affected tissue. For example, the effects of eosinophilic inflammation in the skin can result in a wide spectrum of diseases ranging from atopic dermatitis to eosinophilic fasciitis. Eosinophilic inflammation in the nasal mucosa is associated with increased mucous production, which is why the measurement of nasal eosinophilia can be used as a diagnostic tool for allergic rhinitis, as described below.

Although peripheral eosinophilia is often appreciated in patients with allergic diseases, it is not a specific diagnostic tool. Peripheral eosinophilia is also found in patients with malignancies, infectious diseases and primary eosinophilic disorders (O'Sullivan and Bochner 2018). A serum eosinophil count of 1,500 cells/microliter or greater should prompt an evaluation of hyper-eosinophilic syndrome, a potentially life-threatening cause of eosinophilia (Curtis and Ogbogu 2016). Furthermore, peripheral eosinophil count does not always correlate with the number of eosinophils in tissue. The absence of peripheral eosinophils cannot exclude the presence of tissue eosinophilia or the presence of allergic disease.

Biologic therapies targeting IL-5 that drastically reduce eosinophil counts are effective in the treatment of certain atopic diseases, including eosinophilic asthma and chronic rhinosinusitis with nasal polyposis (Mukherjee et al. 2014). However, these therapeutics are not approved for allergic rhinitis or food allergies. Therefore, although peripheral eosinophilia can be used as a potential signifier of allergic disease, it is not sufficiently sensitive or specific for diagnosis and does not guide therapy among patients with environmental and/or food allergies alone.

Nasal Eosinophils

Eosinophilia in nasal secretions has been correlated with allergic rhinitis since the early 1900s when Eyermann documented in a case series of 92 allergic rhinitis patients that 72% of these patients showed eosinophils in their nasal swab samples (Eyermann 1927). The presence of eosinophilia in nasal secretions can aid in the diagnosis of allergic rhinitis. It may also differentiate allergic from non-allergic rhinitis, as the increasing severity of allergic rhinitis symptoms has been correlated with higher amounts of nasal smear eosinophilia (Amperayani and Kuravi 2011).

Nasal eosinophils are measured by obtaining a scraping of the mucous membrane in the inferior meatus of the nasal passage with a cotton applicator (Crobach et al. 1996). The collected secretion is then dried, stained, rinsed in tap water and examined under the microscope in oil immersion. Like skin prick testing, swabbing for nasal eosinophilia is relatively inexpensive, and one can obtain results within minutes if appropriate equipment is available. It is also less invasive than serum testing. The nasal mucosa swabs of a normal control should contain few, if any, eosinophilic or basophilic cells, making this test quite specific for pathology.

On the other hand, the diagnostic utility of nasal eosinophilia is limited by its relatively low sensitivity, and the presence of nasal eosinophils has not been shown to distinguish between allergic rhinitis, non-allergic rhinitis or eosinophilic non-allergic rhinitis any better than obtaining a thorough history alone (Crobach et al. 1996). Prior research demonstrates incongruent results with regard to whether nasal eosinophilia correlates to disease type. Some studies have shown a strong correlation between nasal eosinophilia and allergic rhinitis, while others have been unable to distinguish between different subtypes of rhinitis with the use of nasal eosinophil counts (Sood 2005; Jacobs et al. 1981). Therefore, it is not widely utilized in clinical practice.

The low sensitivity of nasal eosinophil testing is often attributed to variability in obtaining an adequate sample of nasal secretions and variability in the distribution of eosinophils in the sample. Moreover, there is no standardized approach to grading nasal eosinophilia, as some practitioners use a qualitative assessment and calculate the number of eosinophils per high-power field and others use a semi-quantitative assessment by calculating the percentage of eosinophils per 100 leukocytes (Pal et al. 2017). As opposed to skin prick testing, serum-specific IgE testing, or NPC, checking for nasal eosinophils must be done when the patient is symptomatic to ensure the accuracy of the test (Pederson et al. 1981). Furthermore, concomitant viral or bacterial rhinosinusitis and the use of topical corticosteroids can lead to false negatives (Crobach et al. 1996). Although taking several nasal samples on different occasions has been shown to markedly improve the reliability and sensitivity of the test, this also makes it less convenient for the patient (Mygind 1979).

Serum IgE

Immunoglobulin E (IgE) is the major immunoglobulin involved in atopic disease. When the CD4+ T cells of susceptible individuals are exposed to certain allergens, such as pollens or food proteins, it results in the production of various chemokines that stimulate plasma cells to produce IgE against those proteins (Bernstein et al. 2016). Upon re-exposure to the offending allergen, the antigen-specific IgE binds to IgE receptors on the surface of primarily mast cells and basophils and the receptors crosslink, leading to the release of mediators that cause the downstream effects that result in the clinical symptoms of allergy. Laboratory testing includes total IgE level and serum-specific IgEs to specific allergens, including environmental and food proteins, as well as select other antigens like microbes and medications.

Prior studies have noted statistically significantly higher levels of total IgE among patients with atopic diseases compared to healthy controls (Stone et al. 2010). The elevations of serum IgE are often higher among patients with multiple comorbid allergic diseases (Omenaas et al. 1994). In addition, an elevated total IgE is useful in the diagnosis of the TH2 high phenotype of asthma and can be used to guide long-term treatment with anti-IgE biologic therapies. However, when evaluated to determine its utility in diagnosing seasonal allergies specifically, research shows the total serum IgE does not reliably correlate to reactivity demonstrated on skin prick testing (Burrows et al. 1989). A serum IgE within normal limits cannot exclude allergies, particularly in a patient with a convincing clinical history (Bernstein et al. 2008). Furthermore, an elevation of total IgE is sensitive to allergic diseases but not specific. Therefore, it is important to rule out other causes of elevated serum IgE, including certain malignancies, parasitic diseases, immune disorders and ABPA with a thorough history and physical exam.

In addition to measuring a total serum IgE, serum-specific IgE measurements can be measured against foods and aeroallergens to aid in the diagnosis of food allergy and allergic rhinitis, respectively. Although more clinically useful than total IgE measurements, serum-specific IgE testing has a significantly lower sensitivity (approximately 44%) when compared to skin prick testing (approximately 68%) for the diagnosis of allergic rhinitis (Tschopp et al. 1998). Therefore, IgE testing is often done in lieu of skin testing for patients only for those patients who cannot undergo skin prick testing due to dermographism or inability to stop antihistamine use. Otherwise, skin prick testing remains the optimal diagnostic test for environmental allergies.

Latex Allergy

Latex is a natural rubber material commonly used in the manufacture of several commercial products. Hypersensitivity reactions to several proteins found in latex have been widely reported and have limited its use for certain purposes, such as medical gloves and condoms. Most of the allergenic proteins found in latex come from the rubber tree *Hevea brasiliensis,* the sap of which is used to make latex products (Jacob et al. 1993). The most common proteins that may induce hypersensitivity reactions are named Hev b 1 through Heb v 15 and represent various structural proteins of the sap (Poley and Slater 2000). Susceptible patients can be sensitized through direct contact on body surfaces or through aerosol exposure. The most common cutaneous reaction to latex-containing products is contact dermatitis, which results in localized xerosis and erythema that may develop papular or ulcerated lesions. This could be irritant contact dermatitis or allergic contact dermatitis in response to chemicals used in manufacturing these products rather than to latex itself (Sussman and Beezhold 1995). However, susceptible patients may develop IgE-mediated type I hypersensitivity reactions to latex proteins, causing localized urticaria and pruritus, rhinoconjunctivitis symptoms and/or wheezing (Sussman and Beezhold 1995). Repeated exposure to latex products, in an occupation setting for example, is a significant risk factor for the development of latex allergy (Kelly and Sussman 2017).

The diagnosis of latex allergy is made based on the clinical history and evidence of sensitization to latex with serum-specific IgE testing. Allergenic proteins from the sap of *H. brasiliensis* structurally resemble several fruit proteins, such as kiwi, banana and avocado (Sicherer 2001). Therefore, the presence of IgE antibodies alone is not sufficient for a diagnosis of latex allergy without a history of clinical reaction to latex. This similarity is also why patients with latex allergy may experience oral pruritus or irritation after eating fruit such as kiwis or bananas. A history of irritation, pruritus, rhinoconjunctivitis or wheezing associated with latex exposure, but no evidence of sensitization on specific IgE testing may be due to an alternate allergen or alternate diagnosis. Although skin testing for common latex allergens is widely performed in Canada and Europe, there are no commercially available latex extracts in the United States. Puddle testing can be performed using an aqueous solution of commercial gloves soaked in saline. However, this method of puddle testing of undetermined accuracy, as the allergen content of commercially available latex gloves is widely variable (Yunginger et al. 1994). Avoidance of latex products is the mainstay of treatment for latex allergy.

Glossary of Abbreviations

ASPT – Allergy Skin Prick Testing
BAU – Bioequivalent Allergy Units
IDST – Intradermal Skin Testing

IL – Interleukin
NPC – Nasal Provocation Challenge
PNU – Protein Nitrogen Units
TNSS – Total Nasal Symptom Score

References

Adinoff, A. D., Rosloniec, D. M., McCall, L. L. and Nelson, H. S. 1990. Immediate skin test reactivity to Food and Drug Administration-approved standardized extracts. Journal of Allergy and Clinical Immunology 86(5): 766–774.

Amperayani, S. and Kuravi, N. 2011. Correlation of nasal smear eosinophilia with class of allergic rhinitis. Indian Pediatrics 48(4): 329–334.

Ansotegui, I. J., Melioli, G., Canonica, G. W., Caraballo, L., Villa, E., Ebisawa, M. and Zuberbier, T. 2020. IgE allergy diagnostics and other relevant tests in allergy, a World Allergy Organization position paper. World Allergy Organization Journal 13(2): 100080.

Bernstein, I. L., Li, J. T., Bernstein, D. I., Hamilton, R., Spector, S. L., Tan, R. and Weber, R. 2008. Allergy diagnostic testing: an updated practice parameter. Annals of Allergy, Asthma and Immunology 100(3): S1–S148.

Bernstein, D. I., Schwartz, G. and Bernstein, J. A. 2016. Allergic rhinitis: mechanisms and treatment. Immunology and Allergy Clinics 36(2): 261–278.

Blackley, C. H. 1873. Experimental Researches on the Causes and Nature of Catarrhus Aestivus (Hay-Fever or Hay-Asthma). Baillière, Tindall and Cox.

Burrows, B., Martinez, F. D., Halonen, M., Barbee, R. A. and Cline, M. G. 1989. Association of asthma with serum IgE levels and skin-test reactivity to allergens. New England Journal of Medicine 320(5): 271–277.

Calabria, C. W. and Hagan, L. 2008. The role of intradermal skin testing in inhalant allergy. Annals of Allergy, Asthma and Immunology 101(4): 337–347.

Canbaz, P., Üskudar-Teke, H., Aksu, K., Keren, M., Gulbas, Z. and Kurt, E. 2011. Nasal eosinophilia can predict bronchial hyperresponsiveness in persistent rhinitis: evidence for united airways disease concept. American Journal of Rhinology and Allergy 25(2): 120–124.

Crobach, M., Hermans, J., Kaptein, A., Ridderikhoff, J. and Mulder, J. 1996. Nasal smear eosinophilia for the diagnosis of allergic rhinitis and eosinophilic non-allergic rhinitis. Scandinavian Journal of Primary Health Care 14(2): 116–121.

Curtis, C. and Ogbogu, P. 2016. Hypereosinophilic syndrome. Clinical Reviews in Allergy and Immunology 50(2): 240–251.

Dirksen, A., Mallinc, H. J., Mosbech, H., Søborg, M. and Biering, I. 1985. HEP versus PNU standardization of allergen extracts in skin prick testing: a comparative randomized *in vivo* study. Allergy 40(8): 620–624.

Dolen, W. K. 2001. Skin testing techniques. Immunology and Allergy Clinics of North America 21(2): 273–279.

Dos Santos, R. V., Magerl, M., Mlynek, A. and Lima, H. C. 2009. Suppression of histamine- and allergen-induced skin reactions: comparison of first- and second-generation antihistamines. Annals of Allergy, Asthma and Immunology 102(6): 495–499.

Downie, S. R., Andersson, M., Rimmer, J., Leuppi, J. D., Xuan, W., Akerlund, A. and Salome, C. M. 2004. Symptoms of persistent allergic rhinitis during a full calendar year in house dust mite-sensitive subjects. Allergy 59(4): 406–414.

Eyermann, C. H. 1927. LXXIII. Nasal manifestations of allergy. Annals of Otology, Rhinology and Laryngology 36(3): 808–815.

Fulkerson, P. C. and Rothenberg, M. E. 2013. Targeting eosinophils in allergy, inflammation and beyond. Nature Reviews Drug Discovery 12(2): 117–129.

Hendrick, D. J., Davies, R. J., D'souza, M. F. and Pepys, J. 1975. An analysis of skin prick test reactions in 656 asthmatic patients. Thorax 30(1): 2–8.

Horsmanheimo, L., Harvima, I. T., Harvima, R. J., Ylönen, J., Naukkarinen, A. and Horsmanheimo, M. 1996. Histamine release in skin monitored with the microdialysis technique does not correlate with the weal size induced by cow allergen. British Journal of Dermatology 134(1): 94–100.

Isik, S. R., Celikel, S., Karakaya, G., Ulug, B. and Kalyoncu, A. F. 2011. The effects of antidepressants on the results of skin prick tests used in the diagnosis of allergic diseases. International Archives of Allergy and Immunology 154(1): 63–68.

Jacobs, R. L., Freedman, P. M. and Boswell, R. N. 1981. Nonallergic rhinitis with eosinophilia (NARES syndrome): clinical and immunologic presentation. Journal of Allergy and Clinical Immunology 67(4): 253–262.

Jacob, J. L., d'Auzac, J. and Prevot, J. C. 1993. The composition of natural latex from *Hevea brasiliensis*. Clinical Reviews in Allergy 11(3): 325–337.

Jang, T. Y. and Kim, Y. H. 2015. Nasal provocation test is useful for discriminating allergic, nonallergic, and local allergic rhinitis. American Journal of Rhinology and Allergy 29(4): e100–e104.

Kanthawatana, S., Maturim, W., Fooanan, S. and Trakultivakorn, M. 1997. Skin prick reaction and nasal provocation response in diagnosis of nasal allergy to the house dust mite. Annals of Allergy, Asthma and Immunology 79(5): 427–430.

Kelly, K. J. and Sussman, G. 2017. Latex allergy: where are we now and how did we get there? The Journal of Allergy and Clinical Immunology: In Practice 5(5): 1212–1216.

Litvyakova, L. I. and Baraniuk, J. N. 2001. Nasal provocation testing: a review. Annals of Allergy, Asthma and Immunology 86(4): 355–365.

Mukherjee, M., Sehmi, R. and Nair, P. 2014. Anti-IL5 therapy for asthma and beyond. World Allergy Organization Journal 7: 32.

Mygind, N. 1979. Clinical investigation of allergic rhinitis and allied conditions. Allergy 34(4): 195–208.

Nelson, H. S., Rosloniec, D. M., McCall, L. I. and Iklé, D. 1993. Comparative performance of five commercial prick skin test devices. Journal of Allergy and Clinical Immunology 92(5): 750–756.

Nelson, H. S., Oppenheimer, J., Buchmeiera, A., Kordash, T. R. and Freshwaterc, L. L. 1996. An assessment of the role of intradermal skin testing in the diagnosis of clinically relevant allergy to timothy grass. Journal of Allergy and Clinical Immunology 97(6): 1193–1201.

Nolte, H. and Stahl Skov, P. 1988. Inhibition of basophil histamine release by methotrexate. Agents and Actions 23(3): 173–176.

Omenaas, E., Bakke, P., Elsayed, S., Hanoa, R. and Gulsvik, A. 1994. Total and specific serum IgE levels in adults: relationship to sex, age and environmental factors. Clinical and Experimental Allergy 24(6): 530–539.

Oppenheimer, J. and Nelson, H. S. 2006. Skin testing: a survey of allergists. Annals of Allergy, Asthma and Immunology 96(1): 19–23.

O'Sullivan, J. A. and Bochner, B. S. 2018. Eosinophils and eosinophil-associated diseases: an update. Journal of Allergy and Clinical Immunology 141(2): 505–517.

Pal, I., Babu, A. S., Halder, I. and Kumar, S. 2017. Nasal smear eosinophils and allergic rhinitis. Ear, Nose and Throat Journal 96(10-11): E17–E22.

Patel, G. and Saltoun, C. (2019, November). Skin testing in allergy. In Allergy and Asthma Proceedings (Vol. 40, No. 6).

Pedersen, P. A. and Weeke, E. R. 1981. Allergic rhinitis in Danish general practice: prevalence and consultation rates. Allergy 36(6): 375–379.

Peebles Jr, R. S. and Hartert, T. V. 1997. *In vivo* diagnostic procedures: skin testing, nasal provocation, and bronchial provocation. Methods 13(1): 14–24.

Ramirez, G. A., Yacoub, M. R., Ripa, M., Mannina, D., Cariddi, A., Saporiti, N. and Dagna, L. 2018. Eosinophils from physiology to disease: a comprehensive review. BioMed Research International, 2018.

Sicherer, S. H. 2001. Clinical implications of cross-reactive food allergens. Journal of Allergy and Clinical Immunology 108(6): 881–890.

Sood, A. 2005. Diagnostic significance of nasal eosinophilia in allergic rhinitis. Indian Journal of Otolaryngology and Head and Neck Surgery 57(1): 13–16.

Stone, K. D., Prussin, C. and Metcalfe, D. D. 2010. IgE, mast cells, basophils, and eosinophils. Journal of Allergy and Clinical Immunology 125(2): S73–S80.

Sussman, G. L. and Beezhold, D. H. 1995. Allergy to latex rubber. Annals of Internal Medicine 122(1): 43–46.

Tschopp, J. M., Sistek, D., Schindler, C., Leuenberger, P., Perruchoud, A. P., Wüthrich, B. and SAPALDIA Team. 1998. Current allergic asthma and rhinitis: diagnostic efficiency of three commonly used atopic markers (IgE, skin prick tests, and Phadiatop®) Results from 8329 randomized adults from the SAPALDIA study. Allergy 53(6): 608–613.

Wood, R. A., Phipatanakul, W., Hamilton, R. G. and Eggleston, P. A. 1999. A comparison of skin prick tests, intradermal skin tests, and RASTs in the diagnosis of cat allergy. Journal of Allergy and Clinical Immunology 103(5): 773–779.

Yunginger, J. W., Jones, R. T., Fransway, A. F., Kelso, J. M., Warner, M. A. and Hunt, L. W. 1994. Extractable latex allergens and proteins in disposable medical gloves and other rubber products. Journal of Allergy and Clinical Immunology 93(5): 836–842.

Chapter 3B

Diagnosis of Allergies and Asthma

Sundeep Salvi,[1,2,*] *Deesha Ghorpade*[1] and *Monica Barne*[1]

ROLE OF SPIROMETRY IN THE DIAGNOSIS AND MANAGEMENT OF ASTHMA

Introduction

Spirometry is the "gold standard" objective diagnostic test for obstructive airways diseases, including asthma. The hallmark feature of asthma is expiratory airflow limitation and its variability with time, either with or without treatment. Spirometry helps in documenting both of these features. The spirometer was invented by Sir John Hutchison from the UK who used a water seal drum connected to a calibrated scale. This spirometer measured the volume of air exhaled by the patient after taking a full inhalation. Hutchison called this volume as vital capacity (VC) because he was able to show through research that this volume of air was vital for survival and strongly predicted life span. When this volume of air was removed slowly, it was called slow vital capacity (SVC) and when removed with force, it was called forced vital capacity (FVC). For almost a century, this was the only parameter that was measured using spirometry. In 1945, Robert Tiffeneau from France gave a time component to the VC, measuring the volume of air exhaled in unit time. The volume of air exhaled in the first one second was called FEV_1 or forced expiratory volume in the first 1 second. Subsequently, the volume of air removed in 2 seconds was called FEV_2 and so on.

In the presence of airflow obstruction, the volume of air removed in the first 1 second (FEV_1) is lower and therefore the ratio between FEV_1 and FVC reduces. A ratio of FEV_1/FVC < 0.75 in adults and < 0.85 in children (up to 18 years) indicates airflow obstruction that could be suggestive of asthma.

There are two flow rates that are measured by the flow sensor-based spirometers, PEFR and $FEF_{25\%-75\%}$. The PEFR is the highest flow rate achieved during a forced exhalation maneuver and $FEF_{25\%-75\%}$ is the average flow rate between 25% of the FVC to 75% of the FVC. The PEFR value indicates obstruction in the total respiratory tract, while the $FEF_{25\%-75\%}$ represents flow in the smaller airways.

The five key parameters in spirometry are the two volumes (FEV_1 and FVC), the ratio between the two volumes (FEV_1/FVC) and the two flows (PEFR and $FEF_{25\%-75\%}$). The earlier spirometers used volume displacement methods to measure lung volumes. They were more accurate for measuring FEV_1 and FVC. But they could not give the two flow rate values easily, were huge and

---

[1] Pulmocare Research and Education (PURE) Foundation, Pune, INDIA.
[2] Symbiosis International (Deemed University), Pune, INDIA.
* Corresponding author: sundeepsalvi@gmail.com

VOLUME – TIME GRAPH

FLOW-VOLUME LOOP

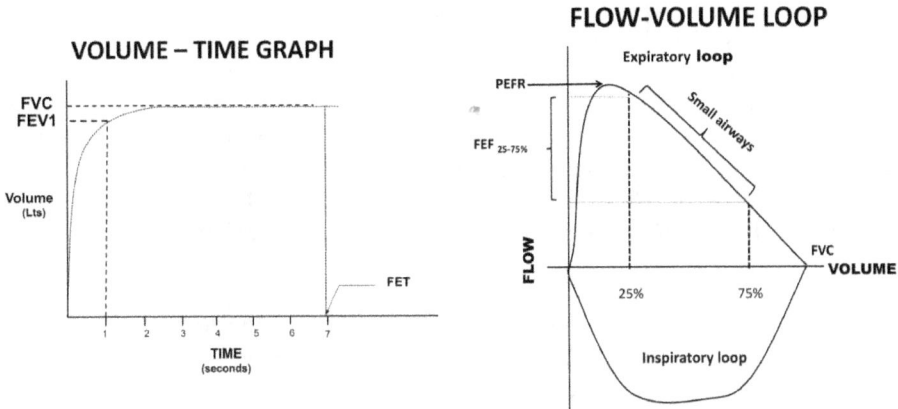

Figure 1. Normal spirometry graphs.

bulky, were not portable and were even difficult to maintain. They were therefore replaced by flow sensor-based spirometers, which were small and portable, gave both the volume time and flow volume curves, were easy to maintain and were cheaper. Various flow sensors are used to measure flow, including pneumotachographs, turbines, anemometers and ultrasonic flow sensors. Flow is converted into volume by multiplying it with time.

The two basic graphs that we get in spirometry are the volume time Graph and the Flow Volume Loop (Figure 1).

In the volume time graph (Y-axis is volume, X-axis is time), we see a sharp increase in the volume in the first one second, which reaches the highest point at around 2–3 seconds and then settles down as a plateau. The plateau is a flat line which indicates that all the air has come out from the lungs and there is no more left to come out. In healthy individuals, this plateau is reached within the first 2 to 3 seconds. The highest point on the Y-axis is called the FVC. The volume of air exhaled in the first 1 second is the FEV_1. The volume time graph also gives the Forced Expiratory Time (FET), which indicates when the flow stopped. This is an important quality assurance criterion.

In the flow volume loop, the flow is plotted on the Y-axis and the volume on the X-axis. When the patient starts exhaling, the flow rate suddenly increases to reach a peak, after which it shows a slow and smooth decline until it reaches the X-axis to give the FVC value. The highest flow rate achieved is called the Peak Expiratory Flow Rate (PEFR), which is also obtained from a peak flow meter (PFM). The flow rate when 50% of volume was exhaled is called the Forced Expiratory Flow at 50% ($FEF_{50\%}$). Similarly, values for $FEF_{25\%}$ and $FEF_{75\%}$ are also obtained. The average of flow values from $FEF_{25\%-75\%}$ is called as $FEF_{25\%-75\%}$. After the compete exhalation, the subject is asked to again inhale in forcefully. The expiratory maneuver looks like the shape of a triangle and the inspiratory flow rate looks like the shape of a semicircle.

Spirometry Procedure

The maneuver of spirometry can be divided into six steps as below:

1. Exhale out completely
2. Take a deep inhalation and fill up the lungs completely
3. Hold the mouthpiece in between the teeth, clasp it in an airtight manner and seal the lips
4. Blow out air into the mouthpiece with maximum force
5. Continue to blow out the air till a plateau of 1 second is obtained or up to a maximum of 15 seconds
6. Inhale deeply and forcefully

Since this is an effort-dependent test, the instructions that are given to the patients have to be very clear to ensure that the patient understands how to perform each step. A demonstration to the patient will be useful and necessary. The skill of the technician in using voice modulation, effective body language and demonstration is of utmost importance. A few trials runs with only the mouthpiece also help the patient to perform the test correctly. We need to get three acceptable graphs from the patients and of the three, the two best need to be reproducible.

The Criteria for Acceptability Are as Below **(Graham et al. 2019)**

1. Maximal inspiration before exhalation
2. Good start. No delay/hesitation in the start, the BEV (back extrapolated volume) must be $\leq 5\%$ of FVC or 0.100 L whichever is greater; best seen in volume/time graph
3. No evidence of faulty zero-flow setting/no evidence of a leak
4. Maximal effort right from the beginning of the expiratory blast
5. Smooth and continuous exhalation, no cough in the first second of expiration, no glottic closure, and no early termination
6. Must achieve one of these three EOFE (End of Forced Expiration) indicators.
   i. Expiratory plateau (≤ 0.025 L in the last 1 sec of expiration)
   ii. Expiratory Time ≥ 15 sec
   iii. FVC is within the repeatability criteria or is greater than the largest prior observed FVC

The acceptability criteria can be analyzed by looking at the shape of the curves and is beyond the scope of this chapter.

Criteria for Reproducibility

The spirometry test is said to be reproducible or repeatable when the difference between the highest two FVC values and the highest two FEV_1 values is less than 150 mL.

Interpretation of Spirometry for Diagnosis of Asthma

Interpretation begins right from when the participant is performing the spirometry test. If a patient is able to blow out effortlessly for more than 10, 12 or 15 seconds it indicates severe airflow obstruction. Just by looking at the shape of the spirometry graphs, we can deduce the presence of airflow obstruction and also determine its severity. Every graph or rather every spirometry report comes with the pre-plotted predicted values which are derived from the patient's demographics and indicates where the patient's values should ideally be. The Global Lung Initiative (GLI) is now recommended as the predicted equation to use.

By comparing the patient's FEV_1, FVC, PEFR and $FEF_{25\%-75\%}$ values with the predicted values we can diagnose the presence of airflow obstruction. The shape of the curves as mentioned in Figure 2 below depicts the interpretation.

Interpreting the spirometry report by looking at the values given in the algorithm (Figure 3). Before you interpret the report by looking at the shape of the curves, ensure that the X:Y scales are appropriate (For flow volume: X-axis 0.5 Lt to Y-axis 1 Lt; For flow time: X-axis 1 sec to Y-axis 2 Lt). The first value that we look at is the FEV_1/FVC ratio. It is said to be normal if it is more than 0.7. Next, if the FVC percentage predicted is also > 80% then the spirometry report is considered to be normal. But if the FVC percentage predicted is reduced then it indicates presence of restrictive lung disease (RLD), which will then need to be confirmed by body box plethysmography. A new term coined for this is Preserved Ratio Impaired Spirometry (PRISM). 30% show evidence of frank RLD on the body box, 20% revert back to normal and around 50% end up developing frank obstructive airways disease. If the FEV_1/FVC ratio is reduced below 0.7, then it indicates

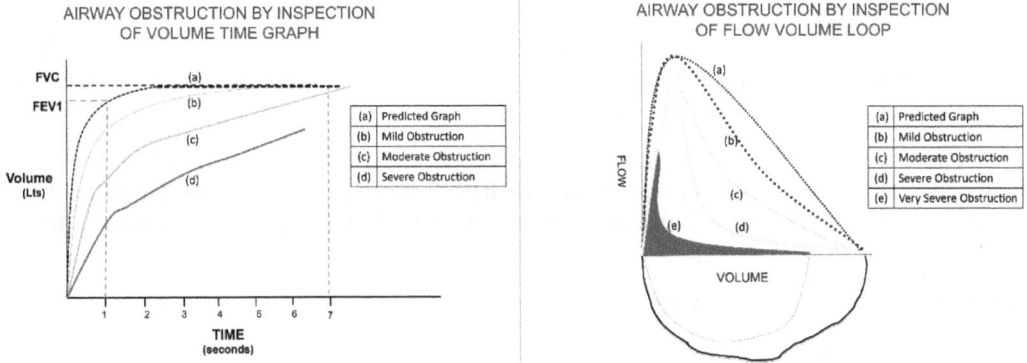

Figure 2. Interpretation by looking at the spirometry graphs.

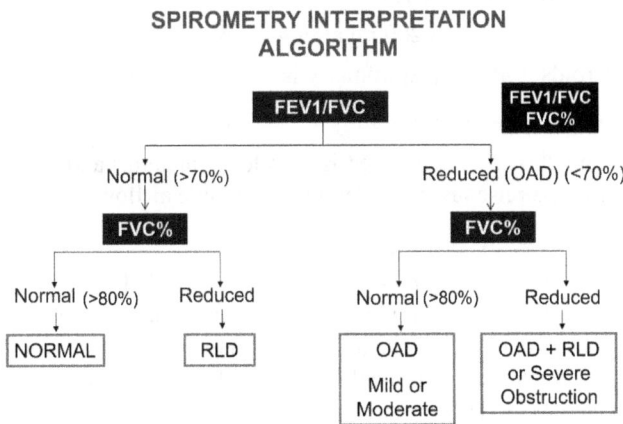

Figure 3. Spirometry interpretation algorithm.

obstructive airway disease (OAD). In this case if the FVC percentage predicted is more than 80%, then it is mild or moderate airflow obstruction. If the FVC percentage predicted is also reduced below 80%, then it indicates either a mixed obstructive plus RLD or a severe airflow obstruction, where the FVC has reduced due to air trapping.

Role of Spirometry in Assessment of Asthma (GINA 2021)

The Global Initiative for Asthma 2021 (GINA 2021) recommends documentation of variable airflow obstruction at the time of diagnosis and before initiation of controller therapy.

To confirm variable expiratory airflow limitation:

- Perform spirometry
- If FEV_1 is reduced and FEV_1/FVC is < 0.75 in adults and < 0.85 in children, it indicates airflow limitation (for COPD a cut-off value of 0.70 is recommended)

To demonstrate bronchodilator response (BDR) variability on spirometry:

A) Reversibility to Bronchodilator

- Record baseline spirometry
- Administer 200 to 400 micrograms of Albuterol (Salbutamol)
- Wait for 15–20 minutes

- Repeat the spirometry
- If the FEV_1 improves by > 12% and > 200 Ml, then it suggests the possibility of asthma. If the FEV_1 increase is to the tune of > 15% and > 400 ml, then it is most certainly asthma. The cut-off for good BDR for children is 12% only.

Note: Before performing bronchodilator reversibility, and if the patient is on a regular inhaled short-acting beta agonist (SABA) or a long-acting beta agonist (LABA), then the following drugs have to be withdrawn before performing the spirometry. Table 1 depicts the optimum bronchodilator withholding time prior to testing.

B) Reversibility to Inhaled Corticosteroid

- Record Baseline spirometry
- Initiate controller therapy with Inhaled Corticosteroids
- Repeat spirometry after 4 weeks of ICS
- If the FEV_1 improves by 12% and 200 ml after 4 weeks of ICS, then it is likely to be asthma
- For oral corticosteroids, follow-up spirometry is to be done 2 weeks later.

C) Positive Exercise Challenge Testing

Fall in FEV1 by 10% and 200 ml after an exercise challenge in adults and fall in FEV1 of > 12% in children indicate positive exercise testing and confirm variable airflow obstruction

D) Positive Bronchial Challenge Testing

Fall in FEV1 by > 20% from the baseline value on challenging the airways with a broncho-provocative agent like methacholine, histamine or mannitol indicates the variable nature of the asthmatic airways. Histamine and methacholine cause direct bronchoconstriction, while adenosine monophosphate activates the inflammatory cells to release histamine and other broncho-constricting substances which simulate the underlying inflammation that happens in asthma.

E) Excessive Variation of Lung Function Between Visits

If in-between visits, the FEV_1 varies between > 12% and > 200 ml, it indicates the likely presence of asthma. In adults, an $FEV_1/FVC < 0.7$ indicates the presence of obstructive airway disease, which could be either asthma or COPD. After giving a short-acting bronchodilator, if the FEV_1/FVC becomes > 0.7, then it indicates a diagnosis of asthma, while if the post-bronchodilator FEV_1/FVC remains < 0.70, it indicates a diagnosis of COPD or asthma with fixed airflow obstruction. As mentioned earlier, for asthma a cut-off of 0.75 is used instead of 0.70.

Instead of the fixed ratio for FEV_1/FVC, the lower limits of normal can also be used, but this is beyond the scope of this chapter. Similarly, FEV_1 and FVC values instead of expressing them as % predicted are now being recommended to be expressed as a z-score (lower 5th percentile value).

Table 1. Bronchodilator medication withholding time.

Bronchodilator Medication	Withholding Time
Short Acting Beta Agonists (SABA) (e.g., albuterol or salbutamol)	4–6 hrs
Short-acting muscarinic antagonist (SAMA) (e.g., ipratropium bromide)	12 hrs
Long-acting Beta Agonists (LABA) (e.g., formoterol or salmeterol)	24 hrs
Ultra-LABA (e.g., indacaterol, vilanterol or olodaterol)	36 hrs
Long-acting muscarinic antagonist (LAMA) (e.g., tiotropium, umeclidinium, aclidinium or glycopyrronium)	36–48 hrs

Spirometry in Children

It is a challenge to do spirometry in children, but trained and experienced technicians with patience, can get children as young as three years to perform spirometry. It is important to have a setup that is child-friendly and equipment that has incentives for the child to perform the test with the best effort. Children may exhale almost all air within the first 1 sec, hence the $FEV_{0.75}$ may be used instead of FEV1 for interpretation. The criteria for repeatability are also lower for children < 6 years of age.

ROLE OF PEAK FLOW METER IN THE DIAGNOSIS AND MANAGEMENT OF ASTHMA

Introduction

Although spirometry is the gold standard diagnostic test for obstructive airways diseases, there are several challenges to using spirometry in clinical practice, i.e., difficulty in getting the test performed, lack of availability of spirometers and difficulty in interpreting the report. These challenges can be overcome by using a simple, easy to perform and easily available tool called the peak flow meter (PFM) (Figure 4). The PFM measures the maximum or peak flow rate that the patient can achieve during maximal exhalation. It measures the airway patency of all the divisions of the airways but is more biased toward the larger airways. The peak flow is achieved at around 200 milliseconds, the test therefore does not need to be performed for more than a second (Dobra 2018).

The PFM is a cylindrical tube of around 10 inches (although there are different sizes and shapes available) that has a slot in the middle for the scale with markings usually from 0 to 800 L/min. One end is for the mouthpiece and the other end is for the air to exit. The marker moves ahead when one blows through the mouthpiece and stops at the maximum flow rate achieved. There are electronic PFMs too that have started becoming available.

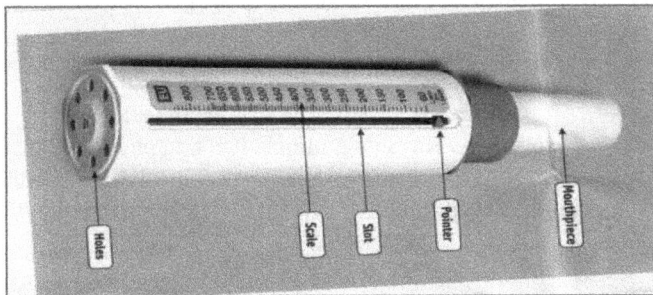

Figure 4. The PFM. The EU represents the European union scale of the markings.

Procedure for Recording the PEFR Value

- Coach the patient
- Fix new mouthpiece to PFM
- Place the indicator at "0" (zero). Hold the PFM in such a way that the fingers are not covering the slot and the indicator can move freely in the slot
- Take a deep breath and fill the lungs with as much air as possible
- Place the PFM in your mouth and seal your lips. Make sure that the tongue is not inserted in the mouthpiece
- Blow out as HARD and as FAST as you can for not more than 1 sec

- Note down the number you get from the scale
- Repeat the above steps two more times
- Record the "highest" of the three values obtained

What Is the Normal PEFR?

Just like spirometry, there are predicted equations for PEFR based on age, height, gender and race. From the equations, we can derive the normal predicted value for an individual. The patient's value is to be compared with this value and a value within 80% of the predicted value is considered to be normal. The predicted equation used is usually the Nunn and Greg equation with or without a correction factor as per the race. There are indigenous predicted equations developed by different countries, which are advisable to be used for the local population, including India (Kodgule R.R. J. Postgrad. Med. 2014).

The PFM has several roles in clinical practice (Dobra 2018):

1. For diagnosis of asthma
2. For daily monitoring of asthma and assisting in asthma self-management plan
3. For evaluating response to treatment
4. For identification of asthma triggers
5. For diagnosis of occupational asthma
6. Severity assessment of acute flare-up of asthma

PFM is comparatively less reliable as compared to spirometry in the diagnosis of asthma in children but may be used in combination with the clinical presentation. For day-to-day monitoring of asthma in children, peak flow readings and Asthma Control Tests are independent of each other and are well correlated (Buzoianu et al. 2014; Chan et al. 2009).

The Global Initiative for Asthma (GINA) 2021 report recommends the use of the peak flow meter to diagnose asthma in three different ways (GINA 2021):

1. *Reversibility to four weeks of inhaled corticosteroids (ICS)*: In patients with a history suggestive of asthma, record the baseline PEFR reading. Initiate ICS treatment with/without a long-acting bronchodilator and continue for four weeks and then repeat PEFR value. Improvement in PEFR by more than 20% after four weeks of ICS treatment indicates a strong likelihood of asthma.

2. *Diurnal variability*: Like many physiological parameters the PEFR also shows diurnal variability with the PEFR values being lower in the mornings and higher in the evenings. However, in healthy subjects, this diurnal variability is not more than 10%. To record diurnal variability, the patient is given a PFM and is asked to record the values in the morning and the evening for two weeks. The daily diurnal variability is calculated by the following formula:

   PEF variability = (Highest PEFR – Lowest PEFR)/Mean of highest and lowest PEFR.

   In adults, if the PEFR variability is > 10% and in children > 13%, it indicates significant diurnal variability, consistent with the diagnosis of asthma.

3. *Negative reversibility to exercise challenge*: If the PEFR value decreases by 15% after an exercise challenge then it indicates the presence of variable airway obstruction, suggestive of asthma.

Day-to-Day Monitoring of Asthma and Prevention of an Acute Exacerbation

The PFM is probably a better tool for the day-to-day monitoring of asthma at home, particularly for patients who are poor perceivers of their symptoms, and consequently is extremely useful for the prevention of an acute exacerbation (Table 2).

Table 2. Zones of asthma control basis the patient's personal best value (Adeniyi and Erhabor 2011).

Green Zone: The patient's peak low reading is between 80–100% of the patient's personal best. This is a zone where the patient's asthma is well controlled, without any symptoms, dietary or activity limitation, no night-time awakenings and no need for reliever medication.
Yellow Zone: In the Yellow zone, the patient's PEFR is reduced to below 80% of the personal best and lies between 50% to 79% of the personal best value. This is an "alert" zone indicating that the asthma is not under control and the patients may develop an acute exacerbation at any time.
Red Zone: When the PEFR reading reduces to below 50% of the patient's personal best, it indicates that the patient is likely having an acute asthma exacerbation and should be managed aggressively.

Concept of Personal Best

A patient with asthma may never achieve his or her predicted value. Hence it is important to identify the individual's own personal best value, which can then be used as the baseline value for comparison of the current PEFR value over time. The personal best value is the highest PEFR value that the patient can attain when his or her asthma is well-controlled on medications and is free of symptoms. This is usually after three weeks of inhaled corticosteroid therapy (Reddel et al. 2004). This value is noted as the baseline value and any decrease by more than 20% of the personal best PEFR should be taken seriously.

A reduction below 80% from the personal best indicates the onset of an impending exacerbation. When detected beforehand, the exacerbation can very well be prevented by either stepping up therapy in the form of a short course of oral steroids or stepping up the dose of ICS.

Monitoring of Asthma Control During Step Down of Treatment

Response to the treatment of asthma can be objectively evaluated by monitoring the improvement in PEFR. The PEFR is also a good tool for daily home monitoring of asthma control and deciding when the medication can be tapered or stopped. This gives the patient and the caregiver a sense of security when the dose is being tapered down and reassuring that after tapering/stopping the medicines the patient is indeed tolerating the regimen.

Trigger Identification

When monitoring the PEFR regularly at home, the observation of a sudden drop in PEFR on a particular day, suggests that it may indicate exposure to a potential trigger on that day.

Diagnosis of Occupational Asthma

The PEFR is the diagnostic tool for occupational asthma as it can be carried to the place of work and the PEFR recording can be obtained as frequently as every 1–2 hours. Ideally, the PEFR value should be taken after waking up and thereafter every 2 hours till the subject returns home. A record of these is kept for at least four weeks. If the tracing shows a reduction in the PEFR values during working days and an improvement on holidays, then this is a strong indicator of occupational asthma.

The PFM is therefore a very useful and handy tool for the diagnosis of asthma, monitoring response to treatment, identifying asthma triggers and diagnosing occupational asthma. More importantly, home-based monitoring with a PFM can help detect an asthma exacerbation several days in advance, especially among the poor perceiver group of asthma symptoms.

ROLE OF FRACTIONAL EXHALED NITRIC OXIDE (FeNO) IN ASTHMA

Introduction

The fractional exhaled nitric oxide or FeNO is a simple, non-invasive, quantitative, reproducible, safe, and easy-to-perform test that helps in detecting type-2 driven eosinophilic airway inflammation that is characteristic of allergic asthma. Several international guidelines recommend this as a useful additional parameter supporting treatment decisions in patients with suspected asthma (Dweik et al. 2011). High FeNO levels in subjects with asthma predict the likelihood of a good therapeutic response to ICS. FeNO can also be used to evaluate compliance and adherence to ICS.

Nitric Oxide and Its Importance in Asthma

Nitric oxide (NO) is a gas produced by different cells in the lung that play an important role in lung biology. Airway epithelial cells are the predominant source, and three different isoforms of the enzyme nitric oxide synthase are responsible for its production. Eosinophils are also an important source of NO, especially in severe asthma. It functions as a vasodilator, bronchodilator, neurotransmitter and inflammatory mediator. FeNO acts locally as an autocoid, paracrine mediator or neurotransmitter. It has bactericidal and viricidal properties and a cytotoxic effect on tumor cells. NO is a highly reactive molecule and has both direct as well as indirect oxidant properties. Under physiological conditions, NO acts as a weak bronchodilator and anti-inflammatory molecule, while at higher levels it acts as a pro-inflammatory mediator in the lung and increases bronchial hyperresponsiveness. Levels of FeNO correlate with the number of eosinophils in the induced sputum or bronchoalveolar lavage and correlate with bronchial inflammation.

Measurement of FeNO

FeNO can be measured using several commercially available analyzers which differ in methods of measurement, complexity or setup. Stationary analyzers measure FeNO by chemiluminescent techniques, while handheld devices measure FeNO using electrochemistry. Ambient NO levels (produced by motor vehicular exhausts and burning of cooking gas) can be high in polluted cities and towns and will therefore interfere with the FeNO measurements. Ideally, FeNO measurements should be performed in a room that has minimal ambient NO levels, but this is quite often not the case. It is important to at least record ambient NO levels at the time of the test, wherever feasible.

Exhaled NO levels from the lower respiratory tract exhibit significant expiratory flow rate dependence, suggesting a characteristic diffusion-based process for NO transfer from the airway wall to the lumen. The higher the flow rate, the higher the FeNO levels, therefore, it is important to use a constant flow rate of 50 mL/sec during exhalation. Breath-holding should be avoided while performing the FeNO test as it will give false high levels. Patients should refrain from eating and drinking for at least 1 hour before the FeNO test. Nitrate-rich foods such as lettuce, spinach and beetroot increase FeNO levels, while caffeine, alcohol and smoking reduce FeNO levels. Viral infections of the upper and lower respiratory tract increase FeNO levels, therefore the presence of these should be recorded while performing the test. If spirometry has to be performed, it should be performed after the FeNO test, as spirometry has been shown to transiently reduce FeNO levels. Nose clips are not recommended as this allows the nasal NO to accumulate and promote leakage via the posterior nasopharynx.

After seating in a comfortable position, the subject should insert the mouthpiece and inhale over 2–3 sec through the mouth to reach total lung capacity, and then exhale immediately without breath hold at a constant mouth flow rate of 50 mL/sec. This back pressure prevents contamination of NO from the nose. Usually, a target mouthpiece pressure or flow rate is displayed on the machine screen or computer screen and the recommended exhalation flow rate should be maintained at around

50 mL/sec. FeNO levels are expressed in parts per billion (ppb), which is equivalent to nanoliters per liter.

Clinical Application of FeNO

Earlier studies showed that FeNO levels increased in asthmatics and decreased in response to ICS, prompting the use of this non-invasive method to diagnose asthma and evaluate its response to treatment. FeNO, therefore, adds a new dimension to traditional clinical tools, such as history, clinical examination and spirometry (Lipworth et al. 2020).

FeNO values less than 25 ppb in adults and < 20 ppb in children (5–12 years) are inconsistent with type-2 allergic asthma. Values greater than 50 ppb in adults and > 35 ppb in children strongly indicate eosinophilic allergic airway inflammation and a greater likelihood of a good therapeutic response to ICS. Persistently high values indicate ongoing exposure to high allergen load and/or non-compliance with the use of ICS. The within-subject variation for FeNO in healthy subjects is 10% or up to 4 ppb. In asthma, the variation is around 20%. A significant response to treatment is indicated by a 20% decrease if the baseline FeNO was > 50 ppb or a 10% decrease if the baseline FeNO was < 50 ppb. A meta-analysis concluded that using FeNo to guide ICS dose adjustment resulted in an overall 42% (24%–55%) reduction in asthma exacerbations (Petsky et al. 2018).

Values that are between 25 to 50 ppb in adults and 20 to 35 ppb in children should be interpreted in conjunction with clinical and spirometry parameters. FeNO values reduce significantly following treatment with monoclonal antibodies, such as dupilumab (anti-IL-4/IL-13), especially among those with baseline values ≥ 50 ppb, and this correlates well with a significant reduction in asthma exacerbations.

There is no strong evidence to use FeNO on its own as an objective diagnostic tool for asthma. Not all asthma is due to eosinophilic airway inflammation. FeNO may help define different preschool wheezing phenotypes and in assessing the risk of later asthma (Busse et al. 2021). In atopic schools, children's presence of respiratory symptoms suggestive of asthma increased FeNO will add confidence to the underlying diagnosis of asthma (Pijnenburg 2019).

COPD is quite often associated with features suggestive of asthma, such as in the asthma-COPD overlap. Some studies have suggested that COPD patients with high FeNO levels respond well to ICS, raising the possibility that FeNO might be used in predicting responsiveness to inhaled steroids in COPD.

THE METHACHOLINE CHALLENGE TEST TO DETECT AIRWAY HYPERRESPONSIVENESS

Introduction

Airway hyperresponsiveness (AHR) is a characteristic feature of bronchial asthma. The airways narrow excessively in response to both direct and indirect external stimuli when compared to normal healthy subjects. The methacholine challenge test (MCT) is used to measure and quantify AHR. It is often used to confirm or exclude a diagnosis of asthma, especially among those with a history suggestive of asthma but with normal or inconclusive spirometry. Direct stimuli such as methacholine or histamine are sensitive to diagnose reactive airway disorders, including asthma, especially if the airway narrowing occurs at a lower dose. Indirect stimuli, such as exercise or adenosine monophosphate (AMP) induce inflammatory mediator changes, which in turn release bronchoconstrictor substances such as histamine and other bronchospastic mediators from mast cells to cause bronchial smooth muscle contraction. Indirect stimuli are more specific for asthma but are less sensitive. Apart from confirming or ruling out asthma, the MCH test is also useful in determining high-risk populations such as commercial divers, submarine services, defense recruits and some occupational exposures.

Inhalation of methacholine at increasing concentrations/doses causes airway narrowing measured on spirometry as a decrease in FEV_1 values. If the FEV_1 drops by $\geq$ 20% at a concentration below, which healthy subjects do not show this effect (16 mg/mL methacholine), it is called positive MCT. The smaller the concentration/dose of methacholine required to cause the 20% drop in FEV_1, the greater the degree of airway hyperresponsiveness.

Contraindications

Conditions That May Compromise the Quality of the Test

Patients unable to perform good quality spirometry tests despite repeated attempts and poorly trained technicians/medical personnel to perform this test are general contraindications for this test. A minimum of 20 supervised tests are required for a person to become proficient in methacholine challenge testing.

Conditions That Will Compromise Safety and Cause Discomfort

FEV_1 < 60% predicted or absolute FEV_1 < 1.5 liters, history of uncontrolled hypertension (systolic > 200 mmHg, diastolic > 100 mmHg), a recent history of eye surgery, myocardial infarction, stroke or ventilation-perfusion mismatch causing arterial hypoxemia are contraindications for performing this test.

Precautions

Sudden bronchospasm to methacholine while performing the test can occur, therefore it is important to ensure that there is a medical doctor performing the test who can manage an acute asthma exacerbation. Drugs such as adrenaline, intravenous corticosteroids, anti-histamine injections, oxygen and a salbutamol inhaler with a spacer/nebulizer should be kept in the MCT room. A stethoscope, sphygmomanometer and pulse oximeter must also be kept handy. In case of acute bronchospasm, nebulized salbutamol or salbutamol via MDI plus spacer should be given immediately. After the MCT test is performed, subjects are often given inhaled salbutamol and made to wait for 30–45 minutes before they can be sent home.

The MCT must be avoided in pregnant and nursing women. Also, patients receiving anti-cholinesterase medications for myasthenia gravis should not undergo MCT.

Method

The MCT must be performed by a well-trained person with all precautions as mentioned above. Provocholine, manufactured in Canada, is the only methacholine agent that is approved by the US FDA. Industrial sources of methacholine are not recommended as they are not approved by the US FDA. Purity, quality and consistency are mandatory as it is a bronchospastic chemical that is inhaled. The methacholine vial is available in a dose of 100 mg and needs to be prepared freshly for the test.

Drugs that need to be discontinued prior to the MCT are salbutamol, salmeterol, formoterol, theophylline and anticholinergic drugs. Smoking and alcohol need to be avoided at least for a day. No discontinuation is required for ICS, antihistamines, cromones, antileukotrienes and oral contraceptive pills (Coates et al. 2017).

Preparation of the methacholine solution should be done according to strict safety standards. Clean and sterile test tubes and pipettes must be used to make the solution. The starting solution should be 6.25 mL of 16 mg/mL made from the stock powder. The 3 mL of this solution should then be mixed with 3 mL diluent (0.9% NaCl) to get a concentration of 8 mg/mL. From this 3 mL should be removed and put into another 3 mL diluent solution to give a concentration of 4 mg/mL. These steps need to be continued until we have the following dilutions in each test tube, i.e., 2 mg/mL, 1 mg/mL, 0.5 mg/mL, 0.25 mg/mL, 0.125 mg/mL, 0.0625 mg/mL and 0.03125 mg/mL. The last tube should have only 0.9% normal saline (Malmberg et al. 2018).

After explaining the test to the patient and obtaining written informed consent, the first step is to perform baseline spirometry on a calibration-checked spirometer. The next step is to administer the plain diluent solution (0.9% normal saline). Tidal breaths are recommended. Deep breathing or reaching TLC is not recommended because deep breathing causes bronchodilation, at least in healthy subjects. FEV_1 values are measured 1 minute and 3 minutes after the end of inhaling the saline (a timer is required for this). The lowest of the two highest FEV_1 values (highest at 1 minute and highest at 3 minutes) is used for calculation. If the drop in FEV_1 is more than 10%, the test is stopped as it indicates hyperresponsiveness to saline.

If the drop is less than 10%, methacholine solutions are administered starting with the lowest concentration and increased step-by-step. FEV_1 values are measured at 1 minute and 3 minutes post and evaluated for any drop. If the drop is more than 20%, the test is stopped. If the drop is less than 20%, it is continued with the next dose and the same steps are applied until the FEV_1 drops by at least 20% or the highest concentration of methacholine (16 mg/mL) is reached.

The method of administering the methacholine should be either a nebulizer (each concentration for 1 minute or more as planned) or a dosimeter which is also a nebulizer that delivers a fixed dose of the methacholine with each breath. The number of breaths need to be standardized and is most often 5 breaths.

Provocative Concentration to Cause a 20% Drop in FEV_1 (PC20) or Provocative Dose to Cause a 20% Drop in FEV_1 (PD20)?

Earlier, PC20 was used as the main endpoint readout. However, more recently, PD20 is accepted universally and is the endpoint that should be used. In PC20, we were measuring only the concentration of the methacholine that caused a 20% drop in FEV1, while in PD20 we measure the actual dose of methacholine that caused the 20% drop. Table 3 compares the PC20 values versus the PD20 values when methacholine was administered by the English Wright nebulizer for two mins.

If the subject shows a 20% drop in FEV_1, before the final concentration of methacholine is reached (16 mg/mL), it is termed the presence of airway hyperresponsiveness (AHR) to methacholine. The lower the concentration at which the 20% drop occurs, the greater the degree of AHR.

The bronchial challenge test requires a fair amount of patient cooperation and patience, as it can take a long period as well as many forceful exhalation blows. The test can be conducted in children as young as 6–7 years of age who are cooperative and the technician is well-versed and experienced in doing the test on these children.

Table 3. Comparing PC20 values versus PD20 values when methacholine was administered by the english wright nebulizer for two minutes (Ref: Coates A.L., et al ERJ 2017; 49: 1601526).

Concentration mg/mL	Dose μg
0.0625	1.425
0.125	2.969
0.25	5.938
0.5	11.875
1	23.75
2	47.5
4	95
8	190
16	380

THE ROLE OF LUNG OSCILLOMETRY IN ASTHMA DIAGNOSIS

Introduction

"Sound" is the major medium through which we all communicate with each other in our day-to-day activities; not only that but there is also a wide range of applications of sound when it comes to diagnosing some of the most important diseases in medical practice. Diagnostic tests such as the heart doppler test, carotid doppler, fetal ultrasound and ultrasound of the abdomen and thorax, all use sound waves as their basic principle for diagnosis. Procedures such as lithotripsy and phacoemulsification use sound for therapeutic purposes.

Sound is also used in lung oscillometry testing for the detection of airway obstruction. The lung oscillometry tests include the forced oscillation technique (FOT) discovered by DuBois in 1956 (Dubois et al. 1956), and the impulse oscillometry system (IOS) developed by Michaelson in 1975 (Michaelson et al. 1975). Oscillometry techniques were developed in the 1950s but have only recently started to gain clinical and diagnostic importance. They measure the mechanical properties of the lungs which act as important determinants to identify several lung diseases. Oscillometry techniques are non-invasive and easy to perform, even in preschool children and relatively more sensitive than spirometry to diagnose obstruction in the airways.

The sound generated through a loudspeaker or any other source (oscillating piston or vibrating mesh) is used to generate pressure waves of different frequencies ranging from 5 Hz to 30 Hz and are then pushed into the lung through a mouthpiece. The FOT emits sound waves as sine waves of a single frequency at a time, whereas IOS emits square-shaped multiple-frequency waves. Sound waves of smaller frequencies, i.e., 5 Hz travel deeper into the lungs while those of higher frequencies such as $\geq$ 20 Hz travel only up to the larger airways. A pneumotach flow sensor attached to the mouthpiece measures the drop in pressure and thereby flows while transmitting the pressure waves. Pressure divided by flow gives us airway/lung resistance (Brashier et al. 2015).

Principle

An oscillating pressure wave generated through sound waves or other sources is forced into the lung at different frequencies (usually from 4–25 Hz) and the resulting Impedance comprising of resistive and reactive forces is derived by measuring the change in pressure and change in flow that gives us the mechanical properties of the lung. Resistance is directly proportional to the change in pressure and inversely proportional to the change in flow, which means if the resistance increases, pressure will increase and flow will decrease. Our lungs are divided into larger airways and distal airways, which further divide into bronchioles and alveoli, just like the branching pattern of trees. Sound waves of smaller frequencies (4 Hz to 5 Hz) travel up to the small airways, whereas sound waves of higher frequencies travel only up to the larger airways. Any obstruction in the larger airways is detected by a change in resistance at 20 Hz also known as R20. Resistance at 5 Hz or R5 represents total airways/lung resistance, and subtracting R20 from R5 (R5–R20), gives us resistance in the smaller airways. Respiratory resistance also denoted as "Rrs" and is found to be generally constant between 5 Hz to 20 Hz, i.e., independent of frequency in healthy adult airways. In children, resistance is dependent on frequency and in case of obstruction, the values obtained will be higher than in adults. The unit used for measuring resistance denoted as "R" is measured in $cmH_2O \cdot L^{-1} \cdot s^{-1}$ or $kPa \cdot L^{-1} \cdot s^{-1}$

Parameters Measured

Along with respiratory resistance (Rrs), respiratory reactance denoted by "Xrs" is also measured, which when added together with Rrs is known as Impedance (I). Respiratory reactance (Xrs) is defined as a combination of Inertance (I) and Capacitance (C). Inertance is the force applied by the air present in the airway column and capacitance represents the elastic property of the small airways or compliance of the lung periphery.

Impedance (Z) = Resistance (Rrs) + Reactance (Xrs)
Impedance (Z) = Resistance (Rrs) + Inertance (I) + Capacitance (C)

In addition to Impedance, resonant frequency also called "Fres" is the frequency at which Inertance and capacitance are equal. The normal range for Fres varies between 8 Hz to 12 Hz and is generally higher in children and decreases with age, but increases with both obstructive and RLD. Another parameter that adds to the importance of lung oscillometry tests is the Area of reactance (Ax) also known as the "Goldman's Triangle," which is the integrated area between a low frequency of 5 Hz and Fres, which is measured in $cmH_2O{\cdot}L^{-1}$ or $kPa{\cdot}L^{-1}$ (Figure 5). The normal AX is usually

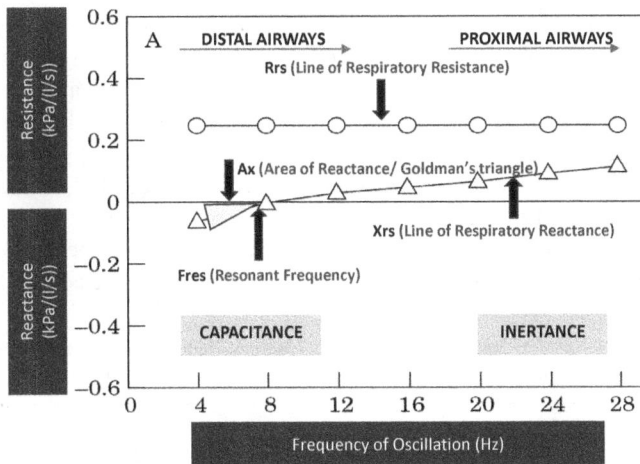

Figure 5. Lung oscillometry parameters.

< 0.33 $kPa.L^{-1}$ and is a good indicator to measure small airway patency along with any changes in terms of obstruction in the peripheral airways, which can be closely related to R5–R20.

How to Perform Lung Oscillometry Test (Figure 6)

1. Explain the procedure to the patients
2. The sitting position is preferred with uncrossed legs to reduce extrathoracic pressure
3. A nose clip should be worn
4. The mouthpiece of the FOT/IOS device should be at a comfortable height
5. Ensure that there is a tight seal between the mouthpiece and lips to prevent air leaks
6. The tongue position should not interfere with the free airflow through the mouthpiece
7. Cheeks to be held firmly
8. Tidal breathing for at least 30–40 sec (120–150 sound impulses are pushed)
9. A minimum of three such readings should be performed (pre- and post-BD each)

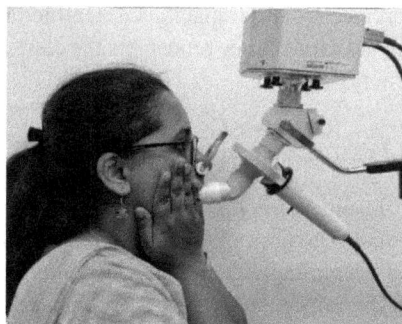

Figure 6. Subject performing lung oscillometry test.

Clinical Applications of Lung Oscillometry

FOT/IOS is useful for the diagnosis of asthma and COPD (in adults and children) (Ahmed et al. 2018). Lung oscillometry parameters are found to be more sensitive when compared to spirometry values (Table 4). Resistance and reactance parameters can also be used as alternatives to spirometry parameters (Nikkhah et al. 2011) (4). Respiratory resistance at 5 Hz is shown to be significantly associated with FEV_1 in COPD patients, whereas respiratory resistance (Rrs) at 20 Hz and respiratory reactance (Xrs) at 5 Hz are found to be significantly associated with FEV_1 in the asthmatic group. Unlike other pulmonary function tests, lung oscillometry parameters are more sensitive to evaluate the functional assessment of peripheral airways. In addition, R20 values can help differentiate between COPD in which case the peripheral airways resistance is increased and asthma in which

Table 4. Showing differences between spirometry and lung oscillometry values (Adapted from Brashier, B. and Salvi, S. 2015. Measuring lung function using sound waves: role of the FOT and IOS. Breathe (Sheff) 11(1): 57–65).

Parameter	Spirometry	FOT/IOS
Principle	Flow sensor/volume displacement helps measure flow rates and lung volumes	Sound waves of multiple frequencies are pushed into the lungs as pressure waves to measure the Impedance
Parameters measured	FEV_1, FVC, PEFR, $FEF_{25\%-75\%}$	Zrs, Rrs, Xrs, Fres, Ax
Patient cooperation	+++	+
Type of breathing maneuvers	Forced exhalation	Tidal breathing
Variability (intra-subject)	3–5%	5–15%
Sensitivity to Airways Location		
Central	+	+++
Peripheral	++	+++
Cut-off for bronchodilator response	12–15% for FEV1	40% for R5 or X5
Cut-off for bronchoconstrictor response	20% for FEV1	50% for R5
Standardized methodology	+++	++
Availability of robust reference values	+++	+

the proximal airways resistance is increased. Therefore, in the case of COPD R5 value will increase and the R20 value will be closer to normal, whereas, in asthma, both R5 and R20 may increase. Bronchodilator reversibility in COPD patients is poor when measured by spirometry, whereas lung oscillometry parameters show significant improvements at follow-up with a decrease in AX by 37% and R5 by 20%. This suggests that lung oscillometry parameters are highly sensitive when it comes to monitoring therapeutic responses in patients with COPD. Lung oscillometry parameters are also useful to evaluate post-lung transplantation surgeries (Cho et al. 2020). A very recent study showed that oscillometry values such as R5, R5–R19, X5 and area of reactance identified graft rejection after 6–9 weeks of lung transplantation, whereas FEV_1 and FVC values remained normal even after three months in the same patients.

Small airways dysfunction (SAD) asthma phenotype is unique, and it predominantly affects small airways (like COPD). This phenotype of asthma is difficult to treat, has recurrent exacerbations, predominant night-time symptoms and is associated with obesity-induced asthma. Diagnosing them accurately will help in prescribing drugs that have ultrafine particles. R5–R20, AX and X_5 are sensitive parameters to detect SAD asthma.

Glossary of Abbreviations

AHR – Airway hyperresponsiveness
AMP – Adenosine Monophosphate
Ax – Area of Reactance
BDR – Bronchodilator Reversibility
BEV – Back Extrapolated Volume
C – Capacitance
$cmH_2O/L/S$ – Centimeters of Water Per Liter Per Second
COPD – Chronic Obstructive Pulmonary Disease
EOFE – End of Forced Expiration
$FEF_{0.75}$ – Forced Expiratory Flow After 0.75 Seconds
$FEF_{25-75\%}$ – Forced Expiratory Flow Between 25% of Forced Vital Capacity to 75% of Forced Vital Capacity
FeNO – Fractional Exhaled Nitric Oxide
FET – Forced Expiratory Time
FEV1 – Forced Expiratory Volume in the First One Second
FEV2 – Forced Expiratory Volume in 2 Seconds
FOT – Forced Oscillation Technique
Fres – Resonant Frequency
FVC – Forced Vital Capacity
GINA – Global Initiative for Asthma
Hz – Hertz
I – Inertance
ICS – Inhaled Corticosteroids
IL – Interleukin
IOS – Impulse Oscillometry
kPa/L/S – Kilopascal Units Per Liter Per Second
L/min – Liters Per Minute
LABA – Long-Acting Beta-Adrenergic Agonist
LAMA – Long-Acting Muscarinic Antagonist
Mcg – Micrograms
MCT – Methacholine Challenge Test
Mg – Milligrams
mmHg – Millimeters of Mercury

NO – Nitric Oxide
OAD – Obstructive Airways Disease
PC20 – Provocative Concentration to Cause a 20% Drop in FEV1
PD20 – Provocative Dose to Cause a 20% Drop in FEV1
PEF – Peak Expiratory Flow
PEFR – Peak Expiratory Flow Rate
PFM – Peak Flow Meter
Ppb – Parts Per Billion
R20 – Resistance at 20 Hertz
R5 – Resistance at 5 Hertz
R5–R20 – Resistance at 5 Hertz Minus Resistance at 20 Hertz
RLD – Restrictive Lung Disease
Rrs – Respiratory Resistance
SABA – Short-Acting Beta-Adrenergic Agonist
SAMA – Short-Acting Muscarinic Antagonist
Sec – Second
TLC – Total Lung Capacity
Type 2 – T-Helper Cellular Type 2
US FDA – United States Food and Drug Agency
VC – Vital Capacity
Xrs – Respiratory Reactance
Zrs – Respiratory Impedance
Z-Score – Lower 5th Percentile Value

References

Adeniyi, B. O. and Erhabor, G. E. 2011. The peak flow meter and its use in clinical practice. Afr. J. Respir Med. 6(2): 5–7.

Ahmed, M. M., Kader, M. A. A. and Mohammed, E. M. 2018. Impulse oscillometry to differentiate between chronic obstructive pulmonary disease and bronchial asthma. Egypt J. Bronchol. (12): 373–378.

Brashier, B. and Salvi, S. 2015. Measuring lung function using sound waves: role of the forced oscillation technique and impulse oscillometry system. Breathe (Sheff) 11(1): 57–65.

Busse, W. W., Wenzel, S. E., Casale, T. B. et al. 2021. Baseline FeNO as a prognostic biomarker for subsequent severe asthma exacerbations in patients with uncontrolled, moderate-to-severe asthma receiving placebo in the LIBERTY ASTHMA QUEST study: a post-hoc analysis. Lancet Respir Med. 9(10): 1165–1173.

Buzoianu, E., Moiceanu, M. and Plesca, D. A. 2014. Asthma control assessment in children: Correlation between asthma control test and peak expiratory flow. Maedica. 9(4): 338.

Chan, M., Sitaraman, S. and Dosanjh, A. 2009. Asthma control test and peak expiratory flow rate: independent pediatric asthma management tools. Journal of Asthma 46(10): 1042–1044.

Cho, E., Wu, J. K. Y., Birriel, D. C., Matelski, J., Nadj, R., DeHaas, E., Huang, Q., Yang, K., Xu, T., Cheung, A. B., Woo, L. N., Day, L., Cypel, M., Tikkanen, J., Ryan, C. and Chow, C. W. 2020. Airway oscillometry detects spirometric-silent episodes of acute cellular rejection. Am. J. Respir Crit. Care Med. 201(12): 1536–1544.

Coates, A. L., Wanger, J., Cockcroft, D. W., Culver, B. H., Bronchoprovocation Testing Task Force: Kai-Håkon Carlsen, Diamant, Z., Gauvreau, G., Hall, G. L., Hallstrand, T. S., Horvath, I., de Jongh, F. H. C., Joos, G., Kaminsky, D. A., Laube, B. L., Leuppi, J. D. and Sterk, P. J. 2017. ERS technical standard on bronchial challenge testing: general considerations and performance of methacholine challenge tests. Eur. Respir J. 49(5): 1601526.

Dobra, R. and Equi, A. 2018. How to use peak expiratory flow rate. Archives of Disease in Childhood-Education and Practice 103(3): 158–162.

Dubois, A. B., Brody, A. W., Lewis, D. H. et al. 1956. Oscillation mechanics of lungs and chest in man. J. Appl. Physiol. 8(6): 587–594.

Dweik, R. A., Boggs, P. B., Erzurum, S. C., Irvin, C. G., Leigh, M. W., Lundberg, J. O., Olin, A. C., Plummer, A. L. and Taylor, D. R. 2011. American Thoracic Society Committee on Interpretation of Exhaled Nitric Oxide Levels (FENO) for Clinical Applications. An official ATS clinical practice guideline: interpretation of exhaled nitric oxide levels (FENO) for clinical applications. Am. J. Respir Crit. Care Med. 184(5): 602–615.

Global Initiative for Asthma. Global Strategy for Asthma Management and Prevention (GINA). May, 2021. https://ginasthma.org/wp-content/uploads/2021/05/GINA-Main-Report-2021-V2- WMS.pdf (accessed Dec 30, 2021).

Graham, B. L., Steenbruggen, I., Miller, M. R., Barjaktarevic, I. Z., Cooper, B. G., Hall, G. L., Hallstrand, T. S., Kaminsky, D. A., McCarthy, K., McCormack, M. C., Oropez, C. E., Rosenfeld, M., Stanojevic, S., Swanney, M. P., Thompson, B. R., Standardization of Spirometry 2019 Update. An Official American thoracic society and european respiratory society technical statement. Am. J. Respir Crit. Care Med. 200(8): e70–e88.

Lipworth, B., Kuo, C. R. and Chan, R. 2020. 2020 Updated Asthma Guidelines: Clinical utility of fractional exhaled nitric oxide (FeNO) in asthma management. J. Allergy Clin. Immunol. 146(6): 1281–1282.

Malmberg, L. P., Kauppi, P. and Mäkelä, M. J. 2018. Standardizing dose in dosimetric bronchial challenge tests. Clin. Physiol. Funct. Imaging 38(5): 903–906.

Michaelson, E. D., Grassman, E. D. and Peters, W. R. 1975. Pulmonary mechanics by spectral analysis of forced random noise. J. Clin. Invest. 56(5): 1210–1230.

Nikkhah, M., Amra, B., Eshaghian, A., Fardad, S., Asadian, A., Roshanzamir, T., Akbari, M. and Golshan, M. 2011. Comparison of impulse osillometry system and spirometry for diagnosis of obstructive lung disorders. Tanaffos 10(1): 19–25. PMID: 25191346; PMCID: PMC4153135.

Petsky, H. L., Cates, C. J., Kew, K. M. and Chang, A. B. 2018. Tailoring asthma treatment on eosinophilic markers (exhaled nitric oxide or sputum eosinophils): a systematic review and meta-analysis. Thorax. 73(12): 1110–1119.

Pijnenburg, M. W. 2019. The role of FeNO in predicting asthma. Front Pediatr. 7: 41.

Reddel, H. K., Marks, G. B. and Jenkins, C. R. 2004. When can personal best peak flow be determined for asthma action plans? Thorax. 59(11): 922–924.

Chapter 3C

Sinus Imaging for Patients with Allergy and Asthma

Mary Beth Cunnane

✕✕

Introduction

Modern imaging allows safe, rapid assessment of the sinuses in patients with allergy and asthma. Computed tomography is the workhorse of sinus imaging, but MRI is useful for problem solving, particularly if there is concern for neoplasm. This chapter presents an introduction to radiographic anatomy of the sinuses and illustrates several classic findings in patients with sinusitis.

Computed Tomography

In modern multi-detector scanners, Computed Tomography (CT) of the sinuses can be performed in less than a minute. The rapidity of scanning, along with dose reduction techniques, has made sinus CT a fast, low-risk procedure for the evaluation of paranasal sinus disease. In many centers, CT has replaced plain films in the initial evaluation of a patient with sinus disease.

Sinus CTs are typically performed without intravenous contrast and images are acquired in the axial plane. Modern scanners allow slice thicknesses of less than 1 mm which results in smooth multiplanar reformations in the coronal and sagittal planes. Images acquired for diagnostic purposes may also be used for intraoperative guidance, should surgery be indicated.

Sinonasal Anatomy and Variants

The nasal cavity typically contains three pairs of turbinates: the inferior, middle and superior (Figure 1). Lateral and inferior to the turbinates are air spaces which are the corresponding superior, middle and inferior meati. The superior meatus drains the ipsilateral posterior ethmoid air cell and the sphenoid sinus (Figure 2). The middle meatus drains the ipsilateral anterior ethmoids, the maxillary sinus via the infundibulum, and the frontal sinus via the fronto-ethmoidal recess (Figure 3). The inferior meati drain the nasolacrimal duct bilaterally.

Knowledge of the drainage pathways allows one to deduce a site of obstruction. For example, opacification of the frontal, anterior ethmoid and maxillary sinuses implies obstruction at the level of the middle meatus into which all of these sinuses ultimately drain. This is an anterior pathway pattern of obstruction. Isolated opacification of the posterior ethmoid and ipsilateral sphenoid sinus implies obstruction at the level of the superior meatus or a posterior pathway pattern of obstruction.

Department of Radiology, Massachusetts Eye and Ear, 243 Charles St. Boston, MA 02114.
Email: MaryBeth_Cunnane@meei.harvard.edu

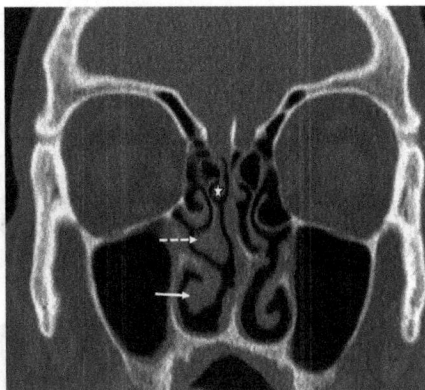

Figure 1. Coronal CT in bone windows demonstrates the superior turbinate (star), the middle turbinate (hatched arrow) and the inferior turbinate (solid arrow). The air spaces lateral and inferior to the turbinates are the corresponding meati.

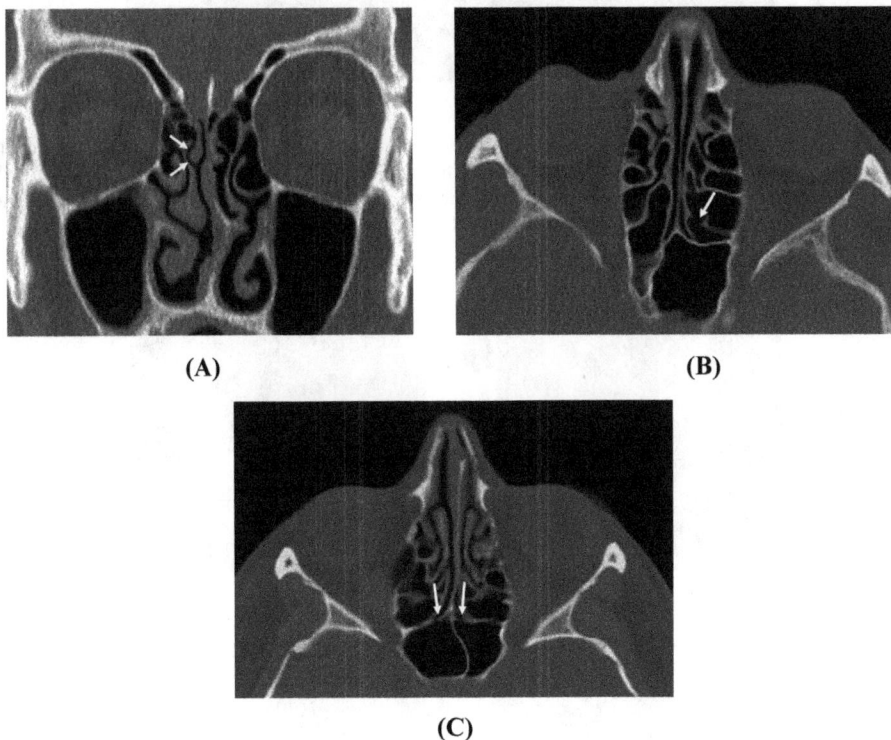

(A)

(B)

(C)

Figure 2. Posterior drainage pathway. (A) The superior meatus is the air space lateral and inferior to the superior turbinate, indicated by white arrows. (B) The posterior ethmoid drainage (arrow) into the superior meatus. (C) The bilateral sphenoethmoidal recesses, along the anterior aspect of the sphenoid sinuses (arrows), drain into the superior meatus.

There are a number of normal anatomic variants in the paranasal sinuses and nasal cavities. Haller cells are ethmoidal air cells that lie within the maxillary sinus, bordering the orbital floor (Figure 4A). Onodi cells are posterior ethmoid cells that extend superior to the sphenoid sinus and border the optic canal (Figure 4B). A concha bullosa is a pneumatized middle turbinate (Figure 4C). Septal deviation is the most common normal variant, seen in over 50% of patients (Figure 4D). Most anatomic variants do not contribute to rhinosinusitis. The exception is a large nasal septal spur that contacts the lateral nasal wall. This may result in headaches. The remaining variants are important

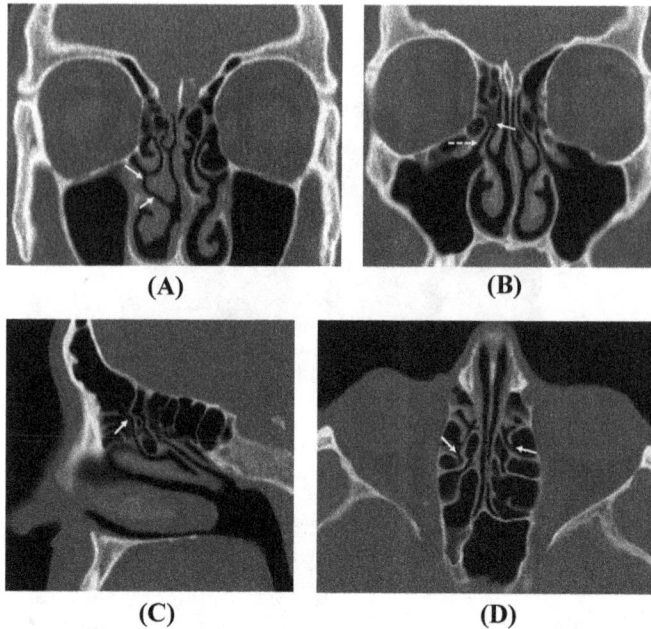

Figure 3. Anterior drainage pathway. (A) The middle meatus is the air space lateral and inferior to the middle turbinate, indicated by white arrows. (B) The maxillary sinus drains into the middle meatus via the infundibulum (hatched arrow) which leads to the hiatus semilunaris at the superior aspect of the uncinate process (solid arrow). (C) The frontal sinus drains via the frontoethmoidal recess (arrow). (D) The anterior ethmoid sinuses each drain directly into the middle meatus (arrows).

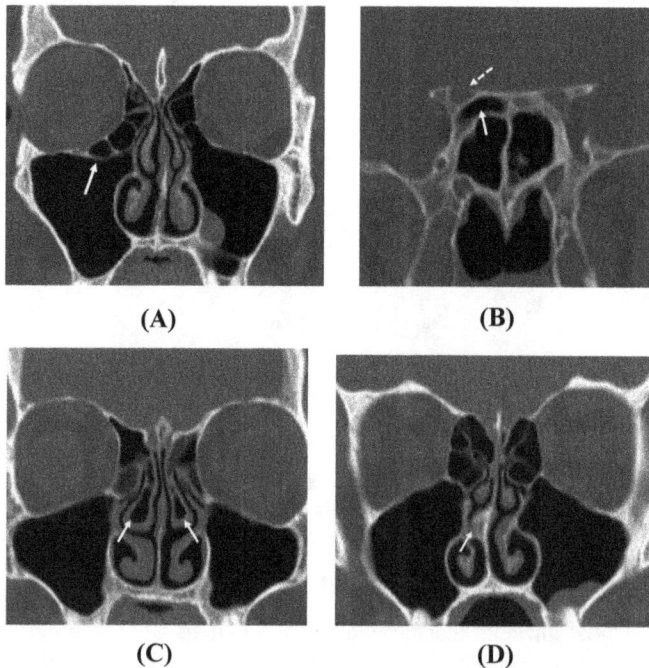

Figure 4. Common normal variants in the nasal cavity and paranasal sinuses. (A) A Haller air cell (arrow) is an ethmoid air cell that lies within the maxillary sinus bordering the orbital floor. (B) An Onodi air cell (solid arrow) is an ethmoid air cell that lies superior to the sphenoid sinus, bordering on the optic canal (dashed arrow). (C) A pneumatized middle turbinate is called a concha bullosa, seen here bilaterally (arrows). (D) Nasal septal deviations are very common variants. In this case, there is a rightward nasal septal deviation with a large nasal septal spur (arrow).

to recognize because many of them are associated with increased complications during Functional Endoscopic Sinus Surgery (FESS) (Shpilberg et al. 2015).

Findings of Sinonasal Inflammation

Though the sinuses are lined by mucosa, the normal non-inflamed mucosa is so thin it is not visualized on CT and the sinuses typically appear to have a bone-air interface at their walls (Figure 5A). Patients with chronic rhinosinusitis will tend to have opacified sinuses. There may be circumferential mucosal thickening (Figure 5B), or a more focal rounded soft tissue density known as a mucous retention cyst (Figure 5C). Air-fluid levels may be recognized by the presence of a dependent meniscus on the axial images (Figure 6). Although air-fluid levels can be seen with acute sinusitis, CSF (in the setting of a leak), and hemorrhage (particularly due to orbital floor fracture) can also result in air-fluid levels.

The density of material in the paranasal sinuses can vary significantly according to the concentration of protein in the sinonasal secretions. Watery secretions will be isodense to muscle on CT (Figure 7A). As mucous becomes thicker and more inspissated, the density will increase (Figure 7B). Ultimately secretions can harden into concretions which may become calcified. Calcification in an opacified sinus may herald the presence of a fungus ball (Ng et al. 2015) (Figure 8).

When a sinus becomes completely obstructed, secretions may continue to accumulate causing pressure to increase within the sinus cavity. This pressure results in the expansion of the sinus with smooth bony erosion of the walls. The expanded sinus is referred to as a mucocele and may exert a mass effect on adjacent structures (Figure 9).

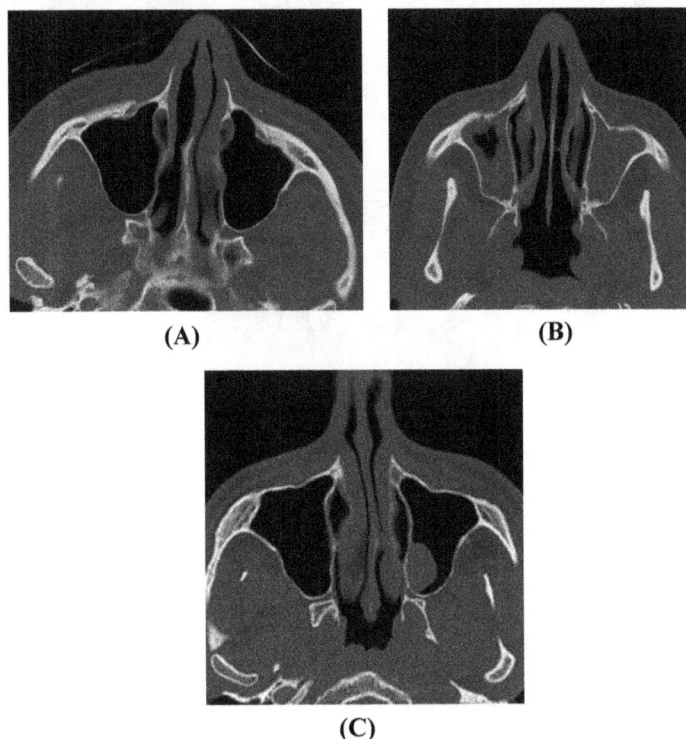

(A)   (B)

(C)

Figure 5. Patterns of opacification of the paranasal sinuses. (A) Axial and coronal images of normal maxillary sinuses. The normal mucosa is imperceptibly thin and there is a bone-air interface at the sinus margins. (B) In this patient there is moderate opacification of the right maxillary sinus but some aeration persists in the center. The left maxillary sinus is nearly completely opacified. (C) Sinus opacification may be more focal as in this case where there is a retention cyst in the left maxillary sinus (arrow).

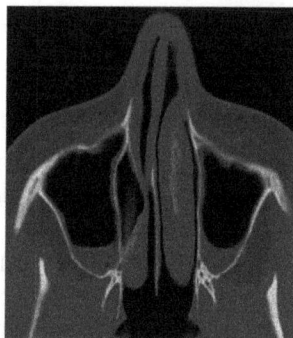

Figure 6. Air-fluid level. In this image, there is mild circumferential mucosal thickening in the bilateral maxillary sinuses. There is also fluid, recognized by the curved meniscus which indicates an air-fluid level (arrows). While air-fluid levels can be associated with acute sinusitis, they are also seen in hemorrhage and CSF leaks.

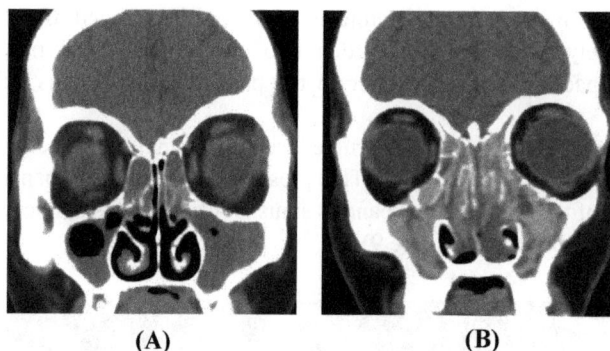

(A)   **(B)**

Figure 7. Differences in attenuation. Sinus secretions may be watery or more proteinaceous. In both (A) and (B), the sinuses are severely opacified; but on soft tissue windows, the opacification in A is isodense to the extraocular muscles in the orbit, whereas in B the secretions are very hyperdense compared with the extraocular muscles.

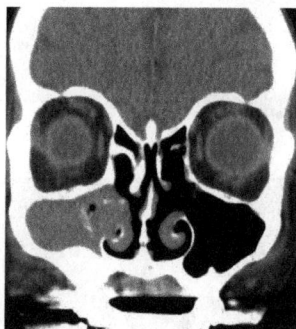

Figure 8. Coronal images through the paranasal sinuses in soft tissue windows show a severely opacified maxillary sinus with curvilinear calcification within it. Calcification within an opacified sinus is more common in patients with fungus balls and this patient was found to have a fungus ball at the surgery.

CT may also demonstrate opacification of the nasal cavity, particularly in patients with nasal polyposis. Nasal polyps appear as soft tissue lobulations within the sinus cavity (Figure 10A). If there are numerous nasal polyps the entire nasal cavity may be opacified (Figure 10B).

History and clinical exams are essential components of accurate diagnosis of inflammatory chronic rhinosinusitis. However, certain imaging patterns can be associated with particular etiologies of chronic rhinosinusitis and can guide the differential. For example, diffuse polyposis with severe

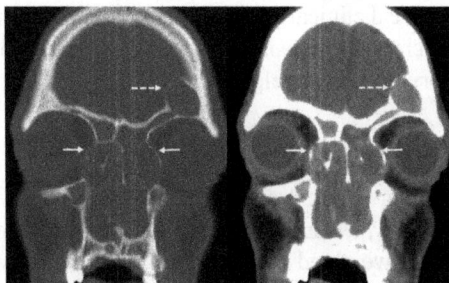

Figure 9. A patient with the severe sinonasal disease and multiple mucoceles. Coronal bone and soft tissue windows demonstrate complete opacification of the nasal cavity and paranasal sinuses by a combination of polypoid soft tissue and hyperdense secretions. There is a smooth bony expansion of ethmoid sinus walls bilaterally (solid arrows). There is a smooth bony expansion of a left supraorbital air cell which is also filled with hyperdense secretions (dashed arrows). This is a typical appearance of allergic fungal rhinosinusitis.

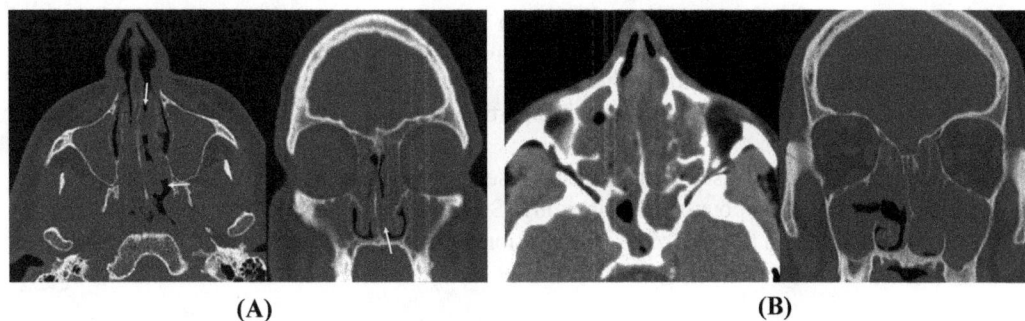

(A)   **(B)**

Figure 10. Nasal polyps. (A) Axial and coronal images through the paranasal sinuses demonstrate lobulated foci of soft tissue (arrows) medial to the turbinates in this patient with nasal polyposis. (B) In this patient with more severe disease, axial soft tissue and coronal bone windows show severe obstruction of the nasal cavity by polyps.

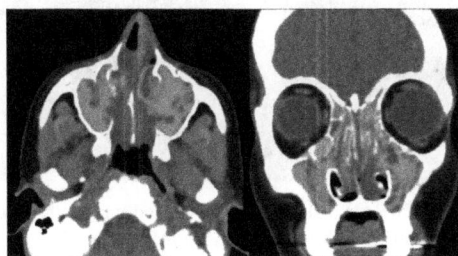

Figure 11. Allergic polyposis. Axial and coronal soft tissue images demonstrate severe opacification of the bilateral nasal cavity, ethmoid sinuses and maxillary sinuses. There are hyperdense secretions filling the maxillary and ethmoid sinuses. At surgery, the patient had thick allergic mucin but there was no evidence of fungal elements in pathology.

pan-sinus opacification can be seen in both NSAID-associated nasal polyposis and allergic fungal rhinosinusitis. Additional findings may include increased density of the sinonasal secretions, bilateral involvement and sinus expansion (Aribandi et al. 2007) (Figure 11). Inflammatory change which predilects the nasal cavity may be seen in Central Compartment Atopic Disease. In CCAD, even opacification of the sinuses has a more central pattern as it tends to occur along the medial walls and floors of the involved sinuses (Roland et al. 2020). CT has poorer contrast resolution than MRI when evaluating soft tissues. For this reason, MRI is an important addition to CT for tumor evaluation and for evaluation of intracranial complications of sinusitis. In addition, many times patients will have had MRIs, which include the paranasal sinuses for other indications (these are most commonly brain MRIs). It is important to recognize that sinonasal opacification in MRIs done for non-sinus indications may reveal clinically unimportant asymptomatic disease (Wani et al. 2001). Nevertheless, for patients with chronic rhinosinusitis who have had MRI imaging, recognition of the typical features of inflammatory disease is helpful.

Characteristics of Sinus Opacification on T1 and T2 Weighted Images

On T1 weighted images free water is relatively hypointense (to muscle). On T2 weighted images, free water is hyperintense. Similarly, watery sinus secretions tend to be low in signal on T1-weighted images and high in signal on T2-weighted images (Figure 12). However, sinus secretions vary in their water content with chronic secretions becoming more inspissated over time. As the secretions become less watery and more proteinaceous, the signal intensity increases on T1-weighted images and can be bright on T1-weighted imaging (Figure 13). As sinus secretions begin to desiccate, signal intensity declines until it is low on both T1 and T2 weighted images. This occurs at approximately a 40% protein concentration (Som et al. 1989).

In addition, the presence of fungal elements may alter the paramagnetic qualities of the sinus secretions. Because of their metabolism, fungi may accumulate iron and manganese in their local environment, resulting in significant loss of signal due to paramagnetic effects (Zinreich et al. 1989). Patients with fungal sinusitis, either allergic fungal rhinosinusitis or fungus ball, may have secretions that are so hypointense, they mimic a partially aerated sinus even when totally opacified (Figure 14).

In addition to air, fungal disease and desiccated secretions, acute hemorrhage and bone or enamel may also result in signal dropout on MRI imaging (Som et al. 1990). Therefore, interpretation of an MRI of the sinuses should be performed with caution and typically a review of a contemporaneous CT is helpful for accurate characterization.

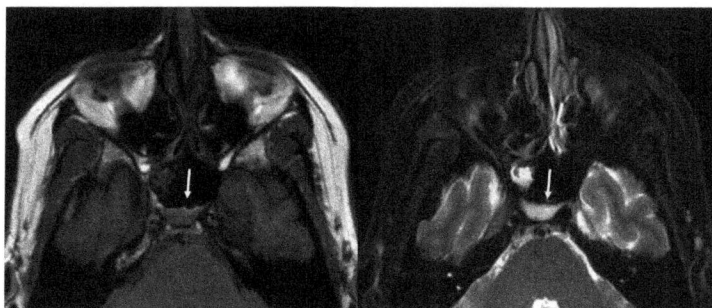

Figure 12. MRI of watery secretions. T1 (left) and T2 (right) weighted images through the sphenoid sinus demonstrate layering fluid with a meniscus (arrow). On the T1 weighted images, the fluid is relatively hypointense. On the T2 weighted images, the fluid is hyperintense. This is typical of watery secretions with low protein content.

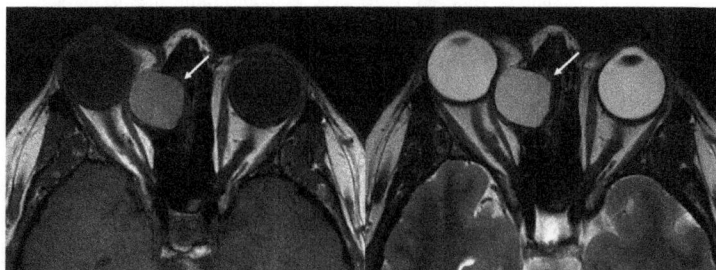

Figure 13. MRI of proteinaceous secretions. T1 (left) and T2 (right) weighted images demonstrate a right ethmoid mucocele with proteinaceous secretions. No contrast was given (note that the nasal mucosa is dark gray and unenhanced) yet the contents of this ethmoid mucocele are hyperintense on T1 weighted imaging. As the protein content of sinus secretions increase, signal intensity increases on T1-weighted imaging until the secretions become densely inspissated.

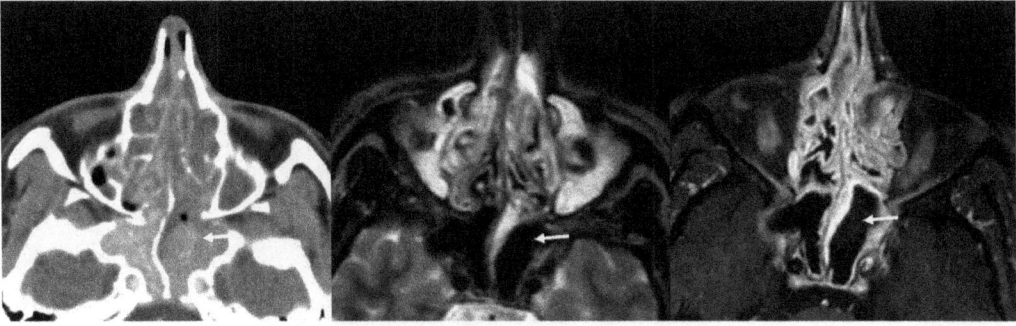

Figure 14. CT and MRI in a patient with AFRS. CT through the sphenoid sinuses clearly demonstrates completely opacified sphenoid sinuses bilaterally with bone thinning posteriorly suggesting mucocele formation. On both T2 weighted images (center image) and post-contrast T1 weighted images (right image), there is a complete signal dropout in these same sinuses with the sinuses almost appearing aerated. This can be seen in fungal sinusitis and is thought to be caused not only by the high protein content of the thick allergic mucin but also by increased concentrations of iron and manganese as a result of fungal metabolism.

Magnetic Resonance Imaging

Characterization of Sinus Enhancement in Benign and Malignant Sinus Disease

After the administration of gadolinium, the intravenous contrast material used for MRI, the highly vascular nasal and paranasal sinus mucosa markedly enhance. A few typical patterns of enhancement are seen in the benign sinonasal disease. There is an avid enhancement of mild mucosal thickening. There can also be polypoid mucosal thickening in the sinuses. In this case, a thin rim of mucosal enhancement may be seen as superficial to more non-enhancing submucosal edema (Figure 15).

In contrast, sinonasal tumors have a more solid pattern of enhancement. Inverted papillomas demonstrate what is termed a cerebriform appearance of enhancement with a heterogeneous enhancement pattern, which has an appearance resembling the gyri and sulci of the brain (Ojiri et al. 2000) (Figure 16). Most malignant tumors enhance to a lesser degree than the adjacent mucosa and can demonstrate the destruction of bony borders and extension outside of the sinus walls (Figure 17) (Agarwal and Policeni 2019).

While an MRI of the sinuses is often performed for evaluation of malignancy, MRI can also be useful for the identification of intracranial complications of benign sinus disease, such as dural inflammation and empyema (Pulickal et al. 2018) (Figure 18).

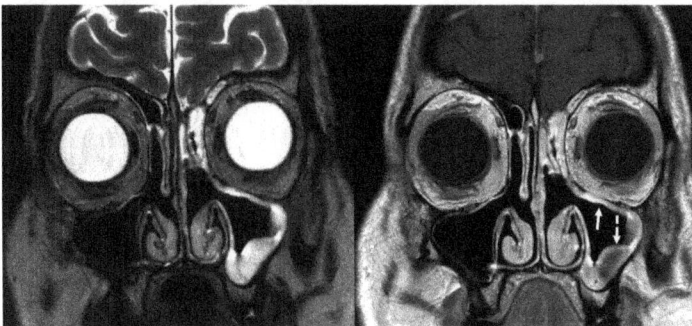

Figure 15. MRI of benign mucosal thickening in the maxillary sinus. T2 weighted image demonstrates T2 hyperintense lobulated thickening in the left maxillary sinus. On post-contrast imaging, we see two different patterns of benign enhancement; along the roof and medial wall of the maxillary sinus, there is an avid enhancement of slightly thickened mucosa (solid arrow). Along the floor of the left maxillary sinus, there is enhancing linear mucosa stretched over non-enhancing submucosal edema (dashed arrow).

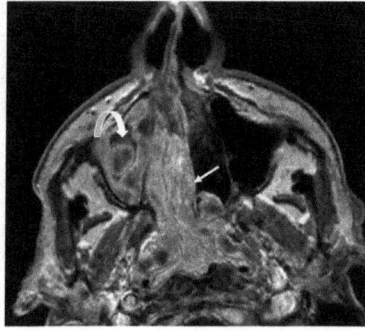

Figure 16. Contrast-enhanced MRI in the axial plane in a patient with an inverted papilloma which involves both the nasal cavity and nasopharynx. Unlike the benign thin linear enhancement surrounding submucosal edema seen in the right maxillary sinus (curved arrow), the inverted papilloma demonstrates heterogeneous solid enhancement (straight arrow) in a pattern reminiscent of the gyri and sulci of the brain, termed "cerebriform."

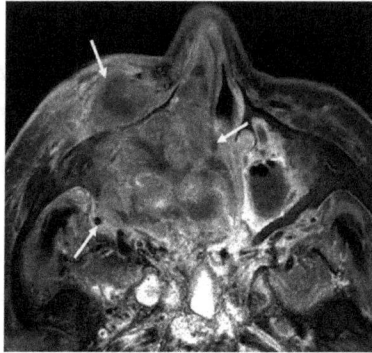

Figure 17. Sinonasal squamous cell carcinoma. Fat-saturated, contrast-enhanced MRI of the sinuses demonstrates a large heterogeneously enhancing, destructive mass in the right maxillary sinus (arrows). Notice how the enhancement is less intense than the benign sinus disease in the left maxillary sinus and sphenoid sinuses. Notice also that the tumor has extended beyond the walls of the maxillary sinus into the premaxillary soft tissues, indicative of the aggressive nature of this tumor.

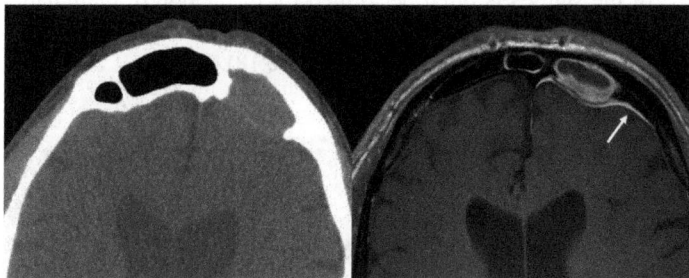

Figure 18. Axial CT and contrast-enhanced T1 weighted MRI images through the frontal sinuses both demonstrate a left frontal mucocele; however, only the MRI also demonstrates the associated dural enhancement (arrow) in the intracranial compartment.

Summary

Both CT and MRI can display abnormalities in patients with chronic sinusitis. Findings can be variable depending on the density of the secretions in the sinuses. CT allows for the best delineation of bony borders and thick proteinaceous secretions. MRI is superior to CT for tumor characterization and evaluation of intracranial complications of sinusitis such as dural thickening or empyema.

Glossary of Abbreviations

CT – Computed Tomography
MRI – Magnetic Resonance Imaging

References

Agarwal, M. and Policeni, B. 2019. Sinonasal neoplasms. Seminars in Roentgenology 54: 244–257.

Aribandi, M., McCoy, V. A. and Bazan, C. 3rd. 2007. Imaging features of invasive and noninvasive fungal sinusitis: a review. Radiographics 27: 1283–96.

Ng, T. Y., Wang, J. Y., Tsai, M. H., Lin, C. C., Tai, C. J. and Ng, Y. K. 2015. Hyperdense findings in sinus computed tomography of chronic rhinosinusitis. Int. Forum Allergy Rhinol. 5: 1181–4.

Ojiri, H., Ujita, M., Tada, S. and Fukuda, K. 2000. Potentially distinctive features of sinonasal inverted papilloma on MR imaging. AJR Am. J. Roentgenol. 175: 465–8.

Pulickal, G. G., Navaratnam, A. V., Nguyen, T., Dragan, A. D., Dziedzic, M. and Lingam, R. K. 2018. Imaging sinonasal disease with MRI: providing insight over and above CT. European Journal of Radiology 102: 157–168.

Roland, L. T., Marcus, S., Schertzer, J. S., Wise, S. K., Levy, J. M. and DelGaudio, J. M. 2020. Computed Tomography findings can help identify different chronic rhinosinusitis with nasal polyp phenotypes. American Journal of Rhinology & Allergy 34: 679–685.

Sahay, S., Gera, K., Bhargava, S. K. and Shah, A. 2016. Occurrence and impact of sinusitis in patients with asthma and/or allergic rhinitis. J. Asthma 53: 635–43.

Shpilberg, K. A., Daniel, S. C., Doshi, A. H., Lawson, W. and Som, P. M. 2015. CT of anatomic variants of the paranasal sinuses and nasal cavity: poor correlation with radiologically significant rhinosinusitis but importance in surgical planning. AJR American Journal of Roentgenology 204: 1255–1260.

Som, P. M., Dillon, W. P., Fullerton, G. D., Zimmerman, R. A., Rajagopalan, B. and Marom, Z. 1989, Chronically obstructed sinonasal secretions: observations on T1 and T2 shortening. Radiology 172: 515–20.

Som, P. M., Dillon, W. P., Curtin, H. D., Fullerton, G. D. and Lidov, M. 1990. Hypointense paranasal sinus foci: differential diagnosis with MR imaging and relation to CT findings. Radiology 176: 777–81.

Wani, M. K., Ruckenstein, M. J. and Parikh, S. 2001. Magnetic resonance imaging of the paranasal sinuses: incidental abnormalities and their relationship to patient symptoms. J. Otolaryngol. 30: 257–62.

Zinreich, S. J., Kennedy, D. W., Malat, J., Curtin, H. D., Epstein, J. I., Huff, L. C. et al. 1988. Fungal sinusitis: diagnosis with CT and MR imaging. Radiology 169: 439–44.

Chapter 3D

Endoscopic Examination of the Upper Airway

Jerald W. Koepke[1,*] and *William K. Dolen*[2,*]

Introduction

In patients presenting with upper airway complaints, the routine examination usually consists of inspection of the anterior nares with an otoscope or nasal speculum and examination of the pharynx with a tongue depressor. The otoscope permits only limited examination of the proximal structures. Such an examination might suffice in patients with uncomplicated chronic rhinitis but will not identify underlying anatomic variants or structural pathology in children or adults that might complicate chronic rhinitis, allergic or nonallergic. The flexible fiberoptic rhinoscope (Figure 1) makes upper airway examination a simple and convenient procedure, permitting comprehensive evaluation of the upper airway. The performance of fiberoptic rhinolaryngoscopy requires a basic understanding of relevant anatomy, physiology and pathology and relatively frequent use of the endoscope.

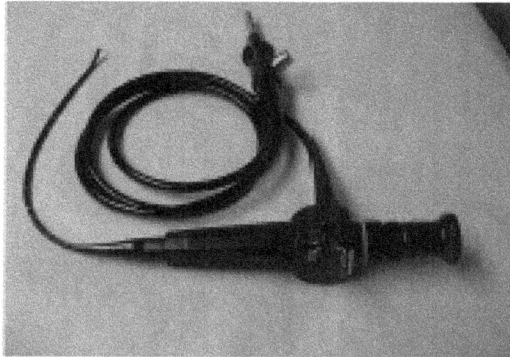

Figure 1. The Olympus ENF-P3 rhinolaryngoscope.

[1] Colorado Allergy and Asthma Centers, Denver, Colorado.
[2] Allergy-Immunology and Pediatric Rheumatology Division, Departments of Pediatrics and Medicine, Medical College of Georgia at Augusta University, Augusta, Georgia 30912.
* Corresponding authors: jwkmlk@gmail.com; bdolen@augusta.edu

An Overview of Normal Upper Airway Anatomy

The upper airway may be divided into regions (Figure 2). In adults, the nasal cavity is a channel approximately 9 to 10 cm in length from the meatus to the posterior choana. The posterior choana separates the nasal cavity from the nasopharynx. The oropharynx, in which the palatine tonsils are located, extends from the inferior margin of the soft palate to the upper edge of the epiglottis. The hypopharynx is located posterior to the aperture of the larynx. The triangular inlet of the larynx (*aditus laryngis*) is formed by the superior margin of the epiglottis, the aryepiglottic folds and the arytenoid cartilages. The larynx becomes continuous with the trachea.

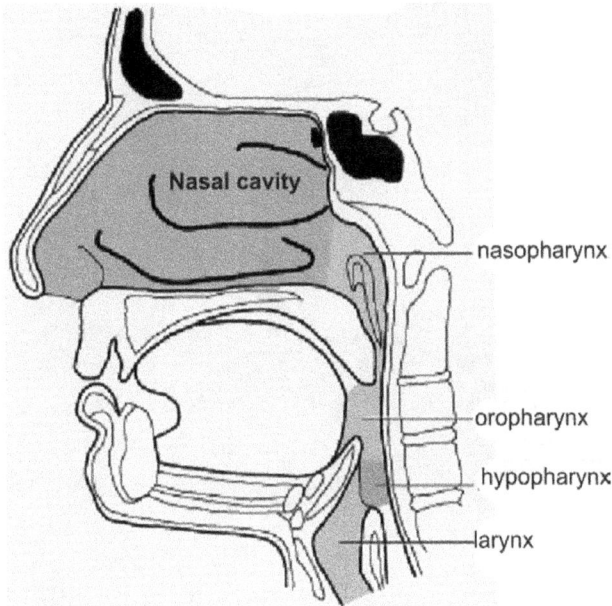

Figure 2. The anatomic divisions of the upper airway; all five divisions may be inspected with a fiberoptic endoscope.

Anterior Nasal Structures

The septum divides the nasal cavity into the right and left chambers. The nasal vestibule is the most anterior and inferior portion of the nasal cavity (Figure 3). It is bounded medially and laterally by the alar cartilages and extends to the inferior border of the lateral nasal cartilage. Above the vestibule and in front of the middle meatus is the nasal atrium, and above this is the *agger nasi*, a prominence that generally contains anterior ethmoid air cells. The nasal floor is formed anteriorly by the maxillary bone and posteriorly by the palatine bone. It is slightly concave and passes horizontally from the vestibule to the choana. The nasal vault narrows superiorly to form the roof of the nose.

Nasal Septum

The nasal septum, rarely straight in normal adults, consists of both cartilaginous and bony components (Figure 4), with mucous membrane overlying the perichondrium or periosteum of the underlying cartilage or bone. The mobile, anterior portion of the septum, is composed of a quadrangular septal cartilage resting in a groove on the maxillary bone and articulating posteriorly with the thin, delicate bone of the perpendicular plate of the ethmoid and inferiorly with the thicker, more rigid bone of the vomer. The vomer forms the medial border of the choanae and rests on the crest of the maxillary

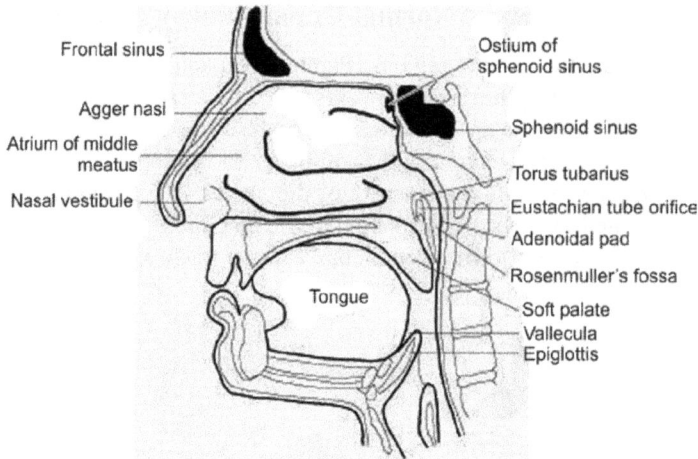

Figure 3. A sagittal section of the head demonstrating lateral structures of the nasal cavity and pharynx.

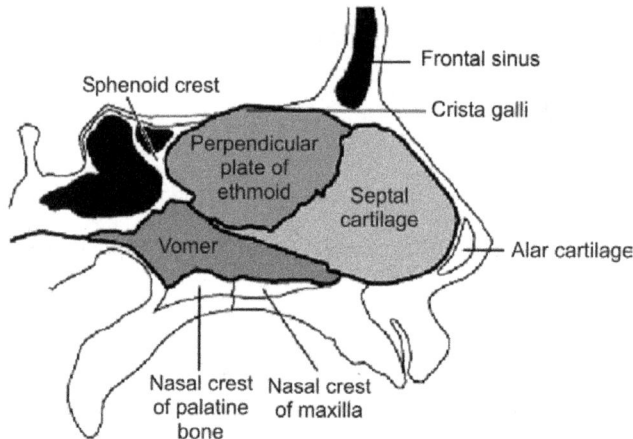

Figure 4. Cartilaginous and bony structures of the Nasal Septum; The Quadrangular septal cartilage and the vomer articulate with bones of the nasal floor; The thin perpendicular plate of the ethmoid extends upward to the cribriform plate.

bone anteriorly and the crest of the palatine bone posteriorly. The perpendicular plate of the ethmoid extends superiorly, attaching to the cribriform plate (*lamina cribosa*). A superior projection of the hard palate, the maxillary ridge (crista nasalis maxillae; the nasal crest of maxilla) often forms a "T" anteriorly at the base of the septum. The lateral wings of the "T" may project into the nasal cavity.

Turbinates

Three or four turbinates provide filtration, heating and cooling and humidification of inspired air and offer resistance to airflow. The turbinates are comprised of a scroll-shaped bony supporting structure, called a concha and overlying mucosa. Clefting or segmentalization of the turbinates may occur both horizontally and sagittally, and clefting of a middle turbinate may be difficult to distinguish from a nasal polyp on anterior examination. The space created by a turbinate and the lateral wall of the nose is called a meatus.

Inferior Turbinate and Inferior Meatus

The inferior concha is a separate bone sitting in an opening in the maxilla and resting in the lateral wall of the nasal passage. It is attached to the palate and maxilla by membranous soft tissue. The turbinate follows the lower lateral wall of the nose in a course parallel to that of the nasal floor. In patients with nasal septal deviation, the inferior turbinates are not the same size. The only structure opening into the inferior meatus is the nasolacrimal duct which drains tears through a large opening in the anterior roof of the meatus (Figure 5), located about 1 cm from the anterior margin of the turbinate. The orifice is rarely seen by fiberoptic rhinoscopy. An opening found in the lateral wall at this location is most likely an antral window surgically placed in the inferior meatus to provide drainage for the maxillary sinus.

Middle Turbinate and Middle Meatus

The middle turbinate, like the superior turbinate, is part of the ethmoid bone and is suspended from the roof of the nose rather than from the lateral wall. The anterior edge is superior and posterior to that of the inferior turbinate.

The semilunar hiatus (*hiatus semilunaris*) is a crescent-shaped cleft located in the middle meatus (Figure 5). The ostium of the nasofrontal duct and the anterior ethmoid sinus ostia typically are located in the anterior and midportions of the hiatus. The nasofrontal duct may have a separate opening anterior to the semilunar hiatus. The maxillary sinuses open into the posteroinferior portion of the semilunar hiatus. The ostium of the maxillary sinus varies in size in normal individuals from pinpoint to several millimeters in diameter and large accessory ostia may be present. The ethmoid bulla (*bulla ethmoidalis*) is a bulge containing anterior and middle ethmoid air cells, located posterior and superior to the semilunar hiatus.

Superior and Supreme Turbinates

The superior turbinate is a short, oblique structure located superior and posterior to the middle turbinate. The posterior ethmoid sinuses drain into the superior meatus (Figure 5). A supreme turbinate medial to the superior turbinate is occasionally noted.

Sphenoethmoidal Recess

The sphenoethmoidal recess is a deep groove located superior, posterior and medial to the superior turbinate. It contains the ostium of the sphenoid sinus (Figure 5).

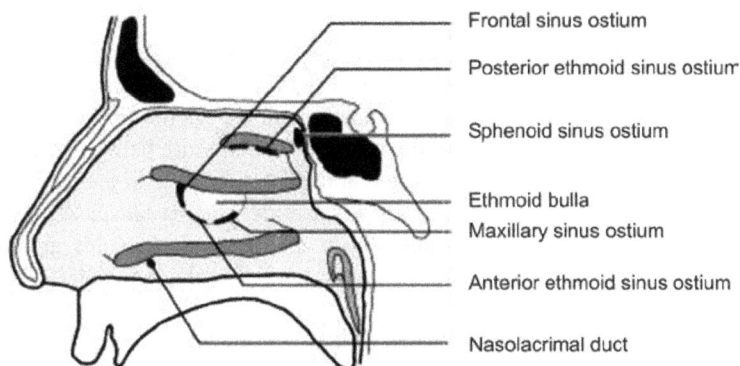

Frontal sinus ostium

Posterior ethmoid sinus ostium

Sphenoid sinus ostium

Ethmoid bulla
Maxillary sinus ostium

Anterior ethmoid sinus ostium

Nasolacrimal duct

Figure 5. A sagittal section of the head with the turbinates removed to demonstrate ostia of the paranasal sinuses and nasolacrimal duct.

Nasopharynx

The torus tubarius is located on the lateral wall of the nasopharynx, defining and protecting the Eustachian tube orifice (Figure 5). Rosenmueller's fossa is a vertical cleft, a potential space, between the posterior lip of the torus tubarius and the adenoidal pad. Many of the insidious malignancies of the pharynx have their origin in this space. The adenoid or pharyngeal tonsil is a primary lymph node of first-line defense against inflammation involving the upper airway.

Oropharynx

The lingual tonsils are located on either side of the dorsum of the tongue anterior to the epiglottis (Figure 6). The median glossoepiglottic fold and the two lateral glossoepiglottic folds attach the epiglottis to the base of the tongue.

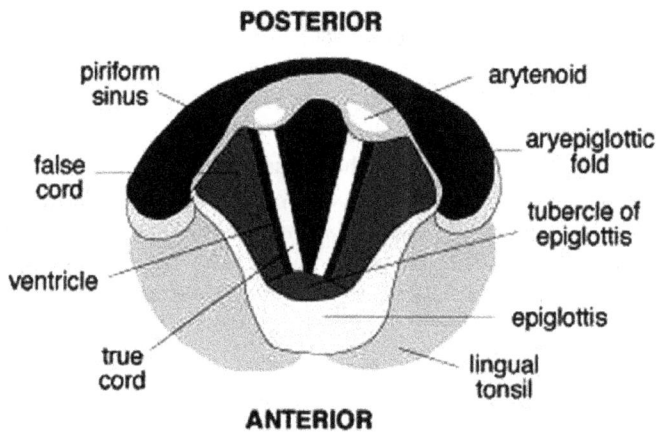

Figure 6. The larynx as viewed from above and oriented as it would be seen with a fiberoptic endoscope.

Hypopharynx

The valleculae are cup-shaped spaces, separated by the median glossoepiglottic fold, posterior to the base of the tongue and anterior to the epiglottis. To the right and to the left of the larynx are the piriform sinuses, gutter-like structures that direct food to the esophagus.

Larynx

The framework of the larynx is formed by the thyroid, cricoid and epiglottic cartilages and by pairs of arytenoid, corniculate and cuneiform cartilages. The aryepiglottic folds and the arytenoids are located immediately behind the epiglottis. The aperture of the glottis (*rima glottidis*) is formed by the true vocal folds (*plicae vocales*) and the posterior commissure between the arytenoids. The anterior ligament of the true vocal folds is located at the anterior angle of the vocal folds. Between the true vocal folds and the false vocal folds (vestibular folds; *plicae ventriculares*) is the laryngeal ventricle. The nodular swellings located medially in the aryepiglottic folds are the corniculate cartilages which sit on top of the arytenoid cartilages. Lateral to the corniculate cartilages are the cuneiform cartilages.

The true vocal folds are anteriorly attached to the thyroid cartilage. The posterior attachment is to the vocal processes of the arytenoid cartilages. The true vocal folds often reflect light in such a manner that they appear whiter than the surrounding mucosa. The strong vocal ligaments are covered by connective tissue and a thin layer of epithelium. Reinke's space is the potential space between the vocal ligaments and the subepithelial connective tissue layer. The mobile arytenoid cartilages move in and out with respiration and phonation.

Examination Procedure

Preparation for Examination

Other than the explanation of the procedure to the patient, the only special preparation usually required is decongestion and anesthesia; the patient is not fasted.

After the procedure has been explained to the patient, the patient is seated in an examining chair, preferably an ENT-type chair with an adjustable headrest. A small child may sit in a parent's lap. The examiner should perform a preliminary nasal examination to determine nasal patency and to identify pathology which might be visible on routine examination.

The patient is asked to clear secretions by the gentle blowing of the nose. If necessary, saline irrigation may be used to clear the nasal passage of mucus and debris.

To shrink the nasal mucosa, topical decongestants, such as phenylephrine or oxymetazoline, may be delivered by a standard nasal atomizer. Xylocaine solution (4%), also delivered by a nasal atomizer, may be used for nasal anesthesia. The examiner should remember that this requires a few minutes to take effect. Pharyngeal and laryngeal anesthesia is not necessary. One or two sprays of each drug should be directed posteriorly, with the same amount directed superiorly and posteriorly at about a 45-degree angle. If desired, the rhinoscope may be lubricated with a water-based lubricant or with 2% viscous xylocaine.

With proper anesthesia, the procedure is not painful. The patient may talk to the examiner during the examination and should be asked to communicate any discomfort (other than pressure) to the examiner so that the endoscope may be withdrawn from that area.

Examination Sequence

The examination should proceed in a consistent, logical sequence that can be varied if needed in individual patients. The examination sequence is the same for children and adults, although a complete examination might not be possible in an uncooperative child. It is usually convenient to examine structures of the anterior nasal cavity first, followed by an examination of the pharynx and larynx. Because the sphenoethmoidal recess and middle meatus are more difficult to examine and may be less well anesthetized than other structures, they are generally examined last.

Examination of the nasal cavity begins with the nasal vestibule. It is usually possible to examine the nasal floor by slowly and gently advancing the endoscope into the nasal cavity. The inferior turbinate, floor of the nose, and septum will be in view (Figure 7). Deformities of the septum include septal spurs (Figure 8). If the endoscope tip is flexed slightly upward, the middle turbinate will be seen in the distance and with upward flexion to 60–90 degrees, the superior portion of the anterior nose can be evaluated. If the inferior turbinate is large or swollen, it may be necessary to advance the tip of the endoscope over the anterior margin of the inferior turbinate in order to view the middle turbinate. To view the anterior portion of the middle turbinate, the tip of the endoscope is directed over the inferior turbinate. In this position, a polyp exiting the middle turbinate might be seen (Figure 9). The endoscope is usually advanced to the choana along the floor of the nose, but this position may be used if the lower route is obstructed. With the endoscope positioned at the posterior choana, it is usually possible to direct the endoscope superiorly and laterally into the middle meatus either at this point in the examination or later after the examination of the larynx and sphenoethmoidal recess.

With the endoscope tip on the nasal floor at the level of the posterior choana, structures of the nasopharynx may be viewed through the choana (Figure 10). Enlarged adenoidal tissue might obscure other structures of the nasopharynx (Figure 11). The endoscope is then advanced into the nasopharynx. The endoscope is advanced into the oropharynx. Structures of the posterior tongue,

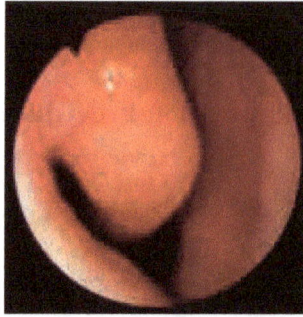

Figure 7. A normal right anterior nasal cavity. The septum is on the right. the inferior turbinate and the inferior meatus are on the left.

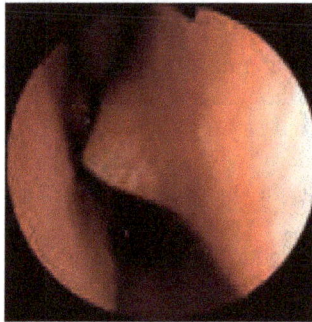

Figure 8. In this view of the superior portion of the mid-nasal passage, a septal spur is seen impinging on the medial surface of the middle turbinate; at some point in the past, this patient had received a direct blow to the nose, causing the posterior portion of the septal (quadrangular) cartilage to displace from its articulation with the bony structures of the septum; this results in facial pain when the patient develops nasal congestion—a symptom complex sometimes called sluder syndrome.

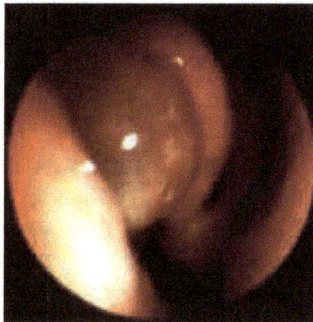

Figure 9. The left middle meatus is occupied by a single ethmoid polyp which displaces the middle turbinate toward the septum located at 9 o'clock; characteristic features of a polyp, distinguishing it from nasal mucosa, include the slightly yellow or translucent coloring of a smooth relatively avascular structure; this polyp can be moved with a cotton-tipped applicator, indicating its origin from the middle meatus.

the epiglottis, the valleculae and glosso-epiglottic and lateral epiglottic folds are examined. Here, the examiner can view abnormalities such as enlarged lingual tonsils (Figure 12) or other enlarged lymphoid structures (Figure 13).

The endoscope tip is kept close to the posterior wall of the pharynx as it is directed into the hypopharynx. The patient is encouraged to breathe quietly and asked not to swallow but reassured that swallowing will merely result in the sensation of attempting to swallow the endoscope, not in discomfort. The endoscope is directed along the posterior pharyngeal wall in the midline, over the

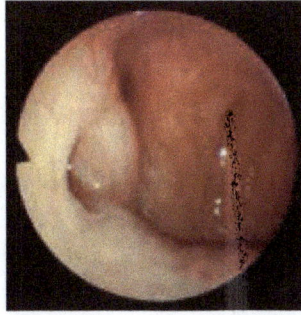

Figure 10. In this view of a normal right posterior nasal passage; the adenoidal pad is seen posteriorly; the eustachian tube orifice; surrounded by the torus tubarius is on the left at 9 o'clock; rosenmüller's fossa is the potential space between the posterior torus and the adenoidal pad.

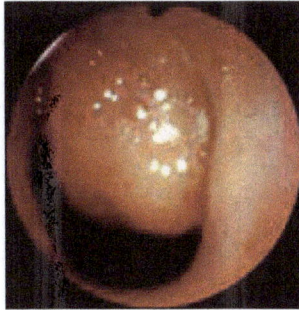

Figure 11. Partial obstruction of the right nasal cavity by adenoidal hyperplasia; the small aperture inferiorly may disappear when the child is sleeping and the palate moves superiorly; this can result in snoring with apnea and mouth breathing with maxillofacial and dental growth abnormalities.

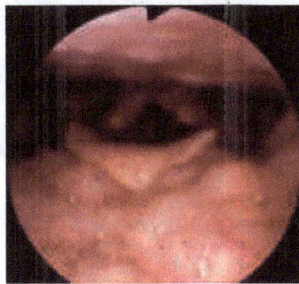

Figure 12. Prominent lingual tonsils.

epiglottis. In this position, the arytenoids, the superior projections of the corniculate and cuneiform cartilages, the aryepiglottic folds, the true and false vocal folds and the ventricles are well visualized (Figure 14). With the endoscope in this position, patients with vocal cord dysfunction syndrome can be identified (Figure 15). Laryngeal edema will also be obvious (Figure 16). Slight rotations of the endoscope in this position will very clearly reveal the piriform sinuses. From this position, the examiner often will see well into the trachea.

To examine the sphenoethmoidal recess, the endoscope is withdrawn under direct visualization to a position just anterior to the choana. As the endoscope is directed superiorly, the anterior margin of the sphenoid bone comes into view.

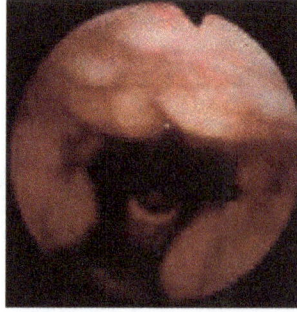

Figure 13. A patient with long standing chronic rhinosinusitis. The tip of the examining scope is in the nasopharynx and is directed inferiorly; at 12 o'clock is the posterior pharyngeal wall. The tip of the epiglottis is seen in the distance in the center of the slide; prominent lymphoid nodularity can be readily visualized on the posterior wall; the palatine tonsils protrude from the lateral walls at 4 o'clock and 9 o'clock.

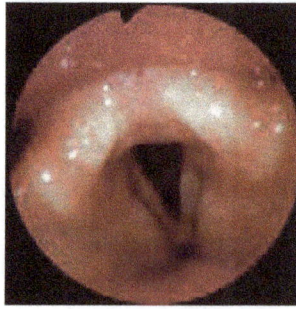

Figure 14. A normal larynx; the true and false vocal folds are clearly seen.

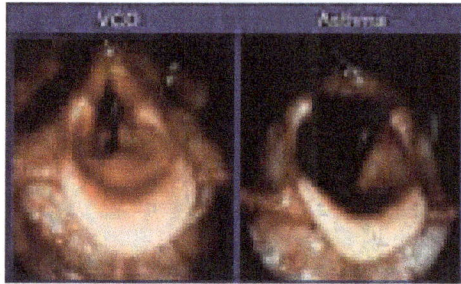

Figure 15. In patients with vocal cord dysfunction syndrome; the vocal folds adduct, forming a posterior diamond-shaped opening as seen on the left figure; this finding is not present in asthma (right figure).

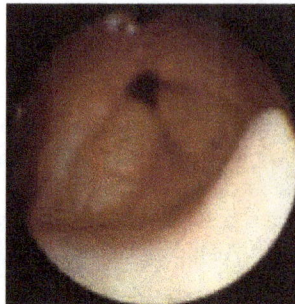

Figure 16. Laryngeal edema.

If structures of the middle meatus were not previously examined, they are studied at this time. It is usually easier to examine the middle meatus from posterior to anterior. Following the withdrawal of the endoscope under direct visualization, an examination of the other side of the nose is carried out. Afterward, the equipment is cleaned and disinfected in preparation for the next examination.

Summary

The endoscopist can quickly and thoroughly examine most areas of the upper airway without discomfort to the patient. Once the endoscopist becomes familiar with the anatomy variations from normal and pathology becomes readily apparent. Examinations may be recorded for permanent record keeping and may be replayed and explained to patients. The use of rhinoscopy will enhance the diagnosis and treatment of upper airway disease.

Acknowledgments

Text, illustrations, and photographs in this chapter are from Selner J.C., Dolen W.K., Spofford B., Koepke J.W. Rhinolaryngoscopy. 2nd ed. Denver, CO; Allergy Respiratory Institute of Colorado; 1989. An updated online version of the text, images and instructional videos may be found at http://www.augusta.edu/mcg/pediatrics/allergy/rhino/. Used with permission. In memoriam, John Canty Selner, MD (1936–2006).

Chapter 3E

Bronchial Thermoplasty

Nishil Dalsania, Sandeep Jewani and *Ali Musani**

Introduction

Severe uncontrolled asthma in patients maximized on pharmacologic therapy accounts for a majority of morbidity and mortality associated with asthma. Bronchial Thermoplasty (BT) is a non-pharmacological FDA-approved bronchoscopic intervention that delivers thermal energy via endobronchial radio frequency wave catheter to the bronchial airways. BT was designed prior to the advent of biologic therapy to assist in controlling severely uncontrolled asthmatics. The principal goal of this procedure is to reduce airway smooth muscle in the bronchial airways. The benefits of bronchial thermoplasty can be in reducing airway hyper-responsiveness, optimizing asthma control, decreasing asthma exacerbations, and stepping down on asthma therapy, including steroids. A crucial component prior to relegating a patient to the procedure is ensuring appropriate patient selection in efforts to maximize benefits and minimize risks associated with the procedure. Complications after bronchial thermoplasty are often seen and predominately involve exacerbation of underlying asthma, atelectasis, respiratory tract infection, and hemoptysis.

Principals of Bronchial Thermoplasty

Bronchial Thermoplasty (BT) is a non-pharmacological FDA-approved bronchoscopic intervention that delivers thermal energy via endobronchial radio frequency (RF) wave catheter to the bronchial airways. The principal goal of this procedure is to reduce airway smooth muscle (ASM) in the bronchial airways (Facciolongo et al. 2018). The benefits of BT can be in reducing airway hyper-responsiveness, optimizing asthma control, decreasing asthma exacerbations and stepping down on asthma therapy, including steroids.

Overview of Asthma and BT

There are a growing number of patients worldwide affected by asthma. More than 235 million patients suffer from asthma, of which only approximately 5% have severe uncontrolled disease and are on maximal conventional inhaled therapy with a high dose inhaled corticosteroid and long-acting inhaled beta agonist. This minority of asthmatics with severely uncontrolled patients have continued symptoms that affect their daily activity and life choices. However, they account for the majority

Division of Pulmonary Sciences and Critical Care Medicine, University of Colorado, 12700 East 19th Avenue, 9C03, Aurora, CO 80045.
Emails: nishil.dalsania@cuanschutz.edu; sandeep.jewani@cuanschutz.edu
* Corresponding author: ali.musani@cuanschutz.edu

of morbidity and mortality associated with asthma. Chronic obstructive disease caused by severe asthma is due to the remodeling and thickening of the airway wall via various mechanisms. Asthma treatment is mainly pharmacological based on relaxing ASM and reducing airway inflammation. Bronchothermoplastic intervention was designed prior to the advent of biologic therapy to assist in controlling severe asthmatics on maximal therapy with the intent to decrease the morbidity and mortality associated with severely uncontrolled asthmatics. BT is carried out by controlled RF thermal energy to the airway wall to reduce ASM, decreasing oral or inhaled glucocorticoid dose and decreasing long-term morphological changes associated with asthma.

Rationale/Data

Clinical trials on bronchial thermoplasty as a treatment for severe uncontrolled asthma began with a single-arm, prospective feasibility study to evaluate the safety of BT in 16 patients with mild to moderate asthma (Cox et al. 2006). Results demonstrated that BT was well tolerated, and all procedure-related adverse events occurred within one week of the procedure. Most of these events are commonly seen in asthmatics after any bronchoscopic procedures. All adverse events resolved spontaneously with antibiotics or a temporary increase in asthma medications.

A randomized controlled trial (AIR Trial) from 2002–2010 was conducted on 112 patients to evaluate the efficacy and safety of BT in moderate to severe asthma (Cox et al. 2007). The primary outcome of this study was the frequency of mild exacerbations, calculated during three scheduled two-week periods of abstinence from LABA at 3, 6 and 12 months. In patients treated with inhaled corticosteroids alone, BT reduced the frequency of mild exacerbations (-0.16 ± 0.37 vs. 0.04 ± 0.29; $P = 0.005$) at a rate equivalent to ten exacerbations per subject per year and provided 86 additional symptom-free days per patient per year. There was no significant difference in FEV_1 or airway hyper-responsiveness by methacholine challenge. The adverse events noted were more common in BT than control group immediately after treatment and at less than six weeks; however, were similar from 6 weeks to 12 months after treatment.

Concomitantly, the non-blinded randomized controlled RISA (Research In Severe Asthma) Trial from 2004–2019 was conducted with 32 patients to assess safety, reduction in medications and asthma symptoms in severe refractory asthmatics (Pavord et al. 2007). In this trial, BT resulted in a transient worsening of asthma symptoms. Seven hospitalizations for respiratory symptoms occurred in 4 of 15 BT subjects during the treatment period. BT was associated with a short-term increase in asthma-related morbidity. Also noted in this trial was a slight improvement in FEV_1 (14.9 ± 17.4 vs. 0.9 ± 22.3; $P = 0.04$) at 22 weeks, although non-significant improvement in FEV_1 at 52 weeks.

After safety analysis from the AIR Trial, the AIR2 Trial (2005–2019), a prospective, randomized multi-site, double-blind, sham-controlled trial with 288 patients, assessed the effectiveness and safety in severe persistent asthma of BT vs. sham procedure (Castro et al. 2010). The primary outcome was the difference in Asthma Quality of Life Questionnaire (AQLQ) scores from baseline at 6, 9 and 12 months, which showed improvement from baseline in the BT group compared with sham (1.35 +/– 1.10 vs. 1.16 +/– 1.23 [PPS, 96.0% ITT and 97.9% per protocol]). Seventy-nine percent of BT and 64% of sham subjects achieved changes in AQLQ of 0.5 or greater (PPS, 99.6%). Six percent more BT subjects were hospitalized in the treatment period (up to 6 weeks after BT).

From 2011–2018 the PAS2 Trial, a prospective open-label observational multi-site trial with 190 patients, assessed the effectiveness and safety of BT in clinical practice (Chupp et al. 2017). At three years, patients had a reduction in severe exacerbations, ED visits and hospitalizations by 45%, 55%, and 40%, respectively. FEV_1 remained unchanged. Although, the mean daily ICS dose was reduced to 2070 from 2300 µg/day ($p = 0.003$), and the percentage of subjects taking daily OCS reduced from 18.9% to 10.2% ($p = 0.0004$).

A meta-analysis published in 2015 reviewed the five years follow-up of patients who had undergone BT (Zhou et al. 2015). This review consolidated an unchanged FEV_1 in BT patients between years 1 and 5 ($p = 0.57$, $p = 0.65$), significance for a reduced frequency of asthma exacerbations (RR = 3.41, 95% CI: 2.96–3.93, p < 0.00001), unchanged rate of emergency department visits (RR = 1.06, 95% CI: 0.77–1.46, p = 0.71), and no increase in hospitalization (RR = 1.47, 95% CI: 0.69–3.12, p = 0.32).

A further multi-center prospective follow-up (BT10+) with 136 BT-treated patients (52% of a total of 260 patients) and 56 sham patients (33% of a total of 169 patients) of the randomized control trials AIR, AIR2 and RISA trial was completed to determine safety and effectiveness of BT at greater than ten years (Chaudhuri et al. 2021). The median follow-up was 12.1 years post-BT. This trial showed similar rates of severe asthma exacerbation in patients treated with BT at ten years (25%) compared to five years (22%) and one year (24%). Similar quality of life measurements and spirometry were measured at ten years, five years, and one year.

Indications and Contraindications

A crucial component prior to relegating a patient to the procedure is ensuring appropriate patient selection in efforts to maximize benefits and minimize risks associated with the procedure. Currently, BT is FDA-approved for adult patients 18 years and older with severe persistent asthma that is uncontrolled on therapy with inhaled corticosteroids and long-acting beta-agonists. Additional patient selection criteria are often utilized, many based on the AIR2 trial. These include pre-bronchodilator $FEV_1 \geqslant 60\%$ predicted, post-bronchodilator FEV_1 within 10–15% of best value, methacholine $PC_{20} < 8$ mg/mL, AQLQ $\leqslant 6.25$, nonsmokers for $\geqslant 1$ year and < 10 pack year prior history (Castro et al. 2010).

Precautions should be taken in patients with other respiratory diseases, such as emphysema, cystic fibrosis, vocal cord dysfunction or upper airway obstruction; and among patients at increased risk for bronchoscopic procedures and anesthesia administration. Temporal contraindications include patients with an active respiratory infection or exacerbation of symptoms in the preceding 2–4 weeks. BT should also be avoided in patients with $\geqslant 4$ lower respiratory tract infections, $\geqslant 3$ hospitalizations for respiratory symptoms, or $\geqslant 4$ oral corticosteroid treatments for asthma within the past 12 months. Finally, absolute contraindications to bronchial thermoplasty include the presence of implanted electronic devices and previously treated patients with BT due to concerns of airway scarring and stricture formation.

Patient Selection

Indications/FDA Approval

$\geqslant 18$ year old
Severe persistent asthma
Uncontrolled on ICS and LABA

Patient Selection

Pre-Bronchodilator $FEV_1 \geqslant 60\%$ Predicted
Post-Bronchodilator FEV_1 within 10–15% of Best Value
Methacholine PC20 < 8 mg/mL
AQLQ $\leqslant 6.25$
Non-Smoker for $\geqslant 1$ year
< 10 Pack Year History

Precautions

Other Respiratory Diseases:
    Emphysema
    Cystic Fibrosis
    Vocal Cord Dysfunction
    Upper Airway Obstruction

High Procedural Risks:
    Bronchoscopic Procedure Risk
    Anesthesia Administration Risk

Relative Contraindications

Active Respiratory Infection
Asthma Exacerbation
⩾ 4 lower respiratory tract infections (last 12 months)
⩾ 3 hospitalizations for respiratory symptoms (last 12 months)
⩾ 4 oral corticosteroid treatments for asthma (last 12 months)

Absolute Contraindications

Implanted Electronic Devices
Prior Treated Patients with BT

Procedure

Bronchoscopic thermoplasty is delivered by Alair BT System (Boston Scientific). The procedure entails three separate bronchoscopic procedures, once every three weeks, by an experienced bronchoscopist under moderate sedation or general anesthesia. Typically, patients are given peri-procedural prednisone 50 mg daily for three days prior to the procedure and until on-day post-procedure. The Alair System uses an, RF controller (Figure 1) and catheter (Figure 2) with thermal energy transfer to bronchial airway walls. The catheter has an expanding basket at the tip similar to those used for foreign body retrieval (Figure 3). The target temperature controlled at the airway wall is approximately 65°C given in 10 seconds at 18 watts. This energy is delivered at

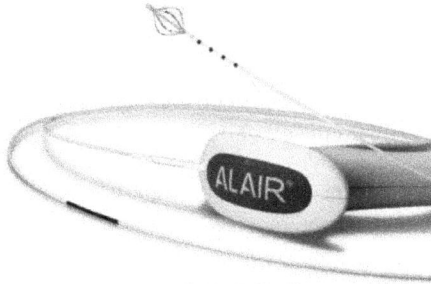

Figure 1. Alair catheter.

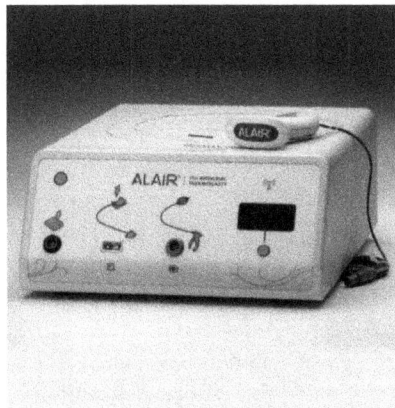

Figure 2. Alair controller.

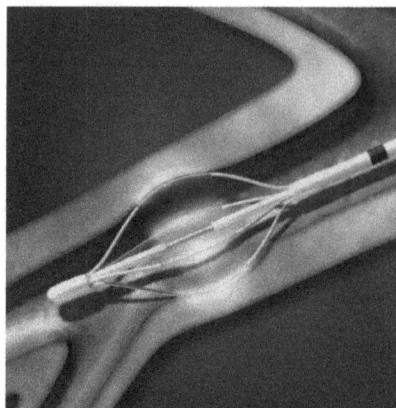

Figure 3. Alair catheter expanding basket.

airways of size 3–10 mm and distal to the main stem bronchi. The airways are treated once, starting with the most distal and moving the catheter a few millimeters proximal each time. This process usually entails 50 to 100 activations during each procedure. The first bronchoscopic procedure is typically the right lower lobe, followed by the left lower lobe, and finally, bilateral upper lobes (Figure 4). This is conducted in three separate procedures to minimize the side effects associated with treating large swaths of the bronchial tree. The right middle lobe is typically not treated due to the theoretical risk of right middle lobe syndrome as a result of smaller airways and increased risk of airway obstruction from post-procedure inflammation. However, many institutions have forgone this rationale.

Complications

Complications after BT are often seen and predominately involve exacerbation of underlying asthma, atelectasis, respiratory tract infection and hemoptysis. Acute exacerbation of asthma appears to be the most frequently reported complication, with one study (Vijayan et al. 2022) reporting it in 53% of patients post-procedure. Heat activation from the procedure almost ubiquitously causes a drop in the FEV_1, which indicates hyper-reactivity within the bronchi and the onset of symptoms. The direct effect of thermal energy on the mucosa can result in the development of bronchial wall edema, increased mucous production and bronchospasm. Additionally, heat activation can initiate an inflammatory reaction with resultant inflammatory mediator release, micro-vascular alterations and fibrin plug formations. This can influence the development of atelectasis due to airway plugging and subsequently the development of respiratory tract infections and pneumonia. The disruption of the vasculature can trigger bleeding with hemoptysis seen in approximately 3% of patients post-procedure (Castro et al. 2010).

Professional Guidelines

BT comes with benefits for those who have few other options; however, there is a chance of significant morbidity associated with its utilization. Currently, several organizations have vocalized their stance and provided guidelines on the role of BT in patient care. The British Thoracic Society (BTS), in their 2019 guideline, stated that BT can be considered in poorly controlled asthmatics; however, assessment and treatment should be undertaken at specialized centers and long-term follow-up is recommended. The Global Initiative for Asthma (GINA) vocalized similar recommendations. It emphasized the importance of patient selection as long-term effects are still poorly understood and the need for large cohort studies. Finally, the European Respiratory Society (ERS) and American

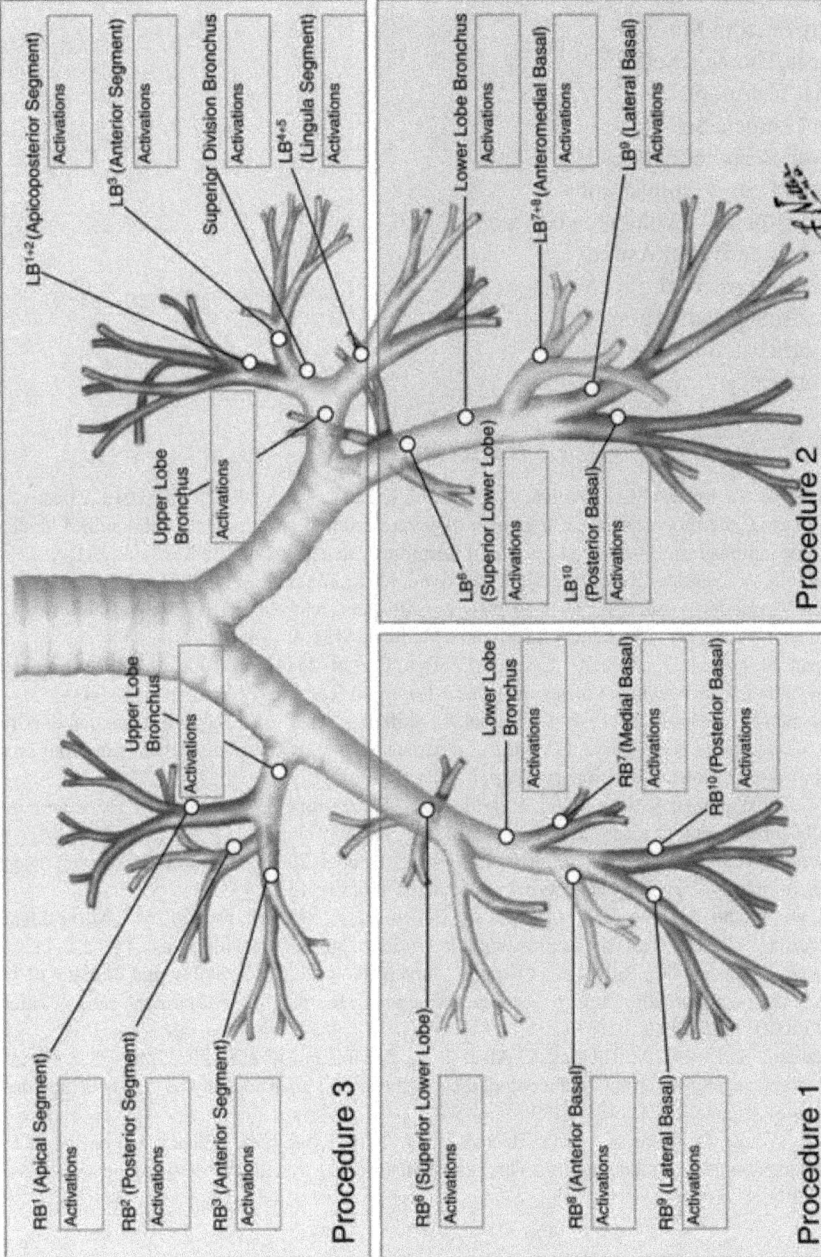

Figure 4. Bronchial thermoplasty map.

Thoracic Society (ATS) released a joint guideline with the most restrictive use of BT. They recommended its use only in the context of institutional review board-approved systematic review or clinical study, citing poor quality evidence available for its current use (Chung et al. 2014).

Glossary of Abbreviations

AQLQ – Asthma Quality of Life Questionnaire
ASM – Airway Smooth Muscle
ATS – American Thoracic Society
BT – Bronchial Thermoplasty
BTS – British Thoracic Society
ERS – European Respiratory Society
FDA – Food and Drug Administration
FEV_1 – Forced Expiratory Volume in one second
GINA – Global Initiative for Asthma
ICS – Inhaled Corticosteroid
LABA – Long-Acting Beta Agonist
OCS – Oral Corticosteroid
RF – Radio Frequency

References

Castro, M., Rubin, A., Laviolette, M., Fiterman, J., De Andrade Lima, M., Shah, P. et al. 2010. Effectiveness and safety of bronchial thermoplasty in the treatment of severe asthma: a multicenter, randomized, double-blind, sham-controlled clinical trial. American Journal of Respiratory and Critical Care Medicine 181(2): 116–124.

Chaudhuri, R., Rubin, A., Sumino, K., Lapa e Silva, J., Niven, R., Siddiqui, S. et al. 2021. Safety and effectiveness of bronchial thermoplasty after 10 years in patients with persistent asthma (BT10+): a follow-up of three randomised controlled trials. The Lancet Respiratory Medicine 9(5): 457–466.

Chung, K., Wenzel, S., Brozek, J., Bush, A., Castro, M., Sterk, P. et al. 2014. International ERS/ATS guidelines on definition, evaluation and treatment of severe asthma. European Respiratory Journal 43(2): 343–373.

Chupp, G., Laviolette, M., Cohn, L., McEvoy, C., Bansal, S., Shifren, A. et al. 2017. Long-term outcomes of bronchial thermoplasty in subjects with severe asthma: a comparison of 3-year follow-up results from two prospective multicentre studies. European Respiratory Journal 50(2).

Cox, G., Miller, J., McWilliams, A., FitzGerald, J. and Lam, S. 2006. Bronchial thermoplasty for asthma. American Journal of Respiratory and Critical Care Medicine 173(9): 965–969.

Cox, G., Thomson, N., Rubin, A., Niven, R., Corris, P., Siersted, H. et al. 2007. Asthma control during the year after bronchial thermoplasty. New England Journal of Medicine 356(13): 1327–1337.

Facciolongo, N., Di Stefano, A., Pietrini, V., Galeone, C., Bellanova, F., Menzell, F. et al. 2018. Nerve ablation after bronchial thermoplasty and sustained improvement in severe asthma. BMC Pulm. Med. 18(1): 1–11.

Pavord, I., Cox, G., Thomson, N., Rubin, A., Corris, P., Niven, R. et al. 2007. Safety and efficacy of bronchial thermoplasty in symptomatic, severe asthma. American Journal of Respiratory and Critical Care Medicine 176(12): 1185–1191.

Vijayan, K., Karakattu, S., Bansal, A., Thomas, A., Alazzeh, A., El Minaoui, W. et al. 2022. Immediate complications and flow volume changes during treatment phases of bronchial thermoplasty: a single-center descriptive study. Journal of Asthma 59(7): 1433–1437.

Zhou, J., Feng, Y., Wang, Q., Zhou, L., Wan, H. and Li, Q. 2016. Long-term efficacy and safety of bronchial thermoplasty in patients with moderate-to-severe persistent asthma: a systemic review and meta-analysis. Journal of Asthma 53(1): 94–100.

Chapter 4A

Food Challenges

Soh Jian Yi* and *Hugo Van Bever*

Introduction

Proper preparation, pre-challenge assessment and execution of a food challenge require understanding key principles underpinning allergy. Building on these principles and others, this chapter goes on to detail the entire process including setup, assessment, counseling and use (and customization) of challenge protocols to follow up. Frequently asked questions are answered at the end of the chapter to address controversial points raised over the years by trainees and practicing specialists in allergy.

Indications

There are two main indications for a food challenge. The doctor decides that the patient:

- is unlikely to have an allergy to the food or
- may have, at most, a moderate chance of having an allergy to the food; and confirming/excluding these matters greatly to the patient.

Proper assessment, setup and interpretation of a food challenge for any indication are based on the Fundamental Principles underpinning allergy.

Fundamental Principles

The three key principles are:

- Sensitization versus disease;
- Threshold of Reactivity;
- This in turn explains the "dose-dependent" relationship of the allergic reaction.

Principle 1: Sensitization Versus Disease

Development of allergic disease requires two steps: (1) sensitization and (2) inability to regulate the immune response to prevent allergic disease.

Principle 2: Threshold of Reactivity

Nurmatov et al. (2017) used the term "Threshold of Reactivity" (ToR) in their paper on the results of oral immunotherapy for food allergy. The ToR represents the quantity of the allergen that the patient must encounter at a single time point (or within a short period) to incite an allergic reaction.

National University of Singapore.

* Corresponding author: paesjy@nus.edu.sg

Principle 3: Dose-Dependent Relationship of the Allergic Reaction

Similar to Principle 2, the ToR provides the basis for a certain quantity of exposure needed to incite a reaction; this principle builds on the ToR, which is the more the exposure exceeds the patient's ToR, the worse the reaction will be. This principle was deduced from examples in the literature such as pancake syndrome, concomitant triggers in food-allergic patients which seem to reduce the ToR to incite or worsen allergic reactions, the author's experience where patients consistently described their reactions in a dose-dependent fashion, and the author's experience with and observations of, food challenges. It is also important to recognize that the chance of developing a severe reaction is based on how much the quantity of exposure exceeds the patient's ToR itself as a "proportionate/relative" excess, rather than a fixed quantity.

For example, a patient with a ToR of 1 mg of peanut protein, develops anaphylaxis on exposure to 10 mg of peanut protein; though the "exceeding" in absolute terms is a tiny 9 mg to most lay people, the 10 mg exposure is ten times the ToR.

In patients who only react to higher doses of allergen (i.e., those with "mild" allergy), severe reactions are extremely rare. With a high ToR, the quantity of exposure required to develop anaphylaxis is very high; so high that no sensible patient who knows they have symptoms on taking that food at a particular dose will deliberately try to take more (see Figure 2 below; note that the X-axis quantity is nearly a 100-fold increase over a patient with low ToR in Figure 1).

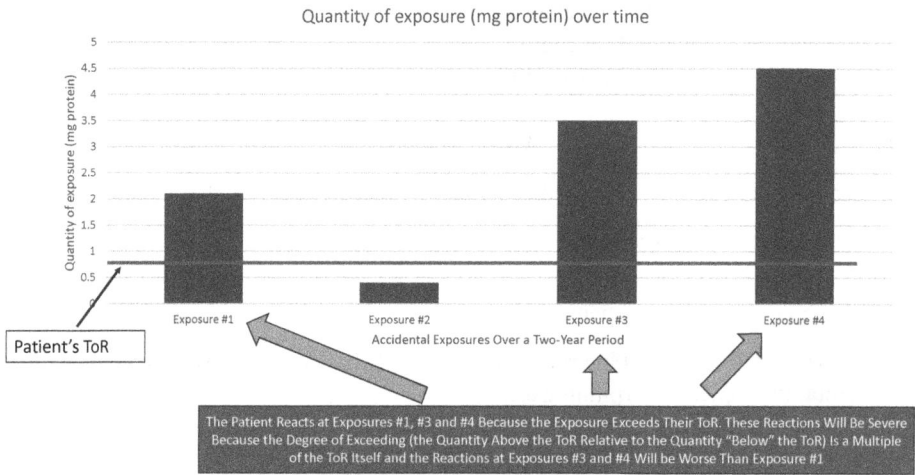

Figure 1. Patient with low threshold of reactivity (TOR).

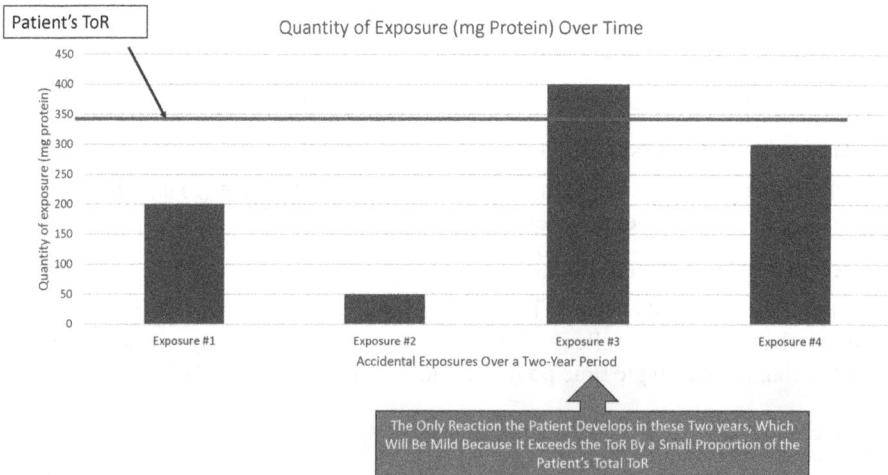

Figure 2. Patient with a high threshold of reactivity (TOR).

The same relationship is seen when a patient's history suggests they are "outgrowing" the allergen. Namely, the reactions they develop on exposure to the same quantity of allergen, diminish over time and eventually do not occur. This is because their ToR is rising over time (see Figure 3 below).

Patients who react on exposure to smaller amounts of the allergen (e.g., inhalation alone induces symptoms) have more severe reactions on exposure to greater doses (ingestion).

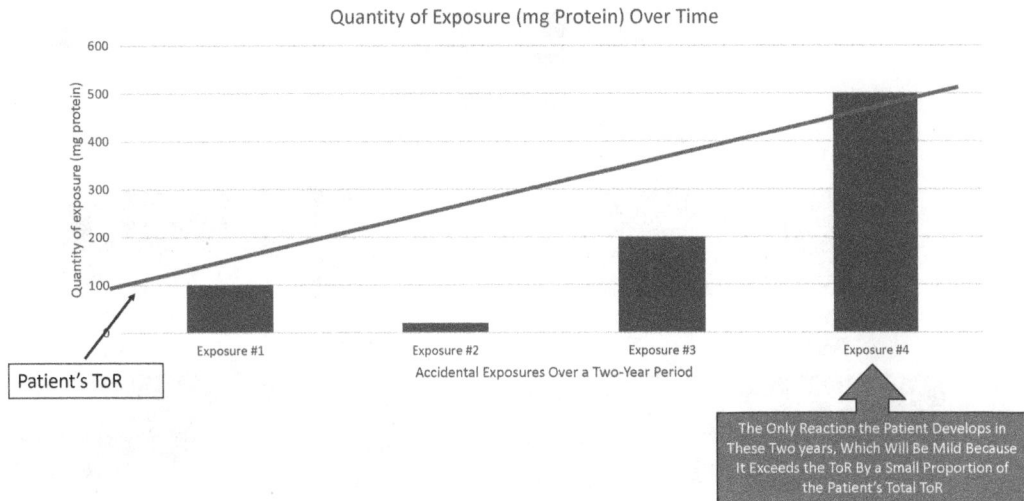

Figure 3. Patient with rising threshold of reactivity (TOR) (Outgrowing Allergy).

Assessment Before a Challenge

Assessment of the patient before deciding on a food challenge should cover four areas:

- The current probability of reacting to the suspect food
- If the patient reacts, the risk of the allergic reaction being severe or fatal
- The presence of any co-morbid conditions that further endanger the patient during a challenge
- The importance of the suspect food to the patient's lifestyle

The bulk of the information above will come from clinical history. A brief physical examination and previous allergy test (SPT, specific IgE, component-resolved diagnostics [CRD] and the most recent failed food challenge to the same allergen) results complete this assessment.

Area 1: Current Probability of Reacting to the Suspect Food

Key questions you must answer in decreasing order of importance for weighting current probability:

- When was the patient's most recent allergic reaction, which can be reasonably attributed to the allergen you are considering a challenge?
- If the patient has had recurrent exposures to the allergen over the past few years, does the history suggest he/she is outgrowing the allergy? (i.e., The ToR is increasing, as suggested by the allergic reactions diminishing in severity on exposure to the same quantities over time, and/ or increasingly higher doses are needed to elicit a mild reaction)

- If there are surrogate allergy tests performed (SPT, specific IgE and/or CRD), has the trend of the results diminished over time to a fraction of the last result obtained when the patient had an allergic reaction at the time of that result?
- What is the natural history of allergy to that particular food, in your population?

At the end of the assessment, decide the current likelihood of failing the food challenge:

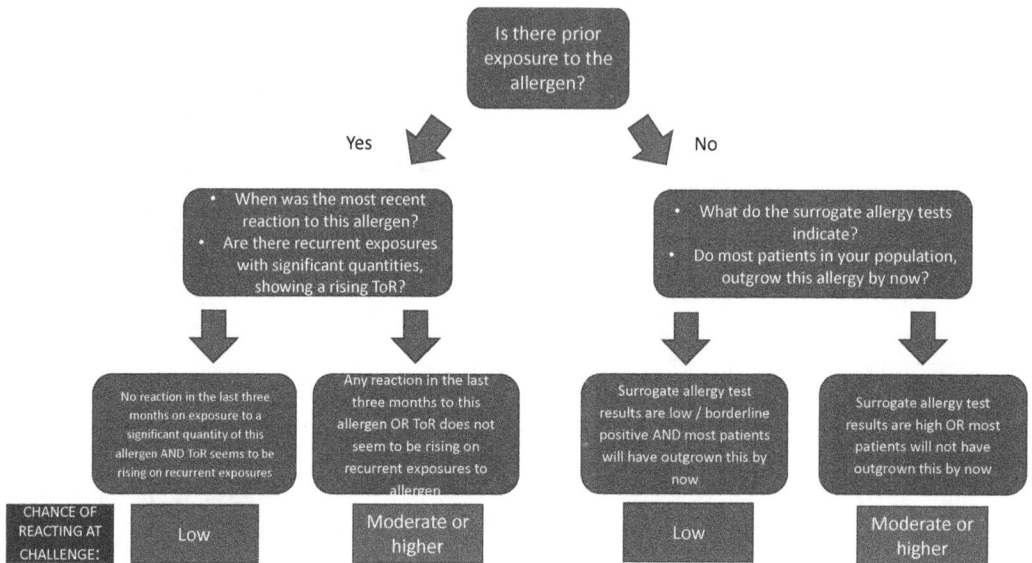

Figure 4. Assessment of the "RISK OF REACTIVITY".

The order of priority of these questions reflects the accuracy of current and trending clinical information over surrogate test results and population-level natural history. The patient-specific clinical history has always been more important and accurate than general indirect information (not just in allergy, but also in other diagnoses); you will see this illustrated repeatedly throughout this chapter.

Area 2: If the Patient Reacts, What Is the Risk of the Reaction Being Severe or Fatal?

This requires Principles 2 and 3 in the preceding section, the ToR and the dose-dependent nature of (food) allergic reactions. Key questions you must answer, in decreasing order of importance for weighting current probability:

- How severe was the patient's most recent allergic reaction, which can be reasonably attributed to the allergen you are considering a challenge?
- Were there any symptoms upon exposure to tiny amounts of the allergen?
- What was the most severe reaction the patient ever had to that allergen?
- How high is the most recent result of surrogate allergy tests?
- What is the usual severity of the allergy to that particular food, in your population?

Decide the danger level of the challenge.

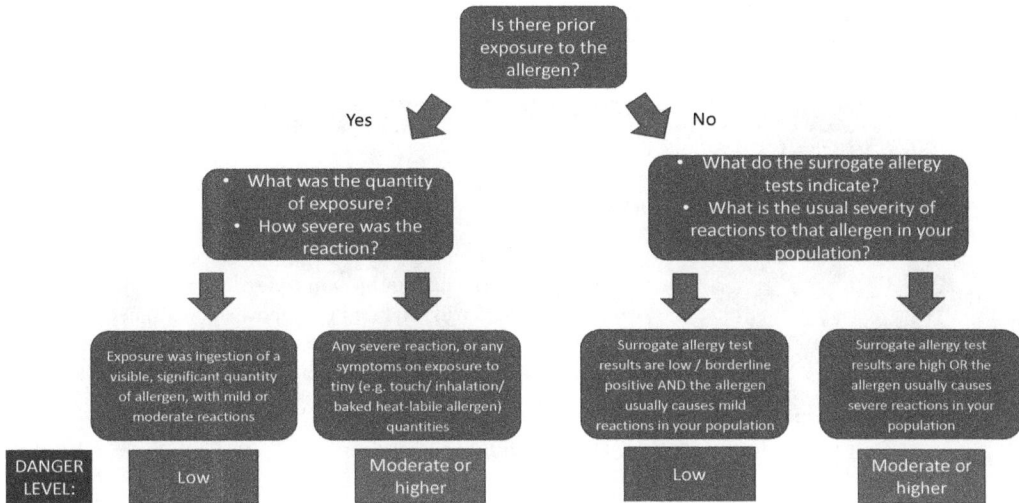

Figure 5. Risk stratification for food oral challenge.

This conclusion decides the appropriate setting for a challenge and the need to customize the challenge protocol.

Area 3: Are There Any Co-morbid Conditions That Further Endanger the Patient During a Challenge?

The co-existence of asthma in a patient with a food allergy is by itself a risk factor for anaphylaxis and death.

Area 4: How Important Is the Suspect Food to the Patient's Lifestyle?

The motivation for the patient to undergo a challenge, with the attendant cost in time, money and risk to themselves, is important to determine. This guides your counseling when proposing a challenge, especially if the challenge has a moderate risk of failing, and/or has a moderate level of danger.

Consider the cultural setting, food preferences of the family and commonality of the suspect food in that locale.

Counseling Prior to the Challenge

Grounding the patient in realistic expectations from the challenge is useful to avoid disappointment (and complaints from the patient subsequently). Since every choice comes with consequences (such as costs, risks, potential benefits, etc.), you should discuss (in this order):

- your recommendation to challenge (or not)
- the appropriate setting for the challenge
- the estimated chance of reacting during the challenge
- the danger level: the likelihood of a severe reaction if the patient reacts (the likelihood is "never" zero)
- the path moving forward if the patient reacts versus the patient not reacting
- the cost in time and money for the challenge (and check if this is feasible for the patient and where relevant, parents of the patient)
- the pros and cons of not undergoing a challenge

If the patient does decide to undergo the challenge, your counseling should anticipate and address common questions patients have for challenges, such as:

QUESTION	ANSWER (AND BASIS)
What can I do during the challenge?	Suggest bringing a book, homework or other entertainment (to avoid boredom; challenges usually take a few hours at a minimum)
Can I eat other food during the challenge?	Usually "yes" unless the patient has multiple other food allergies, and the challenge will start and end between mealtimes (In such a patient, there is the concern of potential cross-contamination in the "outside food" triggering a rection during the food challenge)

Figure 6. Oral food challenge instructions.

Counseling for medications and patient wellness on the challenge day includes:

- The patient should be well for the two days prior to and on the day of the challenge. There should be no symptoms of intercurrent illness, such as cough, fever, rash or breathlessness, to name a few examples. The reason is that ongoing symptoms of illness may interfere with the accurate interpretation of an allergic reaction during a challenge and can endanger the patient if it is difficult to figure out whether the patient is developing symptoms suggestive of anaphylaxis. In addition, intercurrent illness can decrease the ToR in the patient.

- Medications such as oral antihistamines should be stopped for 3–7 days prior to the challenge; the length of time depends on the pharmacokinetics of the specific antihistamine. The reason is that antihistamines can treat and therefore, theoretically can "mask" a mild allergic reaction. This can be dangerous if attempting a challenge, especially in a young child or where the danger level is moderate or higher. However, some patients do require antihistamines on a chronic basis (e.g., those with chronic idiopathic urticaria or allergic rhinitis); if so, this must be discussed with the patient. In a challenge with a low danger level, I would usually continue the antihistamines if the patient absolutely needs the antihistamines.

Setting for the Challenge

There are two settings for a supervised food challenge:

- Community: office or clinic
- Hospital bed (can be inpatient or outpatient ward; this varies according to the style of practice in different countries)

Community Setting: Office/Clinic

Food challenges suitable for the community setting are those with a low danger level. Challenges with a higher danger level, if attempted, require healthcare staff proficient in handling severe reactions and should have the equipment meeting the requirements as per an in-hospital challenge (see below).

A food challenge in the community setting requires at a minimum:

- At least one trained healthcare professional familiar with allergic reactions, handling anaphylaxis and performing cardiopulmonary resuscitation
- Medications for treating allergic reactions; at least one oral nonsedating antihistamine and intramuscular adrenaline

- Basic monitoring equipment including blood pressure measurement and pulse oximetry
- A comfortable bed
- A comfortable space around the bed, with at least one chair, for an accompanying adult for the patient (usually, when the patient is a child)

Hospital

In contrast to the community setting, an in-hospital challenge may be more suitable for challenges with a danger level of moderate or higher. To facilitate a food challenge of moderate or higher danger level, the in-hospital facility should be equipped to handle the anaphylactic shock. This requires (in addition to everything else in the community setting):

- Intravenous cannulation and infusion supplies
- Equipment for intubation of the airway and a bag-valve-mask
- Access to an in-hospital intensive care unit with mechanical ventilators is ideal

How about trying the suspect food at home (i.e., unsupervised challenge)? Suggesting the option of "take the food yourself at home" is only viable when all of the following criteria are fulfilled:

- You are confident the patient has outgrown the food allergy or is about to outgrow the allergy based on the clinical history
- Surrogate allergy test results are negative, correlating with the clinical impression above
- The risk of a severe reaction, in the event you are wrong, is almost zero (see Area 2 in the preceding Section)
- The patient is aware of the option of the supervised food challenge and has declined
- All of the above points are documented in the medical record

If the patient is nervous enough to counter-propose trying the food while sitting in front of your clinic or outside the Emergency Department, you should recommend a supervised challenge.

Steps in a Challenge

Key Points:

- Start with a tiny dose; the exact dose depends on the estimated ToR and danger level of the challenge
- Increments should be a multiple of the previous dose; the exact multiple depends on the Danger level of the challenge (and sometimes on the chance of reacting)
- Increment units – use protein content (especially if transitioning from one form to another)
- The time interval between increments depends on the danger level of the challenge (and sometimes, on the chance of reacting)
- The final dose should approach or equal a meal-size quantity the patient would want to take or encounter

Start With a Tiny Dose

Given the principles of ToR and dose-dependent reactions and that any food challenge carries "some" risk, the challenge should always begin with a tiny dose. It would be disastrous to insist that the patient only needs one step—a meal-size portion–and then have to deal with a significant allergic reaction because you were over-confident. The quantity of the starting dose depends mainly on the ToR you estimate from the clinical history and also on the danger level of the challenge for this patient. A third (minor) factor affecting the quantity of starting doses is the probability of failing the challenge. This initial, tiny dose can be as little as one drop, or a few specks (depending on whether the form of the food is solid or liquid).

Subsequent doses should be at least a doubling of the previous dose. The exact multiple (up to ten times the previous dose in most regimes) mainly depends on the danger level you have determined for this patient; the higher the danger level, the smaller the increments should be (but each step should still be at least double the previous dose). A moderate chance of failure may also indicate using smaller increments. See the table below:

Example of Viable Increments in Food Challenge to Cow's Milk in a Three-Year Old Child			
Low Chance of Reacting; Low Danger Level	Low Chance of Reacting; Moderate Danger Level	Moderate Chance of Reacting; Low Danger Level	Moderate Chance of Reacting; Moderate Danger Level
0.3 ml	0.1 ml	0.3 ml	0.1 ml
2 ml	0.5 ml	2 ml	0.3 ml
10 ml	2 ml	6 ml	1 ml
40 ml	5 ml	15 ml	3 ml
150–200 ml	10 ml	40 ml	6 ml
	30 ml	150–200 ml	15 ml
	60 ml		30 ml
	150–200 ml		60 ml
			150–200 ml

Figure 7. Build-up of food challenge doses based upon the risk stratification.

Notice the difference between the scenarios; the danger level has the largest impact on the starting dose and the size of the increments, which in turn affects the number of steps and total duration of the challenge. A higher danger level means a smaller starting dose and smaller increments in contrast to another patient with a lower danger level.

Why not use even smaller increments (say, just a 30% increase over the prior dose rather than a 100% increase) in a patient whose danger level is moderate or higher?

The answer is small increments can induce desensitization instead of demonstrating the ToR has been exceeded. This means the patient does not react during the challenge because of your desensitization. This is a potential disaster, because the aim of a supervised challenge is to provide accurate information that the doctor and patient will act upon, including the ascertainment of presence and sometimes, the ToR of the food allergy. The desensitization will wear off within the next few days; meaning, the next time the patient takes the (big) dose they appeared to tolerate after your apparently-reassuring challenge, the unexpected reaction will be an unpleasant surprise to them. And to you, once they make their displeasure known after the shock of the unexpected reaction.

Increment Units: Use Protein Content Especially If Transitioning From One Form to Another)

If you are using only one form of food throughout the challenge, in most situations, the dry weight of the food should suffice for measuring and calculating the increments. However, there are two situations where you should use the estimated protein equivalent as your unit of each increment, instead of the dry weight. Both involve using more than one form of the food containing that allergen, either during the challenge or afterward:

Situation 1: You are transitioning between forms of food during the challenge. For example, you are executing a wheat challenge and need to use wheat flour for the initial small doses; then use pasta for the last few doses (because huge amounts of wheat flour are unpalatable). You need to calculate the protein-equivalents for the dry weight of wheat flour you are using for each dose, then do the same for the dry weight of the pasta at the later doses, to get accurate increments at each step. Thus, the increment units are the protein dose being administered.

The dry weight is needed to physically measure out the food being administered. See Figure 8, below, for one example:

FORM	PROTEIN DOSE^	DRY WEIGHT DOSE
Wheat flour*	10 mg	100 mg
Wheat flour	40 mg	400 mg
Wheat flour	100 mg	1 gram
Wheat flour	200 mg	2 grams
Wheat flour	500 mg	5 grams
Pasta**	1,200 mg	24 grams
Pasta	3,000 mg	60 grams
Pasta	9,000 mg	180 grams

*Wheat Flour: 10% Protein by Weight

**Brand Z Pasta: 5% Protein by Weight

^The Protein Dose Is Used to Decide the Increment Sizes

Figure 8. Wheat oral challenge.

Situation 2: You are performing immunotherapy for food allergy. This high-risk procedure requires meticulous precision in measuring and administering the doses, as well as counseling patients on the foods and doses of those foods, they can take after immunotherapy. The time interval between increments depends on the danger level. In most (low danger level) food challenges, a 15-min interval is usually sufficient to notice any reactions and safely stop the challenge.

If the danger level is moderate or higher, a longer observation time for reactions (usually 30 min) between increments is advisable. This is because of the ToR and dose-dependent reaction principles. By knowing your patient has a significant chance of a moderate (or severe allergic reaction) during the challenge, lengthening the observation interval allows more time for symptoms of a mild reaction to appear before you administer the next (much higher) dose.

The final dose should approach or equal a meal-size quantity the patient would want to take or encounter. Since the ToR dictates that the patient will only react when exposed to at least that quantity of allergen, your "final dose," not the cumulative sum of all doses given, should be sufficient to ensure the patient really does not have an allergy to that food at the amount they intend to take or encounter if they pass the challenge.

Niggeman et al. (2012) demonstrated how patients who seemed to pass a food challenge on Day 1, then had reactions the next day when given a higher dose than the final dose administered on Day 1. How did this occur?

The doses reported in the paper had large increments; far too large to induce desensitization in so many subjects. The reactions induced on Day 2 with the very large dose were mostly mild, exactly as expected if the ToR was just exceeded by a bit. This lends strength to the assertion that the ToR should be considered similar to the final dose given, "not" the cumulative dose.

Last of all, the sum total of all the doses given on Day 1 often matched or exceeded the single dose given on day 2, adding more strength to the assertion above about the ToR being similar to the final dose given.

Taking all of these into account, it seems more accurate (and safer) to use the single final dose of the challenge instead of the cumulative dose as the assumed quantity the patient can tolerate. Some protocols suggest a 2-gram protein-equivalent dose for preschool children (less than 5 years of age), and at least a 4-gram protein-equivalent dose for older children/adults.

Challenge: Open-Label or Double-Blind Placebo-Controlled?

Open-label challenges are the mainstay of food challenges. The patient undergoes a single food challenge, both patient and healthcare professionals knowing the challenge is to that food. The double-blind placebo-controlled food challenge (DBPCFC) consists of the patient undergoing two challenges; once to a placebo and once to the suspect allergen. "Double-blind" means that both the patient as well as the healthcare professionals handling the challenge, do not know during these challenges, which one is the placebo and which one is the allergen. To achieve this double-blinding, the placebo and the allergen's taste, smell and texture must be masked in a vehicle, i.e., another food or viscous drink. Given the indications requiring a DBPCFC for clinical care and given the small (but real) possibility of delayed reactions to an allergen after the challenge, each of the two challenges should be conducted on a separate day. DBPCFC is indicated when the clinical history includes "odd" non-IgE-mediated symptoms or when the patient is visibly anxious. Thus, the blinding ensures that both the healthcare professionals as well as the patient do not inject their subjectivity into their actions (and interpretation) during the challenge.

What Reaction Decides Stopping a Challenge

The criteria to stop the challenge is based on both the pre-challenge likelihood of reacting and the danger level. The actual criteria to stop the challenge lie on a spectrum where the physician must balance the pre-challenge likelihood of reacting and the danger level of the challenge. There are two sets of criteria.

In a patient who is unlikely to react and has a low danger level, waiting until the patient has three or more hives, or more objective signs before stopping the challenge, may be justifiable; they are unlikely to have anaphylaxis anyway.

What Reaction Decides Stopping a Challenge?	
Low Chance of Reacting; Low Danger Level	**Either Moderate or Higher Chance of Reacting or Moderate or Higher Danger Level**
Three or more hives	One hive
Abdominal pain/vomiting, globus sensation	Any nausea, abdominal pain, throat pain or globus sensation
Any other sign of an allergic reaction; e.g. wheezing, cough, hypotension	Any other sign of an allergic reaction
*Decrease in energy level / mood, especially in a child <5 years old; look for any signs of allergic reaction	*Decrease in energy level/mood (e.g. more quiet or lethargic), especially in a child <5 years old; look for other signs, consider stopping the challenge
	**skin, throat, tongue or palate itch with no other signs or symptoms; extend the observation period before giving the next increment

Figure 9. Risk stratification to stop the oral food challenge.

What If the Patient Passes the Challenge?

After administering the final dose of the food, the patient should be observed for at least one hour before being discharged. Usually, 2 hours is the observation period for suspected IgE-mediated food allergy. You should follow up on the patient (usually a phone call) in the next 1–2 days to ensure there were no reactions after discharge.

Glossary of Abbreviations

CRD – Component-Resolved Diagnosis
DBPCFC – Double-Blind Placebo-Controlled Food Challenge
SPT – Skin Prick Test
ToR – Threshold of Reactivity

References

Bock, S. A., Muñoz-Furlong, A. and Sampson, H. A. 2001. Fatalities due to anaphylactic reactions to foods. J. Allergy Clin. Immunol. 107(1): 191–3.

Bock, S. A., Muñoz-Furlong, A. and Sampson, H. A. 2007. Further fatalities caused by anaphylactic reactions to food, 2001–2006. J. Allergy Clin. Immunol. 119(4): 1016–8.

Di Palmo, E., Gallucci, M., Cipriani, F., Bertelli, L., Giannetti, A. and Ricci, G. 2019. Asthma and food allergy: which risks? Medicina (Kaunas) 55(9): 509.

Foong, R. X. and Santos, A. F. 2021. Biomarkers of diagnosis and resolution of food allergy. Pediatr Allergy Immunol. 32(2): 223–233.

Niggemann, B. 2010. When is an oral food challenge positive? Allergy 65(1): 2–6.

Niggemann, B., Lange, L., Finger, A., Ziegert, M., Müller, V. and Beyer, K. 2012. Accurate oral food challenge requires a cumulative dose on a subsequent day. J. Allergy Clin. Immunol. 130(1): 261–3.

Nurmatov, U., Dhami, S., Arasi, S., Pajno, G. B., Fernandez-Rivas, M., Muraro, A. et al. 2017. Allergen immunotherapy for IgE-mediated food allergy: a systematic review and meta-analysis. Allergy 72(8): 1133–1147.

Pouessel, G., Turner, P. J., Worm, M., Cardona, V., Deschildre, A., Beaudouin, E. et al. 2018. Food-induced fatal anaphylaxis: From epidemiological data to general prevention strategies. Clin. Exp. Allergy 48(12): 1584–1593.

Shek, L. P., Soderstrom, L., Ahlstedt, S., Beyer, K. and Sampson, H. A. 2004. Determination of food specific IgE levels over time can predict the development of tolerance in cow's milk and hen's egg allergy. J. Allergy Clin. Immunol. 114: 387–391.6+.

Chapter 4B

Oral Immunotherapy

Soh Jian Yi

Indications

There are two main indications for oral immunotherapy (OIT). The patient has an IgE-mediated food allergy:

- with a high risk of anaphylaxis on accidental exposure or
- which significantly impairs their happiness, lifestyle or quality of life

Fundamental Principles

The key principles set out in the food challenge section underpin the basis for OIT and its safe, effective provision.

Format

OIT comprises a series of food challenges in patients who are usually at moderate (or high) Danger Levels for challenges. The timeline involves:

- Pre-treatment assessment and counseling
- First visit procedure
- Up dosing visits
- Follow-up visit during the maintenance phase

Pre-Treatment Assessment and Counseling

At the first visit, a face-to-face session is important (a video call, phone call or another medium of communication is not advisable). The doctor providing OIT should meet with the child, the child's parents and any other stakeholders who are expected to supervise the child's OIT (in some cultures, this can include the grandparents).

Assessment

The doctor must undertake the same assessment as per a food challenge, as well as check for the patient's (and family's) expectations, co-morbid asthma, eczema and familiarity with the adrenaline

National University, Singapore.
Email: paesjy@nus.edu.sg

auto-injector device. Checking in with the family's expectations and addressing these with the counseling (see below) is crucial to avoid unrealistic expectations and subsequent disappointment.

Co-morbid asthma must be controlled (preferably, "completely" controlled) prior to commencing OIT; some studies also recommend ensuring the FEV1 is at least 70% as a requirement. Eczema should be controlled because OIT can cause flares; in addition, the waxing and waning of the symptoms in uncontrolled eczema can cause confusion during OIT. Both of these reasons may prompt a patient to withdraw from OIT. Adrenaline auto-injectors and Emergency Plans should be provided to patients while on OIT because this is a high-risk procedure.

Counseling

The doctor must cover:

- *Expectations*: OIT is a time-intensive, expensive procedure that entails the patient continuing to ingest the allergen in the dose and form they prefer, indefinitely. The primary goal is to raise the patient's Threshold of Reactivity (ToR) enough to protect against accidental exposure to small amounts (such as cross-contamination). To be able to ingest the allergen in meal-size amounts and be "similar" to the patient's peers is a secondary, bonus goal.
- *Work involved*: OIT requires frequent (usually daily) dosing of the allergen initially. Upon completion, the frequency of intake may be decreased, depending on the side effect profile the patient demonstrates. Where the patient is a child, the child should be supervised at each OIT dose intake, usually at mealtime.
- *Side effects*: Describe the common side effect profile in your practice. Acknowledge the risk of anaphylaxis, hence the need for precautions (see below) to be followed. Describe the necessary action for the common side effects as well as anaphylaxis. The usual side effect profile with prudent OIT regimes involves transient oral symptoms (e.g., tingling of lips/tongue), hives and sometimes abdominal pain. Training of the patient and all caregivers responsible for caring for the patient during OIT, in recognizing and handling allergic reactions, must be completed before commencing OIT. Eosinophilic esophagitis should be mentioned and explained.
- *Precautions*: Certain co-factors decrease the ToR transiently. The main triggers are intercurrent infections (e.g., catching a cold), exercise within 1 hour before the dose and to up to 2–4 hours after taking the dose, tiredness (e.g., lack of sleep, end of a long busy day) and ingestion of the dose on an empty stomach. Other co-factors include anaphylaxis (for any reason), menstruation and hot showers (taken within 1 hour before and up to 1 hour after the dose).
- The need for full compliance with dosing, precautions and any other instructions you provide because this is a high-risk procedure. The doctor can unilaterally withdraw the patient from treatment if the patient (or parents in the case of a child) is endangered unnecessarily.
- *Flexibility*: The doctor's setting (office/hospital) should be able to accommodate unexpected changes in the patient's schedule such as intercurrent illness and school hours. This means being able to delay updoses.
- *Contactability*: The doctor should be able to respond to patient queries (the bulk of which will revolve around side effects that occur) through email, phone or video calls. This helps allay the patient's anxiety as well as builds trust. Accurate counseling and contactability will supplement and vindicate assuring statements like: "I'm going to be there for you during this journey."

As all this information is overwhelming to absorb, provide a hardcopy, black-and-white summary of the points with brief explanations to the patient. Give the patient enough time to absorb all the information and read through the hardcopy supplement. Furthermore, give them time to ask any other questions they have. It is useful to obtain a signed consent for the OIT. This signed consent should include the patient acknowledging that the patient has seen, understood and asked any questions they have after going through your counseling.

Checklist: Oral Immunotherapy - Counselling

Dear (insert name of patient),

Please read this through. Should there be any questions or un-addressed areas, please let us know at once. We will not proceed with the Oral Immunotherapy until we have ensured your understanding of the key points (see the signature fields at the end of this document)

--

By signing this document, I declare:

1. I have been counseled on the following key points:

   • Immunotherapy increases my child's ability to tolerate some amount of this food. There are limits to how much my child can take at one sitting.

   • I and my child are required to follow the doctor's advice during and after the treatment. Flouting the precautions increases the chance of an allergic reaction to my child during the treatment, especially anaphylaxis.

   • The minimum interval between updoses is (insert interval) apart. Updoses should be performed when the child is well. I am required to notify (insert name and contact means) in advance if I am aware my child is unlikely to be able to come for an updose.

   • In the event of frequent or significant reactions, my principal doctor will discuss the options of slowing down the size and/or frequency of updoses, or stopping the immunotherapy altogether. My doctor will be balancing the dual concerns of the child's safety and the likely success of proceeding with immunotherapy, for my child. My doctor does not require my agreement to stop immunotherapy for my child, if the reactions persistently disturb my child or endanger my child's life and I refuse to agree to stop the treatment despite such a situation. This is because my doctor must act in my child's best interests.

Figure 1. Sample of start of consent document.

These provisions—hardcopy information supplement, signed consent acknowledging they have understood—are important when the empathic doctor knows the patient (and family) often do not remember everything that was said. See Figure 1 for an example.

Who is Not Suitable for Immunotherapy?

Non-compliance to the dosing regime and precautions is the most dangerous issue in these high-risk patients. A patient who has a track record of non-compliance with important health issues and chronic conditions is not suitable for OIT because the process demands a lot from the patient. Non-compliance emerging during OIT is a big concern that must be addressed, and the patient can be withdrawn from OIT if this persists. Highly anxious patients with subjective symptoms are often unsuitable for OIT. These manifestations of anxiety often emerge at the baseline food challenge.

Setting

As with food challenges, OIT can be performed in either the community or hospital setting:

• Community: Office or clinic
• Hospital bed (can be inpatient or outpatient ward; this varies according to the style of practice in different countries)

Given that these are patients who are at least moderate-danger level or higher, the facilities and training of staff should be as per hospital-level-setting as far possible. The only unfeasible requirement for an office setting is the presence of an adjacent Intensive Care Unit. Wasserman et al. (2021) have published an excellent summary of office-based OIT (see References).

Setup

Preparations for OIT include:

- Sourcing suitable allergen-containing foods
- Training of staff in the basics of OIT
- Training of staff in communications: weighing and handling queries

Sourcing Suitable Allergen-Containing Foods

All allergen sources should be free of cross-contamination from other allergens as far as possible. Palatability, long shelf-life, measurability in tiny amounts and supplier reliability are key priorities. Most doctors providing OIT employ a variety of flours, powders and milk to administer the initial doses of OIT. Provide a list of common foods (often with allergen-protein-equivalent doses) the patient can take once the patient reaches a higher ToR that allows eating these foods.

Training of Staff in Basics of OIT

The doctor may have assistants like other doctors, nurses and so on. The clinical staff must accept that reactions do occur in OIT and be able to stay calm, react and escalate as appropriate if asked by the patient.

Training of Staff in Communications: Weighing and Handling Queries

The doctor will usually have a team or pharmacy helping to weigh out tiny doses of the allergen-containing food to administer as OIT. Given the high-risk patients and the consequence of anaphylaxis/death, strict communications discipline and training are mandatory. One important rule is to always communicate about the doses being weighed (spoken and written) in terms of protein content first (how many milligrams of protein), and then mention the dry weight of the food to be used.

Being contactable through the office/clinic line and/or email helps with rapport and reassuring patients that you will be there for them. This does mean that any staff who are helping with OIT should be trained to do so appropriately and notify the primary doctor as well. The staff may answer the query itself—this being part of the training the OIT doctor should provide to them—but notification of the primary doctor is still required.

Routes

There are two major routes for OIT: the slow route and the rush route. A third route, the sub-lingual (slow) route, is used for patients with the lowest ToR (and thus, have the highest risk). These are compared in Figure 2.

Slow Route

The slow route is the most commonly used, and the "gold standard" for performing immunotherapy for food allergies. The first visit is a baseline food challenge to establish the ToR. Most patients will be at least moderate or high danger levels. This means the willingness to stop the challenge promptly and 30-minute intervals (at least) between increments. After the patient has reacted and has been treated, a dose that is a fraction of the ToR (usually one-quarter or less) and should be lower than the highest, apparently tolerated dose prior to reacting, is thereafter chosen as the starting dose. For example, if the challenge steps were 1, 5, 25 and 75 mg protein and the patient reacted at the 25 mg step, the starting dose must be less than 5 mg protein. The reason is the way the ToR and dose-dependent relationship work: the patient may have had a mild, delayed reaction to the 5 mg step, but you never got the chance to see that because administering the 25 mg protein dose, 30

ORAL (Slow): The Most Common Route, Suitable for Most Patients	SUB-LINGUAL	RUSH ROUTE

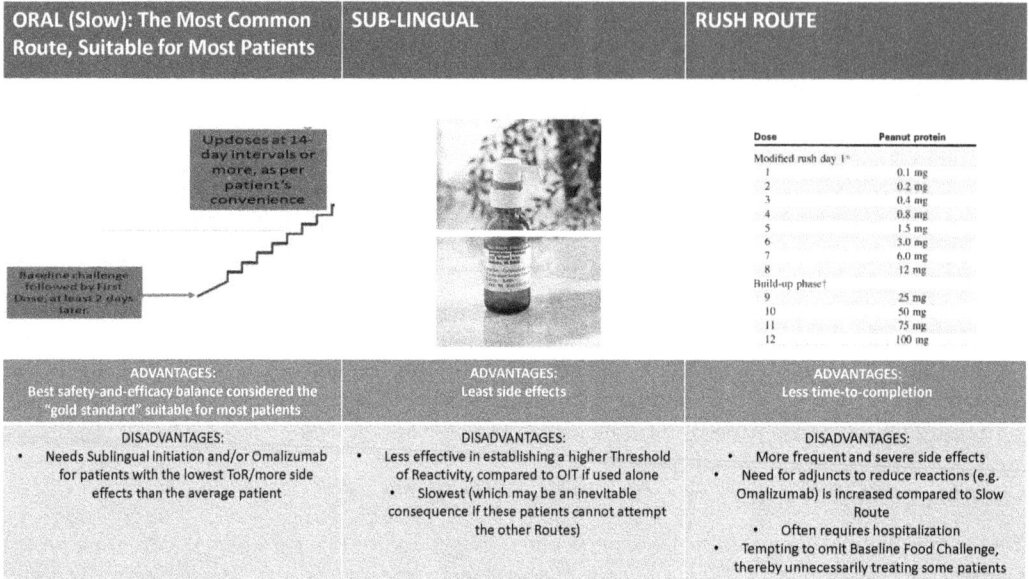

Dose	Peanut protein
Modified rush day 1°	
1	0.1 mg
2	0.2 mg
3	0.4 mg
4	0.8 mg
5	1.5 mg
6	3.0 mg
7	6.0 mg
8	12 mg
Build-up phase†	
9	25 mg
10	50 mg
11	75 mg
12	100 mg

ADVANTAGES: Best safety-and-efficacy balance considered the "gold standard" suitable for most patients	ADVANTAGES: Least side effects	ADVANTAGES: Less time-to-completion
DISADVANTAGES: • Needs Sublingual initiation and/or Omalizumab for patients with the lowest ToR/more side effects than the average patient	DISADVANTAGES: • Less effective in establishing a higher Threshold of Reactivity, compared to OIT if used alone • Slowest (which may be an inevitable consequence if these patients cannot attempt the other Routes)	DISADVANTAGES: • More frequent and severe side effects • Need for adjuncts to reduce reactions (e.g. Omalizumab) is increased compared to Slow Route • Often requires hospitalization • Tempting to omit Baseline Food Challenge, thereby unnecessarily treating some patients

Figure 2. Routes.

minutes later, triggered a more rapid, obvious reaction. A doctor unaware of this relationship, may mistakenly think the ToR was exceeded by the 25 mg protein dose, instead of realising the 5 mg dose may have already exceeded the ToR.

The next visit to ingest the first dose should take place at least 2 days after the baseline challenge. There are two key reasons:

- to ensure the patient has fully recovered from the initial reaction mentally and physically
- to give your weighing team enough time to weigh out the doses the patient must ingest daily at home

Once the patient has tolerated the first dose, the patient is to continue taking the same dose, weighed out before this visit, every day. Many regimes do this once daily; some, twice daily. This frequent gastrointestinal exposure is important for OIT to succeed. The patient returns only for the next increment (also called "updose"), which should take place at least 14 days late. Much shorter intervals—7 days or less—tend to result in more failed doses; the ToR takes some time to increase. Thus, this overall pattern resembles a "staircase" pattern of escalation all the way to the end-of-OIT, as shown in Figure 2.

The baseline food challenge is often the most anxiety-inducing step in OIT. Though it is tempting to skip the challenge, there are patients who have a history of convincing allergic reactions and positive surrogate allergy test results, who then pass the baseline challenge. Confirming the presence of food allergy is a secondary, but important priority; never treat without being sure of the disease being present. Some studies suggest a combination of convincing clinical history and very high surrogate allergy test results can replace a food challenge for confirming food allergy. If the patient wishes to omit the baseline challenge after having been properly counseled, you can follow their wishes. However, you must then start at the lowest possible dose in your protocol since you do not know the patient's ToR.

Sub-Lingual (SLIT) Route

The sub-lingual route allows the smallest amounts of an allergen to be absorbed slowly into the patient and thus is suitable for patients with the lowest ToRs' who may not tolerate even the first dose of traditional, slow-route OIT. However, this same mechanism of SLIT also means that a reaching significant ToR—enough to be of practical use to the patient—is much harder to achieve compared to the slow OIT route over the same period.

There are two ways SLIT is employed:

- As a standalone route. Various studies have shown that taking even a low dose of the allergen regularly for years does raise the ToR
- As a "bridge" to slow-route OIT, for the highest-risk patients. SLIT is begun, and on completion of SLIT, the patient is transitioned to slow-route OIT (there may be a baseline-challenge-pre-slow-OIT to determine the patient's ToR while on the maintenance SLIT dose)

Rush Route

The patient is usually admitted to the hospital ward to try to "rush" to a high ToR in as short a time as possible. Studies generally reported higher dropout and more severe side effect rates. It is tempting to omit the baseline food challenge to determine the ToR and just conduct the "rush" protocol itself; however, this would mean treating some patients who do not have a food allergy.

Blumchen et al. (2010) demonstrated that if the ToR is determined, and a rush protocol is then attempted; most patients do not get beyond their ToR anyway. All of these factors make the rush route unfavorable compared to the "gold standard" slow route.

Baseline Challenge: Open-Label or Double-Blind Placebo-Controlled?

Patients with clear, IgE-mediated food allergy are suitable for OIT and thus the open-label challenge suffices. If a patient is highly anxious or has bizarre symptoms, they are often unsuitable for OIT and this will emerge during the baseline challenge. In theory, a double-blind placebo-controlled challenge will further affirm this suspicion—but will not address the subsequent odd symptoms the patient often reports during OIT. This leaves the doctor in a dilemma about whether to take them seriously and slow down/stop the OIT; or ignore the reported symptoms, potentially endangering the patient by doing so.

Adjuncts for OIT

These are patients with the lowest ToRs' and thus may not tolerate even the first dose of traditional OIT. Omalizumab is an adjunct that decreases side effect rates and severity (Bégin et al. 2014; MacGinnitie et al. 2017). This leads to improved success rates in the highest-risk patients and translates into the same results if attempting forms of OIT where failure and higher side effects are expected, such as the rush route and multi-unrelated-allergen-OIT. Unless the patient is in a hurry and willing to go through the regular Omalizumab injections, however, the most appropriate use of this adjunct should be for the highest-risk patients attempting single-allergen OIT. The probiotic, *Lactobacillus rhamnosus GG*, has shown benefits in peanut OIT by reducing the rate of side effects (Tang et al. 2015). Clinical practitioners report patients mentioning that omission of the daily dose of this probiotic results in the appearance of mild symptoms such as abdominal pain.

Increments During OIT

Older and current studies on OIT that used 100% increments compared to the previous dose have higher dropout (failure) rates and more severe side effect profiles than more recent studies that used smaller increments. Thus, the overall trend of side effect severity and frequency seems to decrease with smaller increments. Increments for OIT, regardless of route, should generally be between 30–80% of the previous dose. The disadvantage of smaller increments is that it will take longer to reach the final, target dose the patient desires. OIT for cow's milk allergy seems to have a higher rate of significant side effects than the other allergens; thus, lean toward using smaller increments if performing cow's milk OIT.

One Allergen or Multi-Allergen OIT?

When commencing OIT, start with one allergen at a time. Record the side effect frequency and severity for the foods you commence OIT, before deciding whether you should attempt multi-allergen OIT (mOIT).

mOIT has two types:

- two-related-allergen OIT whereby the allergens are strongly cross-reactive
- multi-unrelated-allergen OIT, where the allergens are ingested simultaneously, have virtually zero cross-reactivity

Two-related allergen OIT involves food dyads where most patients with an allergy to one, also have an allergy to the other because of strong cross-reactive patterns. Examples include the cashew-pistachio and walnut-pecan dyads. Performing this type of OIT saves the patient time and money compared to doing each separately at a little extra burden to the OIT practitioner because the side effect profile is similar to performing OIT to just one of the dyads. Multi-unrelated-allergen OIT requires significant caution because the chance of developing side effects that slow or derail the entire OIT process is about the same as adding up the side effect profiles of each food if performing one at a time. In addition to the higher chance of failure, more confusion often results; when the patient reacts while taking multiple allergens at once, no one knows which allergen(s) caused the reaction. Multi-unrelated-allergen-OIT can be attempted by practitioners seasoned with single-allergen OIT using regimes with low side effect rates, because the mathematical addition of a low rate of side effects, added up across several foods, should still be a small number.

Missed Doses and Lower-ToR Situations

The ToR increases gradually over time with OIT. This ToR likewise drops gradually over time in a similar fashion upon abstaining from regular allergen ingestion. A summary of studies on "sustained unresponsiveness" demonstrates this (Figure 3); the longer the period of abstinence, the greater the decrease in the ability to tolerate a significant quantity of the allergen regardless of the specific allergen. This is the basis for advice for missed doses and situations where the precautions were flouted:

- If dosing is missed for 1–2 days, the ToR may have dropped slightly. Resume the OIT at half the tolerated dose prior to missing doses, for up to 3 days, then return to the full tolerated dose.
- If the dosing is missed for a week or more, out of the blue (there was no prior discussion with the doctor and the omission was not due to illness), the first reaction is not to resume OIT at a lower dose. Instead, have the patient return promptly for a consultation to review their safety and understanding of OIT. Compliance is the most crucial aspect of safe and effective OIT, and patients unwilling to comply strictly with safety precautions should be withdrawn from treatment.
- If the precautions are flouted, the tolerated dose should be halved, for 3–7 days. In some situations, such as severe gastroenteritis with profuse vomiting, it is more prudent to omit the dose during the 3–7 days.
- Patients may go on a trip with significant exertion (e.g., school camp, mountaineering, trekking in the forest). It may be safer to omit the dose during the period of exertion (which should not be more than a week at most). The patient should then resume their dose at one-quarter or one-half of the previous tolerated dose; taking the dose under medical supervision is recommended if the omission period is a week or longer.

First Author; Journal (Year)	Food Type	Abstinence Period Before Challenge (Weeks)	Rate of Passing Challenge %
Keet CA, JACI (2012)	Milk	1, then 6	86, then 60
Manabe T. Allergol Int (2019)	Egg, milk, wheat	2	77
Tang ML, JACI (2015)	Peanut	2	82 (with LactoGG)
Nagakura Kl. Int Arch Allergy Immunol (2020)	Peanut	2	68
Vickery BP, JACI (2014)	Peanut	4	31
C. Escudero, Clin Exp Allergy (2015)	Egg	4	37
Burks W, NEJM (2012)	Egg	8	28
Kim EH, JACI (2020)	Egg (*subjects had to be tolerant to baked egg)	8-10	43 (egg) 11 (baked egg)
Wood RA, JACI (2016)	Milk	8	48 (with Omalizumab) 36 (no Omalizumab)
Nowak-Wegrzyn, JACI (2018)	Wheat	8-10	30
Syed A, JACI (2014)	Peanut	12, then 24	35, then 15
Chinthrajah RS, Lancet (2019)	Peanut	13, then 26	35, then 20

The longer the abstinence period, the lower the chance of passing a challenge to an arbitrary quantity of food

Figure 3. Sustained unresponsiveness vs. length of abstinence.

The Final Dose for OIT

The patient often will not know whether they like foods containing the allergen until they are completing OIT. Since allergen ingestion must continue (at least twice a week in many patients) indefinitely, the final dose should be sufficient to protect the patient from accidental exposures and be a dose the patient is willing to take indefinitely. The patient can take this allergen in different forms if desired.

Thus, the possible final dose depends on whether the patient:

- *Likes the food*: Let the patient choose a meal-size quantity; the patient can ingest this quantity (often up to 50% above that quantity without expecting problems);
- *Is neutral to the food*: A smaller meal-size quantity is a fair target because being compelled to regularly ingest large quantities may induce a dislike of the food;
- *Dislikes the food*: Choose a quantity sufficient for protection against accidental exposure, as this patient is unlikely to sustainably take a bigger quantity long-term. An example would be 1–2 whole peanuts in a patient who dislikes the taste of peanut.

Maintenance Regime

How long must the patient take their daily dose of OIT? The literature describes multiple regimes with the daily "maintenance phase" spanning anything from 2 weeks to 4 years. Current evidence does not support a longer maintenance phase, because there is no significant benefit to the patient thereafter. Jones et al. (2016) demonstrated how a longer duration of OIT, even at 4 years of daily intake, does not yield significant benefits to most patients in a practical sense. Practically, having the patient take the daily dose of OIT for years often induces weariness and dislike of the food, in addition to having to continue complying with the precautions for every day they take the allergen. Many patients eventually stop OIT if told to continue the daily intake indefinitely.

Thus, some practitioners deliberately have the patient decrease the frequency of intake after a period as short as 2–4 weeks. The patients who generally had minimal or no side effects during OIT, and preferably have zero symptoms at the point of the attempt to reduce their intake frequency, usually tend to be able to decrease their frequency of intake. There is controversy over the utility of

IgEs' and other surrogate allergy tests being biomarkers to predict tolerability of decreased intake frequency, as these tests were not designed for this and the evidence as of the end of 2022 also does not support using surrogate allergy tests to decide which patient is suitable to reduce the frequency of intake.

Arguably, some patients' bodies might not be able to "maintain" their ToR once their intake of the allergen drops below a certain threshold. Since the ToR drops slowly over time, the implication is that any reduction of intake frequency must entail a longer observation period than a mere few days. One method of handling this is to have the totally-asymptomatic patient halve their intake from 7 days a week (once daily) to 4 days a week, and observe for the next 4 weeks. If their body cannot maintain the ToR, mild symptoms will usually emerge over the next 4 weeks. If the 4-week observation is "passed" with no symptoms, the frequency of intake can be halved again, and so on. Though some patients can maintain their ToR with ingestions of once a month or less often (which matters to patients who dislike the food), any stepwise decrease must be carefully discussed.

End-of-OIT Challenges

End-of-OIT challenges to determine "sustained unresponsiveness" (omit ingestion of the allergen for a varying interval of weeks, then have the subject ingest a large quantity of that allergen weeks later) in research, have shown that OIT usually induces desensitization; the effect wearing off over time if abstinence is continued.

Thus, performing end-of-OIT challenges for clinical care generally adds no value to the individual patient. Since the effect does wear off if all allergen intake is stopped for a long enough time, the patient has to consume the allergen regularly regardless of the outcome. Nor does artificially choosing a challenge dose far greater than the patient's preferred long-term dose of OIT (which the patient will not voluntarily take anyway after that challenge), benefit the patient.

Follow Up

Check in with the patient at the expected end of maintenance, and 1–3 months after initiation of reducing the intake frequency. Thereafter, if all is well, annual follow up will suffice.

Is An Adrenaline Auto-Injector Still Needed Post-OIT?

This needs to be discussed on a case-by-case basis. The main indication for an adrenaline auto-injector for every patient is that unique patient is at significant risk of anaphylaxis. This assessment is based on several factors, including the patient's ToR, risk-taking behavior and so on. Even if the patient does not want to carry the adrenaline auto-injector pen and seems to be careful, it may be sensible to suggest carrying the adrenaline auto-injector for at least the first year post-OIT-maintenance, to see how they handle that period of reducing intake frequency and altering their lifestyle—and then reassess again at the end of that year.

Glossary of Abbreviations

FEV 1 – Forced Expiratory Volume in First One Second
OIT – Oral Immunotherapy
SLIT – Sub-Lingual Immunotherapy
ToR – Threshold of Reactivity

References

Bégin, P., Dominguez, T., Wilson, S. P., Bacal, L., Mehrotra, A., Kausch, B. et al. 2014. Phase 1 results of safety and tolerability in a rush oral immunotherapy protocol to multiple foods using Omalizumab. Allergy Asthma Clin. Immunol. 10(1): 7.

Blumchen, K., Ulbricht, H., Staden, U., Dobberstein, K., Beschorner, J., de Oliveira, L. C. et al. 2010. Oral peanut immunotherapy in children with peanut anaphylaxis. J. Allergy Clin. Immunol. 126(1): 83–91.e1.

Burks, A. W., Jones, S. M., Wood, R. A., Fleischer, D. M., Sicherer, S. H., Lindblad, R. W. et al. 2012. Oral immunotherapy for treatment of egg allergy in children. N. Engl. J. Med. 367(3): 233–43.

Chinthrajah, R. S., Purington, N., Andorf, S., Long, A., O'Laughlin, K. L., Lyu, S. C. et al. 2019. Sustained outcomes in oral immunotherapy for peanut allergy (POISED study): A large, randomised, double-blind, placebo-controlled, phase 2 study. Lancet 394(10207): 1437–1449. Erratum in: Lancet. 2020 Aug 8;396(10248): 380.

Escudero, C., Rodríguez Del Río, P., Sánchez-García, S., Pérez-Rangel, I., Pérez-Farinós, N., García-Fernández, C. et al. 2015. Early sustained unresponsiveness after short-course egg oral immunotherapy: A randomized controlled study in egg-allergic children. Clin. Exp. Allergy 45(12): 1833–43.

Jones, S. M., Burks, A. W., Keet, C., Vickery, B. P., Scurlock, A. M., Wood, R. A. et al. 2016. Long-term treatment with egg oral immunotherapy enhances sustained unresponsiveness that persists after cessation of therapy. J. Allergy Clin. Immunol. 137(4): 1117–1127.e10.

Keet, C. A., Frischmeyer-Guerrerio, P. A., Thyagarajan, A., Schroeder, J. T., Hamilton, R. G., Boden, S. et al. 2012. The safety and efficacy of sublingual and oral immunotherapy for milk allergy. J. Allergy Clin. Immunol. 129(2): 448–55, 455.e1-5.

Kim, E. H., Perry, T. T., Wood, R. A., Leung, D. Y. M., Berin, M. C., Burks, A. W. et al. 2020. Induction of sustained unresponsiveness after egg oral immunotherapy compared to baked egg therapy in children with egg allergy. J. Allergy Clin. Immunol. 146(4): 851–862.e10.

MacGinnitie, A. J., Rachid, R., Gragg, H., Little, S. V., Lakin, P., Cianferoni, A. et al. 2017. Omalizumab facilitates rapid oral desensitization for peanut allergy. J. Allergy Clin. Immunol. 139(3): 873–881.e8.

Manabe, T., Sato, S., Yanagida, N., Hayashi, N., Nishino, M., Takahashi, K. et al. 2019. Long-term outcomes after sustained unresponsiveness in patients who underwent oral immunotherapy for egg, cow's milk, or wheat allergy. Allergol. Int. 68(4): 527–528.

Nagakura, K. I., Yanagida, N., Sato, S., Nishino, M., Takahashi, K., Asaumi, T. et al. 2020. Low-dose-oral immunotherapy for children with wheat-induced anaphylaxis. Pediatr Allergy Immunol. 31(4): 371–379.

Nowak-Węgrzyn, A., Wood, R. A., Nadeau, K. C., Pongracic, J. A., Henning, A. K., Lindblad, R. W. et al. 2019. Multicenter, randomized, double-blind, placebo-controlled clinical trial of vital wheat gluten oral immunotherapy. J. Allergy Clin. Immunol. 143(2): 651–661.e9.

Nozawa, A., Okamoto, Y., Movérare, R., Borres, M. P. and Kurihara, K. 2014. Monitoring Ara h 1, 2 and 3-sIgE and sIgG4 antibodies in peanut allergic children receiving oral rush immunotherapy. Pediatr Allergy Immunol. 25(4): 323–8.

Ogura, K., Yanagida, N., Sato, S., Imai, T., Ito, K., Kando, N. et al. 2020. Evaluation of oral immunotherapy efficacy and safety by maintenance dose dependency: A multicenter randomized study. World Allergy Organ J. 13(10): 100463.

Sugiura, S., Kitamura, K., Makino, A., Matsui, T., Furuta, T., Takasato, Y. et al. 2020. Slow low-dose oral immunotherapy: Threshold and immunological change. Allergol Int. 69(4): 601–609.

Syed, A., Garcia, M. A., Lyu, S. C., Bucayu, R., Kohli, A., Ishida, S. et al. 2014. Peanut oral immunotherapy results in increased antigen-induced regulatory T-cell function and hypomethylation of forkhead box protein 3 (FOXP3). J. Allergy Clin. Immunol. 133(2): 500–10.

Tang, M. L., Ponsonby, A. L., Orsini, F., Tey, D., Robinson, M., Su, E. L. et al. 2015. Administration of a probiotic with peanut oral immunotherapy: A randomized trial. J. Allergy Clin. Immunol. 135(3): 737–44.e8.

Varshney, P., Jones, S. M., Scurlock, A. M., Perry, T. T., Kemper, A., Steele, P. et al. 2011. A randomized controlled study of peanut oral immunotherapy: clinical desensitization and modulation of the allergic response. J. Allergy Clin. Immunol. 127(3): 654–60.

Vickery, B. P., Scurlock, A. M., Kulis, M., Steele, P. H., Kamilaris, J., Berglund, J. P. et al. 2014. Sustained unresponsiveness to peanut in subjects who have completed peanut oral immunotherapy. J. Allergy Clin. Immunol. 133(2): 468–75.

Wasserman, R. L., Factor, J., Windom, H. H., Abrams, E. M., Begin, P., Chan, E. S. et al. 2021. An approach to the office-based practice of food oral immunotherapy. J. Allergy Clin. Immunol. Pract. 9(5): 1826–1838.e8.

Wood, R. A., Kim, J. S., Lindblad, R., Nadeau, K., Henning, A. K., Dawson, P. et al. 2016. A randomized, double-blind, placebo-controlled study of omalizumab combined with oral immunotherapy for the treatment of cow's milk allergy. J. Allergy Clin. Immunol. 137(4): 1103–1110.e11.

Chapter 4C Part I

Food Allergy
Specific IgE

Hugo Van Bever

◇◇◇

Determination of Specific IgE

Since the purification of total and specific IgE in 1967, serological testing has become a commonly used test in the evaluation of food allergy (FA). The first immunometric assay, called the radioallergosorbent test (RAST), was patterned after the RIST (radioimmunosorbent) assay for total IgE, except that instead of coupling anti-human IgE to activated paper disks (for determining total IgE), allergen was directly coupled to make an allergosorbent (solid-phase allergen) reagent (Wide 1967). Since then, through the progressive introduction of high-performance laboratory-based IgE methods, such as the production of recombinant allergens, many assays were developed to determine specific IgE against a large variety of allergens with high diagnostic accuracy. The measurement of specific IgE can be achieved both through the usage of single reagents (singleplex) or with a pre-defined panel of several allergens to be tested simultaneously (multiplex).

Like any other serological test—no test is 100% specific or sensitive—every specific IgE test has certain characteristics, related to its methodology (i.e., the structure of the solid phase, the amount of allergen in the tube, the time and conditions for the incubation, the characteristics of the specific anti-IgE and the behavior of the labeled antigen that the detection method used). An overview of the different methods identifying specific IgE can be found in a WAO paper (Ansotegui 2020).

Nowadays, the most common technique and "golden standard" for specific IgE identification is the CAP (Thermo Fisher Scientific) assay (Ewan 1990). Age-related cut-off values for specific IgE to a number of foods have been established, especially in young children, to provide $\geq 95\%$ confidence in patients with a confirmed FA re-confirmed by a food challenge (OFC) (see Table 1 below) (Sampson 2001; Benhamou et al. 2008; Du Toit et al. 2009).

National University, Singapore.
Email: paevbhps@nus.edu.sg

Table 1. Positive predictive values (≥ 95%) for specific IgE (U/ml) (Du Toit et al. 2009).

EGG	**7**
Infants ≤ 2 years	**2**
COW'S MILK	**15**
Infants ≤ 2 years	**5**
PEANUT	**15**
TREE NUTS	**15**
FISH	**20**

Reliability

As specific IgE is the key antibody in allergic reactions, determining specific IgE to allergens in the blood of the patient is therefore of high value in diagnosing the existence of allergy. Nowadays, there are more than 400 characterized allergens available for *in vitro* determination of specific IgE.

The reliability of specific IgE determination varies depending on the type of allergen. In general terms, for inhalant allergens, the specificity and sensitivity of the methods are good, and within the range of 85–95%. However, specificity decreases in the case of food allergens, and they even become lower when the allergen is a drug, such as a beta-lactam antibiotic. Moreover, there is a good correlation between clinical history and specific IgE against inhalant allergens and a lower correlation in the case of food allergens.

Specific IgE vs. SPT

The results achieved with *in vitro* specific IgE measurement and skin testing are nearly comparable with a good correlation (about 90%) between SPT and specific IgE and with some well-known advantages and disadvantages for each diagnostic approach (Frati et al. 2018) (Table 2).

Table 2. Skin prick testing vs. specific IgE.

Skin Prick Testing (SPT)	Specific IgE
More sensitive than specific IgE	More specific and quantitative than SPT
Inexpensive	Expensive
Child-friendly (almost painless)	Blood draw
Results are known after 15–20 minutes	Depends on the lab but can take days before the results are known
SPT reaction can be experienced by the patient (and shown to the parents)	Results are shown on a report
Can cause side effects in specific patients (see below)	No side effects, except blood drawing
Suppressed by antihistamines or other medication	Not suppressed by antihistamines or other medication
Can be performed with virtual all allergens (see "prick to prick" method)	Limited, though extensive, number of allergens available
Dependent on the sensitivity of the skin (influences by hypo reactivity vs. hyperreactivity – dermographism)	Not dependent on skin sensitivity

Indication for Specific IgE Determination

Most allergists consider SPT the test of choice in diagnosing an IgE-mediated disease. Serum IgE determination, which entails no risk to the patient other than a blood draw, is preferable over SPT in the following conditions:

1. If the patient has an unstable or uncontrolled medical condition
2. If there's a high risk of anaphylaxis
3. If essential medication is taken (such as antihistamines) that interferes with SPT
4. If there's a skin condition that limits the reliability of SPT (such as severe eczema)
5. As a follow-up tool of oral immunotherapy (OIT) but still a subject of intense research
6. Some researchers use specific IgE to determine the start dose for food challenges

The development of screening tests with multiple allergens or multiplex tests that identify multiple specific-IgEs with a small blood volume makes this testing more appealing to very young children. However, food allergy panels need to be adapted and improved in order to be cost-effective and more specific.

Remark on total IgE

- While specific IgE is directed against specific allergens, total IgE is the sum of all IgE present in the blood, not only against allergens but also against micro-organisms, such as viruses or parasites. The value of determining total IgE, via RIST, in diagnosing allergy is "limited," as it only gives an idea about the potential of the patient to produce IgE. Although many allergic patients have a raised total IgE, this can also be found in non-allergic patients; for instance, in children after viral or parasitic infections. Therefore, total IgE determination is considered a rough method for screening allergic diseases, though its actual value is controversial because normal values of total IgE do not exclude the existence of the allergic disease, and high values of total IgE are not specific to allergy on itself.

In conclusion, for specific indications, specific IgE is considered the test of choice in diagnosing allergies being a reliable test.

References on Specific IgE (Part: I)

Ansotegui, I. J., Melioli, G., Canonica, G. W., Caraballo, L., Villa, E., Ebisawa, M. et al. 2020. IgE allergy diagnostics and other relevant tests in allergy, a World Allergy Organization position paper. WAO Jour 13: 100080. http://doi.org/10.1016/j.waojou.2019.100080.

Benhamou, A. H., Zamora, S. A. and Eigenmann, P. A. 2008. Correlation between specific immunoglobulin E levels and the severity of reactions in egg-allergic patients. Pediatr Allergy Immunol. 19: 173–9. 53

Du Toit, G., Santos, A., Roberts, G., Fox, A. T., Smith, P. and Lack, G. 2009. The diagnosis of IgE-mediated food allergy in childhood. Ped. Allergy Immunol. 20: 309–19

Ewan, P. W. and Coote, D. 1990. Evaluation of a capsulated hydrophilic carrier polymer (the ImmunoCAP) for measurement of specific IgE antibodies. Allergy 45(1): 22–29.

Frati, F., Incorvaia, C., Di Cara, C. G., Marcucci, F., Esposito, S. et al. 2018. The skin prick test. J. Biol. Regul. Homeost Agents 32(1 Suppl): 19–24.

Sampson, H. A. 2001. Utility of food-specific IgE concentrations in predicting symptomatic food allergy. J. Allergy Clin. Immunol. 107: 891–6.

Wide, L., Bennich, H. and Johansson, S. G. 1967. Diagnosis of allergy by an *in-vitro* test for allergen antibodies. Lancet. 2(7526): 1105–1107.

Chapter 4C Part ll

Component-Resolved Diagnostics (CRD)

Hugo Van Bever

◇◇

Allergens are composed of a large number of specific proteins to which specific IgE is produced. Allergen component-resolved diagnostic testing (CRD) is a method able to dose specific IgE to purified or recombinant allergens that induce specific IgE, thereby identifying specific molecules causing sensitization or clinical allergy. CRD has become of growing importance in clinical research of both IgE-mediated inhalants and food allergies (Eiringhaus et al. 2019). The advantage of CRD is "a more specific diagnosis" (identifying which proteins of the allergens are involved in the allergic reactions), better knowledge of mechanisms of the allergic reaction, detecting cross-reactivity and allowing a more specific treatment (such as specific immunotherapy) and a better prediction of the prognosis of the allergy. In other words, CRD offers important additional information regarding the patient's sensitization pattern, especially in complex clinical cases such as polysensitization or idiopathic reactions, thus avoiding the overuse of *in vitro* and *in vivo* IgE diagnostics. CRD may help the clinician to identify the cause of an allergy and, in the case of complex polysensitization, uncover possible cross-reactivity. CRD is less useful in making the diagnosis of an allergy.

In daily clinical practice, the value of CRD is viewed differently by physicians. Today's most widely applied diagnostic approach starts with the patient's clinical history, followed by an SPT or extract-based IgE testing, and uses CRD only as an additional source of information (Eiringhaus et al. 2019).

In many types of allergy (such as allergy to pollen, food and insects) CRD allows discrimination between clinically significant and irrelevant specific IgE, and the establishment of sensitization patterns with particular prognostic outcomes. Further promising improvements in diagnostics are expected from additional, not yet commercially available, recombinant allergen diagnostics identifying molecules of risk. Overall, CRD may decrease the need for provocation testing and may also improve the specificity of immunotherapy.

Technique of CRD

A currently well-established and frequently used method for measuring IgE sensitization to components is again the ImmunoCAP assay, which is a singleplex immunoassay. Another possibility is the multiplex ImmunoCAP ISAC® 112 (Thermo Fisher Scientific) assay, a microarray currently including 112 allergenic molecules from 51 allergen sources, thus providing a broad sensitization

National University. Singapore.

profile for each patient with a serum or plasma sample of only 30 μL. The Microtest Allergy System (Microtest Diagnostics), another automated microarray platform for allergy diagnostics, has recently become available. Using a 100 μL serum or plasma sample, specific IgE against 19 extracts and 16 components of 22 common allergen sources can be identified (Williams et al. 2016; Onell et al. 2017).

In clinical practice, when CRD is performed, it is usually through single test assays, and clinicians decide which allergen component should specifically be looked at. While CRD by means of microarrays is reprimanded to be too complex and detailed. SPT, on the other hand, is advantageous in terms of providing information on the biological function of the antibody in question.

In recent years, the development of allergen panels oriented to different types of allergies (e.g., food vs. respiratory allergy), age (e.g., pediatric vs. adult), and geographic region (e.g., northern vs. southern Europe) has become the subject of discussion. Such an approach has already, to some extent, been adopted by commercial providers, although mainly focusing on extracts rather than individual molecular components.

Indications of CRD

CRD is of little use when there is a convincing history of IgE-mediated allergy and a positive SPT or specific IgE to the relevant whole food allergen, as this information is already enough to make a diagnosis. However, CRD is useful in the following situations:

1) when there are low abundant and/or labile food proteins in conventional allergy tests;
2) to provide information on risk or severity associated with molecules;
3) to provide indicators of food-related cross-reactivity;
4) markers of genuine (species-specific) sensitization;
5) to predict the outcome of oral immunotherapy for food (under research).

Other indications in which CRD may be useful include idiopathic anaphylaxis, delayed red meat anaphylaxis and wheat-dependent exercise-induced anaphylaxis to differentiate between high versus low-risk molecules from foods giving rise to food-induced anaphylaxis (peanuts, nuts, shrimps, etc.), baked egg or milk allergy (ovomucoid, casein), etc.

The European Academy of Allergy and Clinical Immunology (EAACI) recently proposed the so-called "U-shaped" approach: start with the patient's clinical history, physical examination, and SPT or specific extract-based IgE testing. CRD should be performed for allergen components of sources to which the previous diagnostics have detected a clinically relevant sensitization. Additionally, when IgE sensitization to highly cross-reactive allergens had been found, (a) CRD diagnostics should be broadened to include molecules of the same family and (b) clinical history should be expanded by actively investigating for the presence of possible symptoms caused by other allergen sources of the index protein family (EAACI 2016).

CRD in Food Allergy

CRD has been used in the diagnosis of FA and in specific cases, like soy, peanut and hazelnut allergy, CRD is able to determine the risk of severity of an allergic reaction. Commonly used food proteins that have been identified are in the TABLE below.

Table 3. Commonly used CRP in food allergy.

Food	Component	Cut-Off Level
COW'S MILK	Cow's milk Bos d 8 (casein)	> 24 kU/L for reactivity to baked milk > 6.6 kU/L for reactivity to baked milk
EGG WHITE	Egg white Gal d 1 (ovomucoid) Gal d 2 (ovalbumin)	> 30.7 kU/L for reactivity to boiled egg > 7.3 kU/L for reactivity to raw egg > 10.8 kU/L for reactivity to boiled egg > 5.2 kU/L for reactivity to raw egg > 29.3 kU/L for reactivity to boiled egg > 9.8 kU/L for reactivity to raw egg
PEANUT	Peanut Ara h 2 Ara h 6	> 14.9 kU/L > 1.0 kU/L for severity pf reaction* > 0.8 kU/L for the severity of reaction

* Predicts a severe reaction

Other Examples

- Ovomucoid and omega-5 gliadin seem to be good diagnostic markers for egg allergy and wheat allergy respectively.
- The severity of the allergic reaction can be predicted in peanut allergy with Ara h 2.
- In tree nut allergy it was found that other storage proteins, such as Jug r 1 (walnut), Ana o e (cashew), Ses I 1 (sesame), and Fag e 3 (buckwheat) seem to be better markers of allergic reactions than the whole allergen extract (Sato et al. 2018).

However, age and geographic differences affect CRD results, and they should always be utilized in the context of clinical history. In the future, clinical phenotypes may be differentiated with larger prospective studies utilizing food challenges (Tuano 2015).

Limitations of CRD in Food Allergy

However, in daily practice, CRD has some limitations and is still mainly a research subject. The main limitations include:

a) Not all allergenic molecules of food proteins are commercially available.

b) Positive results for certain allergenic molecules only suggest the severity of a potential reaction, but it does not predict it with certainty.

c) Testing positive for specific allergenic molecules does not imply a certain clinical reaction. As for high positive SPT or high specific IgE for a certain food, the results are only associated with a higher probability of an allergic reaction after an oral food challenge but do not predict the results of the challenge.

d) Diagnostic methods can yield different results. The singleplex method provides quantitative results and it tends to be more precise with respect to the multiplex ones. The latter provides semi-quantitative results, that could be conflicting, depending on the methodology used (Calvani 2020).

Conclusion

At present, allergy diagnostics largely rely on clinical history, physical examination, and *in vivo* SPT. However, although still a subject of intense research, CRD testing is currently finding its way into the clinical routine and can offer additional information on the patient's sensitization profile, prediction of outcome and treatment responsiveness, mainly on specific immunotherapy.

Glossary of Abbreviations

SPT – Allergy Skin Prick Test
CRD – Component-Resolved Diagnosis
RIST – Radio-Immunosorbent
FA – Food Allergy
RAST – Radio-Allergosorbent Test
WAO – World Allergy Organization
OFC – Office Food Challenge
OIT – Oral Immunotherapy
Ku/L – Kilo Units Per Liter

References on CRD (Part: II)

Calvani, M., Anania, C., Caffarelli, C., Martelli, A., Miraglia del Giudice, M., Cravidi, C. et al. 2020. Food allergy: an updated review on pathogenesis, diagnosis, prevention, and management. Acta Biomed. 91(Supplement 11): e202001.

Eiringhaus, K., Renz, H., Matricardi, P. and Skevaki, C. 2019. Component-resolved diagnostics in allergic rhinitis and asthma. J. Appl. Lab Med. 03(05): 883–898.

European Academy of Allergy and Clinical Immunology. EAACI molecular allergology user's guide. Pediatric allergy and immunology. Zurich (Switzerland): EAACI; 2016.

Onell, A., Whiteman, A., Nordlund, B., Baldracchini, F., Mazzoleni, G., Hedlin, G. et al. 2017. Allergy testing in children with persistent asthma: comparison of four diagnostic methods. Allergy 72: 590–597.

Sato, S., Yanagida, N. and Ebisawa, M. 2018. How to diagnose food allergy? Curr. Opinion Allergy Clin. Immunol. 18: 214 0–221.

Tuano, K. S. and Davis, C. M. 2015. Utility of Component-Resolved Diagnostics in food allergy. Curr. Opinion Allergy Clin. Immunol. 15(6): 32.

Williams, P., Onell, A., Baldracchini, F., Hui, V., Jolles, S. and El-Shanawany, T. 2016. Evaluation of a novel automated allergy microarray platform compared with three other allergy test methods. Clin. Exp. Immunol. 184: 1–10. 32.

Chapter 4D

Eosinophilic Oesophagitis

Marion M. Aw

Introduction

Eosinophilic oesophagitis (EoE) is a chronic disorder of the oesophagus first described in the mid-1990s. Published data from the West has shown a significant increase in prevalence over the last two decades with current estimates of 1/2,000 and a male predominance of approximately 3:1 (Mansoor 2016). While EoE is not as prevalent in Asia, there is emerging evidence that EoE would also be a clinically important condition here.

Pathogenesis

EoE is believed to be triggered by environmental factors in a genetically predisposed individual. Familial studies demonstrate that concordance in monozygotic twins is 58%, whereas the figure is closer to 36% in dizygotic twins and only 2.4% in non-twin siblings (Alexander et al. 2014). Twin cohort analysis reveals a more significant contribution by environmental factors (81%) compared to genetics (14.5%) (Alexander et al. 2014).

As the normal oesophagus is devoid of eosinophils, EoE is believed to result from a trigger which leads to inflammation and the migration of eosinophils into the oesophagus. It is not surprising that genes involved in allergen sensitisation and disruption of epithelial barrier function have been implicated in this process. Here Th2 cytokines (IL-5 and IL-13), TSLP (thymic stromal lymphopoietin) and CAPN14 (calpain 14) are thought to have key roles (Kitajima et al. 2011; Litosh et al. 2017; O'Shea et al. 2018).

EoE has also been seen in association with genetic conditions, such as connective tissue disorders with hypermobility (e.g., Ehlers-Danlos syndrome, Loeys-Dietz syndrome), autoimmune conditions (e.g., Hashimoto's thyroiditis, coeliac disease) and a number of other syndromes (e.g., Hyper-IgE syndrome, severe atopy associated with metabolic wasting (SAM) syndrome, Netherton's syndrome) (O'Shea et al. 2018). The oesophageal inflammation in EoE leads to remodelling and fibrosis, resulting in oesophageal rigidity and dysfunction. Untreated, EoE is a progressive fibro stenotic condition with stricture formation as a complication (Dellon et al. 2014).

Clinical Presentation

The diagnosis of EoE is a clinicopathological one (Dellon et al. 2018). That is the presence of histologic criteria in a child with clinical features consistent with the disease. Symptoms

National University, Singapore.
Email: paesawm@nus.edu.sg

experienced are a result of oesophageal dysfunction. Typical clinical symptoms are similar to that of gastroesophageal reflux disease (GERD) with vomiting and pain. Infants and young children may also present with feeding difficulties, feed refusal and failure to thrive. The older child and adolescent may manifest with dysphagia, epigastric or chest pain and PPI-dependent or resistant GERD. The clinical presentation in the adolescent patient is closer to what one may encounter in adult patients with EoE (Liacouras et al. 2005).

Often, one would need to take a careful feeding and/or eating history, as symptoms of dysphagia may be subtle in children. These include selective or picky eating in order to avoid troublesome foods, taking a long time to chew and swallow food and having to drink a fair amount of water or liquid at mealtimes. As EoE is an immunologic disease associated with food allergy, the presence of a personal history of atopy or a family history of atopic and allergic disease (such as eczema, asthma, and allergic rhinitis) should raise the suspicion that EoE could be the underlying cause of what may otherwise appear to be GERD in an infant or child. The physical examination in children with EoE is often normal. Features of atopy (eczema and allergic rhinitis) and nutritional consequences (pallor and poor growth) should be actively looked for.

Investigations for EoE

Discussions and referral to a paediatric gastroenterologist would be useful. As EoE is a clinicopathological diagnosis, endoscopy with biopsy should be performed in any child suspected to have EoE. There are typical endoscopic features of EoE. These include the appearance of white exudates, linear grooves or furrows and concentric rings in the oesophagus (Hirano et al. 2013). As the endoscopic appearance of the oesophagus may be normal in as many as 10–25% of children with EoE and the histologic involvement patchy, multiple biopsies are usually taken. The endoscopist would usually take biopsies from the lower, mid and upper oesophagus (Liacouras et al. 2011). The presence of ≥ 15 eosinophils per high-power field, seen only in the oesophagus, is required to make a diagnosis of EoE. Additional supportive histological features include eosinophilic micro-abscesses, surface layering of eosinophils, extracellular eosinophilic granules, basal cell hyperplasia, dilated intercellular spaces and lamina propria fibrosis (Liacouras et al. 2011). There are a number of other clinical conditions that can result in oesophageal eosinophilia. These include parasitic infections, hyper-eosinophilic syndrome and inflammatory bowel disease to name a few (Dellon et al. 2018). In most instances, the clinical presentation and features would be distinguishable from those of EoE.

Management

Treatment aims to induce remission of inflammation and prevent long-term complications. As food allergy is thought to be a key trigger of EoE in children, elimination of the offending food would be the mainstay of treatment. Other modalities include pharmacological therapy. When complications of strictures occur, mechanical dilation of the oesophagus would be required.

Diet

There are several strategies for food elimination in children with EoE. These include the use of an elemental diet, an empiric elimination diet or a targeted elimination diet. Infants in whom milk can be the sole source of nutrition could be placed on an amino acid-based milk formula. Doing so can achieve a high rate of clinical, endoscopic and histological improvement (Arias et al. 2014). The challenge thereafter would be maintaining this remission when solids and other food are reintroduced back into the diet.

The first food eliminated is usually cow's milk protein. However, a six-food elimination diet (dairy, soy, eggs, wheat, peanuts/tree nuts and fish/shellfish) or a four-food elimination diet (dairy, eggs, wheat and soy) can also be considered in infants and older children (Arias et al. 2014) in whom there is no clear-cut offending food. In instances when a diet history may shed some light as to possible offending foods, skin prick tests (SPT) and atopy patch tests (APT) may be performed to help guide a targeted elimination diet approach. The choice of foods for the six- and four-food elimination diets are based on the most common food triggers in Caucasian populations. As the spectrum of food allergens may differ between countries and populations, the empiric elimination diet would need to be tailored to take that into account. For example, in Spain, legumes were found to be the fourth most common food allergen (Lucendo et al. 2013). Hence the four-food elimination diet in Spain would include diary, eggs, wheat and legumes (which comprise beans, peas, peanuts and soy). A study from Iran demonstrated that the most common sensitised foods on SPT were sesame and walnut (Momen et al. 2018).

Drugs

The first line of pharmacology therapy would be the use of a Proton Pump Inhibitor (PPI), which induces clinical and histologic remission in over 50% of patients (Lucendo et al. 2016). PPI-responsive EoE (previously known as PPI-responsive oesophageal eosinophilia) is now considered a sub-phenotype of EoE.

Other pharmacologic options include the use of topical corticosteroids (fluticasone propionate delivered via metered dose inhaler or oral viscous budesonide) (Table 2) (Furuta and Katzka 2015). A recent meta-analysis demonstrated the effectiveness of topical steroids in providing symptom resolution and decreasing oesophageal eosinophilia (Murali et al. 2016). Patients should be counselled not to eat or drink for 30–60 minutes following swallowing the medication. As symptoms often recur on stopping medications, treatment is generally long-term. The principles for long-term treatment include the use of the lowest possible doses of topical steroids with periodic endoscopic assessment. A number of biologic agents (monoclonal antibodies against various cytokines) have been trialled. However, none are sufficiently effective to be considered part of the therapeutic armamentarium currently.

Table 1. EoE diagnostic criteria (Dellon et al. 2018).

1. Clinical symptoms of oesophageal dysfunction
2. Presence of concomitant atopic features
3. Typical or suggestive endoscopic appearance
4. ≥ 15 eosinophils per high-power field, seen only in the oesophagus
5. Exclusion of other causes of oesophageal eosinophilia

Table 2. Steroid therapy in EoE.

Topical Corticosteroid	Age group	Dose
Fluticasone via MDI	Child	220–440 mcg bd
	Adolescent	440–880 mcg bd
Oral viscous budesonide	Child	0.25–0.5 mg bd
	Adolescent	1–2 mg bd

Endoscopic Dilatation

Endoscopic dilation is reserved for when complications of oesophageal stenosis and stricture are present. This would need to be coupled with management to prevent ongoing inflammation of the oesophagus.

Disease Monitoring

Symptom resolution usually indicates a reduction in oesophageal inflammation. However, this may not always be so, and endoscopic assessment with biopsies would invariably be required to determine the histologic resolution of oesophageal eosinophilia and inflammation. Children with EoE often undergo multiple endoscopies. In order to maximise the clinical information obtained at each procedure, the indication and timing would need to be discussed carefully between the managing clinicians (paediatric gastroenterologist and allergist) as well as parents/patient.

Coeliac Disease in Children

Clinical Presentation

Coeliac disease (CD) is an immune-mediated chronic condition that occurs in genetically predisposed individuals (Husby et al. 2020). It presents in many different ways with gluten exposure being a prerequisite. Traditionally, children with CD manifest features of malabsorption dominated by diarrhoea, steatorrhea, weight loss or failure to thrive. However, CD can also present with gastrointestinal (GI) symptoms similar to that of irritable bowel syndrome (IBS) as well as non-GI symptoms (Table 3).

The diagnostic challenge for clinicians is to distinguish CD from other gluten-related conditions (Figure 1), particularly when the symptoms are not classic or typical. In addition, CD would also need to be distinguished from children with functional bowel disorders (i.e., IBS). In general, children with CD have more extra-intestinal manifestations (EIMs) (62%) than those with functional disorders (33%). The most common EIMs in children with CD are poor growth (27%) and anaemia (18%) (Nurminen et al. 2019).

Table 3. Symptoms of CD and indications for testing.

GI Symptoms	Extra-Intestinal Symptoms	Others
Typical	**Typical**	First-degree relatives with CD
Chronic diarrhoea	Faltering growth	Autoimmune conditions
Recurrent abdominal pain	Short stature	IgA deficiency
Less Typical	**Other Symptoms**	Down syndrome
Chronic constipation not	Dermatitis herpetiformis	
responding to usual treatment	Iron deficiency anaemia	
Recurrent nausea, vomiting	Delayed puberty	
Aphthous ulcers	Fatigue	
	Headaches	
	Irritability	
	Abnormal liver tests	
	Dental enamel defects	

Gluten Related Disorders

Coeliac Disease (Autoimmune) — Wheat Allergy (IgE and non-IgE) — Non-coeliac Gluten Sensitivity (Non-immunologic)

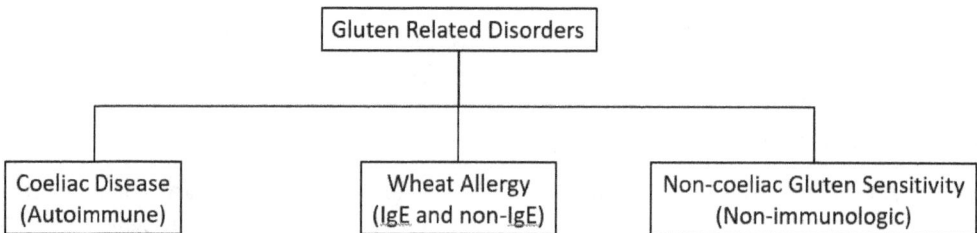

Figure 1. Gluten-related disorders.

Investigations for CD

Updated guidelines for the diagnosis of CD in children were published in 2020 (Husby et al. 2020). Indications to considering testing for CD are shown in Table 1. First-line investigation (regardless of symptoms) would be total IgA and anti-tissue transglutaminase (TGA) IgA, done whilst the child is still taking a gluten-containing diet. Children, who have a high serum TGA-IgA ($\geq$ 10x ULN) and a positive Endomysial antibody (EMA)-IgA in a second blood sample, may be diagnosed to have CD without the need to undergo a small bowel biopsy. This diagnostic approach without tissue biopsy should be discussed with the parent/patient.

In children who are IgA deficient, an IgG-based test (DGP, deamidated gliadin peptide, EMA, TGA) can be performed. Children with an elevated TGA-IgA (< 10x ULN) and IgA deficient children with IgG-positive serological tests should undergo a small biopsy in order to make an accurate diagnosis.

HLA-typing is not recommended as a test to "rule in" the diagnosis of CD. A negative HLA-DQ2/DQ8 means the risk of CD is very low, whereas a positive result does not confirm the diagnosis.

Management

The treatment for children with CD would be a gluten-free diet. Parents and patients need to be taught to read food labels. Advice from a dietician would be helpful to ensure nutritional adequacy. Follow up for children with CD is life-long.

Glossary of Abbreviations

ATP – Atopy Patch Tests
CD – Coeliac Disease
DGP – Deamidated Gliadin Peptide
EoE – Eosinophilic Oesophagitis
EMA – Endomysial Antibody
EIM – Extra-Intestinal Manifestations
GERD – Gastro-Oesophageal Reflux Disorder
HLA – Human Leucocyte Antigen
IBS – Irritable Bowel Syndrome
PPI – Proton Pump Inhibitor
SPT – Skin Prick Test
TGA – Transglutaminase
ULN – Upper Limits of Normal

References

Alexander, E. S., Martin, L. J., Collins, M. H., Kottyan, L., Sucharew, H., Hua He, M. S. et al. 2014. Twin and family studies reveal strong environmental and weaker genetic cues explaining heritability of eosinophilic esophagitis. J. Allergy Clin. Immunol. 134: 1084–92.

Arias, A., Gonzalez-Cervera, J., Tenias, J. M. and Lucendo, A. J. 2014. Efficacy of dietary interventions for inducing histologic remission in patients with eosinophilic esophagitis: a systematic review and meta-analysis. Gastroenterology 146: 1639–48.

Dellon, E. S., Kim, H. P., Sperry, S. L., Rybnicek, D. A., Woosley, J. T. and Shaheen, N. J. 2014. A phenotypic analysis shows that eosinophilic esophagitis is a progressive fibrostenotic disease. Gastrointestinal Endoscopy 79: 577–85.

Dellon, E. S., Liacouras, C. A., Molina-Infante, J., Furuta, G. T., Spergel, J. M., Zevit, N. et al. 2018. Updated International Consensus Diagnostic Criteria for Eosinophilic Esophagitis: Proceedings of the AGREE Conference. Gastroenterology 155: 1022–1033.

Furuta, G. T. and Katzka, D. A. 2015. Eosinophilic esophagitis. N Engl. J. Med. 2015 October 22; 373(17): 1640–1648.

Hirano, I., Moy, N., Heckman, M. G., Thomas, C. S., Gonsalves, N. and Achem, S. R. 2013. Endoscopic assessment of the oesophageal features of eosinophilic oesophagitis: validation of a novel classification and grading system. Gut 62: 489–495.

Husby, A., Koletzko, S., Korponay-Szabo, I., Kurppa, K., Mearin, M. L., Ribes-Koninckx, C. et al. 2020. European society paediatric gastroenterology, hepatology and nutrition guidelines for diagnosing coeliac disease. J. Pediatr Gastroenterol. Nutr. 70: 141–157.

Kitajima, M., Lee, H. C., Nakayama, T. and Ziegler, S. F. 2011. TSLP enhances the function of helper type 2 cells. Eur. J. Immunol. 41: 1862–71.

Liacouras, C. A., Spergel, J. M., Ruchelli, E., Ruchelli, E., Verma, R., Mascarenhas, M. et al. 2005. Eosinophilic esophagitis: A 10-year experience in 381 children. Clin. Gastroenterol. Hepatol. 3(12): 1198–1206.

Liacouras, C. A., Furuta, G. T., Hirano, I., Atkins, D., Attwood, S. E., Bonis, P. A. et al. 2011. Eosinophilic esophagitis: Updated consensus recommendations for children and adults. J. Allergy Clin. Immunol. 128: 3–20.

Litosh, V. A., Rochman, M., Rymer, J. K., Porollo, A., Kottyan, L. C. and Rothenberg, M. E. 2017. Calpain-14 and its association with eosinophilic esophagitis. J. Allergy and Clin. Immunol. 139(16): 1762–1771.

Lucendo, A. J., Arias, A., Gonzalez-Cervera, J., Yagüe-Compadre, J. L., Guagnozzi, D., Angueira, T. et al. 2013. Empiric 6-food elimination diet induced and maintained prolonged remission in patients with adult eosinophilic esophagitis: A prospective study on the food cause of the disease. Journal of Allergy and Clinical Immunology 131(3): 797–804.

Lucendo, A. J., Arias, A. and Molina-Infante, J. 2016. Efficacy of proton pump inhibitor drugs for inducing clinical and histologic remission in patients with symptomatic esophageal eosinophilia: a systematic review and meta-analysis. Clin. Gastroenterol. Hepatol. 14: 13–22.

Mansoor, E. and Cooper, G. S. 2016. The 2010–2015 prevalence of eosinophilic esophagitis in the USA: A population-based study. Dig Dis Sci. 61: 2928–34.

Momen, T., Saneian, H. and Amini, N. 2018. Demographic, clinical, and allergic characteristics of children with eosinophilic esophagitis in Isfahan, Iran. Iran J. Allergy Asthma Immunol. 17(6): 533–539.

Munoz-Persy, M. and Lucendo A. J. 2018. Treatment of eosinophilic esophagitis in the pediatric patient: an evidence-based approach. Eur. J. Pediatr 2018 May; 177(5): 649–663.

Murali, A. R., Gupta, A., Attar, B. M., Ravi, V. and Koduru, P. 2016. Topical steroids in eosinophilic esophagitis: systematic review and meta-analysis of placebo-controlled randomized clinical trials. J. Gastroenterol. Hepatol. 31(6): 1111–9.

Nurminen, S., Kivela, L., Huhtala, H., Kaukinen, K. and Kurppa, K. 2019. Extraintestinal manifestations were common in children with coeliac disease and were more prevalent in patients with more severe clinical and histological presentation Acta Paediatr. 2019 Apr; 108(4): 681–687.

O'Shea, K. M., Aceves, S. S., Dellon, E. S., Gupta, S. K., Spergel, J. M., Furuta, G. T. et al. 2018. Pathophysiology of eosinophilic esophagitis. Gastroenterology 154(2): 333–345.

Chapter 5

Acute and Chronic Urticaria/Angioedema

Vinay Mehta

⬦⬦⬦

Introduction

Urticaria is a common disorder with a lifetime prevalence of approximately 20% in the general population (Greaves 1995). Acute urticaria (lasting < 6 weeks) is more common in children and adolescents whereas chronic urticaria (lasting > 6 weeks) is more common in adults (Bernstein et al. 2014). Chronic urticaria affects up to 1% of the general population, with women affected twice as frequently as men, and the onset typically in the third to fifth decades of life (Zuberbier et al. 2010). It is a potentially disabling condition that can lead to substantial impairment of quality of life (O'Donnell et al. 1997). Furthermore, psychosocial factors such as anxiety, depression and poor sleep are present in half of the population (Ben-Shoshan et al. 2013).

Hives are pruritic, circumscribed, raised, erythematous lesions, often with central pallor (Photo 1). They can vary in size and shape. Hives are transient in duration, usually appearing over minutes to hours, then disappearing within 24 hours. They may appear flattened if the patient is taking antihistamines. Although there is a predilection for pressure-prone areas such as the waist, axilla and groin, hives can occur anywhere on the skin.

Concurrent angioedema may occur and is characterized by subcutaneous or submucosal swelling affecting nondependent areas, most commonly the lips, cheeks, eyelids, extremities and genitals (Photo 2). Angioedema typically develops over minutes to hours and resolves over one to three days. Affected areas typically feel painful, numb or tingling (Zuberbier et al. 2022).

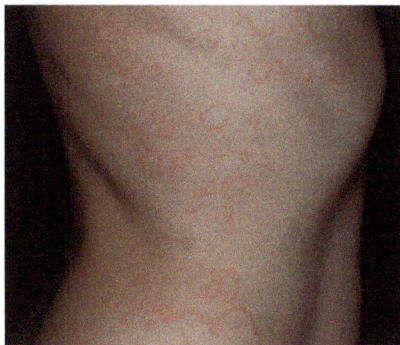

Photo 1. Hives. Source: Attribution details, CC BY 4.0 via Wikimedia Commons; https://commons.wikimedia.org/wiki/File:Chronic_spontaneous_urticaria.jpg.

Allergy & Asthma Associates of Southern California, Irvine, CA, USA and Mission Viejo, CA, USA.
Email: drvinaymehta@gmail.com

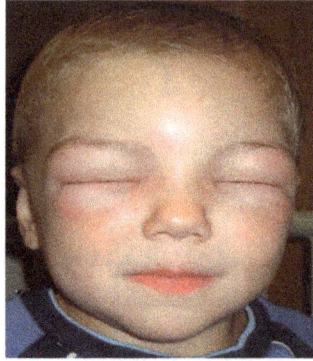

Photo 2. Angioedema. Source: James Heilman, MD, CC BY-SA 3.0 via Wikimedia Commons; https://commons.wikimedia. org/wiki/File:Angioedema2010.JPG.

Classification

Urticaria is categorized by its chronicity. Acute urticaria is defined by hives lasting less than 6 weeks, whereas chronic urticaria is defined by hives that recur most days for 6 weeks or longer (Figure 1) (Kaplan et al. 2009). Approximately 40% of patients with chronic urticaria have accompanying angioedema, whereas 10% have angioedema as their sole manifestation (Saini 2014). The average duration of chronic urticaria is 2–5 years but can last longer if there is concurrent angioedema (Zuberbier et al. 2010).

Approximately 25% of patients with chronic urticaria have an underlying physical trigger which is termed chronic inducible urticaria (CIndU). This type of urticaria is further categorized according to the nature of the inciting stimulus. In the remaining 75% of cases, no specific trigger can be identified, and is termed chronic spontaneous urticaria (CSU). Of these, approximately 30–40% have serological evidence of IgG autoantibodies against IgE or the high-affinity IgE receptor (FcεR1) or circulating IgE autoantibodies to various self-antigens, including thyroid peroxidase (TPO) (Kaplan et al. 2009). Consequently, it is sometimes referred to as "chronic autoimmune urticaria."

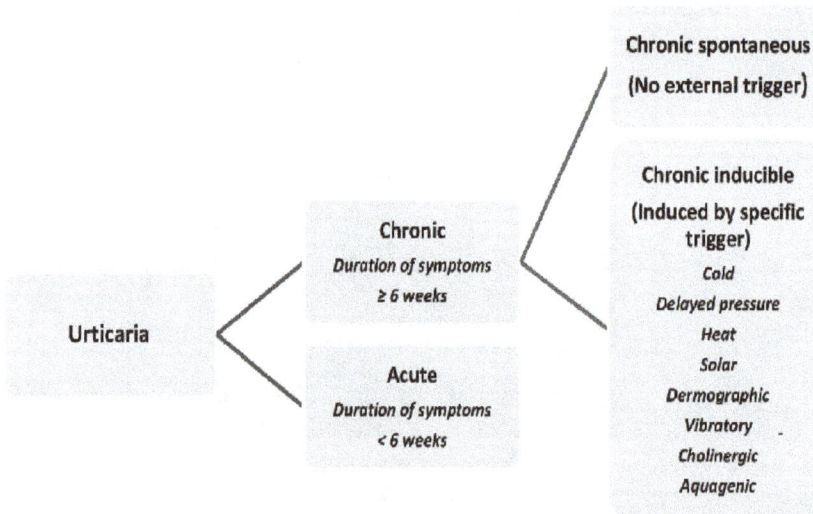

Figure 1. Classification of Urticaria According to EAACI/GA2LEN/WAO 2013 Guideline. Source: Murat Borlu, Salih Levent Cinar and Demet Kartal. (2017). Chronic Inducible Urticaria Part I. DOI: 10.5772/68069 CC BY 3.0 via Wikimedia Commons.

More than two-thirds of cases of new-onset urticaria prove to be acute. However, the lesions of acute and chronic urticaria are identical in appearance, therefore it is not possible to differentiate between the two at the onset (Kaplan 2002).

Pathophysiology

Urticaria is mediated by the degranulation of cutaneous mast cells in the superficial dermis and, to a lesser extent, by basophils. When mast cells and basophils are activated through IgE or non-IgE-mediated mechanisms, they release histamine and vasodilatory mediators, such as prostaglandins, leukotrienes, tryptase, platelet-activating factor and kinins. Within 4–8 hours of mast cell activation, inflammatory cytokines are secreted, resulting in a delayed inflammatory response. Consequently, a skin biopsy typically shows a perivascular infiltrate of cells comprised of CD4+ lymphocytes, monocytes, neutrophils, eosinophils and basophils, similar to the infiltrate seen in late-phase IgE-mediated reactions (Ying et al. 2002). Angioedema associated with urticaria is also mediated by cutaneous mast cells, but it involves mast cells in deeper tissue layers, including the deep dermis and subcutaneous tissues.

Etiology

Acute Urticaria

Acute urticaria is more likely to have an identifiable etiology compared with chronic urticaria. Common etiologies include infections, drugs, foods, insect stings/bites and latex (Table 1). Acute urticaria may develop during or following a viral (e.g., upper respiratory infection) or bacterial infection (e.g., urinary tract infection), particularly in children. In fact, infections are associated with over 80% of cases of urticaria in some pediatric series (Sackesen et al. 2014; Mortureux et al. 1998; Imbalzano et al. 2016; Minciullo et al. 2014) and likely involve the immune complex formation and/or complement activation. Parasitic infections can also result in acute urticaria and are usually associated with prominent eosinophilia.

Urticaria caused by allergic (IgE-mediated) reactions typically occurs within minutes to 2 hours of exposure to the culprit allergen. Among drugs, beta-lactam antibiotics (penicillin and cephalosporin) are the most common culprits. Among foods, cow's milk, egg, peanut, tree nuts, soy and wheat are frequently implicated in children, whereas shellfish, tree nuts and peanuts are most often implicated in adults (Wang and Sampson 2011). Allergic reactions to insects can involve either their stings, such as Hymenoptera (bees, wasps, hornets, and imported fire ants) or their bite, such as Triatoma (kissing bug). On the other hand, the bite of bedbugs, fleas and mites can result in papular urticaria, characterized by clusters of pruritic papules that persist for days to weeks. Exposure

Table 1. Common etiologies of acute urticaria.

Type	Examples
Infections	Viral (upper respiratory tract), bacterial (urinary tract), fungal and parasitic
Drugs (IgE-mediated)	Penicillin and cephalosporins
Foods	Children: cow's milk, egg, peanut, tree nuts, soy and wheat Adult: shellfish, tree nuts and peanut
Insect bites/stings	Hymenoptera: bees, wasps, hornets and imported fire ants Triatoma: kissing bug Bedbugs, fleas and mites (papular urticaria)
Latex	Healthcare and rubber industry workers, patients with spina bifida and patients with multiple surgeries
Drugs (non-IgE-mediated)	Narcotics, muscle relaxants, beta-lactam antibiotics, vancomycin, and radiocontrast media
NSAIDs	Pseudoallergic and allergic

to latex may cause urticaria in sensitized individuals, namely healthcare and rubber industry workers, patients with spina bifida or those who have undergone multiple surgeries (Sussman and Beezhold 1995).

Drugs can also cause mast cell degranulation through non-IgE-mediated mechanisms. Commonly implicated drugs include narcotics, muscle relaxants, beta-lactam antibiotics, vancomycin and radiocontrast media.

NSAIDs can cause urticaria by two distinct mechanisms: pseudoallergic and allergic. Pseudoallergic reactions are nonimmunologic reactions related to the drug's cyclooxygenase-1 (COX-1)-inhibiting properties (Grattan 2003). As a result, affected individuals will react to both aspirin and COX-1 NSAIDs. Allergic reactions, on the other hand, are IgE-mediated. They are elicited by a specific NSAID in a susceptible individual. Of note, there have been no known cases of IgE-mediated reactions to aspirin.

Chronic Urticaria

Chronic Inducible Urticaria

Chronic inducible urticaria (CIndU) is a type of chronic urticaria that occurs in response to specific triggers, such as heat, cold, friction, pressure, exercise, vibration and sunlight (Magerl et al. 2016). The duration of individual wheals is often brief (minutes to hours), except for delayed-pressure urticaria. Current evidence suggests that IgE binding to the high-affinity IgE receptor (FcεRI) on skin mast cells plays important in the pathogenesis of CIndU (Maurer et al. 2018). Moreover, symptoms can be passively transferred through serum IgE to healthy individuals in cold urticaria, solar urticaria and symptomatic dermatographism. Mast cells may also be activated through IgE-independent pathways. A recent area of interest is the role of transient receptor potential (TRP) channels, a group of ion channels that serve as cellular sensors for a variety of physical and chemical stimuli (Freichel et al. 2012).

Symptomatic dermatographia is the most common CIndU (Maurer et al. 2018). Individuals with this condition develop itchy, linear wheals after firm stroking the skin (Photo 3). Symptomatic dermatographia is clinically distinct from the more common "simple" dermatographia, which involves linear wheals without the itch.

Cold urticaria is the second most frequent CIndU (Maurer et al. 2018). It is characterized by pruritic wheals and/or angioedema after exposure to cold temperatures (Photo 4). Triggers include contact with cold objects, cold liquids and cold air. Wheals typically appear within minutes and can last for one hour. Extensive cold contact (i.e., swimming in cold water) may result in anaphylaxis.

Cholinergic urticaria is characterized by small, 1–3 mm punctate wheals (Photo 5). It is induced by an elevation of core body temperature. Exercise and hot environments are the most common triggers. The lesions are typically short-lived and localized to the trunk and extremities. Cholinergic urticaria must be differentiated from exercise-induced urticaria/anaphylaxis, in which exercise is the only trigger, and passively raising the core body temperature does not induce symptoms.

Exercise-induced urticaria/anaphylaxis is a disorder in which symptoms occur only in association with physical exertion. Symptoms range from flushing and mild hives in the early stage of exercise to life-threatening laryngeal edema and vascular collapse. In a subset of patients, symptoms develop only if exercise takes place within a few hours of eating; in most cases, only if a specific food to which the patient is sensitized to is eaten. This unique disorder is termed food-dependent, exercise-induced anaphylaxis. The foods most implicated are wheat, other grains, shellfish and tree nuts (Beaudouin et al. 2006). Cofactors that can precipitate exercise-induced urticaria/anaphylaxis include infections, NSAIDs, alcohol and stress.

Delayed-pressure urticaria/angioedema is characterized by erythematous swelling of the skin approximately 4–6 hours after the application of pressure. The amount of pressure needed to

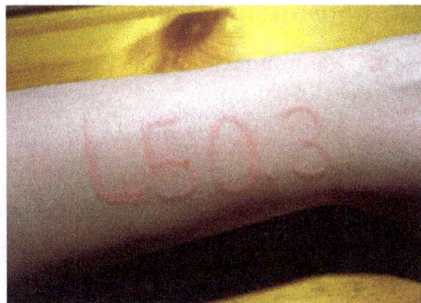

Photo 3. Symptomatic Dermatographia. Source: Mysid, Public domain, via Wikimedia Commons; https://commons. wikimedia.org/wiki/File:Dermatographic_urticaria.jpg.

Photo 4. Cold urticaria. Source: Templeton8012, CC BY-SA 3.0 via Wikimedia Commons; https://commons.wikimedia. org/wiki/File:Cold_urticaria3.jpg.

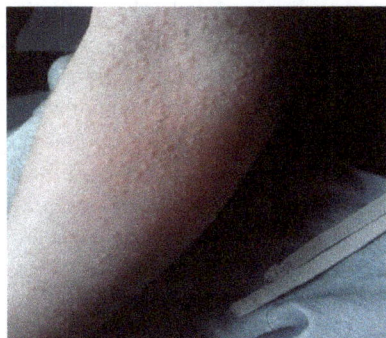

Photo 5. Cholinergic Urticaria. PKeMcG, CC BY 3.0, via Wikimedia Commons; https://commons.wikimedia.org/wiki/ File:WP_20120924_8.jpg.

induce symptoms varies among individuals. Symptoms are often described as burning and pain instead of pruritus, and the swelling may be accompanied by arthralgias (Greaves 2000). Common triggers include wearing tight clothing, sitting for prolonged periods on a hard surface and carrying heavy bags.

More rare forms of CIndU include vibratory, solar and heat. Vibratory urticaria/angioedema involves itching and swelling following a vibratory stimulus. Common triggers include lawn mowing, power tools and horseback riding. Solar urticaria involves urticaria following direct exposure to sunlight. Limited exposure provokes only itching while more prolonged exposure leads to wheals. Heat urticaria involves urticaria following direct contact with a warm stimulus.

Chronic Spontaneous Urticaria

The etiology of CSU is unknown. Two prominent hypotheses are the autoimmune theory and the cellular defect theory.

Autoimmune Theory

Approximately 30–40% of individuals with CSU have serological evidence of IgG autoantibodies against IgE, the high-affinity IgE receptor (FcεR1) or circulating IgE autoantibodies to various self-antigens, such as thyroid peroxidase (TPO) (Kaplan and Greaves 2009). In 1986, Grattan et al. reported a case series of seven out of 12 patients with chronic urticaria in whom autologous serum injected intradermally produced a wheal-and-flare response (Grattan et al. 1986). This became known as the autologous serum skin test (Sabroe et al. 1999). Further evidence in support of the autoimmune theory is based on the increased prevalence of autoimmune disorders among patients with CSU, in particular thyroid disease, vitiligo, rheumatoid arthritis, systemic lupus erythematosus, Sjogren syndrome, celiac disease and Type 1 diabetes mellitus. Antinuclear antibodies are also more prevalent than in the general population.

Cellular Defect Theory

The cellular defect theory proposes that individuals with CSU have defects in basophil trafficking, signaling and function. For example, it has been shown that blood basophils are reduced in patients with CSU, a finding attributed to increased migration of basophils to the skin (Saini 2009). In addition, blood basophils in CSU patients have a reduced ability to release histamine upon IgE receptor activation (Kern and Lichtenstein 1976).

Differential Diagnosis

Several dermatologic conditions can be confused with urticaria. Common mimickers include drug eruptions, atopic dermatitis, contact dermatitis, insect bites, erythema multiforme, bullous pemphigoid, mastocytoma, pityriasis rosea and viral exanthems. A skin punch biopsy should be obtained to rule out urticarial vasculitis whenever individual urticarial lesions persist beyond 24 hours, are painful, have accompanying petechial or purpuric characteristics or leave residual pigmentation (Zuberbier et al. 2022). An elevated CRP/ESR or the presence of systemic symptoms, such as fever or arthralgias, should also raise suspicion for vasculitis.

Urticaria pigmentosa presents with brownish-red cutaneous lesions that become erythematous, pruritic and edematous within 5 minutes after gentle stroking (Photo 6). This physical finding is called Darier's sign (Soter 2000). Urticaria pigmentosa is commonly associated with cutaneous mastocytosis in children, whereas it is commonly associated with systemic mastocytosis in adults.

In patients with isolated angioedema without urticaria, bradykinin-mediated angioedema should be considered. Measurement of complement component 4 (C4) constitutes a good screening test. Low C4 levels should prompt further evaluation for hereditary or acquired C1 inhibitor deficiency.

Diagnostic Investigations

Prior to any investigations, one should first verify that the lesions are truly urticarial in nature, preferably through direct observation, or high-quality photographs. Once the diagnosis of urticaria is confirmed, the duration of symptoms determines the next steps of evaluation.

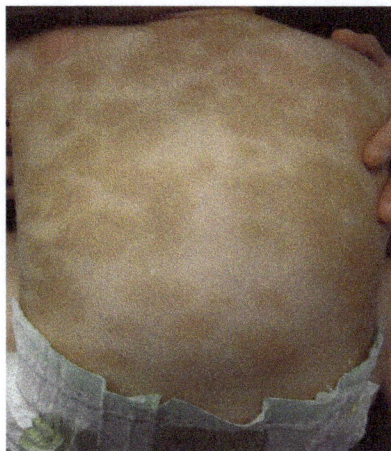

Photo 6. Urticaria Pigmentosa. Source: James Heilman, MD, CC BY-SA 3.0 via Wikimedia Commons; https://commons. wikimedia.org/wiki/File:UriticariaPigmentosa.jpg.

Acute Urticaria (< 6 Weeks)

The evaluation of acute urticaria consists primarily of careful history taking, with an emphasis on trying to identify triggering factors. Routine investigations are "not" recommended due to the short duration and self-limiting nature of the disease. One notable exception is when the clinical history is highly suggestive of an IgE-mediated reaction; in this case, skin testing or allergen-specific IgE testing (if commercially available) of the suspected culprit is appropriate.

For foods, commercial extracts of cow's milk, egg, peanut, tree nuts, soy, fish and shellfish are generally reliable for skin prick tests; in contrast, extracts to fruits and vegetables are often inadequate because the allergen can be labile and altered during processing. In such cases, prick-by-prick testing with fresh foods yields more accurate results. Intradermal skin testing on foods should "never" be performed, as it carries a risk of inducing anaphylaxis.

Unfortunately, the diagnosis of drug allergy is more challenging, as validated skin testing has been established for only a limited number of drugs (penicillin, other beta-lactam antibiotics, neuromuscular blockers and local anesthetics) and *in vitro* tests remain investigational. When interpreting skin tests or allergen-specific IgE tests, one must be mindful that a positive test is only indicative of sensitization, not the allergy. Therefore, obtaining an accurate clinical history is critically important.

Although infections constitute a common cause of acute urticaria, obtaining cultures or serologies is generally not recommended. One notable exception is when a parasitic infection is suspected, in which case stool examination for ova and parasites may be warranted.

Chronic Urticaria (> 6 Weeks)

Chronic Inducible Urticaria

Although clinical history will often suffice to establish the diagnosis of chronic inducible urticaria, provocation testing (Figure 2) and threshold testing (Figure 3) can help confirm the diagnosis and assess disease severity. Prior to testing, oral antihistamines should be discontinued for the appropriate withholding period.

Provocation tests for inducible urticaria

Symptomatic dermographism (Urticaria factitia)

Testsite:	Volar forearm or upper back
Test:	Moderate stroking of the skin with a blunt smooth object (e.g. closed ballpoint pen tip, wooden spatula), dermographic tester (36 g/mm^2), or *FricTest* (longest pin)
Reading time:	10 minutes after testing

W	I

Date / Time _____   Test done by _____

Positive test = wheal & itch: Test trigger strength threshold →

Cold urticaria

Testsite:	Volar forearm
Test:	Melting ice cube in thin plastic bag, *TempTest* (4-44°C) for 5 minutes
Reading times:	10 minutes after testing

W

Date / Time _____   Test done by _____

Positive test = wheal: Test temperature threshold →

Heat urticaria

Testsite:	Volar forearm
Test:	Heat source, *TempTest* (44-4 °C) for 5 minutes
Reading times:	10 minutes after testing

W

Date / Time _____   Test done by _____

Positive test = wheal: Test temperature threshold →

Delayed pressure urticaria

Testsite:	Shoulder or upper back or thighs or volar forearm
Test:	Suspension of weights over shoulder (7 kg, shoulder strap width: 3 cm) for 15 min or weighted rods (1.5 cm diameter: 2.5 kg; or 6.5 cm diameter: 5 kg) for 15 min. Dermographic tester at 100 g/mm^2 for 70 sec
Reading times:	≈6 hours after testing

A	E

Date / Time _____   Test done by _____

Positive test = angio-edema & erythema: Test trigger strength threshold →

Solar urticaria

Testsite:	Buttocks
Test:	UVA 6 J/cm^2 & UVB 60 mJ/cm^2 (e. g. Saalmann Multitester SBC LT 400) & visible light (projector)
Reading times:	10 min after testing

	W
UVA	
UVB	
Visible light	

Date / Time _____   Test done by _____

Positive test = wheal: Test trigger strength threshold (UVA / UVB) →

Vibratory angio-edema

Testsite:	Volar forearm
Test:	Vortex vibrator for 5 minutes, 1000 rpm
Reading times:	10 minutes after testing

A	W

Date / Time _____   Test done by _____

Positive test = angio-edema or wheal

Cholinergic Urticaria

Test 1:	Exercise machine, e.g. bicycle trainer or treadmill. Exercise for 30 min, increase pulse rate by 3 beats/min every minute, **positive test = wheals. If positive, wait > 24 hours and perform**
Test 2:	42 °C bath, monitor body temperature. Continue bath for 15 min after body temperature has increased by ≥ 1°C over baseline
Reading times:	During test as well as immediately and 10 minutes after end of test

Test 1. Exercise	W	How long after begin of test?		Test 2. Hot bath	W
		_____ minutes	→		

Figure 2. Chronic inducible urticaria provocation tests. Source: Magerl et al. 2016.

Symptomatic Dermographism

Provocation testing is commonly performed by stroking the skin with a clean, firm object such as a wooden tongue blade. Commercially available dermographometers provide a more uniform method of testing using defined pressure settings. The FricTest [Moxie, Berlin (Germany)] can simultaneously test four trigger strengths (Photo 7). A test is considered positive if a wheal develops within 10 minutes of provocation.

Threshold tests for inducible urticaria

Symptomatic dermographism (Urticaria factitia)

Testsite: Volar forearm or upper back
Test: Use a dermographometer (e.g. dermographic tester or Fric*Test*)
Reading time: 10 minutes after testing
Threshold: Lowest trigger strength that results in wheal and itch

Fric*Test*	W	I
Pin 1 (shortest)		
Pin 2		
Pin 3		
Pin 4 (longest)		

Dermographic tester	W	I
Minimum trigger strength in g/mm²	___ g/mm²	___ g/mm²

Test done by _____
Date / Time _____

Cold urticaria

Testsite: Volar forearm
Test: Use Temp*Test* for 5 minutes
Reading time: 10 minutes after end of testing
Threshold: Highest temperature that results in wheal

Wheal from 4°C to _____ °C

Test done by _____
Date / Time _____

Heat urticaria

Testsite: Volar forearm
Test: Use Temp*Test* for 5 minutes
Reading time: 10 minutes after end of testing
Threshold: Lowest temperature that results in wheal

Wheal from 44°C to _____ °C

Test done by _____
Date / Time _____

Delayed pressure urticaria

Testsite: Volar forearm (rod) or upper back (dermographic tester)
Test   DPU test device, 15 minutes, diameter of applicator: 6.5 cm,
Reading times: ≈6 hours after testing
Threshold: Rod with lowest weight that results in angio-edema and erythema

kg	A	E
1		
2		
3		
4		
5		

Test done by _____
Date / Time _____

Solar urticaria

Testsite: Buttocks
Test: UVA / UVB irradiation (e.g. Saalmann Multitester SBC LT 400)
Reading times: 10 minutes after testing
Threshold: Lowest dose of irradiation that results in wheal

UVA (J/cm²)	W		UVB (mJ/cm²)	W
2.4			24	
3.3			33	
4.2			42	
5.1			51	
6.0			60	

Test done by _____
Date / Time _____

Figure 3. Chronic inducible urticaria threshold tests. Source: Magerl et al. 2016.

Cold Urticaria

Provocation testing involves placing an ice cube melting in a plastic bag on the volar surface of the forearm for 5 minutes. The test is considered positive if there is a wheal 10 minutes after the removal of the ice cube. Patients with a positive test should subsequently undergo threshold testing

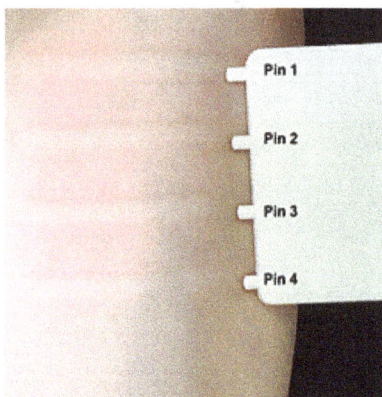

Photo 7. FricTest Dermographometer. Source: https://medelink.ca/product/frictest-4/.

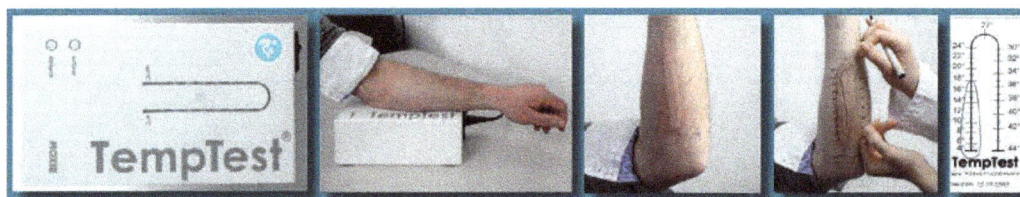

Photo 8. TempTest. Source: https://medelink.ca/allergy/sub-page-temptest/.

if possible. This is performed via the TempTest [Courage and Khazaka in Cologne (Germany)], an element-based temperature exposure device that provides a continuous gradient of temperatures ranging from 4 to 44°C (Photo 8).

Cholinergic Urticaria and Exercise-Induced Urticaria/Anaphylaxis

Provocation testing helps confirm the diagnosis of cholinergic urticaria and distinguish it from exercise-induced urticaria/anaphylaxis. The first step involves an exercise challenge (treadmill or stationary bicycle) sufficiently intense to cause sweating for at least 15 minutes. The test is considered positive if it results in hives. In such a case, the next step is to perform a passive heat challenge to exclude exercise-induced anaphylaxis. The patient's body is placed in a hot water bath (42°C) until the core body temperature rises by 1°C. A positive test for both the exercise challenge and passive heat challenge is diagnostic of cholinergic urticaria, whereas a positive test for only the exercise challenge is diagnostic of exercise-induced urticaria/anaphylaxis.

Delayed-Pressure Urticaria/Angioedema

The traditional provocation test is the "sandbag test," where a 15-lb sandbag is attached to a strap and hung from the shoulder for 15 minutes. The site is then observed for the next 24 hours for evidence of erythematous swelling. In research settings, weighted rods or a dermographometer are used instead.

Heat Urticaria

Provocation testing is conducted by applying a test tube containing warm water at 44°C to the volar forearm for 5 minutes. The test is considered positive if a wheal develops within a few minutes after the removal of the heated object.

Solar Urticaria

Provocation testing involves placing light sources that emit specific wavelengths of ultraviolet A and ultraviolet B 10 to 15 cm from the patient's back or buttocks. Clinical response is assessed every 10 minutes for up to an hour. Most patients with solar urticaria react to a specific wavelength.

Vibratory Urticaria/Angioedema

A vortex mixer is placed in contact with the patient's forearm for 5 minutes at 1,000 rpm. The test is considered positive if the area becomes erythematous, pruritic and edematous.

Chronic Spontaneous Urticaria

A comprehensive clinical history is crucial to the diagnostic evaluation of CSU. This includes associated signs and symptoms, duration of individual lesions and accompanying angioedema. Before establishing the diagnosis of CSU, one must exclude the possibility of a more serious systemic disease. Potential red flags include fever, weight loss, arthralgias, abdominal pain and bone pain.

Certain triggers can aggravate CSU in a subset of patients. These include physical factors, NSAIDs, alcohol, stress and concomitant infections. In addition, some patients report aggravation of symptoms with spicy or fermented foods. This may be related to the histamine content or histamine-releasing properties of these foods.

Considering that the etiology of CSU is unknown in most cases, extensive investigations are not recommended. Nonetheless, a limited workup consisting of CBC with differential, ESR/CRP and TSH may be considered to rule out certain underlying causes (Zuberbier et al. 2022; Bernstein et al. 2014). For example, eosinophilia should prompt evaluation for a parasitic infection. Significant elevations in ESR or CRP should prompt investigation for a rheumatological, infectious or neoplastic disease. An abnormal TSH should prompt evaluation for thyroid disease. In contrast to acute urticaria, skin testing and allergen-specific IgE testing are not indicated, as chronic urticaria is rarely caused by IgE-mediated reactions.

Investigational Tests

Investigational tests include the autologous serum skin test (ASST), tests of basophil activation and assays for antibodies to IgE or the high-affinity mast cell receptor (FcεR1α). The validity of these tests has not been fully established, therefore they are not recommended outside of research settings.

ASST

The ASST is an *in vivo* test to detect basophil histamine-releasing activity from the patient's serum. It involves intradermally injecting a patient with his/her serum. A wheal-and-flare reaction at the site of injection within 30 minutes constitutes a positive test (Grattan et al. 1986). However, its clinical usefulness remains doubtful. For example, one study found positive ASSTs in 56% of healthy controls (Taskapan et al. 2008). In addition, the positivity of the ASST persists in patients with CSU, even when their disorder is in clinical remission (Fusari et al. 2005). Finally, the ASST has not demonstrated clinical utility in identifying patients who respond differently to treatment (Lapolla et al. 2012).

Basophil Histamine Release Assay (BHRA)

The basophil histamine release assay is an *in vitro* test in which a patient's serum is incubated with donor basophils. The cells are centrifuged, and the supernatant is recovered. Using a quantitative enzyme immunoassay, histamine released into the supernatant is measured and compared to normal control. A greater histamine release implies that the patient has an autoimmune basis for the urticaria.

Basophil Activation Test (BAT)

The basophil activation test is an *in vitro* test that uses flow cytometry to assess donor basophil activation markers (CD63 or CD203c) in response to stimulation with the patient's serum. A positive basophil test has been linked to longer disease duration, higher disease activity and a poor response to both antihistamines and omalizumab (Iqbal et al. 2012). However, the utility of this test is limited by several technical challenges. First, basophils from individual donors vary in response to the same serum over time. Second, different laboratories using different basophil donors will yield different results. Third, there are no standardized procedures for handling basophils.

Assessment of Disease Activity, Impact and Control

Urticaria, both acute and chronic, can be debilitating. Therefore, periodic assessments should be made to evaluate disease activity, its impact on quality of life and disease control. Validated patient-reported outcome measures, such as the Urticaria Activity Score (UAS7), the Angioedema Activity Score (AAS), the Urticaria Control Test (UCT) and the Angioedema Control Test (AECT) can be used for this purpose.

UAS7 is a daily personal assessment of both wheals and pruritus measured on a scale of 0–3 over seven consecutive days. AAS assesses daily angioedema activity, scored from 0–15. Patients who experience hives and angioedema should use UAS7 and AAS in combination (Figure 4).

To assess disease control, the UCT is used in patients who experience hives (Figure 5A). It is a four-item questionnaire scored 0–4 with a recall period of 4 weeks. A score of < 12 is indicative of poor control whereas a score of ≥ 12 is indicative of good control. For patients who experience angioedema, the AECT should be used (Figure 5B). A score of < 10 is indicative of poor control

Urticaria activity score (UAS)		
Score	**Wheals**	**Pruritus**
0	None	None
1	Mild (<20 wheals/24 h)	Mild (present but not annoying or troublesome)
2	Moderate (20–50 wheals/24 h)	Moderate (troublesome but does not interfere with normal daily activity or sleep)
3	Intense (>50 wheals/24 h or large confluent areas of wheals)	Intense (severe pruritus, which is sufficiently troublesome to interfere with normal daily activity or sleep)
Angioedema Activity Score (AAS)		
Score	**Dimension**	**Answer options**
–	Have you had a swelling episode in the last 24 h?	No, yes
0–3	At what time(s) of day was this swelling episode(s) present? (please select all applicable times)	Midnight–8 a.m., 8 a.m.–4 p.m., 4 p.m.–midnight
0–3	How severe is / was the physical discomfort caused by this swelling episode(s) (eg, pain, burning, itching?)	No discomfort, slight discomfort, moderate discomfort, severe discomfort
0–3	Are / were you able to perform your daily activities during this swelling episode(s)?	No restriction, slight restriction, severe restriction, no activities possible
0–3	Do / did you feel your appearance is / was adversely affected by this swelling episode(s)?	No, slightly, moderately, severely
0–3	How would you rate the overall severity of this swelling episode?	Negligible, mild, moderate, severe

Note: For the UAS7, the sum of the score (0–3 for wheals +0–3 for pruritis) for each day is summarized over one week (7 days) for a maximum of 42. For the AAS, scores are summed up to an AAS day sum score (0–15). 7 AAS day sum scores to an AAS week sum score (AAS7, 0–105), and 4 ASS week sum scores may be summed up to an AAS 4-week sum score (AAS28, 0–420). Copyright for UAS: GA²LEN; copyright for AAS (UK version): MOXIE GmbH (www.moxie-gmbh.de).

Figure 4. The urticaria activity score (UAS) and AAS for assessing disease activity in CSU. Source: Zuberbier et al. 2022.

(A) **Urticaria Control Test**

Patient name: ______________________ Date: (dd mmm yyyy): ___ ___ ___

Date of birth (dd mmm yyyy): ___ ___ ___

Instructions: You have urticaria. The following questions should help us understand your current health situation. Please read through each question carefully and choose an answer from the five options that *best fits* your situation. Please limit yourself to *the last four weeks. Please don't think about the questions for a long time*, and do remember to answer *all questions* and to provide *only one answer to each question.*

1. How much have you suffered from the **physical symptoms of the urticaria (itch, hives (welts) and/or swelling)** in the last four weeks?

   O very much   O much   O somewhat   O a little   O not at all

2. How much was your **quality of life** affected by the urticaria in the last 4 weeks?

   O very much   O much   O somewhat   O a little   O not at all

3. How often was the **treatment** for your urticaria in the last 4 weeks **not enough** to control your urticaria symptoms?

   O very often   O often   O sometimes   O seldom   O not at all

4. **Overall**, how well have you had your urticaria **under control** in the last 4 weeks?

   O not at all   O a little   O somewhat   O well   O very well

(B) **Angioedema Control Test**

(AECT)

Patient name: ______________________ Date: (dd mmm yyyy): ___ ___ ___

Date of birth (dd mmm yyyy): ___ ___ ___

Instructions: You have recurrent swelling referred to as angioedema. Angioedema is a temporary swelling of the skin or mucous membranes which can occur in any part of the body but most commonly involves the lips, eyes, tongue, hands and feet and which can last from hours to days. Some patients develop abdominal angioedema, which is often not visible but painful. Some forms of swelling can also be associated with hives also known as urticaria.

The following four questions assess your current state of health. For each question, please choose the answer from the five options that *best fits your situation*. Please answer *all questions* and please provide *only one answer to each question.*

1. In the last 4 weeks, how often have you had angioedema?

   O very often   O often   O sometimes   O seldom   O not at all

2. In the last 4 weeks, how much has your quality of life been affected by angioedema?

   O very much   O much   O somewhat   O a little   O not at all

3. In the last 4 weeks, how much has the unpredictability of your angioedema bothered you?

   O very much   O much   O somewhat   O a little   O not at all

4. In the last 4 weeks, how well has your angioedema been controlled by your therapy?

   O not at all   O a little   O somewhat   O well   O very well

Figure 5. (A) The UCT and (B) The AECT. Source: Zuberbier et al. 2022.

whereas a score of ≥ 10 is indicative of good control. Patients who experience both hives and angioedema should use UCT and AECT in combination.

Treatment

Basic Considerations

The treatment of acute and chronic urticaria is the same, regardless of whether hives, angioedema or both are involved. The primary goal is to achieve complete symptom control and normalize the quality of life. This is achieved by first providing reassurance and education. It is important to convey to patients that urticaria and angioedema are self-limited in most cases and rarely associated with a serious underlying disease. Although there is no definite cure, symptoms can be adequately controlled with pharmacotherapy in most cases. Triggering or exacerbating factors should be minimized to the extent possible. These include physical factors, NSAIDs, alcohol, stress and concomitant infections.

Pharmacotherapy

Current EAACI/GA²LEN/EDF/WAO guidelines propose a stepwise treatment algorithm (Figure 6) (Zuberbier et al. 2022). The overall goal of these treatments is to achieve complete symptom control. Consequently, pharmacological treatment should be continuous rather than on demand. However, symptoms should be reassessed at least once every 3–6 months, and treatment adjusted accordingly.

Second-Generation H1-Antihistamine

Initial treatment consists of a nonsedating, second-generation H1 antihistamine at a standard therapeutic dose. Examples include loratadine, desloratadine, fexofenadine, cetirizine and levocetirizine. Individual responses to a given antihistamine may vary. First-generation antihistamines are no longer recommended, as they possess anticholinergic and sedative effects, and can negatively impact REM sleep and school/work performance.

If the standard dose is not effective after 2–4 weeks of continuous use, a four-fold dose escalation is recommended before other treatments are considered. In this situation, twice-daily dosing is preferred. Combining different second-generation H1-antihistamines is not recommended. Although medications are best avoided during pregnancy and breastfeeding, there have been no reports to date of second-generation antihistamines causing birth defects.

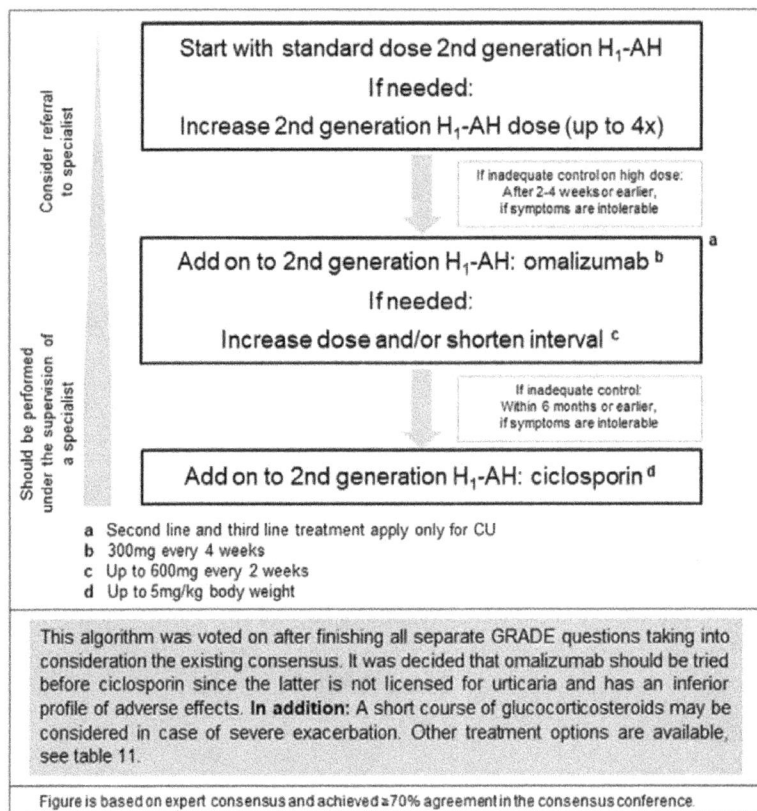

Figure 6. Recommended treatment algorithm for urticaria. Source: Zuberbier et al. 2022.

Omalizumab

Omalizumab, a monoclonal anti-IgE antibody, is approved in most countries for the treatment of chronic urticaria in patients ≥ 12 yrs of age who experience insufficient benefit from 2nd generation H1-antihistamine therapy. A meta-analysis of seven randomized trials involving 1,312 patients demonstrated a significant reduction in weekly itch and wheal scores with omalizumab relative to placebo in patients unresponsive to H1-antihistamines (Zhao et al. 2016). Analyses of different doses showed that 300 mg every 4 weeks was the most effective dose, at which 36% of patients achieved a complete response (UAS7 score of 0). However, omalizumab does not have long-term disease-modifying properties, therefore patients may relapse when omalizumab is tapered or discontinued.

The recommended initial dose is 300 mg subcutaneously every 4 weeks, independent of total serum IgE and body weight. Second-generation H1 antihistamine therapy is continued but may be tapered if the patient responds well to omalizumab. As omalizumab carries a small risk of anaphylaxis (0.2%), patients are advised to carry an epinephrine autoinjector, and the first three doses are administered in a medical facility where patients are generally monitored for 2 hours.

Patients who are inadequately controlled at the licensed dose of 300 mg every 4 weeks can be treated with higher doses, shorter intervals, or both. Studies support the use of omalizumab treatment at doses of up to 600 mg every 2 weeks (Metz et al. 2020). The use of omalizumab in pregnancy appears to be safe, and to date, there is no indication of teratogenicity.

Cyclosporine

For patients who do not achieve adequate disease control with a combination of high-dose H1 antihistamines and omalizumab or for patients who do not have access to omalizumab, the calcineurin inhibitor cyclosporine is the preferred next step. It acts by blocking the calcium-dependent release of histamine, leukotrienes and other mast cell mediators. Advantages include a rapid onset of action, a degree of efficacy comparable with systemic corticosteroids and the possibility of lasting remission after treatment is discontinued. Disadvantages include the potential for hypertension, renal insufficiency, hirsutism and gingival hyperplasia, although these side effects are less common at lower doses.

The recommended dose is 3.5–5 mg/kg per day. Blood pressure, blood urea nitrogen and creatinine should be monitored monthly, while cyclosporine and fasting lipids should be obtained at baseline and then yearly. After 3 months of complete or near-complete control of symptoms, the dose of cyclosporine is generally tapered over several months. In most cases, 6–9 months of treatment is adequate. Although not teratogenic, cyclosporine is embryo-toxic in animal models and is associated with preterm delivery and low birth weight in human infants. Therefore, the benefits vs. risks in pregnant women need to be considered on a case-by-case basis.

Systemic Corticosteroids

Systemic corticosteroids may be used short-term to gain temporary control of symptoms during severe exacerbations, especially if the quality of life is significantly affected. The typical dose of Prednisone is 20–50 mg daily for 5–10 days. Long-term corticosteroid use is discouraged due to potential side effects. Topical corticosteroids have not been shown to be beneficial.

Other Treatments

The level of evidence for leukotriene receptor antagonists, H2-antagonists and Doxepin is low and therefore is no longer included in the EAACI/GA²LEN/EDF/WAO guidelines. However, these drugs may still be of value to individual patients in the appropriate clinical context.

Glossary of Abbreviations

AAS – Angioedema Activity Score
ASST – Autologous Serum Skin Test
AECT – Angioedema Control Test
BAT – Basophil Activation Test
BHRA – Basophil Histamine Release Assay
CIndU – Chronic Inducible Urticaria
COX-1 – Cyclooxygenase-1
C4 – Complement Component 4
CSU – Chronic Spontaneous Urticaria
EAACI – European Academy of Allergology and Clinical Immunology
EDF – European Dermatology Forum
FcεR1 – High-Affinity IgE Receptor
GA²LEN – Global Allergy and Asthma European Network
NSAID – Non-Steroidal Anti-Inflammatory Drug
TPO – Thyroid Peroxidase
TRP – Transient Receptor Potential
UAS7 – Urticaria Activity Score
UCT – Urticaria Control Test
WAO – World Allergy Organization

References

Beaudouin, E., Renaudin, J. M., Morisset, M., Codreanu, F., Kanny, G. and Moneret-Vautrin, D. A. 2006. Food-dependent exercise-induced anaphylaxis—update and current data. Eur. Ann. Allergy Clin. Immunol. 38(2): 45.

Ben-Shoshan, M., Blinderman, I. and Raz, A. 2013. Psychosocial factors and chronic spontaneous urticaria: a systematic review. Allergy 68: 131–141.

Bernstein, J. A., Lang, D. M., Khan, D. A., Craig, T., Dreyfus, D., Hsieh, F. et al. 2014. The diagnosis and management of acute and chronic urticaria: 2014 update. J. Allergy Clin. Immunol. 133: 1270–1277.

Freichel, M., Almering, J. and Tsvilovskyy, V. 2012. The role of TRP proteins in mast cells. Front Immunol. 3: 150.

Fusari, A., Colangelo, C., Bonifazi, F. and Antonicelli, L. 2005. The autologous serum skin test in the follow-up of patients with chronic urticaria. Allergy 60(2): 256.

Grattan, C. E., Wallington, T. B., Warin, R. P., Kennedy, C. T. and Bradfield, J. W. 1986. A serological mediator in chronic idiopathic urticaria—a clinical, immunological, and histological evaluation. Br. J. Dermatol. 114(5): 583–90.

Grattan, C. E. 2003. Aspirin sensitivity and urticaria. Clin. Exp. Dermatol. 28: 123–7.

Greaves, M. W. 1995. Chronic urticaria. N Engl. J. Med. 332: 1767–72.

Greaves, M. W. 2000. Chronic urticaria. J. Allergy Clin. Immunol. 105(4): 664.

Imbalzano, E., Casciaro, M., Quartuccio, S., Minciullo, P. L., Cascio, A., Calapai, G. et al. 2016. Association between urticaria and virus infections: A systematic review. Allergy Asthma Proc. 37(1): 18.

Iqbal, K., Bhargava, K., Skov, P. S., Falkencrone, S. and Grattan, C. E. 2012. A positive serum basophil histamine release assay is a marker for ciclosporin-responsiveness in patients with chronic spontaneous urticaria. Clin. Transl. Allergy 2: 19.

Kaplan, A. P. 2002. Clinical practice. Chronic urticaria and angioedema. N Engl. J. Med. 346(3): 175–9.

Kaplan, A. P. 2004. Chronic urticaria: pathogenesis and treatment. J. Allergy Clin. Immunol. 114(3): 465–74.

Kaplan, A. P. and Greaves, M. 2009. Pathogenesis of chronic urticaria. Clin. Exp. Allergy 39: 777–87.

Kern, F. and Lichtenstein, L. M. 1976. Defective histamine release in chronic urticaria. J. Clin. Invest. 57: 1369–77.

Lapolla, W., Desai, N. and English, J. C. 2012. Clinical utility of testing for autoimmunity in chronic idiopathic urticaria. J. Am. Acad. Dermatol. 66(3): 83.

Magerl, M., Altrichter, S., Borzova, E., Gimenez-Arnau, A., Grattan, C., Lawlor, F. et al. 2016. The definition, diagnostic testing, and management of chronic inducible urticarias - The EAACI/GA²LEN/EDF/UNEV consensus recommendations 2016 update and revision. Allergy 71(6): 780–802.

Maurer, M., Fluhr, J. W. and Khan, D. A. 2018. How to approach chronic inducible urticaria. J. Allergy Clin. Immunol. Pract. 6(4): 1119–1130.

Metz, M., Vadasz, Z., Kocatürk, E. and Giménez-Arnau, A. M. 2020. Omalizumab updosing in chronic spontaneous urticaria: an overview of real-world evidence. Clin. Rev. Allergy Immunol. 59(1): 38–45.

Minciullo, P. L., Cascio, A., Barberi, G. and Gangemi, S. 2014. Urticaria and bacterial infections. Allergy Asthma Proc. 35(4): 295.

Mortureux, P., Léauté-Labrèze, C., Legrain-Lifermann, V., Lamireau, T., Sarlangue, J. and Taïeb, A. 1998. Acute urticaria in infancy and early childhood: a prospective study. Arch Dermatol. 134(3): 319.

O'Donnell, B., Lawlor, F., Simpson, J., Morgan, M. and Greaves, M. 1997. The impact of chronic urticaria on the quality of life. Br J. Dermatol. 136: 197–201.

Orfan, N. A. and Kolski, G. B. 1993. Physical urticarias. Ann. Allergy 71(3): 205.

Sabroe, R. A., Grattan, C. E., Francis, D. M. et al. 1999. The autologous serum skin test: a screening test for autoantibodies in chronic idiopathic urticaria. Br J. Dermatol. 140: 446.

Sackesen, C., Sekerel, B. E., Orhan, F., Kocabas, C. N., Tuncer, A. and Adalioglu, G. 2014. The etiology of different forms of urticaria in childhood. Pediatr. Dermatol. 21(2): 102.

Saini, S. S. 2009. Basophil responsiveness in chronic urticaria. Curr. Allergy Asthma Rep. 9: 286–90.

Saini, S. S. 2014. Urticaria and angioedema. pp. 575–587. *In*: Adkinson, N. F., Bochner, B. S., Burks, A. W., Busse, W. W., Holgate, S. T., Lemanske, R. F. et al. (eds.). Middleton's Allergy: Principles & Practice, 8th Edition. Elsevier, Mosby. Philadelphia, USA.

Soter, N. A. 2000. Mastocytosis and the skin. Hematol. Oncol. Clin. North Am. 14(3): 537.

Sussman, G. L. and Beezhold, D. H. 1995. Allergy to latex rubber. Ann. Intern. Med. 122(1): 43.

Taskapan, O., Kutlu, A. and Karabudak, O. 2008. Evaluation of autologous serum skin test results in patients with chronic idiopathic urticaria, allergic/non-allergic asthma or rhinitis and healthy people. Clin. Exp. Dermatol. 33(6): 754.

Wang, J. and Sampson. H. A. 2011. Food allergy. J. Clin. Invest. Mar; 121(3): 827–35.

Ying, S., Kikuchi, Y., Meng, Q., Kay, A. B. and Kaplan A. P. 2002. TH1/TH2 cytokines and inflammatory cells in skin biopsy specimens from patients with chronic idiopathic urticaria: comparison with the allergen-induced late-phase cutaneous reaction. J. Allergy Clin. Immunol. 109(4): 694.

Zhao, Z. T., Ji, C. M., Yu, W. J., Meng, L., Hawro, T., Wei, J. F. et al. 2016. Omalizumab for the treatment of chronic spontaneous urticaria: A meta-analysis of randomized clinical trials. J. Allergy Clin. Immunol. 137(6): 1742.

Zuberbier, T., Abdul A. H., Abuzakouk, M., Aquilina, S., Asero, R., Baker, D. et al. 2022. The international EAACI/GA²LEN/EuroGuiDerm/APAAACI guideline for the definition, classification, diagnosis, and management of urticaria. Allergy 77(3): 734–766.

Chapter 6

Allergic Contact Dermatitis and Atopic Dermatitis

Luz Fonacier, * *Hope Jin, Jake Rosenblum* and *Sonam Sani*

∞∞

Basics of Patch Testing

PT is the gold standard procedure for diagnosing ACD and identifying the contact allergen responsible for dermatitis. PT involves applying allergens to the patient's back for 48 hours in order to determine if the patient develops a reaction. The use of PT in various clinical scenarios will be discussed. There is much to be learned regarding the epidemiology and pathophysiology of CD; however, this chapter will focus on the procedural aspect of CD, which is the patch test. Indications, protocols, special populations and pearls for PT will be reviewed as well.

Introduction

Overview of Allergic Contact Dermatitis

Contact dermatitis is an inflammatory skin disorder that is characterized by erythema, edema, vesicles, hyperkeratosis and fissuring. Patients may present with complaints of associated pain, itch and swelling. Such clinical manifestations vary depending on the chronicity of dermatitis, as the condition may be acute, subacute or chronic. CD is caused by exposure to an allergen or irritant, leading to ACD and ICD, respectively. ICD accounts for approximately 80% of all occupational dermatitis, whereas ACD is less common (Litchman et al. 2022). ICD is a localized, non-immunologic inflammatory response to a substance that results in direct cellular cytotoxicity; while ACD, in contrast, is classified as type IV cell-mediated delayed hypersensitivity reaction in which prior sensitization to an allergen is needed in order to elicit a reaction upon re-exposure to the allergen (Bolognia 2022). CD is the most common cause of occupational dermatitis and represents a significant amount of physical and psychosocial burden (Nicholson et al. 2010).

Indications for Patch Testing

PT should be considered in patients with acute or chronic eczematous dermatitis with features including erythema, edema, weeping, crusting, scaling or lichenification (Johansen et al. 2015). Avoidance of suspected allergens may lead to improvement in dermatitis; however, identification of the specific allergen can increase options available to patients and lead to improved outcomes

NYU Langone, Mineola NY, USA.
* Corresponding author: luz.fonacier@nyulangone.org

(Fonacier and Noor 2018). Thorough histories should be elicited from each patient in order to determine occupational, environmental and other potential exposures to allergens. Patients with dermatitis and significant exposures should be considered for patch testing. Other indications are patients with dermatitis in generalized or regional areas of interest, such as the face, neck, hands, periumbilical area, and feet and those with dermatitis recalcitrant to conventional therapies (i.e., topical corticosteroids (TCS) and topical non-steroidal immunomodulatory treatments). Consider PT in AD patients who have dermatitis that worsens, changes distribution, fails to improve or immediately rebounds. Other AD considerations that should invoke consideration of PT are atypical distribution, such as head predominance, hand or foot, eyelid predominance, cheilitis/perioral predominance, therapy-resistant hand eczema, adult- or adolescent-onset AD without childhood eczema or severe/widespread dermatitis prior to initiating systemic immunosuppressant or biologics. Thus, the indications for PT are broad and should be considered in patients with localized or diffuse, acute, subacute or chronic, pruritic, eczematous, vesicular or lichenified dermatitis where the clinician has a strong suspicion of ACD.

Special Populations

Children

Children are a particular demographic of interest as one can develop ACD at any age. As with any patient, a thorough history is important and should be tailored to the patient's age (diapers and baby powders in younger children vs. hobbies/sports in older children). Children with persistent AD that worsens despite standard therapy and late-onset AD are candidates for PT. Children with comorbid AD may be sensitized to allergens, such as cocamide DEA, lanolin and TCS found in many eczema treatments (Neale et al. 2021). PT remains the gold standard for diagnosing ACD in children and is a safe procedure for pediatric patients. Currently, there is no FDA-approved PT device for children under the age of 6. However, it has been suggested that in children younger than age 6, if PT is at all needed based on clinical history, certain allergens be diluted to avoid irritation and false positive reactions (Fisher et al. 2019; Jacob et al. 2017). Table 1 lists a recommended limited panel for patch testing in children 6–12 years of age. The limited surface area in pediatric patients translates to a greater emphasis on considering relevance prior to proceeding with PT. Additionally, providers can consider using the thigh or abdominal area to increase the available surface area for PT (Tam and Yu 2020). In general, children over the age of 12 can be tested similarly to adults.

Table 1. Patch test recommendations for children 6–12 years of age (Jacob et al. 2008).

Primary Allergens				Secondary Allergens	
1	Bacitracin	11	Fragrance mix 1	1	Black rubber mix
2	Budesonide	12	Fragrance mix 2	2	Dialkyl thioureas
3	Carba mix	13	Lanolin alcohol	3	Mercaptobenzothiazole
4	Cobalt chloride	14	MCI/MI	4	Para-phenylenediamine
5	Cocamidopropyl betaine	15	Myroxylon pereirae (Balsam of Peru)	5	p-tert Butylphenol formaldehyde resin
6	Colophonium	16	Neomycin sulfate		
7	Compositae mix/dandelion extract	17	Nickel sulfate		
8	Disperse blue	18	Potassium dichromate		
9	Ethylenediamine	19	Quaternium 15		
10	Formaldehyde	20	Tixocortol-1-pivalate		

Jacob, S. E., Brod, B. and Crawford, G. H. 2008. Clinically relevant patch test reactions in children—the United States-based study. Pediatr. Dermatol. 2008 Sep.–Oct.; 25(5): 520–7.*

Pregnancy

While there is no absolute contraindication to PT in pregnancy and breastfeeding, postponing PT until after delivery or completion of breastfeeding is advised (Ingber 2014). However, bothersome symptoms may be, PT is never an emergency and can always wait for more optimal PT conditions.

Biomedical Devices: Metal and Cement Allergy

Metal is a common allergic sensitizer, and nickel is consistently found to be the most common cause of ACD worldwide. Hypersensitivity reactions to implanted prosthetic devices are possible and can have varied presentations including implant failure. More common causes of implant malfunction, such as mechanical failure and infection should always be ruled out prior. Currently, there is a lack of evidence to support the risk-stratification of patients for hypersensitivity to cement or metals. Moreover, there is data to suggest that individuals who have undergone joint implantations have a higher frequency of positive patch tests compared to the general population; yet the connection of positive sensitization to clinical outcome remains unknown (Granchi et al. 2008). Therefore, pre-operative PT is not recommended in those without a history concerning metal, bone cement or adhesive hypersensitivity. Post-implantation PT can be considered in those with dermatitis/rash near the site of prosthetic implantation or after implant failure when more likely etiologies have been ruled out (Pacheco 2019).

Limitations of Patch Testing

Contraindications to Patch Testing

PT is not appropriate in the setting of active generalized exanthematous or erythrodermic eruptions until the underlying dermatitis is controlled. In addition, it is prudent to rule out other potential causes of acute generalized presentations, such as drug eruption or mycosis fungoides. As PT is performed on the patient's back, it is important to be able to discern positive results from background skin changes, including extensive tattoos. Patients, with widely prevalent dermatitis or substantial eczema, compromising the surface area of the back are not good candidates for PT and should first obtain control of their dermatitis. Similarly, patients with significant actinic damage or sunburn on the back may not be ideal candidates for PT. Patients with substantial thick, dark hair on the back need non-irritating hair removal performed 1–2 days prior to the test. PT requires multiple follow-up visits in a specific time frame, thus patients need to work these visits into their schedule. Also, excessive sweating and physical activity must be avoided while the patches are on to prevent dislodging them.

Immunosuppressant agents (such as systemic corticosteroids, cyclosporine or other immunosuppressive agents) can interfere with PT results. Studies have shown that doses of prednisone less than 20 mg per day and low doses of cyclosporine (2–3 mg/kg/day) may still yield clinically relevant PT results (Anveden et al. 2004). It is recommended to avoid the application of TCS and topical calcineurin inhibitors to the PT site for 5–7 days before testing (Prens et al. 1989). In addition, patients should avoid excessive sun exposure 2–4 weeks before the application of a patch test, as ultraviolet radiation can reduce the allergic response (Damian and Halliday 2002).

Special Precautions/Complications of PT

PT is considered to be a generally safe procedure; however, in rare instances, it can be associated with complications. Most adverse effects are due to testing errors, such as using irritant products, too high a concentration of test substance and/or leaving the PT panels on for a prolonged period

(Fisher et al. 2019). Active sensitization, although rare, has been reported (Jensen et al. 2006). Irritant reactions to adhesive tapes are common and tend to resolve quickly. Other complications include a flare of existing dermatitis, as well as hypopigmentation and hyperpigmentation of the skin. Although exceedingly rare, case reports of anaphylactic reactions have been reported after testing with topical antibiotics, nitrogen mustard and latex (Schmidlin et al. 2020).

Utility and Patch Test Methodology

Allergen Sources

There are several PT panels available, including standard panels as well as expanded series. The T.R.U.E. (Thin-layer Rapid Use Epicutaneous) Test® is approved for ages 6 and above and consists of 35 allergens and one negative control preloaded onto chambers. The T.R.U.E. Test® is currently the only FDA-approved PT panel in the United States. While it is easy to apply, its limitation is in the preloaded allergens and so testing cannot be individualized for specific patients. A particular study concluded that 30–40% of causative allergens may be missed with the use of the T.R.U.E. Test® as compared to the use of the North American Contact Dermatitis Group (NACDG) panel described below (DeKoven et al. 2021).

Chamber testing is the alternative to T.R.U.E. Test® and can be done with any number of allergens. The NACDG series consists of 65–80 allergens that are individually loaded into testing chambers. This gives physicians flexibility and the ability to tailor PT to individual patients, potentially adding allergens (such as a metals series) from an extended series if thought to be relevant.

Process of PT

PT is prepared by placing allergens into chambers that can be round or square, mounted on rectangular strips of adhesive in two rows of five chambers each (10 total) per strip of adhesive. Loading chambers come in various sizes, depths and materials. Square chambers and round chambers are comparable, and no chamber is known to be superior to others (Schmidlin et al. 2020). Most allergens are dispersed in a standard concentration petrolatum solution syringe; a small minority are delivered in liquid vehicles packaged in either syringes or dropper bottles (Fisher et al. 2019). The majority of PT allergens should be stored in the refrigerator to maintain the stability of the allergen.

Loading the Chambers

Petrolatum-based allergens are loaded directly into the chamber. The ideal volume is 20 microliters, meaning just greater than 50% of the chamber should be filled with an allergen (Fisher et al. 2019). In an 8 mm Finn chamber, it is about a ribbon of the commercially available standardized allergen from rim to rim. For allergens in liquid form, one drop of mixture is placed into the chamber and is usually sufficient to saturate the chamber (Figure 1). Using a patients own products can optimize the diagnosis of ACD, especially in facial, eyelid and lip dermatitis. Personal products can be placed into individual chambers in suggested concentrations as described in Table 2. PT chambers should ideally be loaded at the time they are applied. Substances in aqueous vehicles should be loaded into chambers as close to the application as possible to prevent drying (Joy et al. 2013). Most allergens in petrolatum vehicles may be prepared 24 to 48 hours before the application if desired. Exceptions include acrylates and fragrances, which should not be preloaded and should be prepared at the time of the visit and applied to the skin immediately.

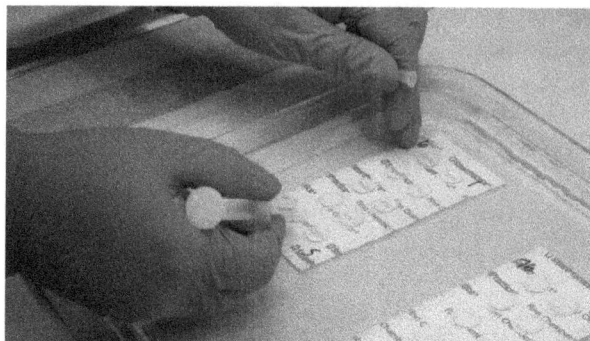

Figure 1. Loading the PT chambers.

Table 2. Guidelines for patch testing selected products.

Product	Concentration	Vehicle
Make-up: nonvolatile (e.g., foundation, powder, eye shadow, eye-liner, moisturizer and antiperspirant)	As is	
Make-up: -volatile (e.g., mascara; after-shave lotion)	Apply to the chamber and wait 5 min before application	dry
Hair spray	As is	dry
Shampoo; soap	Doubtful value, test ingredients	
Perfume; cologne; toilet water	Apply to the chamber and wait 5 min before application	dry
Nail polish	Paint on the chamber as is and allow it to dry for at least 15 min	dry
Skin care preparations (body/hand cream; moisturizers; night cream)	As is	
Baby products (e.g., cream; powder; lotion; oil)	As is	
Topical medications (e.g., antibacterial; corticosteroids)	As is; 20%	
Clothing; shoes; gloves	2 × 2 cm moisten in saline, minimum 10mm punch	
Foods • cauliflower; clove; spice; fruit • garlic	As is; 50%	
Household and industrial products should only be tested after determining their safety from material safety data sheet information and using non-irritating patch test concentrations based on an authoritative text	Refer to Occupational Health Care Professional	

Alternative Techniques

The "use test" may be helpful for leaving on products that are strongly suspicious to be causing ACD. The product is applied the same way as when dermatitis developed albeit in a more limited surface area, such as facial products applied daily to a small area of the face (Fonacier 2014). An additional technique that may be employed for personal care products and cosmetics is the "repeat open application test" (ROAT). This process entails applying a product twice a day for 7–14 days to a select area on the forearm, usually two finger-breadths away from the antecubital fossa, while observing for the development of dermatitis. If dermatitis develops, often between days 2–4, the test can be stopped and considered positive (Schmidlin et al. 2020). The ROAT can be especially helpful in children in which PT is too difficult to perform or has been completed under less-than-ideal conditions (Hannuksela and Salo 1986).

Test Site

Standard allergen concentrations have been determined using the skin of the back as a reference, therefore the upper back is the preferred site for PT (Fonacier 2015). This area also provides a large surface area and the ability for patients to function mostly unimpeded, especially when compared to other body areas. Although not recommended, other areas such as the upper arm can be utilized for the PT if necessary. Importantly, the back must be free from moisture, hair, lesions and other emollients. If necessary, non-irritating hair removal should be performed as mentioned above. Patch tests should not be applied over the vertebrae, as patches can easily be dislodged and are prone to irritant reactions. Proper PT application is shown in Figure 2.

To apply PT, the patient should be facing away from the physician with a slightly hunched-over position. The PT strip should be applied to the patient's upper or mid-back from the bottom-up. Chambers are then pressed from below to expel any air from the chambers and ensure a tight seal. Once the entire strip is on the back, press lightly over each individual chamber (Schmidlin et al. 2020). The patient should be instructed not to wet their back and to limit sweating once the patch tests have been applied.

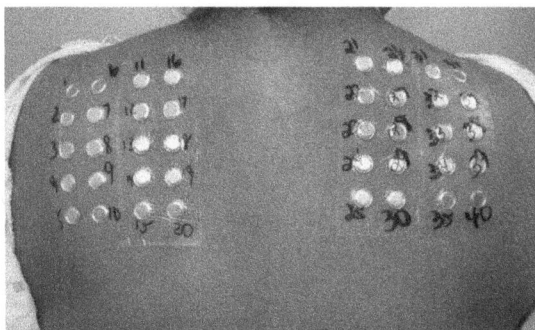

Figure 2. Patch tests applied on the back.

Reading in the PT

The patch test should be removed approximately 48 hours after placement. The first read is conducted at least 30 minutes after removal to allow for irritation to subside. A second read is necessary and usually performed 72–96 hours after placement. This reading is considered the most clinically relevant. A number of allergens, including some metals (gold, potassium dichromate, nickel and cobalt), topical antibiotics (neomycin and bacitracin), PPD and TCS are associated with late peak reactions, warranting a delayed read 7 to 10 days after PT application. It is estimated that up to 30% of sensitization might be missed for these known late-peaking allergens if a third delayed read is not performed (Macfarlane et al. 1989; Isaksson et al. 2000). Irritant reactions tend to peak early, around 48 hours, and fade (decrescendo), whereas allergic reactions tend to increase after first appearing (crescendo). This lends additional importance to the second and third reads to help distinguish irritants from allergic reactions (Fonacier and Noor 2018).

Interpretation of Patch Test Results

Positive Reaction

A standardized grading system should be used at each PT reading. The International Contact Dermatitis Research Group has a widely used and recognized scoring system shown in Figure 3.

	(-) Negative	
	(+/-) Doubtful or indeterminate	Faint macular erythema without infiltration
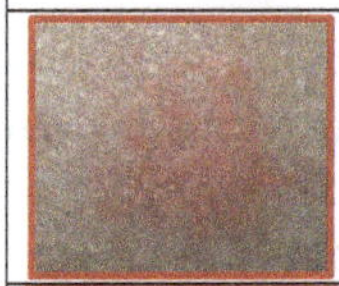	(1+) Weak positive	Non-vesicular erythema, infiltration and possible papules in at least 50% of the area of the patch site
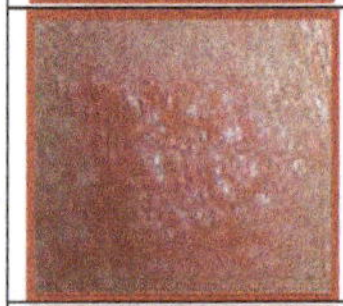	(2+) Strong positive	Vesicular erythema, infiltration and papules over at least 50% of the area of the patch site
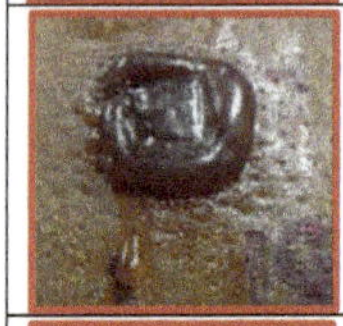	(3+) Extreme positive	Coalescing vesicles, erythema, and infiltration that is confluent
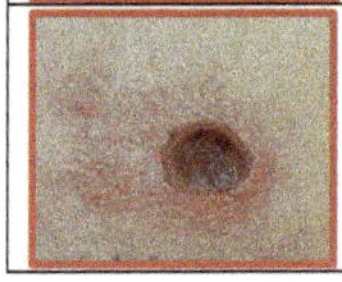	IR Irritant	

Figure 3. Standardized grading system used at each PT reading.

Irritant Reaction

Irritant reactions refer to non-true positive contact allergy reactions and may be confused for a false positive reaction. Potential explanations for false positives include testing with borderline irritants, testing beyond the irritancy threshold and testing patients with a background of dermatitis (Mowad et al. 2016). Irritant reactions present as discrete, patchy or homogenous erythema without infiltration. While discerning between weak positive and irritant reactions may be challenging, certain clinical features may help clarify this distinction. If a reaction fades between the first and second readings, this is most likely an irritant reaction. Conversely, if a reaction continues to develop between the first and second readings, this is known as the crescendo effect and points to a likely allergic reaction (Bolognia 2022).

The angry back syndrome is a severe irritant reaction, which remains incompletely understood. It is thought to arise from hyperirritability in response to a true positive allergen. This causes other tested areas to appear positive when in reality these other areas represent false positives stemming from the single strong true positive reaction. It has also been suggested that angry back syndrome occurs primarily due to another coexisting dermatitis at the time of PT (Bruynzeel and Maibach 1986).

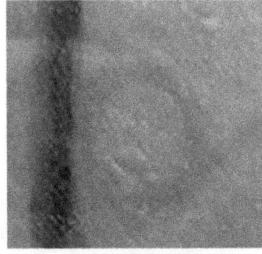

Figure 4. Edge effect in topical corticosteroid patch test.

In addition, a pustular reaction or rim reaction, described as a thin rim of erythema along the edge of the PT chamber, is indicative of an irritant reaction (Fisher et al. 2019) except for corticosteroid allergens. The "edge effect" is a type of irritant reaction where a reaction is noted to be greatest at the periphery rather than the center as demonstrated in Figure 4. This effect tends to dissipate quickly after the removal of the PT. When assessing TCS, the "edge effect" is not a false positive and can represent true allergy due to the anti-inflammatory nature of corticosteroids. The allergic reaction to TCS may be suppressed at earlier readings and may become positive once the anti-inflammatory effect of the corticosteroid decreases; thus, a delayed reading should always be performed.

Determining Relevance

The relevance of a positive PT must be considered for each patient being evaluated. This can be determined with a thorough history and physical examination, including occupational, home and environmental exposures, as well as the distribution of dermatitis. Determining clinically relevant allergens helps patients avoid the appropriate offending allergens and helps clinicians educate patients on irrelevant positive results. Relevance can be divided into four main categories: definite, probable, possible and past (Fonacier and Noor 2018). *Definite* relevance applies to scenarios in which there is a positive PT with the object or product or a positive "use test" with a suspected item. *Probable* relevance is when the suspected allergen is verified in known skin contacts with a consistent clinical presentation; *possible* relevance is if the patient's skin is in contact with materials that likely contain the suspected allergen. All definite, probable and possible relevance are *current* relevance. However, the PT result may have a *past* relevance when the patient no longer has exposure to the positive allergen. In a retrospective study of seven years of PT, 48.6% of patients had definite relevance, 17.1% probable, 24.3% possible and 9.9% no relevance (Morisetty 2011), highlighting the need for standardizing clinical relevance identification.

Treatment

Once an allergen has been identified, it is of utmost importance to counsel patients on the avoidance of any contact with the offending agent. Dispensing a safe list of products that do not contain the identified allergen(s) has been shown to increase patient adherence to avoidance (Fonacier et al. 2015). The American Contact Dermatitis Society (ACDS) operates an online subscription-based database called the Contact Management Allergen Program (CAMP). The CAMP is able to generate a safe list of products for patients based on their positive contact allergens. In addition to avoidance, adjunct medical therapy is appropriate and discussed in greater detail elsewhere.

Selected Allergen Pearls

Cosmetics and Personal Products

Cosmetic ACD should be suspected when there is dermatitis in the areas of the head, neck, face, arms or hands. The main allergens involved have traditionally been fragrance Mix I and II, followed by Balsam of Peru. However, Balsam of Peru is also found in non-cosmetics (spices, food, alcohol and tobacco) and is an overall more common allergen than fragrance mix (Warshaw et al. 2021). Fragrance Mix I and II are composite of a few different chemicals but often produce weak reactions on PT. Thus, positive PT to fragrance is always notable and often relevant.

Metals

Nickel is the most common allergen overall and is known to produce delayed positive reactions. Nickel has also demonstrated cross-reactivity with cobalt (DeKoven et al. 2021). Gold is the most common cause of a persistent positive PT, which ultimately led to its removal from the NACDG standard series some years ago (Chen and Lampel 2015). It is important to note that oral lichenoid, hand, eyelid or facial dermatitis are often presenting signs of gold sensitization.

Textiles

Mercaptobenzothiazole is a rubber accelerator and the leading cause of shoe dermatitis but can also cause glove dermatitis. Thiuram mix is another rubber accelerator that is the number one cause of glove dermatitis and the number one contact allergen in healthcare workers (Bolognia 2022).

Medications

Contact allergy to medications should be considered in patients with worsening dermatitis, despite topical treatment or previously well-controlled dermatitis that is now poorly responsive to medications. Risk factors include older patients with chronic leg ulcers requiring frequent topical treatment (Fonacier and Noor 2018). Neomycin is a typical allergen in this population and is frequently a late reactor as described earlier.

TCS are divided into four different classes (A–D) based on their allergenicity. There are also known cross-sensitivities between groups, notably Class A and D. Class A is the most allergenic and includes Tixocortol. Class B includes Budesonide (also cross-reacts with Class D). Class C includes betamethasone phosphate. Class D includes Hydrocortisone-17-Butyrate (Pratt et al. 2017). Corticosteroid allergens can result in an "edge effect" in the PT read. This describes a reaction that is greatest at the periphery and minimal or absent at the center. Generally, this is thought of as an irritant reaction, however, in the setting of TCS, this is often a true positive result due to the anti-inflammatory nature of corticosteroids. The lower concentration of the TCS at the periphery results in a more traditional positive in those areas, whereas at the center, the higher concentration of TCS leads to a greater anti-inflammatory effect and thus little to no allergenic response. TCS can also result in a false-negative read without any edge effect due to the same mechanism. However, on a delayed read the anti-inflammatory response will fade revealing a positive PT, again highlighting the importance of a delayed (third) read when TCS sensitization is suspected (Sukanto et al. 1981).

Preservatives

Preservatives are often components of topical and cosmetic agents along with wrinkle-free clothing. Methylisothiazolinone (MI) and methylchloroisothiazolinone (MCI) are non-formaldehyde-releasing preservatives found in detergents, wet wipes, bath products and skin care products. MCI and MI in a 3:1 combination (trade names: Kathon CG, Euxyl K 400) is widely used and in the combination, MCI is the more potent allergen. PT to MCI/MI but not MI alone could miss MI allergy in 33–60% of cases, likely because of the low concentration of MI in the MCI/MI PT substance. Testing MI alone at a higher concentration detects contact allergy more reliably. A positive PT result for MCI/MI has high clinical relevance (Castanedo-Tardana and Zug 2013).

Atopic Dermatitis

Atopic Dermatitis: Clinical Features, Diagnosis and Pathophysiology

Atopic dermatitis (AD), also known as atopic eczema, is a chronic, inflammatory pruritic skin disease that most commonly presents in pediatric patients but may also affect adults (Eichenfield et al. 2014; Schneider et al. 2013). It is a relatively common disease, with an estimated prevalence of 15–20% in children and up to 10% in adults (Laughter et al. 2021). Classic AD includes essential features of dry skin and pruritus as well as typical morphology and distribution, a chronic and/or relapsing history and concurrent presence of atopic disease or elevated IgE. Diagnosis of AD is made clinically based on these features, summarized in Table 3. The pathophysiology underlying AD is complex and most likely involves skin barrier dysfunction, genetic factors, immune dysregulation, skin microbial dysbiosis and external environmental triggers of inflammation (Stander 2021).

Table 3. Essential, important and associated-features defining AD.

Essential Features	Important Features	Associated Features
• **Pruritus** • **Eczema** (acute, subacute, chronic) • **Typical morphology** • **Age-specific patterns** Infants/children: Face; neck; extensor Any age group: Current/previous flexural lesions Sparing groin and axilla • **Chronic or relapsing history**	• **Early age** of onset • **Atopy:** Personal and/or family history Elevated total or specific IgE • **Xerosis**	• **Atypical vascular responses** (facial pallor, white dermographism) • **Keratosis pilaris**/pityriasis alba/ hyperlinear palms/ichthyosis • **Ocular/Periorbital** changes • **Other regional** findings (perioral/periauricular, nipple) • **Perifollicular** accentuation Lichen simplex chronicus/ prurigo

Adapted from Eichenfield et al. 2014.

Testing/Differential Diagnosis

The diagnosis of AD is typically made based on clinical history and presentation. However, several disorders may be mistaken for AD and further evaluation may be warranted.

Skin Biopsy

Although there is no substitute for a thorough history and physical exam, histologic information through skin biopsy can be of tremendous value clinically, especially in inflammatory dermatoses. The skin biopsy is a simple in-office procedure with little risk of complication and can provide invaluable information when a diagnosis is uncertain. Histopathologically, many inflammatory eruptions can look similar or overlap, thus both the clinician and the dermatopathologist can refine the clinical diagnosis and guide management.

The most frequently employed biopsy techniques are shave and punch biopsies. Punch biopsies are the preferred modality for the evaluation of most inflammatory conditions, whereas shave biopsies are more often used for the evaluation of neoplastic conditions. Skin biopsy is advantageous in that is a simple procedure that is generally well-tolerated and readily performed. However, biopsy results may sometimes be subtle and nonspecific and repeat biopsy may be required. In addition, performing a biopsy comes with risks such as pain, infection and scarring. Nevertheless, a skin biopsy is a clinically relevant tool that may provide histopathologic findings diagnostic for or suggestive of several other skin conditions and should be considered in patients without typical atopic history or refractory disease.

In cases of eczematous dermatitis presenting in adulthood without a childhood history of AD, the diagnosis of mycosis fungoides (MF) should be considered. MF is a cutaneous T cell non-Hodgkin lymphoma that most commonly presents as persistent skin patches or plaques that are accompanied by pruritus (Pimpinelli et al. 2005). The appearance of skin lesions may be heterogeneous with localized or widespread distribution but can have clinical features that overlap with AD including scale, erythema, alopecia or papules. Ideally, multiple skin biopsies in different locations should be done to diagnose MF. Results suggestive of MF include superficial band-like or lichenoid infiltrates consisting of lymphocytes and histiocytes, epidermotropism without spongiosis and/or lymphoid atypia (Olsen et al. 2007). Additional testing should be performed to assess for immunophenotyping and T-cell receptor gene rearrangement analysis (Fung et al. 2002).

Potassium Hydroxide (KOH) Preparation for Fungal Infections

Some superficial skin infections may present with pruritus and rashes that are similar to those of AD. Suspicion for a fungal etiology of dermatitis can be investigated with KOH preparation of skin scrapings. Diagnosis is confirmed via the presence of segmented hyphae (seen in dermatophyte infections) or budding yeasts, pseudohyphae and septate hyphae (seen in *Candida* infection) (Hainer 2003; Shi and Lio 2013). This test is non-invasive, easily performed, economical and frequently can be performed by the evaluating physician providing rapid results.

Dermoscopy

Infestation of the skin with the mite *Sarcoptes scabiei* can also produce a rash that mimics AD. Skin lesions may include papules, excoriations and vesicles in addition to linear burrows formed by mites as they travel through the epidermis. Pruritus is commonly very intense and can further disrupt skin findings given frequent scratching. Diagnosis is confirmed via the detection of the scabies mite, eggs or fecal pellets through microscopic examination of skin scrapings. Dermoscopy is an office procedure that may allow for visualization of linear burrows, the mite itself, or eggs within burrows (Chandler and Fuller 2019). However, presumptive diagnosis and treatment of scabies infestation are often more common in the clinical setting as many patients have a low mite burden, decreasing the sensitivity of this method and skin scraping/dermoscopy may require specialists trained in such procedures. By contrast, topical permethrin, the most commonly used first-line treatment for scabies infestation, is widely available, completed quickly and well-tolerated with few adverse side effects.

Patch Testing for ACD

ACD may sometimes present similarly to AD, with symptoms of pruritus, burning or stinging, and dermatitis including papules, plaques, vesicles and erythema (Owen et al. 2018). Chronic ACD may also present with lichenification, scaling and fissures. While some patients may have only AD or ACD, diseases with distinct underlying pathophysiology, recent studies have shown that patients who suffer from AD are more likely to also have concurrent ACD (Milam et al. 2019). The proposed pathogenesis for this overlap is likely multifactorial with increased rates of sensitization in AD patients due to the defective skin barrier with augmented antigen presentation and subsequent immune dysregulation. Furthermore, AD patients may have increased exposure to common allergens in topical agents frequently used to treat AD, such as lanolin, fragrances, preservatives and corticosteroids. If there is a concern for ACD or symptoms of AD are refractory to typical therapies, patients may undergo PT to evaluate for possible offending allergens. Please refer to the earlier PT section of this chapter for additional information.

Role of Testing for Other Atopic Diseases

Patients with AD frequently have a concurrent atopic disease, such as asthma, allergic rhinitis or food allergy. Diagnosis of and testing for these overlapping conditions and/or clinical characteristics may aid in the management of AD.

Food Allergen Testing

Patients with AD have an increased risk of IgE-mediated food allergy, particularly those with severe AD. This association may be attributed to cutaneous sensitization via damaged and inflamed skin (as seen in AD), currently the leading hypothesis for the development of food allergy (Lack et al. 2003; Astolfi et al. 2021; Strid et al. 2005). The atopic march, or the progression from AD to food allergy, asthma and allergic rhinitis at certain ages is likely due to shared underlying immune dysregulation and T-helper type 2 inflammation (Hill and Spergel 2018). If there is a clinical history of reaction to specific foods in patients with AD, clinicians may consider pursuing testing to evaluate suspected allergens. Testing for food allergies is discussed in Chapter 4 of this textbook. Most common food allergies seen in infants and children with AD, include egg, milk, peanut, soy, wheat, fish and tree nut and in adults, peanut, tree nuts, fish and shellfish (Hon et al. 2008; Sicherer and Sampson 1999).

While the association between food allergy and AD has been demonstrated clearly, the role of food allergies and their effect on AD disease severity remains controversial. Exposure to allergenic foods may cause *urticarial* reactions in patients with AD, subsequently triggering the itch-scratch cycle. As such, a limited evaluation of IgE-mediated food allergy with subsequent elimination of these foods in the diet may provide some clinical benefit to patients with AD. A second type of dermatologic manifestation reported is food-exacerbated AD in which ingestion of the offending food is thought to trigger flares of AD with symptoms limited to increasing *erythema* and *pruritus* (Werfel and Breuer 2004). However, subsequent studies have shown conflicting data, for example, patients were found to have equal rates of AD exacerbation with both placebo food ingestion and challenge food ingestion in a study conducted by Roerdink et al. (Roerdink et al. 2016). Other considerations to take into account when deciding to test for food allergy are that patients with AD may have increased sensitization to foods without clinically significant reaction on double-blind, placebo-controlled food challenges (DBPCFC) (Eller et al. 2009). Testing for food sensitization without oral food challenge to confirm the diagnosis may have additional pitfalls; in the Eller et al. study (2009), patients with AD were more likely to be sensitized to wheat, while the egg was the most common food to which patients are truly allergic based on a food challenge. Reports of increased rates of IgE-mediated reactions to foods after beginning elimination diets have also been seen in AD patients, highlighting the need to avoid unnecessary food eliminations (Chang et al. 2016). Taking recent data together, testing broadly for food allergy based on moderate to severe eczema alone in absence of clinical immediate hypersensitivity reactions is no longer recommended (Singh et al. 2022).

Environmental Allergen Testing

Allergic rhinitis is also commonly seen in patients with AD. Exposure to environmental allergens has been reported to exacerbate AD and testing for specific allergens with minimization of exposures may help to decrease AD flares (Narla and Silverberg 2020). In AD, special considerations for dust mite allergy may be of clinical relevance as dust mites are the most common aeroallergen sensitization (Ponyai et al. 2008). The atopy patch test (APT) consists of applying a suspected allergen to the skin (via a similar method employed in PT for ACD) to determine sensitization for aeroallergens. Performing the APT for dust mites in patients with AD has shown increased rates of sensitization, even in children who have negative SPT or RAST testing for dust mites (Fuiano et al. 2010). Additionally, few studies have shown that allergen-specific immunotherapy, especially for dust mites, may result in improved management of AD (Darsow 2012; Bae et al. 2013). Other aeroallergen sensitization commonly seen in AD include cat dander, dog dander, pollens and molds (Schafer et al. 1999; Sidbury et al. 2014). Testing for additional aeroallergens is discussed in more detail in Chapters 2 and 3 of this textbook.

Filaggrin

Filaggrin, a major epidermal protein, is found in the stratum corneum of the epidermis and is critical to maintaining the barrier function of the epidermis. Mutations in the gene *FLG,* encoding filaggrin, have been shown to be involved in the pathogenesis of AD as well as other allergic diseases. Filaggrin mutation is the most significant genetic risk factor for AD (Drislane and Irvine 2020). Loss of function mutations in *FLG* has been associated with a distinct AD phenotype with early onset persistent disease, increased severity, palmar hyperlinearity, increased risk of eczema herpeticum, staphylococcal infection, asthma and allergic sensitization. Analysis of the *FLG* gene can be accomplished via genetic sequencing. In addition to genetic studies, measuring filaggrin expression *in vivo* may be relevant to AD patients and can be done via two methods: Raman microspectroscopy (RMS) or stratum corneum tape stripping technique. RMS is an optical method of measuring filaggrin expression *in vivo* though generally more costly and less widely available. In tape stripping, adhesives are placed on the skin surface and when removed, provide components of the epidermis that may be collected for further analysis. High-performance liquid chromatography (HPLC) is then performed to quantify filaggrin degradation products. While the tape stripping method is both easy and quick to perform, the additional HPLC analysis may prolong results. Both genetic sequencing for filaggrin and also measuring *in vivo* filaggrin are not commonly performed for AD patients as they are not widely-accessible, cost-effective and often do not change management course.

Skin Microbiome

Patients with AD have been shown to have altered skin microbiomes and are particularly at increased risk of infection with *Staphylococcus aureus*. The abundance of *S. aureus* is associated with disease severity as it may indicate underlying skin inflammation and deficiencies in innate host immune responses. Testing for *S. aureus* in AD patients can be done via skin cultures, a safe, well-established and inexpensive procedure and may provide clinical benefit as the confirmed presence of the pathogen can be treated with antimicrobial therapies (Hulpusch et al. 2021). Patients found to have *S. aureus* may consider local antiseptics, such as chlorhexidine or the use of bleach baths.

Scoring of Atopic Dermatitis Severity

Multiple tools for the evaluation of AD severity have been created and utilized to monitor the disease and efficacy of therapies. These consist of clinician rating scores, patient-reported symptoms/scoring or a combination of both. This section will address the most commonly used scoring systems in both clinical practice and research protocols. See Figure 5 for a comparison of validated scoring tools incorporating a clinician evaluation component.

Calculation of Body Surface Area

Estimation of the body surface area (BSA) involved in AD patients is important to monitor the severity of the disease and is frequently used in validated scoring tools. A simple method of quickly calculating the percent of BSA affected in both pediatric and adult patients can be accomplished using the palmar method (Figure 6). Each patient's palmar surface area represents approximately 0.5% of their total BSA and including fingers surface area, approximately 1% of BSA (Rhodes et al. 2013). Another frequently utilized system of estimating BSA is the "Wallace Rule of Nines,"

AD Disease Severity Tools Used in Clinical Trials

SCORAD SCORing Atopic Dermatitis	EASI Eczema Area and Severity Index	IGA Investigator's Global Assessment
• **Physician-assessed symptoms**[3] – Erythema – Induration/Papulation/Edema – Excoriation – Lichenification – Oozing/Crusting – Xerosis	• **Physician-assessed symptoms**[1] – Erythema – Induration/Papulation/Edema – Excoriation – Lichenification	• **Physician-assessed symptoms**[6] – Erythema – Induration/Papulation/Edema – Oozing/Crusting
• **Extent of lesions measured using the rule of nines**	• **Extent of lesions calculated by area score for each body region**[1]	• **Extent of lesions not formally measured**
• **Includes patient-assessed symptoms**[3] (pruritus; insomnia)	• **Does not include patient-assessed symptoms**[1]	• **Does not include patient-assessed symptoms**[6]

SCORAD	Mild<25	Moderate 25-50	
EASI	Mild <8	Moderate 8-15	
IGA	Almost clear=1	Mild =2	Moderate =3

1. Hanifin JM et al. *Exp Dermatol.* 2001;10:11–18. 2. Chalmers JR et al. *Br J Dermatol.* 2014;171:1318–1325. 3. European Task Force on Atopic Dermatitis. *Dermatology.* 1993;186:23–31. 4. Willemsen MG et al. *Dermatol Res Pract.* 2009;2009:357046. 5. Foundation for Atopic Dermatitis. www.fondation-dermatitie-atopique.org/en/c/easi.   6. Rehal B et al. *PLoS One.* 2011;6:e17520. 7. HOME III meeting notes. 2013.

NYU Long Island
School of Medicine

Figure 5. Comparison of AD disease severity tools.

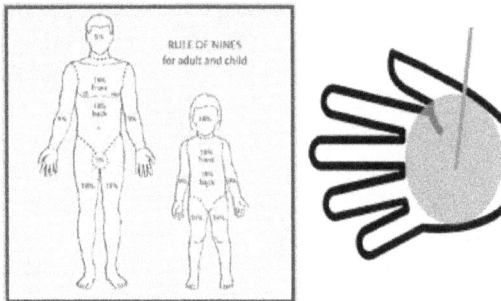

The palmar surface alone equates to 0.5% BSA; including fingers, this equates to 1% BSA

Figure 6. Determining BSA.

in which specific areas of the body are assigned certain percentages. Of note, children and adults have differing distributions due to proportionally larger heads and smaller leg sizes relative to total body size.

Scoring of Pruritus

Patient-reported pruritus scores may be a simple and effective way to monitor symptomatic control and its impact on the quality of life in patients with AD. The Peak Pruritus Numerical Rating Scale (NRS) is a validated tool that asks patients to measure the peak pruritus, or "worst" itch, over the past 24 hours based on the question: "On a scale of 0 to 10, with 0 indicating "no itch" and 10 being "worst itch imaginable," how would you rate your itch at the worst moment during the previous 24 hours?" (Yosipovitch et al. 2019). The Peak Pruritus NRS can be adapted in clinical use as well

In the past 7 days...	No itch 0	1	2	3	4	5	6	7	8	9	Worst imaginable itch 10
how intense was your itch at its worst?	☐ 0	☐ 1	☐ 2	☐ 3	☐ 4	☐ 5	☐ 6	☐ 7	☐ 8	☐ 9	☐ 10
how intense was your itch in general?	☐ 0	☐ 1	☐ 2	☐ 3	☐ 4	☐ 5	☐ 6	☐ 7	☐ 8	☐ 9	☐ 10

0 – No itch
6 – Distracts from activities
8 – Wakes you up from sleep
10 – Worst imaginable itch

Figure 7. NRS for pruritus.

by asking patients to report on average peak pruritus score over seven days compared to the general average pruritus score (Figure 7).

Severity Scoring of Atopic Dermatitis (SCORAD)

The SCORAD index evaluates disease extent (percentage of the area involved) and five clinical characteristics: erythema, edema/papulation, oozing/crusting, excoriation and lichenification. Clinical characteristics are assessed based on an average representative area on a scale of 0 to 3, with 0 indicating the absence of the characteristic and 3 indicating severe intensity. In addition to health care practitioner scoring, SCORAD also incorporates patients' subjective assessments of pruritus and sleep loss (each assessed on a scale of 0–10) (Kunz et al. 1997; "Severity Scoring of Atopic Dermatitis: The SCORAD Index. Consensus Report of the European Task Force on Atopic Dermatitis" 1993). The final score is calculated with the following formula: extent/5 + intensity × 7/2 + subjective items. This scoring tool has been widely used for many years and found to be valid and reliable across many interobserver in many trials (Schmitt et al. 2013).

Eczema Area and Scoring Index (EASI)

EASI was developed as a severity scoring system by adapting the PASI (Psoriasis Area and Severity Index) (Hanifin et al. 2001). This validated scoring tool evaluates AD severity based on the extent of disease at four body sites and measures erythema, induration/papulation, excoriation and lichenification on a scale of 0 to 3 with 3 indicating severe findings. No patient-reported subjective outcomes are included. The final score is determined by adding up the total scores per body region (determined from the sum of severity scores multiplied by the area score multiplied by the corresponding body region constant weighted value). Scores greater than 21 are characterized as severe diseases, while scores ranging from 50.1 to 72 are considered very severe diseases.

Investigators' Global Assessment (IGA)

IGA is a scoring tool that can be used to measure overall disease severity on a scale of 0 (clear) to 5 (very severe disease) based on clinical characteristics of erythema, infiltration, papulation, oozing and crusting as general guidelines. The simple scoring system of the IGA confers an advantage over measures such as SCORAD or EASI, however, has a high variability among observers thus less reproducible (Rehal and Armstrong 2011). Recently, a validated IGA (vIGA-AD) scale for AD was published based on expert consensus with the goal of harmonizing efficacy and outcome assessments in clinical trials for AD (see Table 4) (Simpson et al. 2020). The vIGA-AD is the only

Table 4. Validated IGA.

Instructions:

The IGA score is selected using the descriptors below that best describe the overall appearance of the lesions at a given time point. It is not necessary that all characteristics under Morphological Description be present.

Score	Morphological Description
0 – Clear	No inflammatory signs of atopic dermatitis (no erythema, no induration/papulation, no lichenification, no oozing/crusting). Post-inflammatory hyperpigmentation and/or hypopigmentation may be present.
1 – Almost clear	Barely perceptible erythema, barely perceptible induration/papulation, and/or minimal lichenification. No oozing or crusting.
2 – Mild	Slight but definite erythema (pink), slight but definite induration/papulation, and/or slight but definite lichenification. No oozing or crusting.
3 – Moderate	Clearly perceptible erythema (dull red), clearly perceptible induration/papulation, and/or clearly perceptible lichenification. Oozing and crusting may be present.
4 – Severe	Marked erythema (deep or bright red), marked induration/papulation, and/or marked lichenification. Disease is widespread in extent. Oozing or crusting may be present.

validated IGA scale that is feasible, simple and a good option for use in clinical practice. However, the vIGA-AD does not include the extent of the disease (percentage of body surface area (BSA) affected) and, as a result, fails to capture an important aspect of severity.

Patient-Oriented Eczema Measure (POEM)

The Patient-Oriented Eczema Measure (POEM) was first developed as a tool to monitor symptoms of AD based on patient perspectives (Charman et al. 2004). It determines an overall score based on patient responses to questions assessing the frequency of pruritus, disrupted sleep, the integrity of skin and other characteristics of eczematous skin based on seven questions (Figure 8). Like the IGA, it is relatively straightforward, able to be completed quickly and specifically targets symptoms important to patients, thus it is a useful tool in clinical practice. However, in contrast with SCORAD, EASI and the IGA, POEM is based on patient-reported symptoms only and does not utilize clinician input.

Atopic Dermatitis Control Tool (ADCT)

Atopic Dermatitis Control Tool (ADCT) is a recently validated, brief and easily scored patient self-assessment tool (Pariser et al. 2020; Simpson et al. 2020). It consists of six concise questions to evaluate the different dimensions of AD control identified as relevant by patients and clinicians (Figure 9). ADCT can be self-administered by patients or used in routine consultations. It is designed to help facilitate meaningful patient-physician discussion on the control of AD in every day clinical practice, enabling improvements in disease monitoring.

Special Considerations

Evaluation of Pediatric Patients

Pediatric patients have unique characteristics to consider when treating AD in this population. The distribution of AD lesions in infants and young children (zero to two years of age) may predominantly involve extensor surfaces, cheeks or may be generalized with sparing of the diaper area (Rudikoff and Lebwohl 1998). Pediatric patients also have a higher BSA-to-weight ratio and thus have a higher risk of systemic absorption of topical corticosteroid therapy. Another important consideration for infants and children with eczema, particularly severe and early onset disease,

Please circle one response for each of the seven questions below about your/your child's eczema. If your child is old enough to understand the questions then please fill in the questionnaire together. Please leave blank any questions you feel unable to answer.

1. Over the last week, how many days has your/your child's skin been itchy because of eczema?

No days   1–2 days   3–4 days   5–6 days   Every day

2. Over the last week, how many nights has your/your child's sleep been disturbed because of eczema?

No days   1–2 days   3–4 days   5–6 days   Every day

3. Over the last week, how many days has your/your child's skin been bleeding because of eczema?

No days   1–2 days   3–4 days   5–6 days   Every day

4. Over the last week, how many days has your/your child's skin been weeping or oozing clear fluid because of eczema?

No days   1–2 days   3–4 days   5–6 days   Every day

5. Over the last week, how many days has your/your child's skin been cracked because of eczema?

No days   1–2 days   3–4 days   5–6 days   Every day

6. Over the last week, how many days has your/your child's skin been flaking off because of eczema?

No days   1–2 days   3–4 days   5–6 days   Every day

7. Over the last week, how many days has your/your child's skin felt dry or rough because of eczema?

No Days   1–2 Days   3–4 days   5–6 days   Every day

TOTAL SCORE (Maximum 28): _____

How is the scoring done?

Each of the seven questions carries equal weight and is scored from 0 to 4 as follows:

No days	= 0
1-2 days	= 1
3-4 days	= 2
5-6 days	= 3
Every day	= 4

What does a poem score mean?

To help patients and clinicians to understand their POEM scores, the following bandings have been established (see references below):

- 0 to 2 = Clear or almost clear
- 3 to 7 = Mild eczema
- 8 to 16 = Moderate eczema
- 17 to 24 = Severe eczema
- 25 to 28 = Very severe eczema

Figure 8. POEM Questionnaire.

ATOPIC DERMATITS CONTROL TOOL (ADCT)

Please answer the following questions thinking about your experiences with eczema, sometimes called "atopic dermatitis".

	0 points	1 point	2 points	3 points	4 points
1. Over the last week, how would you rate your eczema-related symptoms (for example, itching, dry skin, skin rash)?	None	Mild	Moderate	Severe	Very Severe
2. Over the last week, how many days did you have **intense episodes of itching** because of your eczema?	Not at all	1-2 days	3-4 days	5-6 days	Every day
3. Over the last week, how **bothered** have you been by your eczema?	Not at all	A little	Moderately	Very	Extremely
4. Over the last week, how many nights did you have **trouble falling or staying asleep** because of your eczema?	No nights	1-2 nights	3-4 nights	5-6 nights	Every night
5. Over the last week, how much did your eczema **affect your daily activities?**	Not at all	A little	Moderately	A lot	Extremely
6. Over the last week, how much did your eczema **affect your mood or emotions?**	Not at all	A little	Moderately	A lot	Extremely

© Atopic Dermatitis Control Tool_Version 1, 27 Nov 2018. Sanofi Group and Regeneron Pharmaceuticals Inc. All Rights Reserved ADCT – US/English

CALCULATING THE ADCT SCORE
Step 1: Each ADCT question is scored 0–4 points, as shown in the table above
Step 2: The sum of the scores from all six ADCT questions forms the ADCT total score
The minimum ADCT total score is 0, and the maximum ADCT total score is 24

INTERPRETING THE ADCT TOTAL SCORE:
POINT-IN-TIME CONTROL STATUS
A higher score indicates lower AD control
A patient's AD may not be well controlled if:
- The ADCT total score is at least seven points or
- One of the patient's answers falls into the blue boxed area in the ADCT table above

CHANGES IN CONTROL STATUS OVER TIME
A change of 5 points is the threshold for meaningful within-person change
- Decrease of 5 points or more: Indication of clinically relevant improvement of atopic dermatitis control
- Increase of 5 points or more: Indication of clinically relevant worsening of atopic dermatitis control
ADCT can be used to detect change over time supporting a patient-physician conversation on sustained control in clinical practice.

Figure 9. ADCT.

is the increased risk for IgE-mediated food allergy. Studies have shown the development of food allergy (FA) may occur via the exposure of potential allergens to the defective skin barrier in AD, a process called transcutaneous sensitization (Lack et al. 2003). Based on the results of the Learning Early About Peanut Allergy (LEAP) trial, infants with severe eczema are now recommended to begin the early introduction of peanuts to decrease the likelihood of developing peanut allergy (Du Toit et al. 2015). Given the increased risk of sensitization and FA in patients with severe AD, it is generally recommended to test for peanut allergy prior to introducing it into the diet (Singh et al.

2022). For patients with mild to moderate eczema, no specific food testing is required prior to the introduction of foods. The role of testing for FA before the introduction is controversial, as some studies have shown that pre-screening is not associated with improved outcomes or preventing more cases of FA (Fleischer et al. 2021). Ultimately, providers and parents should engage in shared decision-making regarding the risks and benefits of testing prior to introduction, to introduce a diverse and complementary diet around 6 months of life once the infant is tolerating other typical weaning foods in accordance with the family and cultural preferences. Newer evidence suggests both early introductions of allergenic foods and aggressive intervention in AD may be beneficial to preventing food allergies; trials to evaluate the role of these interventions are currently ongoing (Mancuso et al. 2021).

Evaluation of Skin of Color

AD assessment may be more difficult in darker skin tones due to differences in clinical presentation. Classic features of AD include erythematous plaques with fine scale found on flexor surfaces; in contrast, studies have shown patients of various ethnic backgrounds may have differences in the distribution of skin lesions as well as appearance (Kaufman et al. 2018). For example, patients of African descent may present with more extensor involvement and patients of Asian descent tend to have more well-demarcated lesions with increased scaling and lichenification (Noda et al. 2015). Other differences reported in darker skin tones include papular AD lesions or a lichen planus-like presentation (Allen et al. 2008). Furthermore, erythema tends to appear more violaceous, brownish or ashy gray in dark-skinned individuals, which can be more difficult to detect. As such, commonly used scoring tools such as SCORAD and EASI, which utilize erythema as a key measure of disease severity, tend to underestimate the degree of disease severity and BSA in darker skin tones. Additional features should be considered in patients with darker skin, such as the presence of skin warmth, edema or scale in order to detect underlying erythema.

Evaluation of Steroid Side Effects

Frequent TCS use in patients with AD is not without side effects and special attention should be given at each visit to evaluate these, particularly in patients with higher burden of corticosteroids (i.e., in moderate to severe cases). The most frequently seen adverse effects of corticosteroids include skin atrophy, striae, rosacea, perioral dermatitis, acneiform eruptions and purpura or telangiectasias (Hengge et al. 2006). Other reported side effects include delayed wound healing, cutaneous infections or contact dermatitis. Systemic absorption, though relatively rare, may also occur especially in children, leading to adrenal suppression, hyperglycemia, hypertension, cataracts and glaucoma (Wood Heickman et al. 2018). The risk of developing side effects with corticosteroid use increases with a higher burden of corticosteroids, i.e., with the use of higher potency ointments, larger area of application, prolonged use, occlusion and application to areas of thinner skin. Furthermore, clinicians should consider the use of corticosteroids for other concurrent diseases, such as inhaled corticosteroids in asthma and intranasal corticosteroids for allergic rhinitis, both conditions commonly seen in patients with AD. Particular attention to the adverse effects of TCS should be given to pediatric AD patients, who have an increased ratio of BSA to weight, and to older patients, who have increased thinness and fragility of the skin.

Treatment of Refractory AD

The first-line treatment of AD consists of topical therapies to improve skin barrier function (emollients to reduce water loss) and decrease inflammation (TCS). Other topical treatments, including calcineurin inhibitors (tacrolimus and pimecrolimus), phosphodiesterase-4 inhibitors (crisaborole) and JAK inhibitors (ruxolitinib) have been approved for mild to moderate AD. These non-steroidal ointments may be utilized as a maintenance therapy to prevent AD flairs given a favorable side effect profile compared to long-term TCS use. However, severe cases of AD may not be controlled with these management strategies, and these patients require additional therapies to control the disease.

Dilute Bleach Baths

Some studies show that a dilute bleach bath can decrease the severity of eczema (Huang et al. 2009). In a full bathtub (~ 40 gallons), one can mix 1/4 to 1/2 cup of common liquid bleach (e.g., Clorox) into the water, making a solution of diluted bleach at ~ 0.005%. Soak in the chlorinated water for about 10 minutes, pat dry and apply topical medication and/or moisturizer as directed. Bleach baths can be done two to three times a week or as prescribed by the physician.

Wet Wraps

The application of wet wraps (also known as wet dressings) has been shown to be successful in treating severe generalized AD flares (Oranje et al. 2006). This therapy consists of applying a medium-potency TCS and/or emollient to the affected skin, covered with a wet layer and finally topped with a dry layer. Either close-fitting cotton clothing or bandages may be used as layers, and specialized garments are available to buy specifically for wet wrap therapy. Wet wraps may be applied once or twice daily and left in place for two or more hours or overnight if tolerated. This occlusive method should be used only as short-term therapy; however, it has been shown to result in increased systemic absorption of the corticosteroid.

Phototherapy

Phototherapy may be an adjunctive treatment for patients with uncontrolled disease. This is done primarily through narrowband ultraviolet B (NBUVB) or ultraviolet A1 (UVA1) phototherapy (Garritsen et al. 2014). Typically, NVUVB is administered two to three times per week with progressive dose increases as tolerated. Phototherapy is generally safe for older children (> six years of age) and adults; however, it should not be used in infants and younger children who cannot cooperate with treatment. Potential adverse effects include erythema, blistering, herpes simplex reactivation and anxiety (Jury et al. 2006). This therapy is generally well-tolerated and widely available, though cost and increased office visits per week may be prohibitive to certain patients. Increased risks are associated with UVA radiation, which has been shown to have a higher risk of developing cutaneous malignancies (Lindelof et al. 1991).

Biologics/Newer Therapies

Newer targeted therapies have emerged in the last several years that have proven to be safe and effective for the treatment of moderate to severe AD. *Dupilumab*, a monoclonal antibody that blocks interleukin (IL) 4 and IL-13 signaling by binding IL-4 receptor alpha, is currently approved for patients who have failed topical prescription therapies. *Tralokinumab* an anti-IL-13 has also been approved for the treatment of moderate to severe AD in adult patients (> 18 years old) whose disease is not adequately controlled with topical prescription therapies or when those therapies are not advisable. The initial dose is 600 mg SQ followed by 300 mg every 2 weeks. Differentiating from Dupilumab, patients below 100 kg who are clear or almost clear after 16 weeks may consider 300 mg every 4 weeks. *Abrocitinib* and *Upacitinib* are oral JAK inhibitors approved in the US for moderate to severe AD in Jan 2022. Ruxolitinib, a topical JAK inhibitor, was approved for mild to moderate AD who have failed topical therapies. Other experimental agents with specific cytokine targets (anti-IL-31, S1P Receptor Modulators, CCR4 and OX40 targets) and other oral JAK inhibitors are currently undergoing clinical trials as are studies on off-label use of biologics such as Omalizumab for the treatment of AD. Chapter 10 discusses Dupilumab and other newer therapies in greater detail.

Other Systemic Immunomodulators

Different types of systemic therapies have been used for the control of pruritus and refractory AD. The most commonly used options include prednisone, cyclosporine, methotrexate, azathioprine or mycophenolate mofetil. These treatment options are associated with significant adverse effects however and should be used only in severe refractory cases in which other standard therapies have failed.

Glossary of Abbreviations

ACD – Allergic Contact Dermatitis
ACDS – American Contact Dermatitis Society
AD – Atopic Dermatitis
ADCT – Atopic Dermatitis Control Tool
APT – Atopy Patch Test
BSA – Body Surface Area
CAMP – Contact Management Allergen Program
CD – Contact Dermatitis
DBPCFC – Double-Blind, Placebo-Controlled Food Challenges
EASI – Eczema Area and Scoring Index
FLG – Filaggrin
HPLC – High-Performance Liquid Chromatography
ICD – Irritant Contact Dermatitis
IGA – Investigators' Global Assessment
IL – Interleukin
JAK – Janus Kinase
KOH – Potassium Hydroxide
MCI – Methylchloroisothiazolinone
MF – Mycosis Fungoides
MI – Methylisothiazolinone
NACDG – North American Contact Dermatitis Group
NBUVB – Narrowband Ultraviolet B
NRS – Numerical Rating Scale
PASI – Psoriasis Area and Severity Index
POEM – Patient-Oriented Eczema Measure
PT – Patch Testing
RMS – Raman Microspectroscopy
ROAT – Repeat Open Application Test
SCORAD – Severity Scoring of Atopic Dermatitis
TCS – Topical Corticosteroids
T.R.U.E. – Thin-Layer Rapid Use Epicutaneous
UVA1 – Ultraviolet A1
vIGA – Validated IGA

References

Allen, H. B., Jones, N. P. and Bowen, S. E. 2008. Lichenoid and other clinical presentations of atopic dermatitis in an inner city practice. J. Am. Acad. Dermatol, 58(3): 503–504. doi:10.1016/j.jaad.2007.03.033.

Anveden, I., Lindberg, M., Andersen, K. E., Bruze, M., Isaksson, M., Liden, C. et al. 2004. Oral prednisone suppresses allergic but not irritant patch test reactions in individuals hypersensitive to nickel. Contact Dermatitis 50(5): 298–303. doi:10.1111/j.0105-1873.2004.00340.x.

Astolfi, A., Cipriani, F., Messelodi, D., De Luca, M., Indio, V., Di Chiara, C. et al. 2021. Filaggrin loss-of-function mutations are risk factors for severe food allergy in children with atopic dermatitis. J. Clin. Med. 10(2). doi:10.3390/jcm10020233.

Bae, J. M., Choi, Y. Y., Park, C. O., Chung, K. Y. and Lee, K. H. 2013. Efficacy of allergen-specific immunotherapy for atopic dermatitis: a systematic review and meta-analysis of randomized controlled trials. J. Allergy Clin. Immunol, 132(1): 110–117. doi:10.1016/j.jaci.2013.02.044.

Bolognia, J. J. and Schaffer, J. 2022. Dermatology (3 ed. Vol. 1). Philadelphia: Elsevier Saunders.

Bruynzeel, D. P. and Maibach, H. I. 1986. Excited skin syndrome (angry back). Arch Dermatol. 122(3): 323–328.

Castanedo-Tardana, M. P. and Zug, K. A. 2013. Methylisothiazolinone. Dermatitis 24(1): 2–6. doi:10.1097/DER.0b013e31827edc73.

Chandler, D. J. and Fuller, L. C. 2019. A review of scabies: an infestation more than skin deep. Dermatology 235(2): 79–90. doi:10.1159/000495290.

Chang, A., Robison, R., Cai, M. and Singh, A. M. 2016. Natural history of food-triggered atopic dermatitis and development of immediate reactions in children. J. Allergy Clin. Immunol. Pract. 4(2): 229–236 e221. doi:10.1016/j.jaip.2015.08.006.

Charman, C. R., Venn, A. J. and Williams, H. C. 2004. The patient-oriented eczema measure: development and initial validation of a new tool for measuring atopic eczema severity from the patients' perspective. Arch. Dermatol. 140(12): 1513–1519. doi:10.1001/archderm.140.12.1513.

Chen, J. K. and Lampel, H. P. 2015. Gold contact allergy: clues and controversies. Dermatitis 26(2): 69–77. doi:10.1097/DER.0000000000000101.

Damian, D. L. and Halliday, G. M. 2002. Measurement of ultraviolet radiation-induced suppression of recall contact and delayed-type hypersensitivity in humans. Methods 28(1): 34–45. doi:10.1016/s1046-2023(02)00208-6.

Darsow, U. 2012. Allergen-specific immunotherapy for atopic eczema: updated. Curr. Opin. Allergy Clin. Immunol. 12(6): 665–669. doi:10.1097/ACI.0b013e3283588cf4.

DeKoven, J. G., Silverberg, J. I., Warshaw, E. M., Atwater, A. R., Reeder, M. J., Sasseville, D. et al. 2021. North American contact dermatitis group patch test results: 2017–2018. Dermatitis 32(2): 111–123. doi:10.1097/DER.0000000000000729.

Drislane, C. and Irvine, A. D. 2020. The role of filaggrin in atopic dermatitis and allergic disease. Ann. Allergy Asthma Immunol. 124(1): 36–43. doi:10.1016/j.anai.2019.10.008.

Du Toit, G., Roberts, G., Sayre, P., Bahnson, H., Radulovic, S., Santos, A. et al. 2015. Randomized trial of peanut consumption in infants at risk for peanut allergy. N Engl. J. Med. 372(9): 803–813. doi:10.1056/NEJMoa1414850.

Eichenfield, L. F., Tom, W. L., Berger, T. G., Krol, A., Paller, A. S., Schwarzenberger, K. et al. 2014. Guidelines of care for the management of atopic dermatitis: section 2. Management and treatment of atopic dermatitis with topical therapies. J. Am. Acad. Dermatol. 71(1): 116–132. doi:10.1016/j.jaad.2014.03.023.

Eller, E., Kjaer, H. F., Host, A., Andersen, K. E. and Bindslev-Jensen, C. 2009. Food allergy and food sensitization in early childhood: results from the DARC cohort. Allergy 64(7): 1023–1029. doi:10.1111/j.1398-9995.2009.01952.x.

Fisher, A. A., Fowler, J. F., Zirwas, M. J. and Fisher, A. A. 2019. Fisher's Contact Dermatitis (7th edition. ed.). Phoenix, AZ: Contact Dermatitis Institute.

Fonacier, L. A. M. 2014. Textbook of Allergy for the Clinician (1 ed.). Boca Raton, FL: CRC Press, Taylor and Francis Group.

Fonacier, L. 2015. A practical guide to patch testing. J. Allergy Clin. Immunol. Pract. 3(5): 669–675. doi:10.1016/j.jaip.2015.05.001.

Fonacier, L., Bernstein, D. I., Pacheco, K., Holness, D. L., Blessing-Moore, J., Khan, D. et al. 2015. Contact dermatitis: a practice parameter-update 2015. J. Allergy Clin. Immunol. Pract. 3(3 Suppl): S1–39. doi:10.1016/j.jaip.2015.02.009.

Fonacier, L. and Noor, I. 2018. Contact dermatitis and patch testing for the allergist. Ann. Allergy Asthma Immunol. 120(6): 592–598. doi:10.1016/j.anai.2018.03.003.

Fuiano, N., Fusilli, S. and Incorvaia, C. 2010. House dust mite-related allergic diseases: role of skin prick test, atopy patch test, and RAST in the diagnosis of different manifestations of allergy. Eur. J. Pediatr. 169(7): 819–824. doi:10.1007/s00431-009-1118-6.

Fung, M. A., Murphy, M. J., Hoss, D. M. and Grant-Kels, J. M. 2002. Practical evaluation and management of cutaneous lymphoma. J. Am. Acad. Dermatol. 46(3): 325–357; quiz, 358–360. doi:10.1067/mjd.2002.121355.

Garritsen, F. M., Brouwer, M. W., Limpens, J. and Spuls, P. I. 2014. Photo(chemo)therapy in the management of atopic dermatitis: an updated systematic review with implications for practice and research. Br J. Dermatol. 170(3): 501–513. doi:10.1111/bjd.12645.

Granchi, D., Cenni, E., Tigani, D., Trisolino, G., Baldini, N. and Giunti, A. 2008. Sensitivity to implant materials in patients with total knee arthroplasties. Biomaterials 29(10): 1494–1500. doi:10.1016/j.biomaterials.2007.11.038.

Hainer, B. L. 2003. Dermatophyte infections. Am. Fam Physician 67(1): 101–108.

Hanifin, J. M., Thurston, M., Omoto, M., Cherill, R., Tofte, S. J. and Graeber, M. 2001. The eczema area and severity index (EASI): assessment of reliability in atopic dermatitis. EASI Evaluator Group. Exp. Dermatol. 10(1): 11–18. doi:10.1034/j.1600-0625.2001.100102.x.

Hannuksela, M. and Salo, H. 1986. The repeated open application test (ROAT). Contact Dermatitis 14(4): 221–227. doi:10.1111/j.1600-0536.1986.tb01229.x.

Hengge, U. R., Ruzicka, T., Schwartz, R. A. and Cork, M. J. 2006. Adverse effects of topical glucocorticosteroids. J. Am. Acad. Dermatol. 54(1): 1–15; quiz 16–18. doi:10.1016/j.jaad.2005.01.010.

Hill, D. A. and Spergel, J. M. 2018. The atopic march: Critical evidence and clinical relevance. Ann. Allergy Asthma Immunol. 120(2): 131–137. doi:10.1016/j.anai.2017.10.037.

Hon, K. L., Leung, T. F., Ching, G., Chow, C. M., Luk, V., Ko, W. S. et al. 2008. Patterns of food and aeroallergen sensitization in childhood eczema. Acta Paediatr. 97(12): 1734–1737. doi:10.1111/j.1651-2227.2008.01034.x.

Huang, J. T., Abrams, M., Tlougan, B., Rademaker, A. and Paller, A. S. 2009. Treatment of *Staphylococcus aureus* colonization in atopic dermatitis decreases disease severity. Pediatrics 123(5): e808–814. doi:10.1542/peds.2008-2217.

Hulpusch, C., Weins, A. B., Traidl-Hoffmann, C. and Reiger, M. 2021. A new era of atopic eczema research: Advances and highlights. Allergy 76(11): 3408–3421. doi:10.1111/all.15058.

Ingber, A. 2014. Contact dermatitis and patch tests in pregnancy. Current Dermatology Reports 3. doi:10.1007/s13671-014-0081-2.

Isaksson, M., Andersen, K. E., Brandao, F. M., Bruynzeel, D. P., Bruze, M., Camarasa, J. G. et al. 2000. Patch testing with corticosteroid mixes in Europe. A multicentre study of the EECDRG. Contact Dermatitis 42(1): 27–35. doi:10.1034/j.1600-0536.2000.042001027.x.

Jacob, S. E., McGowan, M., Silverberg, N. B., Pelletier, J. L., Fonacier, L., Mousdicas, N. et al. 2017. Pediatric contact dermatitis registry data on contact allergy in children with atopic dermatitis. JAMA Dermatol. 153(8): 765–770. doi:10.1001/jamadermatol.2016.6136.

Jensen, C. D., Paulsen, E. and Andersen, K. E. 2006. Retrospective evaluation of the consequence of alleged patch test sensitization. Contact Dermatitis 55(1): 30–35. doi:10.1111/j.0105-1873.2006.00863.x.

Johansen, J. D., Aalto-Korte, K., Agner, T., Andersen, K. E., Bircher, A., Bruze, M. et al. 2015. European Society of Contact Dermatitis guideline for diagnostic patch testing—recommendations on best practice. Contact Dermatitis 73(4): 195–221. doi:10.1111/cod.12432.

Joy, N. M., Rice, K. R. and Atwater, A. R. 2013. Stability of patch test allergens. Dermatitis 24(5): 227–236. doi:10.1097/DER.0b013e3182a0a19d.

Jury, C. S., McHenry, P., Burden, A. D., Lever, R. and Bilsland, D. 2006. Narrowband ultraviolet B (UVB) phototherapy in children. Clin. Exp. Dermatol. 31(2): 196–199. doi:10.1111/j.1365-2230.2006.02061.x.

Kaufman, B. P., Guttman-Yassky, E. and Alexis, A. F. 2018. Atopic dermatitis in diverse racial and ethnic groups-Variations in epidemiology, genetics, clinical presentation and treatment. Exp. Dermatol. 27(4): 340–357. doi:10.1111/exd.13514.

Kunz, B., Oranje, A. P., Labreze, L., Stalder, J. F., Ring, J. and Taieb, A. 1997. Clinical validation and guidelines for the SCORAD index: consensus report of the European Task Force on Atopic Dermatitis. Dermatology 195(1): 10–19. doi:10.1159/000245677.

Lack, G., Fox, D., Northstone, K., Golding, J., Avon Longitudinal Study of, P. and Children Study, T. 2003. Factors associated with the development of peanut allergy in childhood. N Engl. J. Med. 348(11): 977–985. doi:10.1056/NEJMoa013536.

Laughter, M. R., Maymone, M. B. C., Mashayekhi, S., Arents, B. W. M., Karimkhani, C., Langan, S. M. et al. 2021. The global burden of atopic dermatitis: lessons from the Global Burden of Disease Study 1990–2017. Br J. Dermatol. 184(2): 304–309. doi:10.1111/bjd.19580.

Lindelof, B., Sigurgeirsson, B., Tegner, E., Larko, O., Johannesson, A., Berne, B. et al. 1991. PUVA and cancer: a large-scale epidemiological study. Lancet 338(8759): 91–93. doi:10.1016/0140-6736(91)90083-2.

Litchman, G., Nair, P. A., Atwater, A. R. and Bhutta, B. S. 2022. Contact Dermatitis. In StatPearls. Treasure Island (FL).

Macfarlane, A. W., Curley, R. K., Graham, R. M., Lewis-Jones, M. S. and King, C. M. 1989. Delayed patch test reactions at days 7 and 9. Contact Dermatitis 20(2): 127–132. doi:10.1111/j.1600-0536.1989.tb03121.x.

Mancuso, J. B., Lee, S. S., Paller, A. S., Ohya, Y. and Eichenfeld, L. F. 2021. Management of severe atopic dermatitis in pediatric patients. J. Allergy Clin. Immunol. Pract. 9(4): 1462–1471. Doi: 10.1016/j.jaip.2021.02.017.

Milam, E. C., Jacob, S. E. and Cohen, D. E. 2019. Contact dermatitis in the patient with atopic dermatitis. J. Allergy Clin. Immunol. Pract. 7(1): 18–26. doi:10.1016/j.jaip.2018.11.003.

Morisetty, H. M. B. and Michelis M. 2011. Relevance of patch test results to the clinical diagnosis of allergic contact dermatitis-need for standardization. Journal of Allergy and Clinical Immunology 129(2): AB38. doi:https://doi.org/10.1016/j.jaci.2011.12.803.

Mowad, C. M., Anderson, B., Scheinman, P., Pootongkam, S., Nedorost, S. and Brod, B. 2016. Allergic contact dermatitis: Patient management and education. J. Am. Acad. Dermatol. 74(6): 1043–1054. doi:10.1016/j.jaad.2015.02.1144.

Narla, S. and Silverberg, J. I. 2020. The role of environmental exposures in atopic dermatitis. Curr. Allergy Asthma Rep. 20(12): 74. doi:10.1007/s11882-020-00971-z.

Neale, H., Garza-Mayers, A. C., Tam, I. and Yu, J. 2021. Pediatric allergic contact dermatitis. Part I: Clinical features and common contact allergens in children. J. Am. Acad. Dermatol. 84(2): 235–244. doi:10.1016/j.jaad.2020.11.002.

Nicholson, P. J., Llewellyn, D., English, J. S. and Guidelines Development, G. 2010. Evidence-based guidelines for the prevention, identification and management of occupational contact dermatitis and urticaria. Contact Dermatitis 63(4): 177–186. doi:10.1111/j.1600-0536.2010.01763.x.

Noda, S., Suarez-Farinas, M., Ungar, B., Kim, S. J., de Guzman Strong, C., Xu, H. et al. 2015. The Asian atopic dermatitis phenotype combines features of atopic dermatitis and psoriasis with increased TH17 polarization. J. Allergy Clin. Immunol. 136(5): 1254–1264. doi:10.1016/j.jaci.2015.08.015.

Olsen, E., Vonderheid, E., Pimpinelli, N., Willemze, R., Kim, Y., Knobler, R. et al. 2007. Revisions to the staging and classification of mycosis fungoides and Sezary syndrome: a proposal of the International Society for Cutaneous Lymphomas (ISCL) and the cutaneous lymphoma task force of the European Organization of Research and Treatment of Cancer (EORTC). Blood 110(6): 1713–1722. doi:10.1182/blood-2007-03-055749.

Oranje, A. P., Devillers, A. C., Kunz, B., Jones, S. L., DeRaeve, L., Van Gysel, D. et al. 2006. Treatment of patients with atopic dermatitis using wet-wrap dressings with diluted steroids and/or emollients. An expert panel's opinion and review of the literature. J. Eur. Acad. Dermatol. Venereol. 20(10): 1277–1286. doi:10.1111/j.1468-3083.2006.01790.x.

Owen, J. L., Vakharia, P. P. and Silverberg, J. I. 2018. The role and diagnosis of allergic contact dermatitis in patients with atopic dermatitis. Am. J. Clin. Dermatol. 19(3): 293–302. doi:10.1007/s40257-017-0340-7.

Pacheco, K. A. 2019. Allergy to surgical implants. Clin. Rev. Allergy Immunol. 56(1): 72–85. doi:10.1007/s12016-018-8707-y.

Pariser, D. M., Simpson, E. L., Gadkari, A., Bieber, T., Margolis, D. J., Brown, M. et al. 2020. Evaluating patient-perceived control of atopic dermatitis: design, validation, and scoring of the Atopic Dermatitis Control Tool (ADCT). Curr. Med. Res. Opin. 36(3): 367–376. doi:10.1080/03007995.2019.1699516.

Pimpinelli, N., Olsen, E. A., Santucci, M., Vonderheid, E., Haeffner, A. C., Stevens, S. et al. 2005. Defining early mycosis fungoides. J. Am. Acad. Dermatol. 53(6): 1053–1063. doi:10.1016/j.jaad.2005.08.057.

Ponyai, G., Hidvegi, B., Nemeth, I., Sas, A., Temesvari, E. and Karpati, S. 2008. Contact and aeroallergens in adulthood atopic dermatitis. J. Eur. Acad. Dermatol. Venereol. 22(11): 1346–1355. doi:10.1111/j.1468-3083.2008.02886.x.

Pratt, M. D., Mufti, A., Lipson, J., Warshaw, E. M., Maibach, H. I., Taylor, J. S. et al. 2017. Patch test reactions to corticosteroids: retrospective analysis from the North American Contact Dermatitis Group 2007–2014. Dermatitis 28(1): 58–63. doi:10.1097/DER.0000000000000251.

Prens, E. P., Benne, K., Geursen-Reitsma, A. M., van Dijk, G., Benner, R. and van Joost, T. 1989. Effects of topically applied glucocorticosteroids on patch test responses and recruitment of inflammatory cells in allergic contact dermatitis. Agents Actions 26(1-2): 125–127. doi:10.1007/BF02126583.

Rehal, B. and Armstrong, A. W. 2011. Health outcome measures in atopic dermatitis: a systematic review of trends in disease severity and quality-of-life instruments 1985–2010. PLoS One 6(4): e17520. doi:10.1371/journal.pone.0017520.

Rhodes, J., Clay, C. and Phillips, M. 2013. The surface area of the hand and the palm for estimating percentage of total body surface area: results of a meta-analysis. Br J. Dermatol. 169(1): 76–84. doi:10.1111/bjd.12290.

Roerdink, E. M., Flokstra-de Blok, B. M., Blok, J. L., Schuttelaar, M. L., Niggemann, B., Werfel, T. et al. 2016. Association of food allergy and atopic dermatitis exacerbations. Ann. Allergy Asthma Immunol. 116(4): 334–338. doi:10.1016/j.anai.2016.01.022.

Rudikoff, D. and Lebwohl, M. 1998. Atopic dermatitis. Lancet 351(9117): 1715–21. doi: 10.1016/S0140-6736(97)12082-7.

Schafer, T., Heinrich, J., Wjst, M., Adam, H., Ring, J. and Wichmann, H. E. 1999. Association between severity of atopic eczema and degree of sensitization to aeroallergens in schoolchildren. J. Allergy Clin. Immunol. 104(6): 1280–1284. doi:10.1016/s0091-6749(99)70025-4.

Schmidlin, K., Sani, S., Bernstein, D. I. and Fonacier, L. 2020. A hands-on approach to contact dermatitis and patch testing. J. Allergy Clin. Immunol. Pract. 8(6): 1883–1893. doi:10.1016/j.jaip.2020.02.009.

Schmitt, J., Langan, S., Deckert, S., Svensson, A., von Kobyletzki, L., Thomas, K. et al. 2013. Assessment of clinical signs of atopic dermatitis: a systematic review and recommendation. J. Allergy Clin. Immunol. 132(6): 1337–1347. doi:10.1016/j.jaci.2013.07.008.

Schneider, L., Tilles, S., Lio, P., Boguniewicz, M., Beck, L., LeBovidge, J. et al. 2013. Atopic dermatitis: a practice parameter update 2012. J. Allergy Clin. Immunol. 131(2): 295–299 e291–227. doi:10.1016/j.jaci.2012.12.672.

Severity scoring of atopic dermatitis: the SCORAD index. Consensus Report of the European Task Force on Atopic Dermatitis. 1993. Dermatology 186(1): 23–31. doi:10.1159/000247298.

Shi, V. Y. and Lio, P. A. 2013. In-office diagnosis of cutaneous mycosis: a comparison of potassium hydroxide, Swartz-Lamkins, and chlorazol black E fungal stains. Cutis 92(6): E8–10.

Sicherer, S. H. and Sampson, H. A. 1999. Food hypersensitivity and atopic dermatitis: pathophysiology, epidemiology, diagnosis, and management. J. Allergy Clin. Immunol. 104(3 Pt 2): S114–122. doi:10.1016/s0091-6749(99)70053-9.

Sidbury, R., Tom, W. L., Bergman, J. N., Cooper, K. D., Silverman, R. A., Berger, T. G. et al. 2014. Guidelines of care for the management of atopic dermatitis: Section 4. Prevention of disease flares and use of adjunctive therapies and approaches. J. Am. Acad. Dermatol. 71(6): 1218–1233. doi:10.1016/j.jaad.2014.08.038.

Simpson, E., Bissonnette, R., Eichenfield, L. F., Guttman-Yassky, E., King, B., Silverberg, J. I. et al. 2020. The Validated Investigator Global Assessment for Atopic Dermatitis (vIGA-AD): The development and reliability testing of a novel clinical outcome measurement instrument for the severity of atopic dermatitis. J. Am. Acad. Dermatol. 83(3): 839–846. doi:10.1016/j.jaad.2020.04.104.

Singh, A. M., Anvari, S., Hauk, P., Lio, P., Nanda, A., Sidbury, R. et al. 2022. Atopic dermatitis and food allergy: best practices and knowledge gaps-work group report from the AAAAI allergic skin diseases committee and leadership institute project. J. Allergy Clin. Immunol. Pract. doi:10.1016/j.jaip.2021.12.037.

Stander, S. 2021. Atopic Dermatitis. N Engl. J. Med. 384(12): 1136–1143. doi:10.1056/NEJMra2023911.

Strid, J., Hourihane, J., Kimber, I., Callard, R. and Strobel, S. 2005. Epicutaneous exposure to peanut protein prevents oral tolerance and enhances allergic sensitization. Clin. Exp. Allergy 35(6): 757–766. doi:10.1111/j.1365-2222.2005.02260.x.

Sukanto, H., Nater, J. P. and Bleumink, E. 1981. Influence of topically applied corticosteroids on patch test reactions. Contact Dermatitis 7(4): 180–185. doi:10.1111/j.1600-0536.1981.tb04038.x.

Tam, I. and Yu, J. 2020. Allergic contact dermatitis in children: recommendations for patch testing. Curr. Allergy Asthma Rep. 20(9): 41. doi:10.1007/s11882-020-00939-z.

Warshaw, E. M., Voller, L. M., Maibach, H. I., Zug, K. A., DeKoven, J. G., Atwater, A. R. et al. 2021. Eyelid dermatitis in patients referred for patch testing: Retrospective analysis of North American Contact Dermatitis Group data, 1994–2016. J. Am. Acad. Dermatol. 84(4): 953–964. doi:10.1016/j.jaad.2020.07.020.

Werfel, T. and Breuer, K. 2004. Role of food allergy in atopic dermatitis. Curr. Opin. Allergy Clin. Immunol. 4(5): 379–385. doi:10.1097/00130832-200410000-00009.

Wood Heickman, L. K., Davallow Ghajar, L., Conaway, M. and Rogol, A. D. 2018. Evaluation of hypothalamic-pituitary-adrenal axis suppression following cutaneous use of topical corticosteroids in children: a meta-analysis. Horm Res. Paediatr. 89(6): 389–396. doi:10.1159/000489125.

Yosipovitch, G., Reaney, M., Mastey, V., Eckert, L., Abbe, A., Nelson, L. et al. 2019. Peak Pruritus Numerical Rating Scale: psychometric validation and responder definition for assessing itch in moderate-to-severe atopic dermatitis. Br J. Dermatol. 181(4): 761–769. doi:10.1111/bjd.17744.

Chapter 7

Drug Allergy

Saad Alshareef,* William Bermingham, Rashmeet Bhogal, Mohamed Omar and
Mamidipudi Thirumala Krishna

Introduction

Adverse drug reactions occur in around 15% of hospitalized patients and up to 25% of the patients in ambulatory clinics. Drug allergy is less common as it accounts only for less than 10% of all adverse drug reactions (Thong and Tan 2011). The prevalence of penicillin allergy labels has been estimated to be between 5.9% and 10% in the UK and the USA's population studies and up to 15% of hospitalized patients. However, a number of studies have shown that, following comprehensive allergy tests, 90–95% of penicillin allergy labels are inaccurate (West et al. 2019; Macy and Contreras 2014; Lee et al. 2000; National Institute for Health and Care Excellence 2014).

Adverse drug reactions can be broadly classified as either predictable (Type A) or unpredictable (Type B) (Table 1). Predictable reactions are dose-dependent and related to a known pharmacologic action of the drug. Common examples include drug toxicity, side effects and drug interactions. The reaction could be due to an overdose or binding to "off-target" receptors. Whereas unpredictable reactions are dose-independent and are unrelated to known pharmacologic actions of the drug. Unpredictable reactions can be subdivided into drug intolerance, drug idiosyncrasy, pseudoallergic reaction and hypersensitivity reactions (HSRs).

Gell-Coombs' classification of hypersensitivity links the clinical presentation to an underlying immunological mechanism (Table 2). A more recent classification emphasized the importance of other pathomechanisms of delayed HSRs (Pichler 2019). In addition to allergic immune reactions that occur secondary to antigens, there are also p-I (pharmacological interaction with immune receptors) and pseudoallergic reactions (Table 3). In p-I mediated reaction, the drug binds directly to the immune receptor and leads to T-cell mediated reactions, such as maculopapular exanthema, drug

[1] International training fellow, University Hospitals Birmingham NHS Foundation Trust.

[2] MRCP, FRCPath. Specialist trainee in Immunology. University Hospitals Birmingham NHS Foundation Trust.

[3] Antimicrobial and Research Pharmacist Prescriber. Pharmacy department, University Hospitals of Birmingham NHS Foundation Trust.

[4] MRCP, FRCPath. Consultant Allergist and Immunologist. University Hospitals Birmingham NHS Foundation Trust.

[5] FRCP, FRCPath, DNB. Consultant Allergist and Immunologist, University Hospitals Birmingham NHS Foundation Trust. Honorary Professor in Allergy, Clinical Immunology and Global Health Institute of Immunology & Immunotherapy and Institute of Clinical Sciences the University of Birmingham. Head of Postgraduate School of Pathology, West Midlands Health Education England.

Emails: william.bermingham@nhs.net; rashmeet.bhogal@uhb.nhs.uk; Omar.Mohamed@uhb.nhs.uk; Thirumala.Krishna@uhb.nhs.uk

* Corresponding author: saadmd3@gmail.com

Table 1. Types of drug reactions.

Type of Adverse Drug Reactions	Features	Examples
A: Predicable	– Dose-dependent – Due to the pharmacologic actions of the drug – Occurs in healthy individuals	Drug toxicity Side effects Drug interactions

B: Unpredictable	– Dose-independent
	– Unrelated to the pharmacologic actions of the drug
	– Some reactions occur in susceptible individuals
		– Drug allergy
		– Pseudoallergic reactions
		– Drug intolerance:
		  • Example: aspirin-induced tinnitus
		– Drug idiosyncrasy:
		  • Usually due to underlying abnormalities of metabolism, excretion, or bioavailability
		  • Example: primaquine induced hemolytic anemia in G6DP–deficient individuals

Table 2. Gell-coombs classification of drug hypersensitivity.

Classification of Immunologically Mediated Drug Hypersensitivity Reactions (Gell-Coombs Classification)			
Types	Mechanism	Notes/Symptoms	Selected Examples
1	IgE mediated hypersensitivity reactions	Urticarial rash, pruritus, and wheezing. Severe symptoms include hypotension, laryngeal edema, and anaphylaxis. (Within minutes-few hours depending on the route of administration).	→ Anaphylaxis to penicillin, ciprofloxacin, rocuronium, atracurium, etc.
2	Cytotoxic reactions	Antibodies, in this case IgM or IgG, bind to cell bound antigens leading to complement activation leading to cell destruction. Drugs can alter the cell surface, generating new epitopes that could be the target of these antibodies.	→ Haemolysis caused by methyldopa and penicillin. → Thrombocytopenia caused by quinidine. These reactions are very rare and not amenable to skin tests.
3	Immune complex reactions	Antigen-antibody complexes deposition causes complement activation and more damage. Fever, rash, urticaria, lymphadenopathy, and arthralgia. It occurs few weeks after exposure to the offending drug.	→ Phenytoin induced vasculitis. → Penicillin induced serum sickness.
4	Cell mediated reactions	Can be subdivided into four categories depending on the type of effector cells recruited: → monocytes (IVa) → eosinophils (IVb) → CD4 or CD8 T cells (IVc) → neutrophils (IVd)	→ Contact dermatitis. → Allopurinol induced DRESS. → Carbamazepine induced → SJS/TEN. → Quinolones-induced AGEP

rash with eosinophilia and systemic symptoms (DRESS), Stevens-Johnson syndrome SJS/Toxic epidermal necrolysis (TEN), acute generalized exanthematous pustulosis (AGEP) and hepatitis. Some of these are mediated by delayed HSRs (HSRs; Type-4; see Table 2). In pseudoallergic reactions, the drugs bind directly to effector cells or inflammatory cells and induce symptoms depending on the receptor they bind to. For example, when a drug binds directly to the MRGPRX2 receptor on mast cells, it induces stimulation of the mast cells and release of mediators that can cause anaphylaxis-like symptoms without the need for prior sensitization. Several agents are known

Table 3. Immune pathomechanism and classification of drug hypersensitivity.

Type B Drug Reactions	Mechanism	Example
Allergic Immune	– Formation of new antigen by the binding between the drug or drug metabolite to proteins (hapten-protein complex) – "Both" humoral and/or cellular immune responses can be involved	Any type of Coombs and Gell's hypersensitivity classification
p-i	– Drugs bind directly to immune receptors proteins – Results in a **T-cell mediated** reactions which could have features of both hypersensitivity and/or autoimmunity – This is an example of a drug binding an off-target receptor which leads to unwanted T-cell stimulation – Some of these reactions occur in carriers of certain HLA alleles (For example, abacavir-induced severe hypersensitivity in carriers of HLAB*5701 allele)	DRESS SJS/TEN AGEP
Pesudoallergic	– Drug directly activates effector inflammatory cells, and hence the humoral and cellular immune systems are not involved – Dose dependent – Prior sensitization is not required.	– Some drugs can bind and activate the MRGPRX2 on mast cells, which leads to mast cells activation and release of mediators – Examples include some of the NMBA, e.g., atracurium, and fluoroquinolones, e.g., ciprofloxacin

(Pichler 2019)

to cause such reactions, such as opiates, radiocontrast media, some neuromuscular blocking agents and vancomycin.

Drug Hypersensitivity

Drug HSRs are immunologically mediated responses. Most are Type-1 or Type-4 HSRs, and a small proportion is deemed secondary to p-I or pseudoallergic mechanisms (Demoly et al. 2014). The reactions are usually against active ingredients of the drug and rarely to excipients. The reaction typically occurs following prior sensitization, which results in the production of drug-specific antibodies, T cells or both.

History

Most of the available investigations have limited utility due to unknown predictive values, therefore allergists rely on a systematic clinical history and scrutiny of available documentation in the diagnostic process. Standard documentation of the drug reaction should include the following:

1. The name of the medication
2. The clinical indication for the medication
3. How long ago did the reaction occur?
4. The systems (e.g., cutaneous, respiratory and gastrointestinal) involved in the reaction and its characteristics?
5. When during the treatment course did the reaction occur?
6. Was the patient taking concurrent medications at the time of the reaction? If yes, then what are the medications? For how long he has been taking these medications? And is he still taking them?

7. The therapeutic management of the reaction?

8. Had the patient taken the same or a cross-reacting medication before the reaction?

9. Has the patient been re-exposed to the same or similar medication since the reaction?

10. Were any investigations done to evaluate the reaction?

11. Does the patient have an underlying condition (e.g., chronic spontaneous urticaria, mastocytosis) that enhances the risk of reactions to certain medications?

Physical Examination

It is important to document all the physical signs that were observed during the allergic reaction. Different cutaneous manifestations can accompany any drug reaction. Recognizing the pattern, the timing and the morphology of the skin involvement is vital to reach an accurate diagnosis. While urticaria and angioedema are common features of drug HSRs, bullous exanthem, mucosal involvement and systemic symptoms are suggestive of more severe reactions, i.e., SJS and TEN. Non-blanching petechiae or purpura may suggest "drug-induced vasculitis."

Differential Diagnosis

Not every rash that occurs while the patient is taking a drug necessarily represents a drug allergy. Rash that accompanies infections or chronic spontaneous urticaria is frequently misdiagnosed as a drug allergy.

Infection

Different bacterial and viral infections are associated with a rash which could be precipitated by commencing antimicrobials. A typical example is amoxicillin-induced rash in patients with Epstein-Barr virus (EBV) infection. Patients typically lack other symptoms of allergy, pruritus, mucocutaneous swelling, wheezing or hemodynamic instability. The rash is typically mild and self-limiting. This is not an allergic reaction and patients are likely to tolerate future courses of the antibiotic in the future.

Chronic Idiopathic Urticaria

Patients with chronic idiopathic urticaria experience urticarial rash randomly which can be triggered by different factors including infections. Patients may notice urticarial rash when they have an infection and start antibiotics and attribute the rash to drug allergy. Usually, these patients will report similar episodes of spontaneous rash without taking on the drug.

Investigations

Serum Tryptase

An elevated acute serum tryptase level indicates mast cell activation. Samples ideally should be collected within between 15 minutes and 3 hours (levels peak 1–2 hours) after symptoms onset and should be rechecked > 24 hours after initial presentation. Baseline tryptase levels are usually persistently elevated in patients with clonal mast cell disorders (e.g., systemic mastocytosis). Discrimination between mature β-tryptase and total serum tryptase leads to greater specificity in the diagnosis of anaphylaxis. Acute serum tryptase $\geq (2 + 1.2 \times$ baseline tryptase levels) indicates mast cell activation. However, it is worth noting that serum tryptase may not be elevated in a small proportion of patients with anaphylaxis.

Skin Tests

Skin tests are used to investigate Type-1 and Type-4 HSRs. They must always be interpreted in conjunction with clinical history and an understanding of pre-test probability for HSRs. Skin tests should not be used to "screen" patients for an allergy. They should not be used in the context of Type-2 or Type-3 HSRs. Skin tests involve skin prick tests followed by intradermal tests. Intradermal tests are performed when skin prick tests are negative or equivocal. There are published Non-Irritant concentrations for skin tests of common drugs (Brockow et al. 2013; Broyles et al. 2020; Joint Task Force on Practice Parameters 2010). Where non-irritant concentrations are not available skin prick tests and intradermal tests may be considered at "neat"/1:10 and 1:1,000–1:10 of stock solutions. A positive skin prick test indicates the presence of drug (or excipient) specific IgE. Similarly, a positive intradermal test at 15–20 minutes indicates sensitization (IgE) and a delayed positive response (at 48–72 hours) indicates a T-cell mediated or delayed hypersensitivity response (Mirakian et al. 2009). As with other allergens, antihistamines should be temporarily withdrawn for 3–5 days prior to the tests. Concurrent therapy with high-dose corticosteroids and/or immunosuppressive medications may affect delayed intradermal test response.

Immunoassay for Allergen-Specific IgE

Predictive values (sensitivity/specificity) are established only for very few drugs, making these tests less useful when compared to skin testing. In general, they are very useful when tests are positive in the context of a high pre-test probability (positive predictive value); however, negative results do not exclude IgE-mediated allergy as most have poor negative predictive values. In other words, a negative serum-specific IgE test on its own does an exclude an allergy. Antihistamines do not need to be withdrawn prior to specific IgE testing.

The Basophil Activation Test (BAT) and Lymphocyte Transformation Test (LTT)

During BAT, the patient's blood is incubated to the allergen (drug) in question. Basophil activation is determined by flow cytometry using expression of CD63 and/or CD203c and indicates the presence of drug-specific IgE. Whereas in the lymphocyte transformation test, the patient's blood is incubated with the allergen and the drug-specific T-cell proliferation is measured. While BAT can be useful in the investigation of Type-1 HSRs, LTT is used to investigate Type-4 HSRs. Both tests have not made their way into routine clinical practice as they are expensive and require specialist laboratory setup, are labor intensive, require specialist interpretation and are not yet validated (Mirakian et al. 2015).

Drug Provocation Test (DPT)

DPT remains the gold standard in confirming or excluding drug allergies. Indications, contraindications and practical aspects are listed in Table 4. Available protocols have not been validated, and they should be customized to each patient. For example, patients with penicillin allergy labels are stratified as "low risk" and "high risk." Low-risk patients are deemed most unlikely to be truly allergic based on the clinical history and/or review of clinical records. They may be subjected to a "direct oral penicillin challenge" under supervision without undertaking allergy tests or a single dose DPT has undertaken after demonstrating negative tests. On the other hand, those stratified as "high risk" have a clinical history suggestive or either a Type-1 or Type-4 HSRs and/or an associated co-morbidity, such as severe or uncontrolled asthma, COPD, etc., and a 3–4 step graded challenge might be undertaken. An example of an amoxicillin oral challenge is shown in Table 5 (Mirakian et al. 2015; Romano et al. 2020).

Table 4. Indications, contraindications, safety and practical issues of the drug provocation tests.

Drug Provocation Test (DPT)	
Indications	• To exclude allergy in cases where hypersensitivity is unlikely (i.e.: nonspecific or mild symptoms not in keeping with an immune mediated reaction, e.g., refuting an inaccurate label of penicillin allergy) • As a final step in evaluating drug allergy, after demonstrating absent sensitization • As a proof of or reassurance for clinical tolerance to a potential cross-reacting drug. For example, cephalosporin in a patient with a mild index reaction to penicillin, where skin test either cannot be conducted or when skin tests are negative to penicillins and/or cephalosporin
Contraindications	• Strong clinical history (and positive skin test and/or SSIgE) • If the index reaction was a severe cutaneous adverse reaction (e.g., SJS, TEN, etc.) • History suggestive of type-2 or -3 hypersensitivity • General anaesthetic agents (neuromuscular blocking agents, propofol, etc.) • Patient choice
Safety and Practical Issues	• Procedure must be done in a controlled environment with an immediate access to a resuscitation cart and drugs for management of anaphylaxis • Patients must be fit for the procedure; haemodynamically stable, and do not have severe uncontrolled cardiorespiratory diseases • Preferable to withdraw antihistamines for 3-5 days prior where possible • If patient is taking beta blocker*, it should be temporarily withheld for 24 hours prior to the procedure after consulting with a cardiologist and/or patients family physician • Protocol should be customized based on index reaction; longer observations between steps may be undertaken

* In exceptional and/or urgent cases DPT can be undertaken without withdrawal of beta blocker. Glucagon should be available as part of available resuscitation facilities to manage potential refractory anaphylaxis.

Table 5. An example of oral amoxicillin challenge protocol (from our centre).

Time (minutes)	Dose (mg)	Cumulative Dose (mg)	Heart Rate	Blood Pressure	Peak Expiratory Flow Rate	Symptoms
0	5	5				
30	25	30				
60	75	105				
90	150	255				
120	250	505				
180	————	————				

Practical Steps
• Obtain informed consent
• Check baseline HR, BP, and PEFR
• Repeat prior to dose escalations and ensure an allergic reaction has not occurred
• Monitor for 60 minutes post-last dose
• A prolonged dose of 250 mg twice daily is given for 3 days at our center in patients with an indeterminate history or those where index reaction occurred during a course of therapy. This is done to exclude delayed or type-4 hypersensitivity
• Counsel patient regarding the outcome, amend clinical records appropriately and provide a written note

Management

Promptly withdrawing the likely offending drug is the first step in the clinical management of a suspected allergic reaction, in addition to avoiding re-exposure to the drug (or exposure to cross-reacting drugs) in the future. Also, clear and thorough documentation is paramount to avoid further reactions. Referral to allergy services should be considered for the following situations:

1. If the drug is considered indispensable, regardless of the severity of the index reaction

2. Multiple drug allergy/intolerance label

3. Penicillin allergy label, particularly with an infection-related co-morbidity (e.g., hyposplenism, immunodeficiency, immunosuppressed state, COPD, bronchiectasis, diabetes, etc.)

4. Perioperative anaphylaxis

Rapid Drug Desensitization

Rapid drug desensitization involves supervised administration of a drug to a patient with a history of (or suspected history of) Type-1 HSRs, and there are no suitable alternatives (e.g., penicillin in bacterial endocarditis, rifampicin in tuberculosis, cancer chemotherapy, etc.). This procedure is also employed in non-IgE mediated reactions to aspirin in the context of those requiring dual anti-platelet therapy prior to undertaking percutaneous coronary intervention or in the treatment of aspirin-exacerbated respiratory disease (e.g., nasal polyp in Samter's triad). There is some evidence for employing this procedure in Type-4 HSR, in patients reporting mild mucocutaneous HSRs (i.e., not severe cutaneous adverse reactions). The procedure induces a temporary immunological tolerance to the drug, and the state of immunotolerance is maintained as long the treatment is not interrupted for more than 24 hours.

The procedure is undertaken in a clinically supervised environment starting at a very small dose (e.g., 10^{-6} of therapeutic target dose) with dose escalation at 15–20 minutes, usually involving 12–16 steps. Rapid drug desensitization can be undertaken either via oral and/or intravenous routes depending on the formulation available and clinical indication. Baseline vital parameters are checked, and the patient is monitored prior to each dose escalation and for 60 minutes post-final dose. Further details are summarized in Table 6 (Krishna and Huissoon 2011; de Groot et al. 2012; Scherer et al. 2013). Common case scenarios are discussed in scenarios 1 and 2 to put basic principles into clinical perspective. An overall approach to drug allergy is summarized in Flowchart 1 and key messages are in Table 7.

Table 6. Indications, contraindications and practical aspects of rapid drug desensitization.

Desensitization	
Indications	• Confirmed type-1 hypersensitivity to a drug (positive skin test and/or specific IgE) or when there is a strong history of type-1 hypersensitivity. No suitable alternative available and the drug is needed (e.g., penicillin in bacterial endocarditis, rifampicin in TB, cancer chemotherapy drugs etc.) • Can be considered for delayed or type-4 reaction, if the index reaction was mild cutaneous and not a severe cutaneous adverse reaction • Aspirin in the context of aspirin exacerbated respiratory disease/nasal polyps or percutaneous coronary intervention with a need for double antiplatelet therapy (see main text)
Contraindications	• If the index reaction is severe cutaneous reaction such as SJS, TEN, and DRESS. • If the index reaction is likely to represent Gell-Coombs type 2, or type 3 hypersensitivity reaction. • Severe uncontrolled respiratory disease (asthma, chronic obstructive pulmonary disease) • Hemodynamic instability • Poorly controlled cardiovascular diseases
Checklist	• Written informed consent • Inpatient procedure (intensive treatment unit or a regular ward) • 1:1 supervision with availability of a clinician on-site • Immediate access to cardiopulmonary resuscitation and critical care outreach team • Ensure patient's cardio-respiratory status is stable (e.g.: asthma, chronic obstructive pulmonary disease, heart function) • Beta blockers should be discontinued if deemed safe (otherwise keep glucagon ready for treatment of refractory anaphylaxis) • Antihistamine/s should be discontinued where possible • Peripheral vein cannulation for IV access • Check baseline vital parameters including heart rate, blood pressure, and peak expiratory flow rate (PEFR) and prior to each step. • Monitor the patient for symptoms of an allergic reaction.

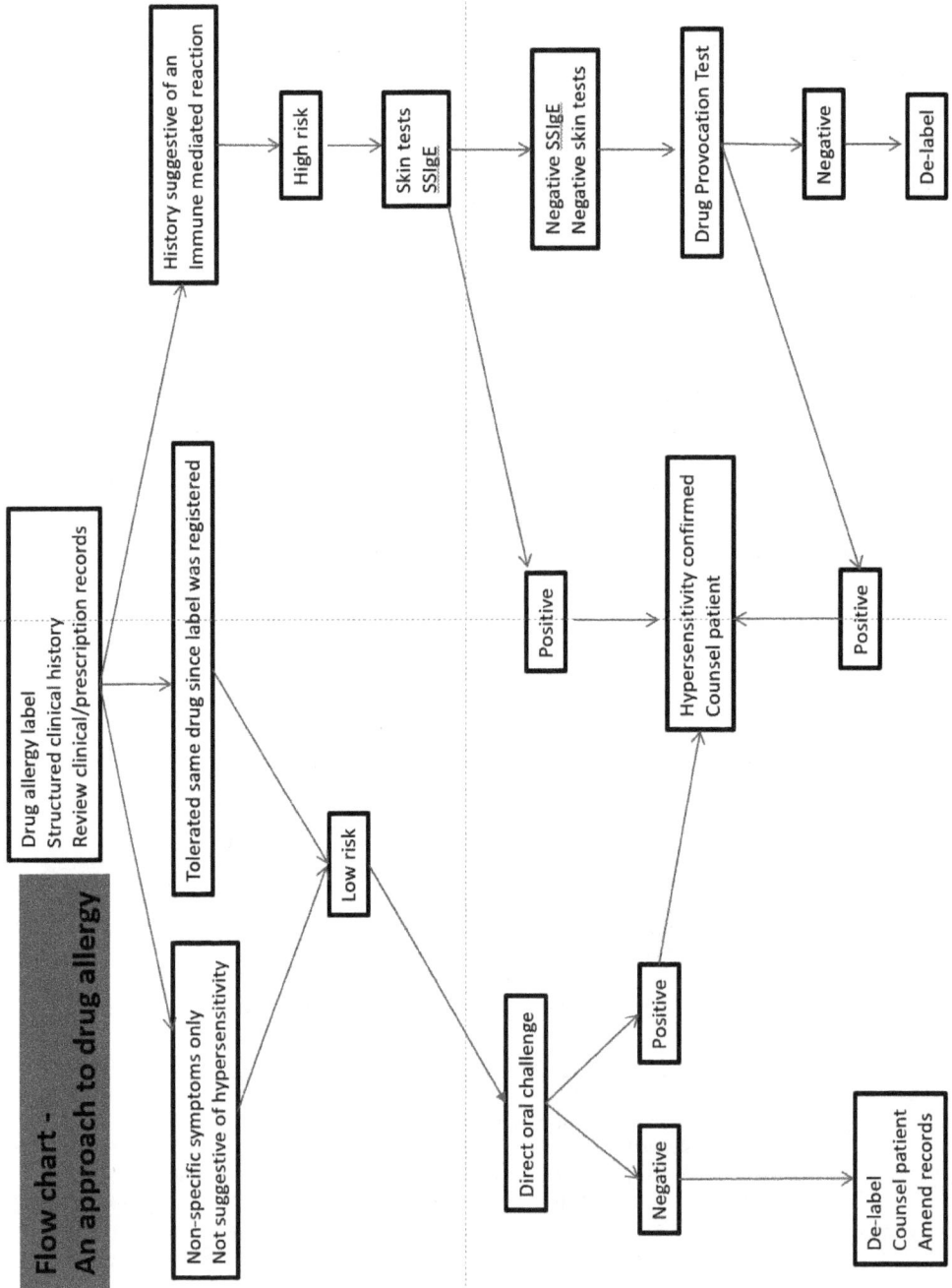

Flowchart 1. A general approach to drug allergy.

Table 7. Drug allergy key messages.

Drug Allergy – 'Clinical Pearls'	• Structured clinical history • Scrutinise clinical/prescription records – drugs, doses, temporal association with symptoms • Evaluate for systemic involvement and characterise clinical presentation • Ask the question – 'Is this a hypersensitivity (HSR) reaction'? consider differential diagnosis • Stop suspected drug/s • Consider referral to a specialist with experience in drug allergy • Consider allergy tests • Bear in mind: Predictive values not known for skin tests and in vitro tests for most drugs not established • Drug Provocative Tests (DPT) is 'gold standard' in diagnosis • Consider DPT when allergy is unlikely and after undertaking a 'risk-benefit analysis' • Ask the Q: 'Is this drug really essential for this patient'? • Basic knowledge of hypersensitivity reactions and immune mechanisms of drug allergy is essential to work your way through!

Conclusion

Key to successful clinical outcomes in drug allergy management is to obtain a systematic clinical history and review of clinical/prescription records. Current best practice involves performing and interpreting skin tests (and specific IgE where available) in the context of the patient's clinical history. Prior knowledge of performance characteristics of allergy tests to individual drug classes is needed in specialist clinical practice.

DPT should be undertaken in a safe clinical environment preferably by trained personnel with immediate access to the management of anaphylaxis and access to critical care management. Furthermore, knowledge of drugs implicated in specific types of non-immediate or Type-4 HSRs and maintaining a broad differential diagnosis is key to underpinning accurate diagnosis and management of serious systemic non-immediate HSRs.

Prospective data collection and characterization of adverse drug reactions and the application of information technology and machine learning might provide a platform to generate more reliable datasets regarding epidemiology and for the application of pharmaco-genomics to pave the way for precision and personalized medicine.

Common Scenarios

1. **A 60-year-old male patient was admitted via the emergency department with a case of neurosyphilis. He has a documented history of anaphylaxis to penicillin 4 years ago. What is the most appropriate approach?**

Intravenous penicillin is the preferred treatment for neurosyphilis. Desensitization is the most appropriate approach for this patient due to the following:

• There are no suitable alternatives to penicillin to treat neurosyphilis

• The initial reaction was an anaphylaxis

• The urgency to start antimicrobial

An example of a penicillin desensitization protocol is shown in Table 8. Desensitization can be offered for patients with confirmed drug allergies or in cases where the drug is needed urgently, and treatment cannot be postponed until the complete evaluation is done. It induces only a temporary tolerance to the drug, so future courses of the drug should be introduced via desensitization. Also, it is important to review the patient carefully for the presence of any contraindications. Please look at Table 6 for the practical aspects of desensitization.

Table 8. Example of Intravenous Penicillin Desensitization Protocol.

Dose Number	Penicillin Concentration (mg/mL)	Infusion Rate (mL/h)	Dose (mg)	Cumulative Dose (mg)	Time	Heart Rate	Blood Pressure	Respiratory Rate	Oxygen Saturation
1	0.01	6	0.015	0.015					
2	0.01	12	0.03	0.045					
3	0.01	24	0.06	0.105					
4	0.01	50	0.125	0.23					
5	0.1	10	0.25	0.48					
6	0.1	20	0.5	1.0					
7	0.1	40	1.0	2.0					
8	0.1	80	2.0	4.0					
9	0.1	160	4.0	8.0					
10	10.0	3	7.5	15.0					
11	10.0	6	15.0	30.0					
12	10.0	12	30.0	60.0					
13	10.0	25	62.5	123.0					
14	10.0	50	125.0	250.0					
15	10.0	100	250.0	500.0					
16	10.0	200	500.0	1000.0					

The time interval between doses should be 15 minutes, and it should 30 minutes before the final dose. Approximate duration of the whole procedure is 4.5 hours. Reproduced with permission from de Groot, H., W. M. Mulder and I. Terreehorst. 2012. Utility of desensitisation for allergy to antibiotics. Neth J. Med. 70(2): 58–62.

2. **A 32-year-old female patient had anaphylaxis during an appendectomy. The acute serum tryptase level was 45 ng/L at 30 minutes post-anaphylaxis and a baseline measurement at 24 hours was 30 ng/L. The patient received atracurium, fentanyl, propofol and ondansetron at induction. Skin test (intradermal) confirmed a positive reaction to atracurium, and there was no demonstrable sensitization to fentanyl, propofol, ondansetron, latex and chlorhexidine. Tests were also undertaken for rocuronium and suxamethonium as alternative NMBAs and these were negative. What is the most appropriate approach?**

This young patient developed anaphylaxis during the procedure, and baseline serum tryptase level was persistently high suggestive of a possible clonal mast cell disorder such as systemic mastocytosis. The key step in long-term management is to avoid certain triggers as far as possible than can induce mast cell activation and these include:

1. *Pharmacological agents with histamine-releasing properties*: radio-contrast medium (RCM), opiates, NMBAs (especially atracurium and mivacurium), vancomycin, amphotericin B and NSAIDs. These drugs are not contraindicated if there is no previous history of an allergic reaction or if the patient has shown clinical tolerance recently. However, it is recommended that the first dose is administered under close clinical supervision with immediate access to the management of anaphylaxis in a hospital setting. Some clinicians prefer to premedicate patients with high-dose antihistamines and/or corticosteroids prior to administration of RCM.

2. Mechanical factors include tourniquet pressure and trauma.

3. Sudden change in temperature; a cold operating room or cold intravenous fluid.

4. Bee and wasp stings.

It is important to be aware of the pharmacological effect of the drugs that are routinely used during the induction or maintenance of anesthesia. A physiological drop in blood pressure after induction can occur because of the vasodilator effect of these agents. Also, reactions related to transfused blood products or colloids, and hypotension or hypoxia secondary to other medical problems (acute myocardial infarction and pulmonary embolism), should not be confused with allergic reactions

When evaluating a patient with a history of perioperative anaphylaxis, it is useful to perform skin testing for the drugs used during the procedure as well as for safe alternatives to consider in the future. In addition, latex, antiseptics, and diagnostic dyes should be included in the evaluation of any perioperative reactions. Because of the intrinsic histamine-releasing activity of neuromuscular blocking agents, it is recommended to use two dilutions for skin prick testing to minimize the risk of false positive results. These are the neat concentration and the 1:10 dilution for skin prick testing. The risk of a false-positive is even greater with intradermal testing, therefore further dilution is needed. A general approach to patients with perioperative reactions is summarized in Flowchart 2 (Garvey et al. 2019; Ewan et al. 2009).

3. **A 53-year-old male patient presented with acute myocardial infarction, and he is planned to receive dual antiplatelets for percutaneous coronary intervention. He has well-controlled asthma and has undergone two operations for nasal polyps. There is documented history of "aspirin allergy"—reports wheezing and a possible throat swelling 30 minutes after the first dose about 5 years ago. What is the most appropriate approach?**

Aspirin is a nonsteroidal anti-inflammatory drug (NSAID). Several phenotypes have been identified for NSAID reactions. This includes:

- Aspirin exacerbated respiratory disease (AERD); as in this patient
- NSAID-exacerbated cutaneous disease (NECD)
- NSAID-induced urticaria and/or angioedema (NIUA) in chronic spontaneous urticaria
- Single NSAID-induced urticaria/anaphylaxis

Aspirin desensitization is indicated for this patient. Successful desensitization protocols have been reported in patients with acute ischemia. Aspirin desensitization is usually done over a few hours, but the protocol can be customized to be over a day or two. An example of a protocol that is adopted in our center (Heartlands Hospital) is shown in Table 9. If the patient develops any allergy symptoms, treat the reaction promptly and go back 2–3 steps in the protocol prior to cautiously repeating the dose that induced the reaction.

4. **A 43-year-old male with no previous medical illness has been admitted with community-acquired pneumonia. The medical team wants to commence amoxicillin, but he has a penicillin allergy label on his record. The patient reports a very mild rash (not urticaria and nothing to suggest vasculitis, desquamation, mucosal or systemic involvement) on day 4 of treatment with amoxicillin for a urinary tract infection 10 years ago. What management options can you provide for this patient?**

Clinical presentation is not suggestive of an immune-mediated reaction (i.e., 'low risk' as described in the previous section). This patient is suitable for a "direct oral penicillin challenge" without undertaking allergy tests. He should be counseled, written informed consent obtained and 500 mg amoxicillin can be administered orally and the patient monitored for an immediate allergic reaction. If Type-1 HSRs are excluded, a full therapeutic dose of amoxicillin is administered, and the patient is monitored for non-immediate HSRs. After the patient confirms clinical tolerance to the therapeutic course, the penicillin allergy label can be removed from his records, and written communication is provided to the patient's family physician. This process is called penicillin allergy de-labeling.

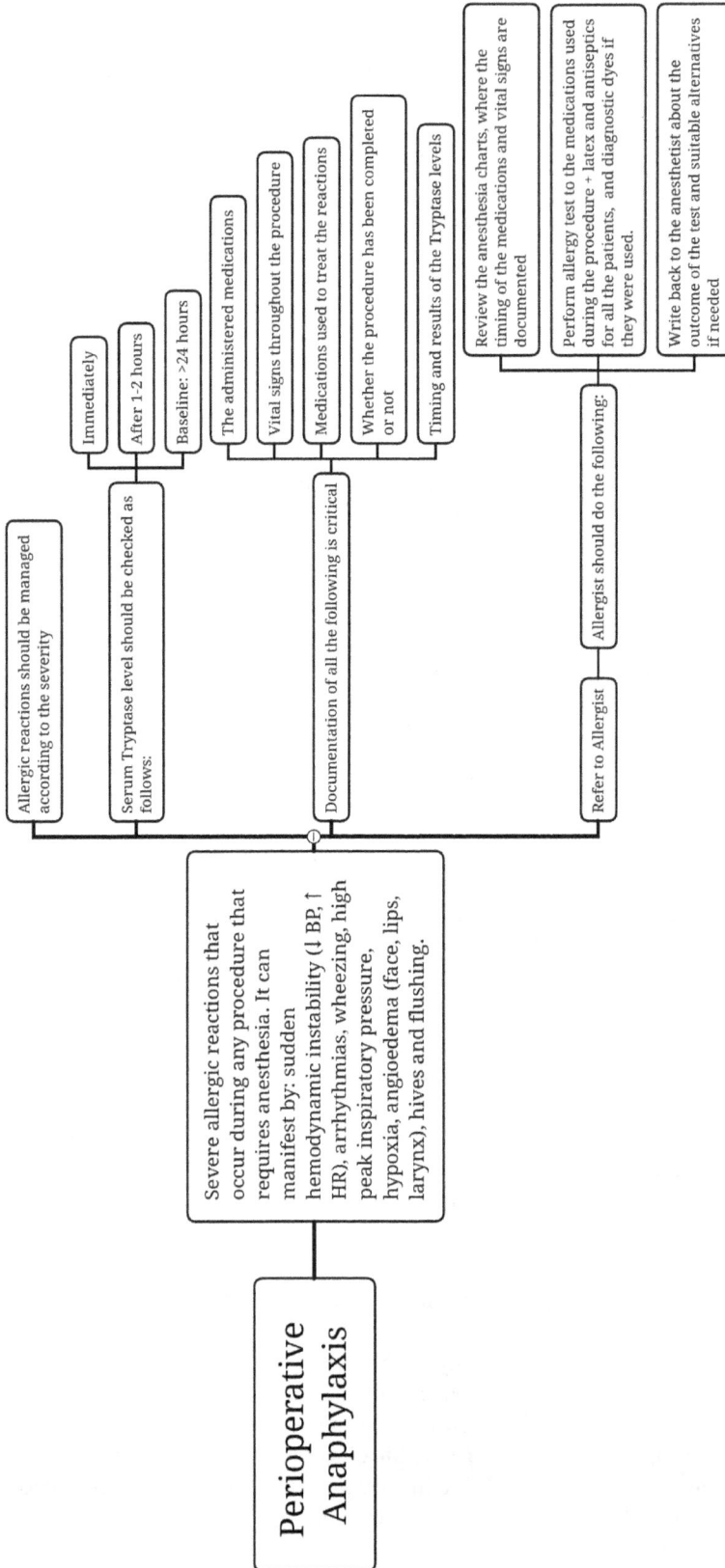

Flowchart 2. A general approach to patients with perioperative reactions.

Table 9. A suggested protocol for aspirin desensitization.

Time (min)	Aspirin Dose (mg)	Volume (ml)
0	1	
30	5	
60	10	
90	20	
210	40	
330	100	

If, on the other hand, the patient reported symptoms suggestive of an immediate or non-immediate HSRs (urticarial, angioedema, wheeze, etc.), the patient is stratified as "high risk," i.e., not suitable for a direct oral penicillin challenge, the current infection is managed with an alternative antibiotic and penicillin allergy de-labeling may be considered electively and this would involve skin tests ± DPT as described in previous sections. Please look at Flowchart 3.

5. **You have received a consultation from the medical ward, regarding a 58-year-old male patient who has just been admitted with pyelonephritis, and the team would like to start ceftriaxone for him. The patient has a penicillin allergy label, and the team is wondering about the safety of introducing cephalosporin to this patient.**

Penicillin and cephalosporin cross-reactivity exists in the context of Type-1 HSRs. The estimated percentage of penicillin-allergic patients that react upon introducing cephalosporin varies in the literature from 0.2% to 8%. Cross-reactivity is expected to be more if the penicillin and cephalosporins share a side chain. These could include amoxicillin and cefadroxil or ampicillin and cephalexin. When considering cephalosporins in a patient with penicillin allergy, consider the approach illustrated in Flowcharts 3 and 4.

Glossary of Abbreviations

AGEP – Acute Generalized Exanthematous Pustulosis
BP – Blood Pressure
EBV – Epstein-Barr Virus
DPT – Direct Provocation Tests
DRESS – Drug Rash With Eosinophilia and Systemic Symptoms
GDP – Glucose-6-Phosphate Dehydrogenase
HR – Heart Rate
HSR – Hypersensitivity Reaction
MRGPRX2 – Mas-Related G-Protein-Coupled Receptor X2
NMBA – Neuromuscular Blocking Agents
PEFR – Peak Expiratory Flow Rate
P-I – Pharmacological Interaction With Immune Receptors
SJS – Stevens-Johnson Syndrome
SSIgE – Serum-Specific Immunoglobulin E
TEN – Toxic Epidermal Necrolysis

Penicillin allergy label needing beta lactam for infection and no immediate access to allergy tests

 # 'High risk' stratification
- History suggestive of type-1 HSR

AVOID:
- **All penicillins**
- **First-second generation cephalosporins**

Consider 1 of the following:
Supervised graded administration of
- Carbapenems
- Supervised graded administration of 3rd–5th generation cephalosporins
- Penicillin desensitisation

 # 'High risk' stratification
- History suggestive of type-4 HSR

AVOID
- **All penicillins**

Consider:
- Carbapenems
- Cephalosporins

 # 'High risk' stratification
- unclear if type-1 or type-4 HSR

AVOID:
- All penicillins
- First-second generation cephalosporins

Consider 1 of the following:
- Supervised graded administration of
- Carbapenems
- Supervised graded administration of 3rd–5th generation cephalosporins
- @Penicillin desensitisation

'Low risk' stratification
- History not suggestive of a HSR**
OR
- patient tolerated penicillin since index reaction
AND
- clinically stable
- No severe cardiorespiratory compromise*
- Not pregnant*
- Capacity to give informed consent and a reliable history

Consider direct oral penicillin challenge (DPT) and de-label

In some cases allergy testing with specialist input may be required for reassurance and formal de-labelling via skin tests

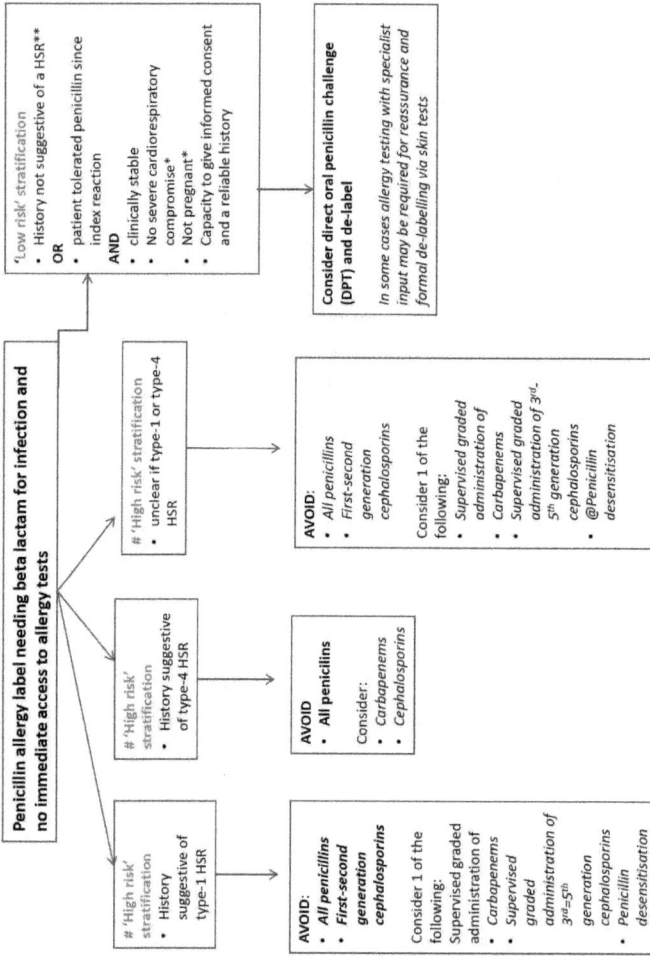

Flowchart 3. A practical approach to penicillin allergy by non-allergy specialist.

* *Switch to 'high risk' algorithm for type-1 HSR in pregnancy, clinically unstable or severe cardio-respiratory compromise, unable to consent or give a reliable history until patient is de-labelled by allergist*

@ *Contraindicated if index reaction is suggestive of Severe Cutaneous Adverse Reactions (SCAR)*

\# *Referral to allergy specialist must be considered at a later time point*

**CRITERIA:
- *Benign rash only*
- *Pruritis only*
- *Non-specific symptoms only (eg: GIT symptoms, headache, dizziness, etc)*
- *History >10years ago with no features of IgE mediated reaction*
- *Based on family history of PenA*

Introducing
Cephalosporins to a
Patient with Penicillin
Allergy Label

Was the initial reaction
to penicillin severe?
was it an anaphylaxis?

Yes —— Perform Skin testing to
Penicillin

Positive —— Skin test the required
Cephalosporin before
introduction

Negative —— Introduce the required
Cephalosporin without
skin testing

No

Introduce the required
Cephalosporin via
graded challenge

OR

Skin testing to
penicillin and proceed
accordingly as
illustrated above

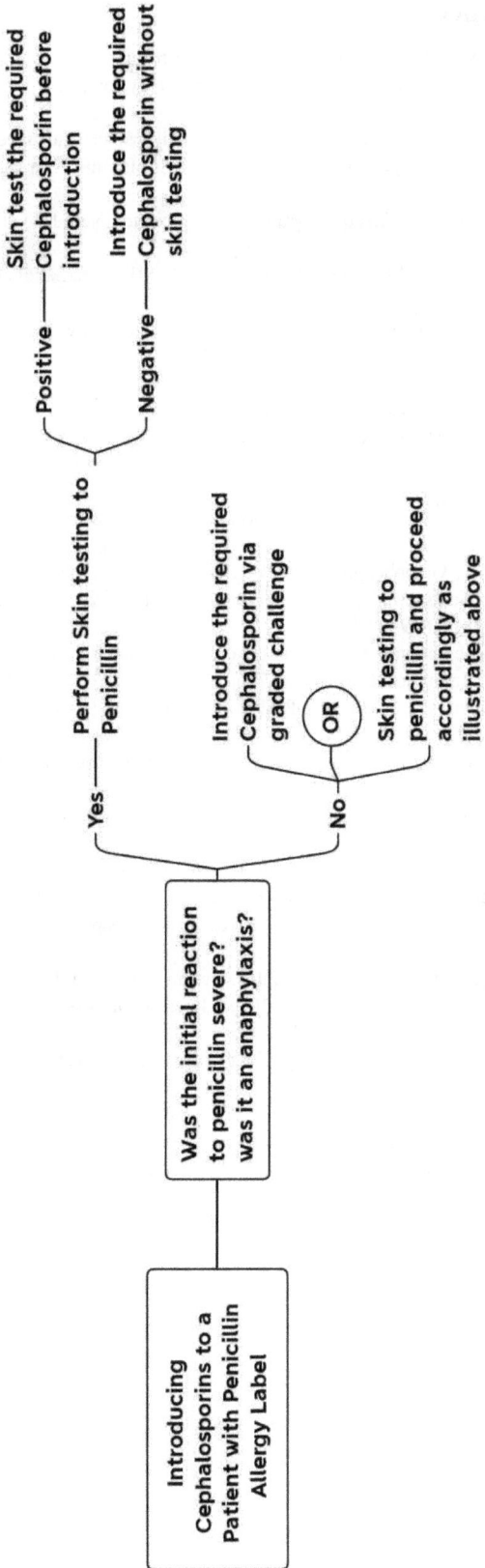

Flowchart 4. Introducing cephalosporins to patients with penicillin allergy.

References

Brockow, K., Garvey, L. H., Aberer, W., Atanaskovic-Markovic, M., Barbaud, A., Bilo, M. B., Bircher, A. et al. 2013. Skin test concentrations for systemically administered drugs—an ENDA/EAACI Drug Allergy Interest Group position paper. Allergy 68(6): 702–712.

Broyles, A. D., Banerji, A., Barmettler, S., Biggs, C. M., Blumenthal, K., Brennan, P. J. et al. 2020. Practical guidance for the evaluation and management of drug hypersensitivity: specific drugs. J. Allergy Clin. Immunol. Pract. 8(9S): S16–S116.

De Groot, H., Mulder, W. M. and Terreehorst, I. 2012. Utility of desensitisation for allergy to antibiotics. Neth J. Med. 2012 Mar; 70(2): 58–62.

Demoly, P., Adkinson, N. F., Brockow, K., Castells, M., Chiriac, A. M., Greenberger, P. A. et al. 2014. International Consensus on drug allergy. Allergy 69(4): 420–437.

Ewan, P. W., Dugué, P., Mirakian, R., Dixon, T. A., Harper, J. N., Nasser, S. M. et al. 2010. BSACI guidelines for the investigation of suspected anaphylaxis during general anaesthesia. Clin. Exp .Allergy 40(1): 15–31.

Garvey, L. H., Ebo, D. G., Mertes, P. M., Dewachter, P., Garcez, T., Kopac, P. et al. 2019. An EAACI position paper on the investigation of perioperative immediate hypersensitivity reactions. Allergy 74(10): 1872–1884.

Joint Task Force on Practice Parameters; American Academy of Allergy, Asthma and Immunology; American College of Allergy, Asthma and Immunology; Joint Council of Allergy, Asthma and Immunology. Drug allergy: An updated practice parameter. Ann. Allergy Asthma Immunol. 105(4): 259–273.

Krishna, M. T. and Huissoon, A. P. 2011. Clinical immunology review series: an approach to desensitization. Clin. Exp. Immunol. 163(2): 131–146.

Lee, C. E., Zembower, T. R., Fotis, M. A., Postelnick, M. J., Greenberger, P. A., Peterson, L. R. et al. 2000. The incidence of antimicrobial allergies in hospitalized patients: implications regarding prescribing patterns and emerging bacterial resistance. Arch. Intern. Med. 160(18): 2819–2822.

Macy, E. and Contreras, R. 2014. Health care use and serious infection prevalence associated with penicillin "allergy" in hospitalized patients: A cohort study. J. Allergy Clin. Immunol. 133(3): 790–796.

Mirakian, R., Ewan, P. W., Durham, S. R., Youlten, L. J., Dugué, P., Friedmann, P. S. et al. 2009. BSACI guidelines for the management of drug allergy. Clin. Exp. Allergy 39(1): 43–61.

Mirakian, R., Leech, S. C., Krishna, M. T., Richter, A. G., Huber, P. A., Farooque, S. et al. 2015. Management of allergy to penicillins and other beta-lactams. Clin. Exp. Allergy 45(2): 300–327.

NICE. 2014. The National Institute for Health and Care Excellence. Drug Allergy: Diagnosis and Management. pp. 5–6.

Pichler, W. J. 2019. Immune pathomechanism and classification of drug hypersensitivity. Allergy 74(8): 1457–1471.

Romano, A., Atanaskovic-Markovic, M., Barbaud, A., Bircher, A. J., Brockow, K., Caubet, J. C. et al. 2020. Towards a more precise diagnosis of hypersensitivity to beta-lactams—an EAACI position paper. Allergy 75(6): 1300–1315.

Scherer, K., Brockow, K., Aberer, W., Gooi, J. H., Demoly, P., Romano, A. et al. 2013. Desensitization in delayed drug hypersensitivity reactions—an EAACI position paper of the Drug Allergy Interest Group. Allergy 68(7): 844–852.

Thong, B. Y. and Tan, T. C. 2011. Epidemiology and risk factors for drug allergy. Br J. Clin. Pharmacol. 71(5): 684–700.

West, R. M., Smith, C. J., Pavitt, S. H., Butler, C. C., Howard, P., Bates, C. et al. 2019. 'Warning: Allergic to penicillin': association between penicillin allergy status in 2.3 million NHS general practice electronic health records, antibiotic prescribing and health outcomes. J. Antimicrob. Chemother, 74(7): 2075–2082.

Chapter 8

Laboratory Analysis of Primary Immunodeficiency

Vijaya Knight[1] and *Mandakolathur R. Murali*[2],*

Introduction

Immunodeficiency is defined as the inability to produce an adequate immune response due to the partial or complete absence of a component of the immune system or it can be caused by functional deficits in one or more components of the immune system. Immunodeficiency generally manifests as increased susceptibility to infection; however, autoimmunity (Schmidt et al. 2017), inflammation (Fodil et al. 2016), allergy (Chan and Gelfand 2015) and malignancy (Pai et al. 2021) are increasingly being recognized as possible initial clinical presentations of immunodeficiency. These clinical presentations may occur at any stage of life, from infancy to adulthood. Therefore, immunodeficiency should have a differential diagnosis when evaluating patients with recurrent, treatment-refractory or unusual infections, autoimmunity, unexplained lymphadenopathy and allergies including food allergies. Immunodeficiency may either be inherited [otherwise known as "Inborn Errors of Immunity (IEI)" or Primary Immunodeficiency (PID)] or acquired due to extrinsic factors (Secondary Immunodeficiency or SID). The causes of secondary immunodeficiency are listed in Table 1.

Inborn Errors of Immunity (IEI)

Inherited immunodeficiency (IEI) is due to pathogenic, germline variants in genes that are responsible for immune development and/or function. To date, 406 distinct IEIs with 430 different gene defects have been identified (Bousfiha et al. 2020). IEI can be autosomal or X-linked with dominant or recessive inheritance patterns. Furthermore, the gene defect may be fully or partially penetrant, leading to severe or milder clinical presentations, respectively. The clinical presentation of IEI is highly variable and includes increased susceptibility to infection, autoimmune manifestations, malignancy and/or inflammatory conditions. Other features include failure to thrive, diarrhea

[1] Associate Professor, University of Colorado School of Medicine, Department of Pediatrics, Section of Allergy and Immunology, Children's Hospital, Colorado, Translational and Diagnostic Immunology Laboratory, 13123 East 16th Avenue, Aurora, Colorado 80045.

[2] Director of Clinical Immunology laboratory, Departments of Medicine and Pathology, Massachusetts General Hospital, Assistant Professor of Medicine, Harvard University, Boston, Massachusetts 02114.
Email: vijaya.knight@childrenscolorado.org
* Corresponding author: murali50@aol.com

Table 1. Causes of secondary immunodeficiency.

Cause	Description	References
Infection	HIV infection is well recognized as a cause of secondary immunodeficiency, leading to the gradual destruction of CD4+ T lymphocytes and extreme susceptibility to opportunistic organisms. Infection with several other pathogens can lead to immunodeficiency, including measles, influenza, HTLV, malaria and Bordetella. Immunodeficiency in some of these cases may be transient	(Chinen and Shearer 2010)
Malnutrition	The most common cause of secondary immunodeficiency, worldwide. A deficiency of micronutrients required for adequate development of the innate and adaptive immune system results in diminished and inadequate immune response and oftentimes a quantitative decrease in immunoglobulins and lymphocyte subsets	(Bourke et al. 2016)
Chemotherapy/ Immunosuppressive – Therapy	Chemotherapy leads to bone marrow suppression biologics, such as rituximab selectively deplete lymphocyte populations, and pathway inhibitors such as JAK inhibitors suppress immune activation. Radiation therapy impairs innate and adaptive immunity	(Henrickson et al. 2016)
Extremes of Age	Neonates are particularly susceptible to infection owing to the immaturity of their immune system and lack of antigenic exposure Older individuals are at a higher risk of infections and malignancy owing to the diminished ability of the immune response to mount an adequate response to foreign antigens	(Goronzy 2019)
Surgery and Trauma	May be accompanied by post-surgical or trauma-related immunosuppression	(Moins-Teisserenc et al. 2021)
Metabolic Diseases	Diabetes mellitus and uremia have deleterious effects on immunity, leading to compromised innate and adaptive immune responses	(Berbudi et al. 2020; Steiger et al. 2022)
Environment	Exposure to ionizing radiation, ultraviolet light, chronic cold or heat exposure can have adverse effects on the immune system	(Lumniczky et al. 2021)

Table 2. The current IUIS classification of IEI.

Category	Examples
Immunodeficiencies affecting cellular and humoral immunity	Severe combined immunodeficiency (SCID), CD40 ligand deficiency and bare lymphocyte syndrome 1 and 2
Combined Immunodeficiency (CID) with Associated Syndromic Features	DiGeorge syndrome, Wiskott Aldrich syndrome, ataxia and telangiectasia
Predominantly Antibody Defects	X-linked agammaglobulinemia and common variable immunodeficiency
Disease of Immune Dysregulation	Familial hemophagocytic lymphohistiocytosis, Chediak-Higashi syndrome, autoimmune lymphoproliferative syndrome, immune dysregulation, polyendocrinopathy, enteropathy and X-linked syndrome (IPEX), autoimmune polyendocrinopathy, candidiasis and ectodermal dystrophy (APECED)
Congenital Defects of Phagocyte Number/Function	Shwachman-Diamond syndrome, chronic granulomatous disease (CGD), leukocyte adhesion deficiency (LAD) I, II and III
Innate Immune Defects	Mendelian susceptibility to mycobacterial disease (IFNγ and IL-12 Pathway Defects)
Auto-inflammatory defects	Inflammasome-associated auto-inflammatory syndromes, such as familial Mediterranean fever (FMF), Muckle-Wells syndrome, etc., and Type 1 Interferonopathies
Complement Defects	Deficiencies in individual complement pathway proteins and Hereditary Angioedema (HAE)
Bone marrow failure	Fanconi anemia and Dyskeratosis congenita
Phenocopies of IEI	Atypical hemolytic uremic syndrome (aHUS), pulmonary alveolar proteinosis (PAP) and adult-onset immunodeficiency with susceptibility to mycobacterial disease

and generalized skin lesions. The International Union of Immunological Societies (IUIS) expert committee on IEI reviews and proposes the classification of IEI every other year, organizing the information into the phenotypic classification of IEI and their associated gene defects. The latest reviews of well-characterized IEIs define ten distinct categories, as shown in Table 2 (Bousfiha et al. 2020; Tangye et al. 2022). A few examples of immune disorders are provided under each category.

Infectious Presentations of IEI

Although the clinical presentation of IEI can be varied, when the infection is the chief clinical complaint, knowledge of the association of certain infectious presentations with specific immune defects may guide the investigation of the immune system. Loss of or compromised function of specific immune cell populations can increase susceptibility to specific groups of pathogens. Therefore, in addition to the IUIS classification of IEI, laboratory workup for IEI may be guided by the infectious presentation. Phenotypically, IEI can be broadly classified into defects affecting T cells, B cells, neutrophils and other innate immune cells, such as monocyte/macrophages and the complement pathway (Table 3).

Table 3. Association of specific immune component with infectious presentation.

Defective Immune Component	Infectious Presentation/Associated Specific Pathogens
T Cell Defects	• Systemic or organ-specific bacterial, fungal, viral or opportunistic pathogen infections. • Severe infections that may be treatment refractory. • Pathogens include *Pneumocystis jirovecii, Candida albicans, Cryptococcus neoformans*, cytomegalovirus, rotavirus, mycobacteria, including atypical mycobacterial species and BCG vaccine, and live viral vaccine strains, such as measles vaccine.
B Cell Defects	• Repeated respiratory tract infections, such as sinusitis and pneumonia. • Common pathogens include encapsulated bacteria, such as *Streptococcus pneumoniae, Haemophilus influenzae, Neisseria and meningitidis*. • Gastrointestinal infections with *Giardia lamblia*.
Neutrophil Defects	• Deep-seated skin or organ infections. • Poor wound healing. • Common pathogens include *Staphylococcus aureus*, gram-negative bacteria, *Candida albicans*, and *Aspergillus* species.
Innate immune defects (monocyte/macrophage)	• Intracellular infections may be localized to an organ or may be disseminated. • Common pathogens include *Mycobacterium tuberculosis*, and non-tuberculous mycobacteria, such as *Mycobacterium avium*, Salmonella species and Varicella-Zoster virus.
Complement Defects	• Sinusitis, pneumonia and meningitis • Autoimmune diseases • Capsulated organisms, such as *Streptococcus pneumoniae* and *Neisseria meningitidis*. Neisserial meningitis is almost exclusively seen in defects of the alternative and terminal complement pathways

T Cell Deficiency

Patients with T cell defects present with a broad range of non-infectious and infectious presentations and are typically susceptible to infection with opportunistic pathogens such as *Pneumocystis jiroveci* and atypical mycobacteria. However, they also suffer serious infections with common viral pathogens (e.g., cytomegalovirus, adenovirus, viral vaccine strains), bacteria and fungi. Because T cell help is required for robust antibody production, these patients also suffer from compromised humoral immunity and may have antibody production deficits and compromised ability to mount an effect antibody response following vaccination or infection. Thus, T cell defects are most often accompanied by some form of depressed B cell immunity and are generally referred to as "Combined

Immunodeficiency." Autoimmune manifestations are not uncommon and include inflammatory bowel disease, cytopenias, eczematous rash and enteropathy.

Severe Combined Immunodeficiency (SCID) is the most severe manifestation of T cell deficiency. SCID occurs due to defects in genes responsible for T cell development and is characterized by < 300 T cells/mcL in peripheral blood. Leaky SCID may occur when the expression of the defective gene is not fully penetrant, resulting in the development of a few T cells that make it to peripheral circulation. However, these aberrant T cells then proliferate and become reactive against self-antigens, therefore leading to autoimmune manifestations including skin rash and enteropathy. Alternatively, maternal T cells may engraft in a patient with SCID, leading to the expansion of these T cells and reactivity against the infant's tissues. Leaky SCID and maternal engraftment can present with features of autoimmunity including skin rash and enteropathy.

While SCID is the most severe of T cell defects, partial or complete lack of thymic tissue may also present as SCID, owing to the fact that T cell precursors cannot complete the thymus-specific final maturation step prior to exiting to the periphery as mature, naïve T cells. Partial or complete lack of thymic tissue results in 22q11.2 deletion or DiGeorge Syndrome (DGS) (McDonald-McGinn et al. 2015). DGS is associated with defective development of the pharyngeal pouch system, caused by chromosomal deletion at 22q11.2. In addition to significant T cell lymphopenia, these patients present with conotruncal cardiac anomalies and hypocalcemia due to parathyroid hypoplasia. Complete DGS is a result of the complete absence of the thymus, whereas, in partial or atypical DGS, a small amount of thymic tissue is present. In such cases, T cells may develop but are frequently oligoclonal and ineffective not only at mounting adequate responses to pathogens but also at assisting B cells to produce robust antibody responses. Complete or partial DGS patients can present clinically similar to patients with SCID, owing to their significantly low T cell numbers.

Other less-severe T cell-related IEI include defects in genes that encode proteins that drive T cell development in the thymus, such as major histocompatibility complexes I and II, that are necessary for the development of CD8 and CD4 T cells respectively (Reith and Mach 2001), or molecules that are necessary for T cell signaling, such as ZAP70 (Walkovich and Vander Lugt 2021). Rare defects in calcium sensor and calcium-release activated channels due to genetic defects in *STIM1* and *ORAI1* are associated with defective T cell activation and T cell deficiency along with myopathy (Feske et al. 2010).

Recognition of the cause of T cell lymphopenia is critical as it impacts the management of these patients. If the defect lies in genes that are integral to the T cells, then these patients may benefit from bone marrow or hematopoietic stem cell transplant to replace defective hematopoietic precursors (Haddad and Hoenig 2019), or from enzyme replacement therapy (e.g., ADA enzyme replacement in ADA-deficient SCID) (Booth and Gaspar 2009), or gene therapy, where the patient's hematopoietic stem cells are transfected with a viral vector carrying the corrected gene (Cicalese and Aiuti 2015; Cicalese et al. 2018). However, if the defect lies in the thymus as in DGS, a thymic implant may be needed depending on the severity of the defect (Davies et al. 2017).

B Cell Deficiency

In contrast to inherited defects of T cells which can manifest with severe, life-threatening infections with opportunistic microorganisms within the first few months of life, B cell developmental defects tend to present clinically after about 6 months of age (Demirdag and Gupta 2021). This is because newborns are protected by maternal immunoglobulins that are at their highest level at birth and wane over the course of the next 5–6 months. If infants are unable to produce adequate levels of immunoglobulins as maternal immunoglobulin wanes, their susceptibility to infection, particularly at mucosal surfaces, increases. Transient hypogammaglobulinemia of infancy (THI) may occur in infants > 6 months of age in whom IgG levels are significantly lower than the expected reference range limit (Dalal et al. 1998). THI generally resolves with age, often within the first 2 years of life, but has also been known to persist into early childhood.

Defects of B cell development leading to antibody deficiency commonly present clinically with increased susceptibility to encapsulated bacteria (e.g., *S. pneumoniae, H. influenzae*) leading to recurrent sinopulmonary infections, otitis media and pneumonia or gastrointestinal infections with organisms, such as *Salmonella* species, *Campylobacter jenuni* and rotavirus or with parasites such as *Giardia lamblia*. More severe infectious presentations include meningitis, infectious arthritis and osteomyelitis due to *Pseudomonas aeruginosa, Staphylococcus aureus* or Mycoplasma (reviewed in Demirdag and Gupta 2021).

The prototypical humoral or antibody deficiency is X-linked agammaglobulinemia (XLA), which occurs due to pathogenic variants of the gene encoding Bruton's Tyrosine Kinase (BTK) (Bruton 1952). BTK is critical for the early development of B cells in the bone marrow. Therefore, lack of BTK leads to severely depressed production of B cells and < 1% of B cells are detectable in the peripheral circulation. As BTK is encoded on the X-chromosome, this disorder manifests in boys who may present after about 6 months of age with bacterial or viral infections, absent or severely decreased B cells in peripheral blood and undetectable serum immunoglobulins (IgG, IgA and IgM).

A few other causes of inherited antibody deficiency include (1) selective IgA deficiency, which is the most common immunodeficiency (Yel 2010); (2) specific antibody deficiency (SAD) which is characterized by generally normal numbers of B cells and normal immunoglobulin levels, but impaired responses to vaccines (Ambrosino et al. 1987); (3) hyper IgM syndrome, which is characterized by high levels of IgM and inability to mount adequate antibody responses to infection (Notarangelo et al. 1992); (4) Common Variable Immunodeficiency (CVID), which is characterized by low IgG, often accompanied by low IgA and/or IgM and even though B cells may be present in normal numbers, they are unable to develop into memory B cells (Bonilla et al. 2016); (5) IgG subclass deficiency which may be associated with impaired responses to pneumococcal polysaccharides (IgG2 deficiency) or with a variety of inflammatory diseases (IgG4-related diseases).

The infectious manifestations of antibody deficiency are managed with appropriate antibiotics, while the underlying immunodeficiency, i.e., low immunoglobulins, is treated with immunoglobulin replacement therapy either in the form of intravenous immunoglobulin (IVIG) or subcutaneous immunoglobulin (SCIG). Hyper IgM syndrome, due to pathogenic variants in CD40 ligand, may require a bone marrow transplant to correct the underlying gene defect.

Neutrophil Defects

Neutrophils comprise the body's initial defense mechanism against infection. Therefore, primary neutrophil defects typically present early in life when the adaptive immune system (T and B cells) is still maturing. Patients with neutrophil defects frequently present with severe, often life-threatening infections with bacteria, such as *Staphylococcus aureus, Nocardia* species and fungi such as *Aspergillus fumigatus* or *Candida albicans*. Infectious presentations can range from mild skin infections to septicemia. Patients may present with skin abscesses, lymph node infections and deep-seated abscesses involving organs, such as the liver or lung infections (reviewed in Dinauer 2020). Secondary neutrophil defects are seen in patients with leukemias, myelodysplastic syndromes and hematopoietic clonal disorders, such as paroxysmal nocturnal hemoglobinuria (PNH) (Toma et al. 2012).

Defects of neutrophils are classified into defects of neutrophil numbers (neutropenia) or defects of neutrophil function. Neutropenia may be mild (1,000–< 1,500 cells/mcL), moderate (500–< 1,000 cells/mcL), or severe (< 500 cells/mcL) and are either due to pathogenic variants of genes that are critical to neutrophil development (e.g., Griscelli syndrome and Chediak-Higashi syndrome) (Donadieu et al. 2017) or due to extrinsic factors such as nutritional deficiency, infections or autoimmunity (Boxer 2012).

Functional neutrophil defects include CGD and LAD, among other, much less frequently encountered, defects. CGD predominantly occurs as an X-linked disease and therefore manifests in boys, often within the first year of life, with severe bacterial or fungal infections of the skin, lymph nodes and lungs. Autosomal recessive (AR) forms of the disease can present in either sex. Infectious presentations in the AR form of the disease are generally milder and tend to present in older children or adults. Patients with CGD have severely decreased or absent neutrophil oxidative burst, which is critical for control of bacterial and fungal infections. Neutrophil oxidative burst is mediated by the NAPDH oxidase complex, which is composed of six proteins—gp91phox, p22phox, p47phox, p67phox and p40phox and Rac-2. X-linked CGD occurs due to defects in gp91phox, whereas AR-CGD occurs due to defects in any one of the other proteins (Yu et al. 2021). LAD is characterized by the inability of leukocytes to exit the vasculature and migrate into tissue spaces. Three LAD syndromes, all inherited in an AR manner, have been identified: LAD I, LAD II and LAD III.

Leukocyte Adhesion Deficiency I (LAD I) occurs due to defects in neutrophil surface proteins known as β2-integrins. This family of surface receptors is essential for enabling neutrophils to arrest the vascular endothelium in response to an infectious stimulus and through diapedesis, enter tissue spaces to clear the infection. Pathogenic mutations of CD18, the beta-chain of the β2 integrin family, lead to severely decreased or loss of β2 integrin expression, leading to an inability of neutrophils to migrate to sites of infection. The classical clinical presentation in LAD I is omphalitis (delayed separation of the umbilical stump). Patients also can present with skin, respiratory tract, perianal or bowel infections. Erosive gingivitis is another feature. Characteristic findings in LAD I include the absence of pus at sites of infection as neutrophils are unable to migrate to these sites and cause a dramatic increase in neutrophils in the peripheral circulation (leukocytosis) (Etzioni 2009).

LAD II occurs due to defective fucosylation of macromolecules. Pathogenic variants of the guanosine diphosphate (GDP)-fucose transporter gene (*SLC35C1*) result in impaired transport of fucose to the Golgi complex, thereby affecting fucosylation of macromolecules. This defect impacts sialyl Lewis X or CD15s, which is the ligand for selectins that are expressed on vascular endothelium. The interaction of CD15s and selectins is essential for neutrophil rolling and tethering to the vascular endothelium, prior to migration into tissue spaces. Thus, LAD II patients' neutrophils are functionally impaired, therefore leading to increased susceptibility to infection. However, these patients tend to have fewer and milder infections compared with LAD I patients. Additionally, defective fucosylation affects H antigen expression. Therefore, LAD II is associated with the rare Bombay (hh) blood type. Non-immune clinical findings include short stature, severe intellectual impairment, microcephaly and distinctive facial features that include a depressed nasal bridge. As with LAD I, neutrophilia is a consistent finding.

LAD III, previously described as the LAD I variant, is characterized by severe infections, leukocytosis and severe bleeding disorder. The underlying defect is in the protein, kindlin-3, encoded by the gene *FERMT3*. Kindlin-3 is an adapter protein that binds the intracellular portions of β-1, β-2 and β-3 integrins and increases their activation and binding to their cognate ligands. As these integrins are found on both neutrophils and platelets, the function of both of these blood components is affected. Clinical features of LAD III included delayed umbilical cord separation, increased susceptibility to infection and severe bleeding episodes that are similar to those seen in patients with Glanzmann thrombasthenia. LAD III is also characterized by marked leukocytosis.

Complement Defects

The complement system comprises serum as well as cell membrane-associated proteins that interact with both innate and adaptive immune systems. By efficiently transporting potential self-reactive nuclear products of apoptotic cells as well as inflammatory immune complexes to the reticuloendothelial system, wherein they are phagocytosed and eliminated, complement proteins and complement receptors maintain immune homeostasis (Shih and Murali 2015). The tightly regulated complement pathways recognize the biochemical divergence of self-structures from structural pathogen-associated molecular patterns (PAMPs), such as lipopolysaccharide of gram-negative bacteria (alternative pathway or AP) or mannose present on fungi and ficolins of some gram-positive bacteria (lectin or mannose pathway or LP). Antigen-antibody complexes activate the Classical Pathway (CP). These events result in activation of distinct early complement proteins and generation of convertases that converge on C3 (C3 convertases), giving rise to the anaphylatoxins C4a and C3a as well as C3b. Besides its opsonic function, C3b functions as an enzyme in the generation of C5a, a potent chemoattract for phagocytic cells. The anaphylatoxins (C3a, C4a and C5a) mediate the vascular phase of inflammation while C5a recruits phagocytic cells. These events integrate the vascular and cellular phases of immune defense and inflammation. Derangements in this cascade of activating and regulatory proteins results in either failure of complement mediated defenses and hence recurrent or severe infections or autoactivation of complement proteins leading to immune inflammation, while defects in complement mediated clearance of immune complexes and apoptotic cells cause autoimmune diseases.

Complement deficiencies account for approximately 0.06% of inherited immune deficiencies in the general population. Complement deficiencies may manifest with primarily autoimmune phenomena (e.g., Systemic Lupus Erythematosus), primarily infectious manifestations (e.g., Neisserial meningitis) or immune dysregulatory defects (e.g., Hereditary Angioedema (HAE), Hemolytic Uremic Syndrome (HUS), or Paroxysmal Nocturnal Hemoglobinuria (PNH)). Fulminant infections with *Neisseria meningitidis*, including septicemia and meningitis, almost exclusively occur in deficiencies of the terminal complement pathway proteins (C5, C6, C7, C8 and C9). HAE is a genetically inherited disease that occurs due to low levels or abnormal function of the complement control protein C-1 esterase inhibitor (C1-INH). C1-INH is responsible for not only regulating activation of the complement pathway but also the regulation of the Hageman, bradykinin and fibrinolytic pathways. This deficiency manifests as spontaneous episodes of angioedema (mediated by bradykinin), which may be localized (hands or feet), involve mucosa of the gut resulting in severe abdominal pain or may manifest as life-threatening laryngeal edema. The trigger for these episodes has not been well defined (Schroder-Braunstein and Kirschfink 2019).

Table 4 depicts some of the congenital complement deficiency diseases and the resulting infections and/or autoimmune manifestations.

Table 4. Congenital complement deficiency states and disease association.

Complement Deficiency	Consequences	Disease Association
C1q, C1r, C1s, C4 and C2	Inability to generate/activate classical C3 convertase or CP	Systemic lupus erythematosus (SLE)
C3	Defective C3b opsonic activity and MAC activity, no activation of AP and decreased inflammation (no C3a activity)	Recurrent childhood infections. *N. meningitidis, S. pneumoniae* and other encapsulated bacteria
Late Components – C5, C6, C7, C8 and C9	Inability to form the MAC	Recurrent, disseminated Neisserial infections
Factor D and Properdin	Inability to generate/activate the AP C3 convertase	Recurrent, disseminated Neisserial infections
Mannose Binding Lectin (MBL) and MASP-2	Decreased or absent activity to activate the LP	Recurrent childhood infections, pyogenic bacteria
Factor H, I, MCP and C3 Nephritic Factors	Lack of regulation of C3 convertases by all pathways of complement activation	Membranoproliferative glomerulonephritis, atypical hemolytic uremic syndrome, age-related macular degeneration.
C1-Inhibitor (C1-INH)	Loss of regulation of C1 and bradykinin activation	Hereditary angioedema
DAF (CD55), Homologous Restriction Factor (HRF) or CD59	Failure to regulate complement activation on autologous cells (particularly red cells)	PNH

Laboratory Workup for Suspected Immunodeficiency

Detailed clinical history of recurrent, difficult-to-treat or unusual infections, family history of similar clinical symptoms and/or early death and a thorough physical examination are crucial when suspicion for immunodeficiency is high. While genetic analysis is becoming increasingly cheaper and more widely available and oftentimes used as the first line of laboratory investigation, it should not replace routine laboratory tests as they provide clinically significant and useful information when working up a patient as well as when monitoring clinical outcomes in patients with immunodeficiency.

General laboratory workup includes complete blood count (CBC) with differential (see Chapter 2), and serum immunoglobulin levels to assess whether the distribution of RBC and RBC parameters, WBC (neutrophils, lymphocytes, monocytes, basophils and eosinophils), platelets and serum immunoglobulins (IgG, IgA and IgM) are within the expected range. It is important to note that these parameters vary considerably with age, therefore interpretation of patients' test results in the context of age-matched reference ranges is critical. Additionally, maternal immunoglobulin G is transferred transplacentally to the fetus and reaches maximal levels at birth. Maternal IgG declines over the first 6 months of life and infant IgG increases, as the newborn begins to synthesize it along with the other immunoglobulin isotypes (IgA, IgM and IgE). Thus, assessment of serum immunoglobulins for evaluation of antibody deficiencies is not reliable within the first 6 months of age.

Responses to the routine vaccine (antibody titers) may be assessed to determine whether the patient is capable of responding to vaccination. The distribution of lymphocyte populations (T cells, B cells and Natural Killer (NK) cells) may be assessed by flow cytometry. Functional analysis of neutrophils and lymphocytes is performed in specialized laboratories when a functional deficit is suspected. Some of the more commonly used laboratory tests for immunodeficiency work up are presented in Table 5 and are discussed in further detail below.

Table 5. Commonly used immunological tests for workup of immunodeficiency.

Test	Utility for Evaluation of Immunodeficiency
TREC analysis by PCR	Newborn screening for SCID
CBC with differential	Evaluation of cytopenias (e.g., anemia, neutropenia and lymphopenia), abnormal cellular morphology (e.g., giant granules in Chediak-Higashi Syndrome)
Serum immunoglobulin levels and serum protein electrophoresis	Hypogammaglobulinemia, selective IgA-deficiency, hyper IgM and hyper IgE syndromes and immunodeficiency due to monoclonal B cell abnormalities
Vaccine response	Specific antibody titers to routinely administered vaccines (e.g., diphtheria, tetanus and pertussis (DTvP2 and DTaP), pneumococcal vaccine (PCV13 and PCV23)
Lymphocyte subset analysis	Abnormal decreases or increases in T cells (CD3, CD4 and CD8), B cells (CD19 and CD20) and NK cells (CD16/CD56). Markers for naïve (CD45RA) and memory (CD45RO) T cells, naïve (IgD+CD27-) and memory (CD27+) B cells, as well as class-switched memory (IgD-CD27+) B cells are useful
Neutrophil oxidative burst	Evaluates the ability of neutrophils to produce reactive oxygen intermediates that are critical for clearance of pathogens
Neutrophil adherence markers	Flow cytometry evaluation of expression of b2-integrins and sialyl Lewis X or CD15s on the surface of neutrophils
Lymphocyte proliferation	Flow cytometry evaluation of the ability of lymphocytes to divide following stimulation with a mitogen or an antigen or after T cell receptor (anti-CD3) and CD28 activation
Complement analysis	Functional testing for the integrity of the classical and alternative complement pathways. Analysis of specific complement proteins, both level and function and complement pathway inhibitors

Abbreviations: TREC; T Cell Receptor Excision Circle; Severe Combined Immunodeficiency (SCID).

T Cell Defects

Newborn Screening for SCID

Newborn screening (NBS) for SCID was developed by the states of Wisconsin and California in 2008. Since then, screening for SCID at birth has been implemented across the United States and several countries across the world. NBS for SCID involves polymerase chain reaction (PCR) amplification of a piece of DNA known as TREC or T Cell Receptor Excision Circle (Puck 2012). TREC is generated in newly developed T cells as they re-arrange their T cell receptor genes in the thymus and emerge as naïve T cells in the peripheral circulation. The starting sample for TREC analysis is DNA extracted from dried blood spots following a heel prick that is routinely collected in newborn babies to screen for a variety of metabolic diseases. Abnormally low TREC levels are indicative of low T cell production and are followed up by analysis of T cells in peripheral circulation by flow cytometry (Figure 1A–C and described under "Lymphocyte Subset Phenotyping").

Newborns who test abnormal on the NBS–SCID screen but have detectable T cells in peripheral circulation, occasionally up to 1,500 T cells/mcL, may have leaky SCID (hypomorphic mutations of SCID-related genes), Omenn Syndrome (hypomorphic gene defects, erythroderma and elevated IgE) or maternal T cell engraftment (Shearer et al. 2014). In these patients, analysis of the proportions of naïve and memory T cells is invaluable in order to clinch the diagnosis (Knight et al. 2020). At birth, the vast majority of a newborn's T cells are antigen-inexperienced, naïve T cells which express the glycoprotein, CD45RA. Over the course of life, as naïve T cells encounter antigen, a percentage turn into CD45RO-expressing memory T cells. The relative proportion of memory T cells increases from infancy to adulthood. Thus, analysis of CD45RA and CD45RO on T cells enables quantification of the relative proportions of naïve and memory T cells. In leaky SCID, Omenn Syndrome or maternal engraftment, the few T cells that are present are reactive memory cells and express CD45RO (Figure 2).

Lymphocyte Subset Phenotyping

Lymphocytes in peripheral blood can be identified by tagging them with fluorescently labeled monoclonal antibodies that are specific for certain cell surface proteins that define specific subsets of lymphocytes. These fluorescently labeled cells can by analyzed by flow cytometry, whereby cells are interrogated by a laser beam that activate the fluorescent molecules. Activation of these fluorescent molecules leads to release of photons whose wavelength is converted into digital signals that are read by specialized software. The technique enables high throughput and rapid analysis of complex mixtures of cells, such as those found in peripheral blood (Figure 3).

Lymphocyte subset phenotyping is performed by flow cytometry analysis of peripheral blood. In brief, whole blood (50–100 mcL) is incubated with monoclonal antibodies that are specific for leukocyte and lymphocyte surface proteins (Table 6). Following a 15–20-minute incubation, blood is washed by centrifugation, RBCs are lysed and the sample is analyzed by flow cytometry.

Leukocytes, which include lymphocytes, monocytes and neutrophils are identified by their expression of CD45 and the variation in their complexity (i.e., smaller, less complex leukocytes are lymphocytes and larger, more complex leukocytes are neutrophils). The lymphocyte population is further analyzed for the percentages of T cells (CD3+, CD4+ and CD8+), B cells (CD19+), NK and CD16+CD56+ cells. Flow cytometry analysis yields relative percentages of these lymphocyte subpopulations. Absolute numbers can be calculated using the absolute lymphocyte count from the corresponding CBC and the percentages from flow cytometry analysis and are useful parameters for clinical follow up rather than relying on just percentages

Lymphocyte subset phenotyping is routinely performed to assess percentages and absolute numbers of T, B and NK cells. A variation of this test is used for CD4 T cell counts for diagnosis

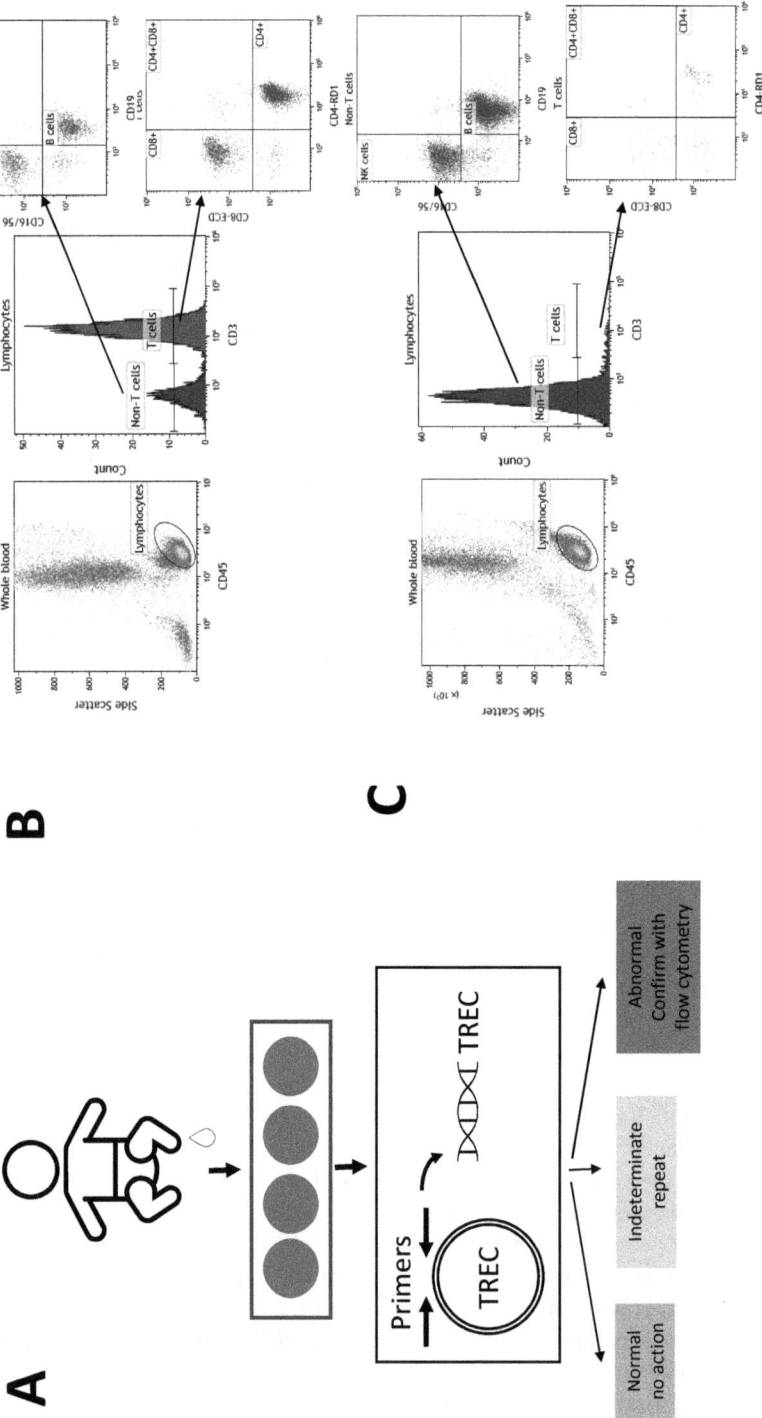

Figure 1. Screening and Confirmatory Testing for Severe Combined Immunodeficiency. (A) Newborn screening for SCID: Blood spots are collected via heel sticks from newborns. A 3 mm punch is taken from a dried blood spot and DNA is extracted. Primers specific for TREC and a housekeeping gene (generally β–actin) are used to amplify a portion of TREC and the β–actin gene, which is used to assess the quality of the extracted DNA. If TREC levels are normal and β–actin is adequate, the result of the screen is "normal," and no further action is required. If TREC levels are low and β–actin amplification is inadequate, the result is "indeterminate" and a repeat PCR and/or DNA extraction is needed. If TREC levels are low and β–actin is adequate, the result is "abnormal" and must be followed by confirmatory flow cytometry. (B) Flow cytometry analysis of peripheral blood for CD3+ T cells, CD3+CD4+ T cells, CD3+CD8+ T cells, CD19+ B cells and CD16/56+ NK cells. The flow cytometry plots show analysis of a normal, healthy adult donor. (C) Flow cytometry analysis of peripheral blood collected from a newborn who had an abnormal SCID screening test result. Note that T cells are barely detectable, whereas B cells and NK cells appear adequate. This flow cytometry result is typical of a T-B+NK+ SCID and may also occur in 22q11 deletion syndrome (DiGeorge syndrome).

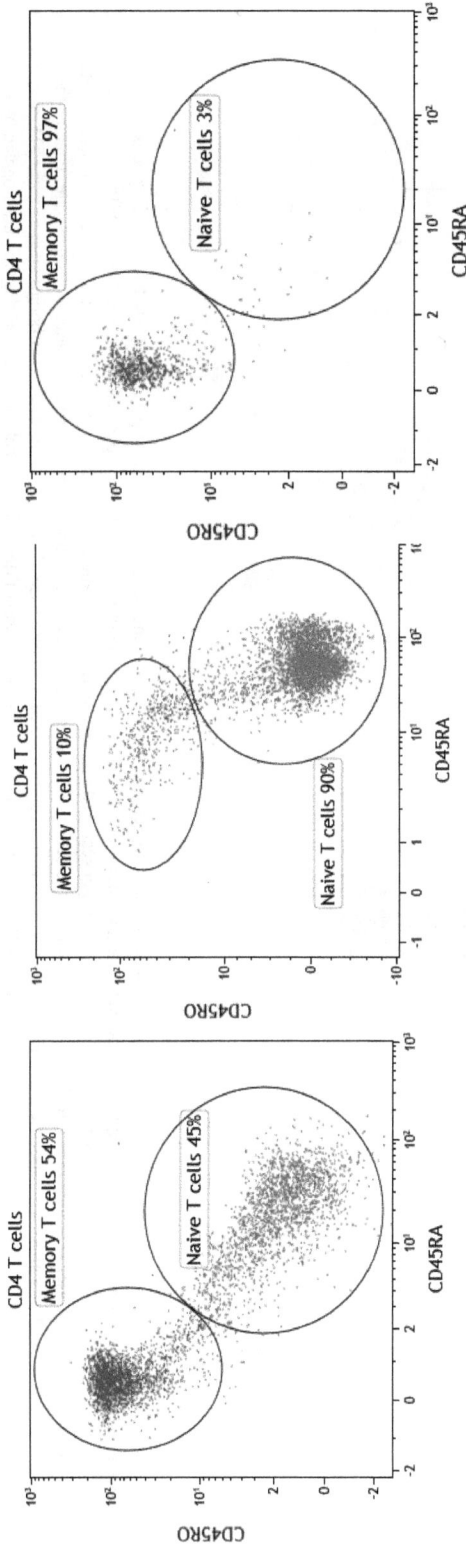

Figure 2. Analysis of Naïve and Memory T Cells. Follow-up testing for SCID includes analysis of naïve (CD45RA+) and memory (CD45RO+) T cells. This is particularly important for the analysis of leaky SCID, Omenn Syndrome, or maternal T-cell engraftment. CD45RO+ memory T cells are generally higher in adults (A) and CD45RA+ naïve T cells are higher in infants and young children (B). In patients with leaky SCID, the few T cells that get to the periphery expand, develop a memory phenotype and may react against self-tissues. Panel C shows an analysis of T cells in leaky SCID, where close to 100% of T cells are CD45RO+.

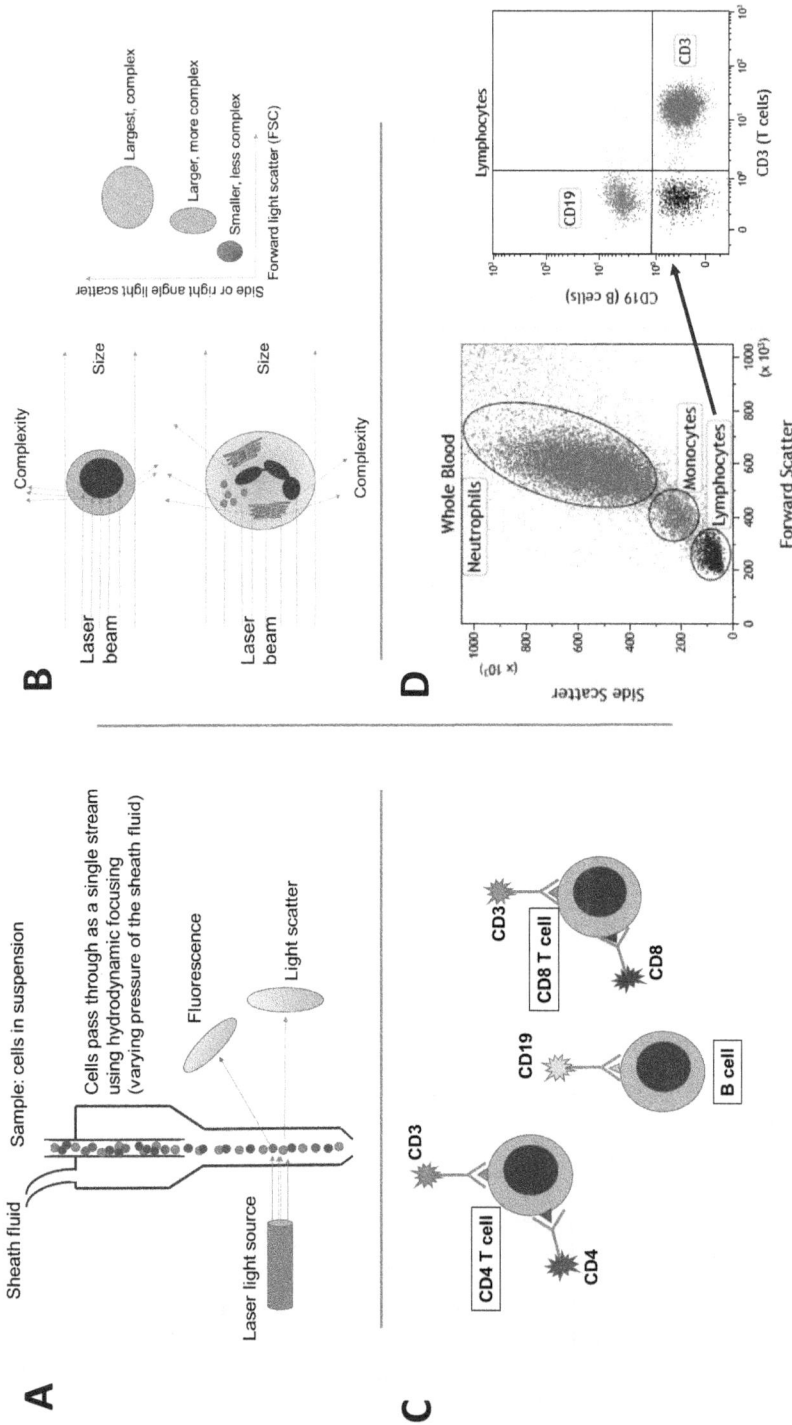

Figure 3. Overview of flow cytometry analysis of peripheral blood. Flow Cytometry is a technique to measure the physical properties of particles, including cells in suspension. Individual cell types in heterogeneous samples, such as peripheral blood can be analyzed and quantified by flow cytometry. (A) Cells in suspension are injected into the flow cell of the flow cytometer. As the cells pass through the flow cell, they are interrogated by a laser beam. Light scattered incident to the laser beam measures the size of the cell (also known as forward scatter; FSC), and light scatter at right angles to the laser beam measures the internal complexity of the cells (side scatter; SSC). (B) The combination of forward scatter and side scatter enables the separation of cells according to these physical properties. (C) Specific molecules on the surface of cells can be tagged with fluorescently labeled monoclonal antibodies such as anti-CD3, anti-CD4 and anti-CD8 antibodies for the detection of T cells, or anti-CD19 for recognition of B cells. The signals from the activation of these fluorescent molecules as they are interrogated by the laser beam can be analyzed by special software to provide relative percentages of the various cell subsets in the sample. (D) Flow cytometry analysis of whole blood: whole blood separates into lymphocytes (low FSC and low SSC), monocytes (moderate FSC and SSC) and granulocytes (high FSC and SSC). Analysis of lymphocytes tagged with anti-CD3 and anti-CD19 enables quantification of CD3+ T cells and CD19+ B cells.

Table 6. Cell surface markers used for routine analysis of peripheral blood lymphocytes.

Cell Surface Marker	Description
CD45	Expressed in all nucleated cells of the hematopoietic lineage.
CD3	Expressed on all T cells. CD3 in association with the T cell receptor is essential for T cell signaling and function.
CD4	Defines "helper" T cells. These cells recognize antigens presented by MHC Class II.
CD8	Defines "cytotoxic" T cells. These cells recognize antigens presented by MHC Class I.
CD19	Highly expressed on B cells at all stages of development.
CD20	Highly expressed on B cells at all stages of development with the exception of antibody-producing plasmablasts and plasma cells.
CD16	Strongly expressed in NK cells. Used along with CD56 to identify NK cells.
CD56	Strongly expressed in NK cells.
CD45RA	Isoform of CD45 that is expressed chiefly on naïve T cells. A subset of terminally differentiated T cells may express CD45RA as well.
CD45RO	Isoform of CD45 that is expressed on memory T cells.
IgD	Expressed on naïve B cells and non-class-switched memory B cells.
CD27	Expressed on memory B cells. Note: Memory B cells are either non-class switched (i.e., express CD27 and IgD) or class-switched (i.e., express CD27 and lose expression of IgD). Class-switched memory B cells express surface IgG, IgM, IgA or IgE and secrete the corresponding antibody isotype).

Abbreviations: Major Histocompatibility Complex (MHC); Natural Killer (NK)

and management of patients with HIV and for HIV staging. T, B and NK lymphocyte analysis form part of the routine workup for suspected cellular immunodeficiency and as a follow-up to an abnormal NBS for SCID. Flow cytometry analysis for abnormal NBS-SCID may yield T-B+NK+, T-B-NK+ or T-B-NK- results, whereby severe T cell deficiency may be accompanied by a deficiency in B and/or NK cells. These results can often provide clues to the underlying genetic defect, i.e., whether T cell development-specific genes alone are affected, whether genes specific to T and B cell development are affected or whether genes specific to the development of all three lymphocyte lineages are affected. B cells are low or absent in inherited defects involving B cell development, a classic example of which is XLA.

It should be noted that lymphocyte subset analyses by flow cytometry provide a quantitative profile and often needs corroborative assessment of their functional state, and this is achieved by proliferation studies as indicated below.

Lymphocyte and/or T Cell Proliferation

The ability of lymphocytes or T cells to proliferate to specific stimuli can be assessed by several methods. The most widely used method to date is the incorporation of tritiated thymidine (^{3}H-Tdr) into the DNA of proliferating cells, and the detection of incorporated radioactivity as a measure of the extent of proliferation. The major caveat to this method is the inability of the assay to discriminate among the various cell populations that proliferate in response to stimulation. Therefore, with this method, an overall reduction in T cell numbers and compromised T cell function yield a similar result, i.e., diminished overall lymphocyte proliferation. Newer methods that use DNA binding dyes or fluorescently tagged nucleotides followed by flow cytometry enable analyses of specific lymphocyte populations, such as T cells.

To assess lymphocyte or T cell proliferation, peripheral blood mononuclear cells are separated from whole blood through density gradient centrifugation. The cells are resuspended in a cell culture medium and stimulated either with mitogens (e.g., phytohemagglutinin (PHA), which is a pan-T cell stimulator) or antigens (e.g., tetanus toxoid, which specifically stimulates memory

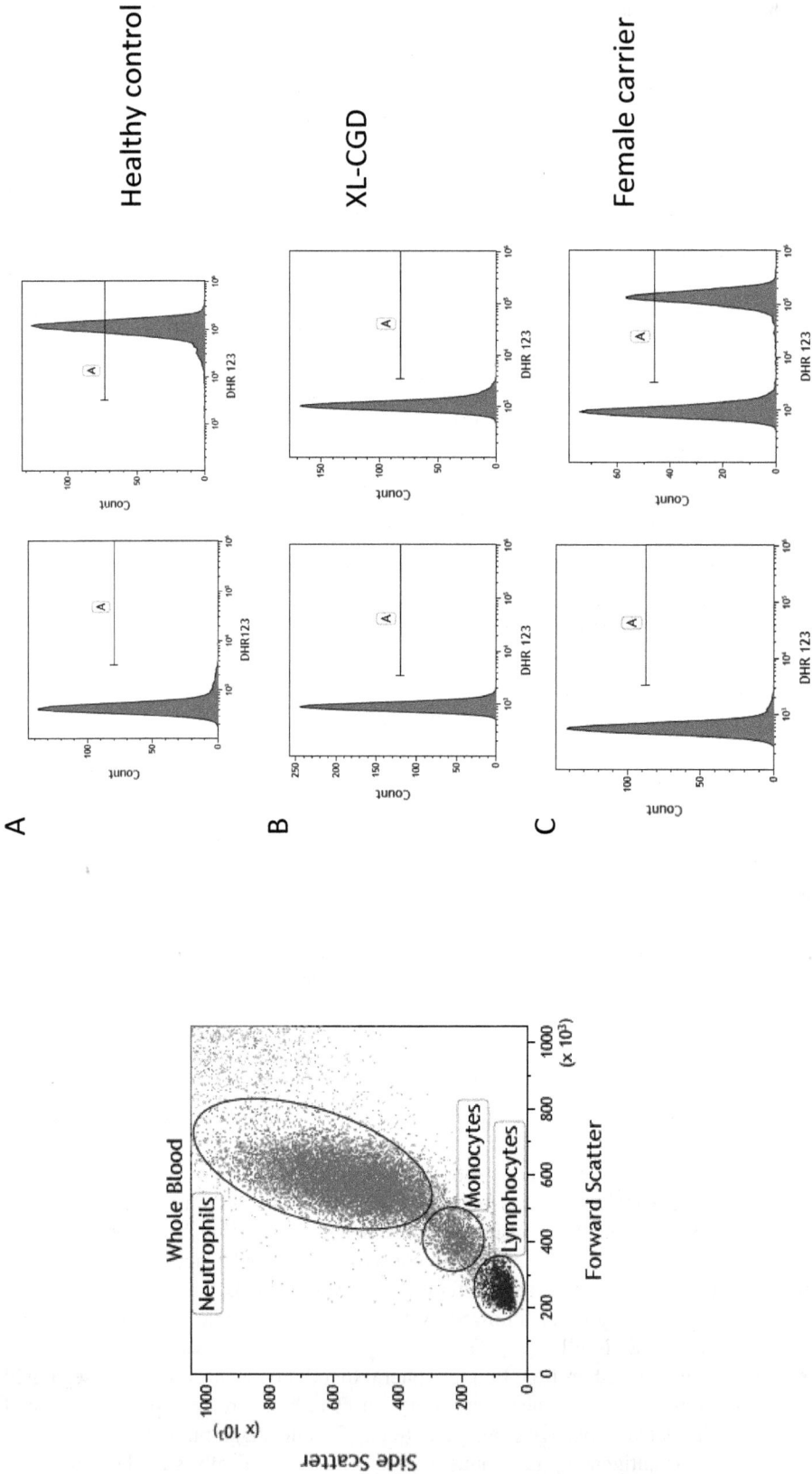

Figure 4.   T Cell Proliferation in Response to PHA Stimulation. To assess T cell proliferation, peripheral blood mononuclear cells are separated from whole blood and stimulated with phytohemagglutinin (PHA) for 3 days. At the end of the stimulation period, a modified nucleoside, 5-ethynyl-2'-deoxyuridine or EdU, is added and is incorporated into proliferating cells. EdU is labeled with a fluorophore and analyzed by flow cytometry. (A) T cells are identified by their expression of CD45 and CD3. Note that when T cells are stimulated, they become larger and more complex as indicated by higher side scatter (SSC). (B) PHA stimulated cells are shown in the blue line and unstimulated cells are shown in red. Proliferating cells have incorporated EdU and therefore, their fluorescence increases as shown by the shift of the blue histogram to the right.

T cells that develop in response to tetanus vaccination). Many labs also utilize solid-phase anti-CD3 and anti-CD28 antibodies for optimal T cell stimulation (Frauwirth and Thompson 2002). These tests are better standardized and more reproducible compared to mitogen stimulation tests (Stone et al. 2009). The cells are cultured for approximately 3 days (PHA or anti-CD3/CD-28) or 5–7 days (tetanus) to allow responding T cells to proliferate. At the end of the culture period, ^{3}H-Tdr or a modified nucleoside (5-ethynyl-2'-deoxyuridine, EdU) that can be tagged with a fluorophore is added. Proliferating cells incorporate these modified nucleotides and proliferation can be measured by either radioactive counts or by analyzing fluorescent cells by flow cytometry (Figure 4 shows an example of flow cytometry data for assessment of T cell proliferation in response to PHA stimulation).

Analysis of lymphocyte or T cell proliferation is performed when suspecting T cell or Combined Immunodeficiency. Some IEI can result in defective T cell function in a setting of relatively normal T cell numbers. Thus, analyzing the ability of T cells to proliferate in response to stimulation can be helpful. PHA stimulation or solid phase anti-CD3 and anti-CD28 antibodies is used to assess global T cell function, whereas the response to tetanus, specifically measures the ability of T cells to make a response to a specific antigen. T cell proliferation measurement is not a diagnostic assay in and of itself, but when used in combination with analysis of T and B cells and their subpopulations (e.g., naïve and memory T or B cells) and NK cell numbers, it can provide useful information when working up a patient for suspected combined or T cell immunodeficiency.

B Cell Defects

Immunological evaluation of B cell defects, similar to T cell disorders, involves quantification of immunoglobulins and B cell phenotypes, both of which also evaluate the functional status of B cells. Analyzes of B cell defects start with the interpretation of serum total proteins (T.P.) and serum albumin levels. The difference between T.P. and albumin denotes the globulin fraction. If the T.P. is decreased and serum albumin is normal, it suggests a decrease in globulin fraction, often noted in an antibody deficiency syndrome, such as T-B-NK+ or T-B-NK-SCID or agammaglobulinemia such as XLA; if the total protein is elevated and serum albumin is normal, it represents an elevated level of globulins. This elevated level of globulins could be polyclonal (as in chronic inflammation, infection or autoimmune diseases) or monoclonal (as seen in B cell monoclonal dyscrasia) and is an indication for serum protein electrophoresis or SPEP. Serum albumin is often low in symptomatic protein-losing enteropathy or proteinuria in renal disease associated with other characteristic changes on the electrophoretogram. Table 7 summarizes the value of SPEP in clinical diagnoses of primary as well as secondary immunodeficiency states.

Table 7. Serum protein electrophoresis profile in immune deficiency diseases.

Clinical Disorders	Total Protein	Albumin	α-1	α-2	β	β-γ bridge	γ
Acute inflammatory pattern	N	↓	↑	↑	N	Not present	N
Chronic inflammatory diseases	↑	↓	↑	↑	↑	Present in chronic mucosal inflammation	↑
Monoclonal or polyclonal gammopathy (IFE recommended)	+/–	+/–	+/–	+/–	+/–	+/–	+/–
Liver disease/cirrhosis	+/–	↓	+/–	+/–	↑	Present	↑
Nephrotic syndrome	↓	↓	+/–	↑	+/–	Absent	↓
Protein-losing enteropathy	↓	↓	↓	↓	↓	Absent	↓
Autoimmune diseases	+/–	+/–	↑	↓	N	Not present	↑
α-1 antitrypsin deficiency	+/–	+/–	↓↓	↑	+/–	Not present	↑
Hypogammaglobulinemia	↓	+/–	N	↑	+/–	Absent	↓↓
Hemolytic anemias/congenital hemoglobin defects	N	N	N	↓	+/–	Absent	+/–

N = Normal ↑ = Increased ↓ = Decreased +/– = Equivocal.

Serum Immunoglobulin Analysis

Immunoglobulins are produced by B cells and are easily measured in a peripheral blood sample. Most tests for immunoglobulin measurement are highly automated and utilize the principle of antigen-antibody reactions. For example, when measuring IgG levels, the test uses an anti-IgG antibody that forms a complex or lattice when in equilibrium with IgG present in serum. Typically, immunoglobulin levels are measured when the reaction reaches equilibrium.

Two techniques, turbidimetry and nephelometry, are used to measure immunoglobulin levels. In both techniques, a light source is projected through the liquid sample in which the antigen-antibody reaction is occurring. Turbidimetry measures a decrease in light intensity when the reaction is in equilibrium, whereas nephelometry measures the scatter of light as it passes through the sample. A decrease in light intensity, or amount of light scatter, is proportional to the amount of immunoglobulin in the sample. A serum immunoglobulin panel usually includes measurement of IgM, IgG and IgA. When necessary, serum IgD and IgE levels, IgG subclasses as well as serum free light chains (Kappa and Lambda) and their ratio (indicated in the evaluation of the spectrum of monoclonal gammopathies) are also measured by either turbidimetry or nephelometry. It is critical that the laboratories report serum immunoglobulin results in reference to appropriate age-specific ranges as immunoglobulin levels are dynamic and change with age from newborn to adult.

Serum immunoglobulin measurement is used widely when assessing a patient for antibody deficiency, which may manifest as increased susceptibility to bacterial or viral infections, particularly of the respiratory tract. Measurement of immunoglobulins in infants less than 6 months of age should be interpreted with caution since the majority of IgG in circulation from newborn to ~ 6 months is of maternal origin. Hypogammaglobulinemia is generally defined as an IgG level that is two standard deviations below the age-matched mean. This value may vary between laboratories and is dependent on the population that the specific laboratory has used to develop its reference ranges. Agammaglobulinemia is defined as an IgG level < 100 mg/dL. Low levels of all three antibody isotypes (G, A and M) define pan hypogammaglobulinemia and is a feature of severe combined immunodeficiencies. While a low IgG level is required laboratory criteria to make a diagnosis of CVID, IgM and/or IgA may be normal. Elevated or normal IgM levels with decreased IgG and IgA levels is a feature of hyper IgM syndrome. Isolated IgA deficiency is relatively common among the human population.

The diagnosis of selective IgG subclass deficiencies can be made with confidence only when there is a significant decrease in the serum concentrations of the specific IgG subclass isotype and clear documentation of an abnormal or suboptimal specific antibody response. Abnormal antibody responses to tetanus and diphtheria vaccines are a feature of IgG1 and IgG3 deficiency, while abnormal antibody responses to pneumococcal and *H. Influenzae* vaccines are a feature of IgG2 and IgG4 deficiency. Isolated IgG4 deficiency is hard to define as IgG4 levels decline with infection and serum IgG4 levels are very low even in healthy individuals. Evidence of recurrent infections along with decreased levels of IgG subclasses and functional derangements of specific IgG antibody production to vaccines define this entity (Buckley 2002).

Vaccine Antibody Titers (Functional Analysis)

Antibody responses to specific antigens, such as vaccines, can be impaired despite normal immunoglobulin levels. Measurement of antibodies to routinely administered vaccines, such as pneumococcal vaccines, or diphtheria and tetanus toxoid vaccines provide information on the ability of B cells to make antibodies to polysaccharide antigens that do not require T cell help (T-independent antigens) or to proteins antigens that do require T cell help (T-dependent antigens), respectively. Antibodies to vaccines are measured by immunoassays, such as ELISA or multiplex bead assays. The ELISA is described below.

Vaccine antigens are coated on microwell plates and uncoated sites are blocked with a non-specific protein, such as bovine serum albumin. The patient's serum is added to the microwells. If antibodies to the vaccine are present, they bind to the vaccine antigen and any unbound antibodies or serum proteins are washed off. These antibodies are detected using anti-human immunoglobulin linked to an enzyme. When the enzyme substrate is added, the color of the substrate changes proportional to the amount of antibody bound to the vaccine antigen. This color change is read by a spectrophotometer and reported either qualitatively as "present/absent" or "positive/negative," or reported as a titer (i.e., 1/80, 1/160, etc.), or may be reported as a concentration in mg/mL, U/mL or IU/mL. The results are referenced both to a normal range and to expected protective concentrations in some cases (e.g., tetanus antibody protective level is defined as > 0.01 IU/mL).

Analysis of vaccine responses is an indirect measure of antibody function, the ability of B cells to raise appropriate antibody responses to an antigen and the ability of B and T cells to collaborate to make an antibody response. Measurement of antibodies to multiple pneumococcal serotypes is used to evaluate the T-independent antibody response and is also used to make decisions regarding immunoglobulin replacement therapy. In Combined Immunodeficiency, immunoglobulins are generally low and responses to both T-independent and T-dependent antigens are defective. SAD is defined as an inadequate response to polysaccharide antigens with intact responses to protein antigens. SAD may occur in isolation or as part of primary immunodeficiencies, such as CVID, or in secondary immunodeficiency. Impaired vaccine responses may also occur in secondary immunodeficiency due to medications, protein loss or malnutrition and is generally accompanied by low immunoglobulin levels. It should be noted that vaccine responses cannot be reliably measured in patients who are on immunoglobulin replacement therapy since these preparations contain antibodies to a variety of vaccines.

Neutrophil Defects

CBC is used for the assessment of neutropenia. The performance and reporting parameters of CBC have been discussed in Chapter 2 and will not be covered here. This section includes descriptions of tests used to assess neutrophil function.

Neutrophil Oxidative Burst

Following an infectious stimulus, neutrophils undergo an oxidative burst response that is mediated by the NADPH oxidase complex. This oxidative burst response results in the release of reactive oxygen species (ROS), including peroxide, which is necessary for the clearance of infection. The dihyrorhodamine123 test (DHR123) is a simple flow cytometry test for neutrophil oxidative burst. In this test, whole blood is loaded with the dye DHR123. Neutrophils take up the dye. Blood is then stimulated to induce oxidative burst and ROS that are released reduce the dye to rhodamine, which fluoresces brightly. This change in fluorescence can be measured by flow cytometry.

In brief, whole blood, 100 mcL is incubated with DHR123 for 15 minutes at 37°C. Phorbol myristate acetate (PMA) is added to stimulate oxidative burst, and blood is incubated for 10 minutes. RBCs are lysed and the sample is analyzed on a flow cytometer.

A normal oxidative burst will result in a shift in the fluorescence of neutrophils which is indicated by the movement of the histogram in Figure 5A from the left to the far right. Decreased oxidative burst will not result in an increase in fluorescence. The data are interpreted using a stimulation index, which is calculated as the mean DHR123 fluorescence of the stimulated sample/mean fluorescence of the unstimulated sample and is referenced to the laboratory's cut-off value.

The DHR123 assay is used for the evaluation of patients with clinical suspicion of CGD. Patients with X-linked CGD have little or no oxidative burst and therefore their neutrophils will show no shift in fluorescence following stimulation (Figure 5B). Consequently, their stimulation index is 1 or close to 1. Patients with autosomal recessive CGD have diminished oxidative burst and may show a marginal to moderate increase in fluorescence but still lower than that of neutrophils from

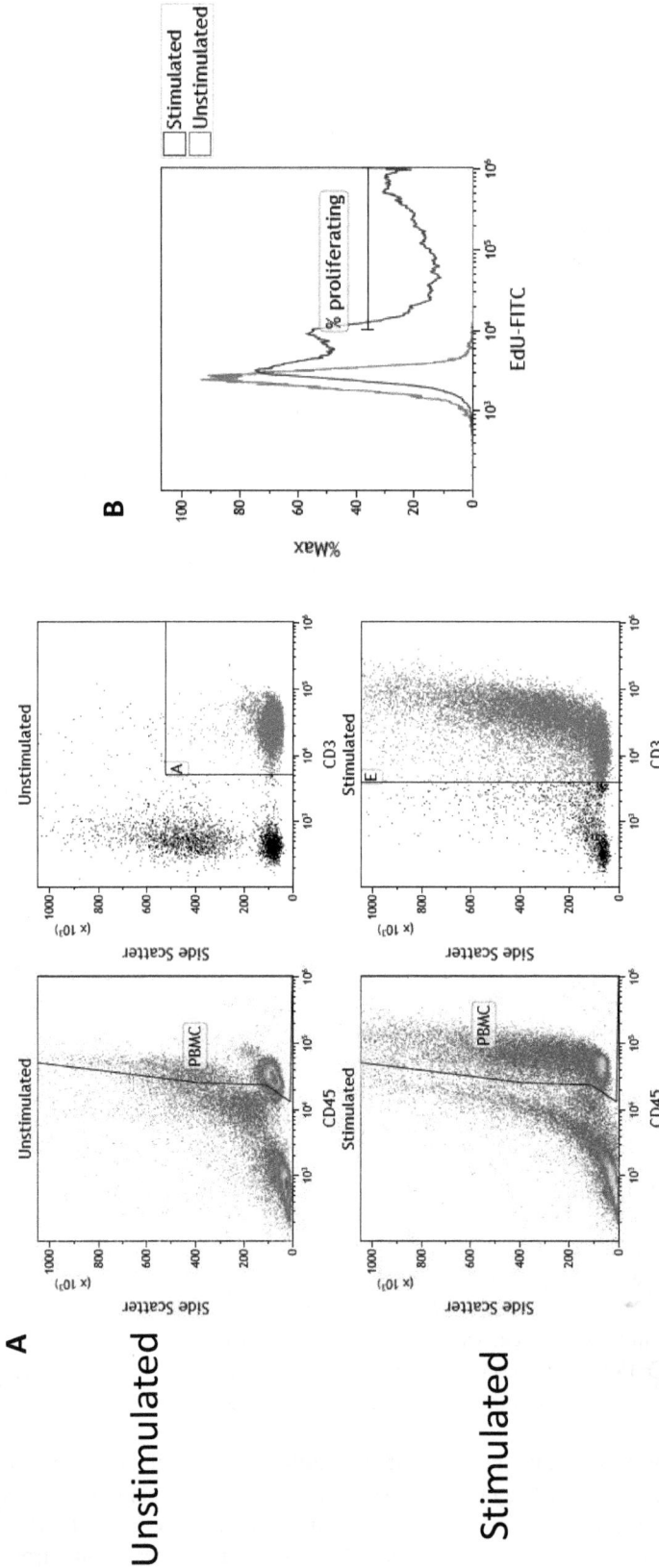

Figure 5. Dihydrorhodamine 123 (DHR 123) Test for Neutrophil Oxidative Burst. The DHR 123 test is used for the evaluation of suspected X-linked or AR chronic granulomatous disease. Whole blood is loaded with the dye, DHR 123 and then stimulated with phorbol myristate acetate (PMA) for 10–15 minutes. PMA induces oxidative burst in neutrophils. Reactive oxygen intermediates that are released during this process reduce DHR 123 to rhodamine which fluoresces brightly. This shift in fluorescence is measured by flow cytometry. (A) Healthy control neutrophils show an increase in fluorescence following stimulation. (B) X-linked CGD neutrophils show no change in fluorescence following stimulation owing to lack of oxidative burst. (C) Female carriers have two populations of neutrophils owing to the mutated *CYBB* gene carried on the defective X-chromosome, and the normal *CYBB* gene carried on the normal X-chromosome.

a healthy control. Carriers of X-linked CGD [mothers or sisters of boys with confirmed X-linked CGD) have two populations of neutrophils: one with normal oxidative burst representing the normal X-chromosome, and the other with a decreased or absent oxidative burst, representing the abnormal chromosome (Figure 5C)]. Thus, this test, which is relatively easy to perform, can be used to make a diagnosis of CGD within a few hours. It can also be used to track the engraftment of neutrophils following bone marrow transplant to correct the underlying genetic defect. As neutrophils tend to start degranulating fairly quickly after blood is collected for analysis, the DHR123 assay should preferably be performed on the day of sample collection to avoid spurious flow cytometry results that could confound the interpretation of results.

Adherence Markers (β2 Integrin Family)

LAD I occurs due to decreased or absent expression of CD18 on the surface of neutrophils. The expression of CD18 can be analyzed by flow cytometry.

For this analysis, whole blood is incubated with fluorescently tagged monoclonal antibodies to CD45, CD18 and CD11a, CD11b or CD11c. After a 15-minute incubation and a wash to remove unbound antibodies, red blood cells are lysed and the sample is analyzed by flow cytometry. Neutrophils are identified by their larger size, increased complexity and lower expression of CD45, and the expression level of CD18 and CD11a, CD11b or CD11c is assessed.

Expression of β2-integrins is reported either qualitatively as "present/absent" or as the mean fluorescence intensity of the molecule and is compared with the laboratory's established reference range.

Flow cytometry analysis of CD18 is a useful initial analysis when suspecting LAD I. Severe forms of LAD I result in little to no expression of CD18, whereas milder forms may have some residual surface expression. As with any other suspected inborn error of immunity, flow cytometry analysis, if abnormal, should be confirmed with genetic analysis. The test can also be used to track engraftment and reconstitution of normal neutrophils following bone marrow transplant to correct severe LAD I.

Surface expression of CD15s can be similarly assessed on neutrophils using flow cytometry for diagnosis of LAD II. Diagnosis of LAD III relies on genetic analysis of the *FERMT3* gene as there are no well-defined functional assays for β-integrin activation.

Laboratory Evaluation of Complement Deficiencies and Complement Activation

It is useful to remember that activation of the complement system by the three pathways (classical, lectin and alternate) culminate in C3 activation, which is an important central point of the activation cascade. Once C3 is cleaved by the C3 convertases to the fluid phase C3a (the anaphylatoxin that activates mast cells and initiates the vascular phase of inflammation) and C3b, the C3b binds to the activating cell surface and promotes C5 cleavage leading to terminal pathway activation and formation of membrane attack complex (MAC) that disrupts the bilipid layer of the target and destroys it. It is to be noted that C4 is utilized by the classical and lectin pathway but not the alternate pathway. On the other hand, the alternate pathway uses factors D and B and properdin to form alternate pathway C3 convertase and does not need C4. Factor B is central to alternate pathway activation. C3, C4 and Factor B can be easily measured in a sample by turbidometry or nephelometry.

Table 8 provides the profile of C3, C4 and Factor B levels in clinical conditions that have preferential pathways of complement activation. These are confirmed by the Classical Pathway CH50 values.

Table 8. Complement levels in clinical disorders based on pathways of complement activation.

Activation Pathways	Complement Levels				Clinical Examples
	C3	C4	Factor B	CH50	
Classical	↓	↓	N	↓	SLE, SS and systemic immune complex diseases.
Alternative	↓	N	↓	↓	C3 nephritic factor GN, aHUS and endotoxemia
Classical and Alternative	↓	↓	↓	↓	SLE, gram-negative septic shock and systemic immune complex diseases
Fluid Phase Response	N	↓	N	↓	HAE, P. vivax infection and cryoglobulinemia
Acute Phase Response	↑	↑	↑	↑	Acute and chronic inflammation; pregnancy.
Sample Mishandling (Sample Collection Problems)	N	N	N	↓	Cryoglobulins. Coagulation associated activation.

Abbreviations: Systemic Lupus Erythematosus (SLE); Systemic Sclerosis (SS); Glomerulonephritis (GN); Atypical Hemolytic Uremic Syndrome (aHUS); Hereditary Angioedema (HAE).

CH50 Hemolytic Assays

Complement hemolytic activity is a functional test of the classical and alternative pathways of complement in plasma or serum. The Classical Pathway method (CH50) is based on lysis of sensitized sheep erythrocytes in the presence of Ca^{++} and Mg^{++}. It is helpful as screening test when complement depletion or deficiency is suspected. The test is sensitive to the reduction, absence and/ or inactivity of any component of the pathway. Complement hemolytic assay activity is expressed as that dilution of serum which supports lysis of 50% of the sensitized sheep erythrocytes, hence called a "CH50 assay." It is a functional assay and is used to evaluate the functional integrity of the complement cascade to cause lysis of target cells (Costabile 2010).

In the evaluation of the Classical Pathway CH50, sheep erythrocytes sensitized with rabbit antibody are incubated with serial dilutions of the patient's serum at 37°C. Activation of the classical complement pathway will result in hemolysis. After incubation the samples are centrifuged to obtain supernatant. The free hemoglobin concentration in the supernatant, which is directly proportional to complement activity, is measured by means of a spectrophotometer at a wavelength of 415 nm. Plotting the dilution factor of serum against the degree of hemolysis allows for the calculation of the CH50 (CH50 denotes the dilution of serum which supports hemolysis of 50% of erythrocytes; 50% represents the steepest straight line of the S shaped curve when plotting hemolysis against serum dilutions). The result is expressed as a titer, which indicates the serum dilution at which 50% of the erythrocytes are hemolyzed. The positive reference is total lysis induced by lysis fluid and the negative reference is obtained after incubation with dilution buffer. The CH50 requires all of the CP and terminal components (C1, C4, C2, C3, C5, C6, C7, C8 and C9). For the assessment of the functional integrity of the AP, rabbit erythrocytes (deficient in sialic acid and hence permits binding of Factor B) is used as the activator as well as indicator of hemolytic activity or AH50. The AH50 requires all of the AP and terminal complement proteins (Factor B, D, properdin, C3. C5, C6, C7, C8 and C9). The combined use of CH50 and AH50 is the most efficient screening method for detecting genetic deficiencies of the complement components. Complete deficiencies will generally result in titers of < 5% in one or both assays. Deficiencies of Factor H, I and nephritic factors often result in very low C3 levels, leading to reduced tiers of both CH50 and AH50.

Lectin pathway dysfunction (and MBL deficiency) is determined using a specific ELISA, in which the patient's serum is added to wells coated with mannan. Binding of MBL and activation of the LP results in the deposition of C4b and C4d that are detected with specific monoclonal antibodies. This is a functional assay, MBL levels can also be determined by antigenic assays.

CH50 Enzymatic Assays [also called Complement AcTivity by Enzymatic methods (CATE)]

The complement cascade acts in a number of ways to eliminate invading organisms with a major function being the lysis of bacteria through the formation of the MAC. The complex interactions of this cascade indicate that the functionality of MAC cannot necessarily be inferred by apparently normal levels of any one complement component. This was the basis of the development of the hemolytic CH50 assay—a gold standard for evaluating the functional integrity of the cascade. However, this method is time-consuming, complicated by lack of automation, and fraught with reagent instability. An alternative method that is automated, with rapid turn-around times and with less batch-to-batch variation, uses turbidimetry to interrogate the CP functional activity as a surrogate for hemolytic activity. The surrogate for microorganisms are liposomes encapsulating the enzyme glucose 6 phosphate dehydrogenase (G6PDH). The reagent contains antibodies to the dinitrophenyl (DNP) groups on the liposome and the addition of the sample (containing complement proteins) to the reagent initiates DNP and anti-DNP antibody complexes that activate complement proteins in the sample (or control) and lyse the liposomes, releasing G6PDH to react with G6PD and nicotinic amide dehydrogenase (NAD). The change in absorbance is then measured and is proportional to the complement activity in the sample (Yamamoto et al. 1995).

Figure 6 depicts the flow chart for the evaluation of inherited complement deficiencies based on the principles of CH50 and AH50 assays.

Some of the clinical indications for comprehensive complement testing are:

1. Recurrent pyogenic infections with normal antibody function
2. Disseminated Neisseria infection

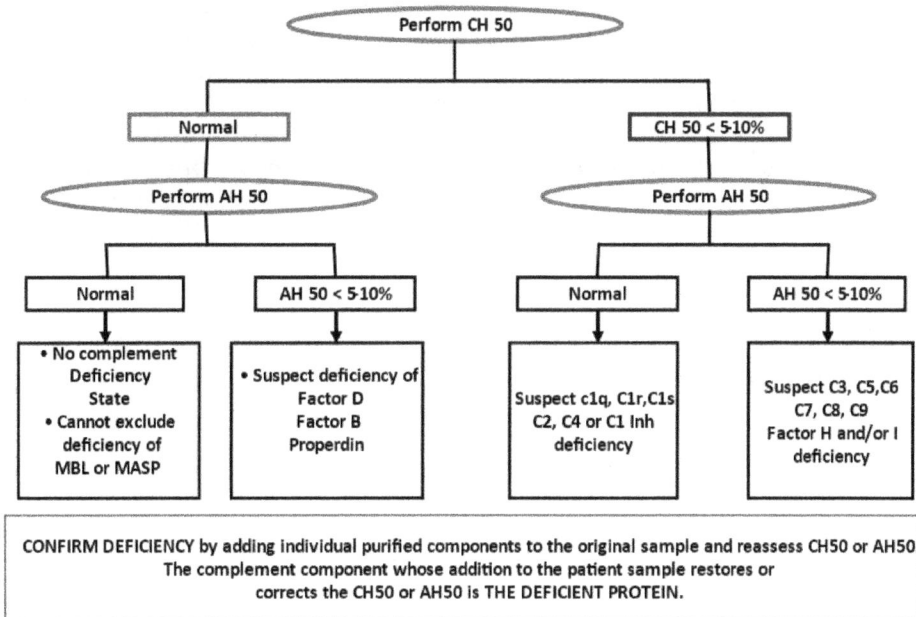

Figure 6. Flow Chart for Evaluating Inherited Complement Deficiencies. The flow chart depicts the clinical diagnostic value obtained by sequential analyses of CH50 and AH50 values obtained from a patient's serum. This algorithm provides an approach to defining complement deficiency or dysregulation.

3. Autoimmune disease with normal antibody function and infections that are not due to therapeutic immunosuppression

4. Family history of complement deficiency.

C1 Inhibitor (C1-INH)—Assay for HAE and AAE

C1 inhibitor (C1-INH) is a serine protease inhibitor or serpin whose function transcends beyond the regulation of the complement system. In fact, this multi-specific protease inhibitor that is present in normal human plasma and serum regulates enzymes of the coagulation, fibrinolytic and kinin-forming systems, besides activated C1, from which it derives the name. The enzymes (proteases) regulated by this protein include the C1r and C1s subunits of the activated first component of complement, activated Hageman factor (factor XIa), kallikrein (Fletcher factor) and plasmin.

A deficiency of functionally active C1-INH causes a spectrum of recurrent but transient attacks of non-pruritic angioedema affecting various tissues of the body. Bradykinin (BK) is the mediator of C1-INH deficiency or gain of function mutations of the Kallikrein-Kinin system (KKS). It consists of a group of three plasma proteins: factor XII (FXII, Hageman factor), prekallikrein (PK) and high-molecular-weight kininogen (HMWK). Since bradykinin is the major mediator of vascular permeability this group of angioedemas is termed "kininergic angioedema," in contrast to mast cell derived histamine that causes allergic urticaria and angioedema. Its manifestations depend upon the organs involved. While the frequent cause of death is from airway obstruction due to laryngeal edema, abdominal attacks lead to a diversity of symptoms ranging from pain, cramps, vomiting and may masquerade as intestinal obstruction. The variable nature of the symptoms at different periods during the course of the disease makes it difficult to make a definitive diagnosis based solely on clinical observation, hence the need for laboratory testing.

Two major forms of C1-INH deficiency have been reported: the congenital form, termed hereditary angioedema (HAE), and the acquired angioedema (AAE), which is associated with a variety of diseases, including lymphoid malignancies.

There are two types of HAE that can be distinguished biochemically. Patients with the more common type (85% of HAE patients) have low levels of functional C1-INH and C1-INH antigen. Patients with the second form (15% of HAE patients) have low levels of functional C1-INH but normal or increased levels of C1-INH antigen that is dysfunctional.

Cicardi et al. (1999) have proposed a classification, which can distinguish on one hand, the angioedema due to C1-INH deficiency, be it hereditary or acquired origin; on the other, the angioedema associated with normal C1-INH function is an important group of unknown biological diagnoses.

Quantitative Measurement of C1-INH

It provides a numerical value of antigenic C1 INH only irrespective of its functional status. It is measured by nephelometry or turbidimetry (described under immunoglobulin measurements). It is decreased in Type I HAE but normal in Type II HAE and many forms of AAE.

Functional Measurement of C1-INH

It is the cornerstone in the diagnoses of HAE, AAE and the rarer variant of angioedema associated with normal C1-INH function. C1-INH function is best performed on plasma or serum, collected and stored appropriately.

1) The most commonly available and reliable functional C1-INH assay is the chromogenic assay. In this assay excess C1 esterase (activated C1s) is added to the test sample or plasma controls (obtained from the World Health Organization (WHO)) resulting in the formation of C1 INH-C1 esterase complexes and free active residual C1s. This residual C1s is then measured by its

activity on a substrate resulting in the formation of para-nitro aniline (p-NA) that is measured at 37°C. The concentration of C1 INH is inversely proportional to the delta absorbance/minute measured as absorbance at 405 nm. The reference range is 70–130% of normal C1-INH (0.70–1.30 IU/mL) (Li et al. 2015).

The assay principle can be stated as follows

STEP 1. Incubate excess C1s with sample or control to form C1-INH-C1s complexes and residual C1s.

STEP 2. Add supernatant after reaction 1 with substrate specific for C1s.

STEP3. Measure the delta absorbance of para-nitroaniline released from the substrate at 405 nm.

2) A new C1-INH function chromogenic assay has been developed providing an enzymatic readout, with the advantage of targeting all KKS proteases responsible for HMWK cleavage and BK production, as opposed to C1s protease in the chromogenic assay commonly used in clinical laboratories and described above (Ghannam et al. 2015).

3) Another approach for C1-INH function was recently proposed in which the ability of C1-INH protein to form complexes with either FXII or plasma kallikrein (Joseph et al. 2015). The assays that used kallikrein-kinins (KK) as a target are more relevant to C1-INH-HAE in line with the regulatory effect of C1-INH on BK generation via the KKS involved in the pathogenesis of angioedema.

Value of Antigenic C4 Measurements

Antigenic C4 is best measured by nephelometry as it is more accurate than immunodiffusion methods. Low C1-INH function leads to uncontrolled activation of the classical complement pathway, with a subsequent reduction in circulating antigenic C4 (Davis 1988). It is important to keep in mind that a low antigenic C4 is suggestive of C1-INH-HAE, but it is not conclusive because of the presence of C4AQO or C4BQO null alleles in healthy individuals with allele frequency values in Anglo-Saxons of 0.169 and 0.185, respectively. Evidence suggests that normal antigenic C4 can be seen in patients with C1-INH-HAE (Gompels et al. 2002; Tarzi et al. 2007). However, measuring antigenic C4 during an HAE attack might improve the sensitivity of the diagnostic in cases where normal antigenic C4 was noted in between attacks. While antigenic C4 has been considered as an initial step in supporting diagnosis, antigenic C1-INH and function must be measured even in the presence of normal antigenic C4 if C1-INH-HAE is suspected (Charest-Morin et al. 2018).

Value of Antigenic C1q Measurements

C1q as measured by nephelometry is the standard assay method and has replaced the more variable immunodiffusion methods of the past. C1q is proximal to activated C1s and is not utilized in HAE and is thus normal. A quantitative or functional C1-INH deficiency with negative family history, and low antigenic C1q is the hallmark of AAE. It is often associated with anti-C1-INH antibodies of significant titer. The screening for anti-C1-INH antibodies must be performed in patients above 50 years with a recent appearance of attacks. C1-INH-AAE is caused by either C1-INH-anti-C1-INH antibody complexes fixing C1q and leading to excessive activation of C1 due to loss of available C1-INH regulatory activity, or secondary to tumor proliferation, dysglobulinemia or autoimmune disease with a proteolytic consumption of C1-INH.

C3 is characteristically normal as the activation of C1 and its regulation by C1-INH is in the fluid phase and not on a membrane that supports C14b2a or C3 convertase formation—an obligate necessity for C3 cleavage. Table 9 summarizes the complement profiles in Hereditary and Acquired angioedema.

Table 9. Complement profile in HAE and AAE.

Clinical Disease	C4	C1q	C3	C1-INH Antigen	C1-INH Functional
HAE Type I	D	N	N	D	D
HAE Type II	D	N	N	N	D
AAE Type I	D	D	N/D	D	D
AAE Type II	D	D	N/D	D/N	D
ACEi Induced AAE	N	N	N	N	N
Autoimmune Diseases SLE; Sjogren	D	D	N /D	D	D

NOTE: D = Decreased; N = Normal and N/D = Could be Normal or Decreased; ACEi induced AAE = Angiotensin inhibitor-induced acquired angioedema.

No role for complement in pathogenesis. Angioedema is due to tissue persistence of bradykinin, which is because of the lack of ACE needed to degrade bradykinin. While C4 is decreased in both remission (asymptomatic) and exacerbation (symptomatic) of C1-INH deficiency, C2 is decreased during an exacerbation only and is normal in remission.

Genetic Testing

Genetic testing is a complementary tool in the diagnosis of C1-INH-HAE or other forms of hereditary angioedema, especially in the case of normal C1-INH HAE syndromes. Pathogenic variants in four different genes have been identified to cause HAE; these genes are serine protease inhibitor G1 (*SERPING1*), factor XII (*F12*), plasminogen (*PLG*) and angiopoietic 1 (*ANGPT 1*) (Banday et al. 2020). These gene variants lead to increased bradykinin two receptor-mediated signaling via increased production of bradykinin except mutations in *ANGPT1* that disturbs the cytoskeletal assembly of vascular endothelial cells.

Genetic analysis of the *SERPING1* gene is helpful to confirm a familial diagnosis or, very rarely, when results from the classical assays are still inconclusive after using samples of poor quality. It is required for patients younger than 1 year of age, where C1-INH expression is variable resulting in serum/plasma values that are hard to interpret, compared to the adult. Next-generation sequencing (NGS) platforms that target the entire *SERPING1* gene offer a powerful approach to the genetic analysis of patients with respect to C1-INH-HAE. A real advantage of NGS when associated with copy number variation analysis is to provide information about the size and localization of recombination fragments.

More than 500 *SERPING1* variants have been reported in the online Human Gene Mutation database HMGD®. New *SERPING1* variants need to be validated for their association with decreased C1-INH function and clinical phenotype. *De novo* mutations within the *SERPING1* gene are not uncommon, requiring further attention to family segregation. Another advantage of genetic testing includes the identification of APP and ACE deficiencies as they could potentially help in identifying patients with more frequent or more severe angioedema attacks (Charignon et al. 2014). Identification of variants within the *F12, PLG* and *ANGPT1* genes (described in normal C1-INH-HAE) and are important when C1-INH-associated angioedema syndromes have to be' excluded in a patient.

Conclusion

Immunodeficiency may be primary (inherited genetic defects), or secondary (e.g., due to infection, malignancy or protein loss). In either case, partial or complete immune deficits can contribute to increased susceptibility to infection, autoimmunity, malignancy or autoinflammation. Primary immunodeficiency can manifest at any age, therefore, recognition of clinical features of primary immunodeficiency and the use of appropriate laboratory testing is essential to guide both the diagnosis and management of such patients.

Glossary of Abbreviations

AAE – Acquired Angioedema
ADA – Adenosine Deaminase
aHUS – Atypical Hemolytic Uremic Syndrome
AP – Alternative Pathway
AR – Autosomal Recessive
BTK – Bruton's Tyrosine Kinase
C1-INH – C1 esterase inhibitor
CBC – Complete Blood Count
CGD – Chronic Granulomatous Disease
CP – Classical Pathway
CVID – Common Variable Immunodeficiency
DGS – DiGeorge Syndrome
DHR123 – Dihydrorhodamine 123
EdU – 5-ethynyl-2'-deoxyuridine
FMF – Familial Mediterranean Fever
HAE – Hereditary Angioedema
HIV – Human Immunodeficiency Virus
HTLV – Human T-Lymphotropic Virus
HUS – Hemolytic Uremic Syndrome
IEI – Inborn Errors of Immunity
IUIS – International Union of Immunological Societies
IVIG – Intravenous Immunoglobulin
JAK – Janus Kinase
LAD – Leukocyte Adhesion Deficiency
LP – Leptin Pathway
MAC – Membrane Attack Complex
MSMD – Mendelian Susceptibility to Mycobacterial Disease
NADPH – Nicotinamide adenine dinucleotide phosphate
NBS – Newborn Screen
PAMP – Pathogen Associated Molecular Complex
PAP – Pulmonary Alveolar Proteinosis
PCR – Polymerase Chain Reaction
PHA – Phytohemagglutinin
PID – Primary Immunodeficiency
PMA – Phorbol Myristate Acetate
PNH – Paroxysmal Nocturnal Hemoglobinuria
RBC – Red Blood Cell
ROS – Reactive Oxygen Species
SAD – Specific Antibody Deficiency
SCID – Severe Combined Immunodeficiency
SCIG – Subcutaneous Immunoglobulin
SID – Secondary Immunodeficiency
SPEP – Serum Protein Electrophoresis
THI – Transient Hypogammaglobulinemia of Infancy
TREC – T Cell Receptor Excision Circle
WBC – White Blood Cell
XLA – X-Linked Agammaglobulinemia

References

Ambrosino, D. M., Siber, G. R., Chilmonczyk, B. A., Jernberg, J. B. and Finberg, R. W. 1987. An immunodeficiency characterized by impaired antibody responses to polysaccharides. N Engl. J. Med. 316(13): 790–793.

Banday, A. Z., Kaur, A., Jindal, A. K., Rawat, A. and Singh, S. 2020. An update on the genetics and pathogenesis of hereditary angioedema. Genes Dis. 7(1): 75–83.

Berbudi, A., Rahmadika, N., Tjahjadi, A. I. and Ruslami, R. 2020. Type 2 diabetes and its impact on the immune system. Curr. Diabetes Rev. 16(5): 442–449.

Bonilla, F. A., Barlan, I., Chapel, H., Costa-Carvalho, B. T., Cunningham-Rundles, C., de la Morena, M. T. et al. 2016. International Consensus Document (ICON): Common variable immunodeficiency disorders. J. Allergy Clin. Immunol. Pract. 4(1): 38–59.

Booth, C. and Gaspar, H. B. 2009. Pegademase bovine (PEG-ADA) for the treatment of infants and children with severe combined immunodeficiency (SCID). Biologics 3: 349–358.

Bourke, C. D., Berkley, J. A. and Prendergast, A. J. 2016. Immune dysfunction as a cause and consequence of malnutrition. Trends Immunol. 37(6): 386–398.

Bousfiha, A., Jeddane, L., Picard, C., Al-Herz, W., Ailal, F., Chatila, T. et al. 2020. Human inborn errors of immunity: 2019 update of the IUIS phenotypical classification. J. Clin. Immunol. 40(1): 66–81.

Boxer, L. A. 2012. How to approach neutropenia. Hematology Am. Soc. Hematol. Educ. Program 2012: 174–182.

Bruton, O. C. 1952. Agammaglobulinemia. Pediatrics 9(6): 722–728.

Buckley, R. H. 2002. Immunoglobulin G subclass deficiency: fact or fancy? Curr. Allergy Asthma Rep. 2(5): 356–360.

Chan, S. K. and Gelfand, E. W. 2015. Primary immunodeficiency masquerading as allergic disease. Immunol. Allergy Clin. North Am. 35(4): 767–778.

Charest-Morin, X., Betschel, S., Borici-Mazi, R., Kanani, A., Lacuesta, G., Rivard, G. E. et al. 2018. The diagnosis of hereditary angioedema with C1 inhibitor deficiency: a survey of Canadian physicians and laboratories. Allergy Asthma Clin. Immunol. 14: 83.

Charignon, D., Ghannam, A., Defendi, F., Ponard, D., Monnier, N., Lopez Trascasa, M. et al. 2014. Hereditary angioedema with F12 mutation: factors modifying the clinical phenotype. Allergy 69(12): 1659–1665.

Chinen, J. and Shearer, W. T. 2010. Secondary immunodeficiencies, including HIV infection. J. Allergy Clin. Immunol. 125(2 Suppl 2): S195–203.

Cicalese, M. P. and Aiuti, A. 2015. Clinical applications of gene therapy for primary immunodeficiencies. Hum Gene Ther. 26(4): 210–219.

Cicalese, M. P., Ferrua, F., Castagnaro, L., Rolfe, K., De Boever, E., Reinhardt, R. R. et al. 2018. Gene therapy for adenosine deaminase deficiency: a comprehensive evaluation of short- and medium-term safety. Mol. Ther. 26(3): 917–931.

Cicardi, M., Bergamaschini, L., Zingale, L. C., Gioffre, D. and Agostoni, A. 1999. Idiopathic nonhistaminergic angioedema. Am. J. Med. 106(6): 650–654.

Costabile, M. 2010. Measuring the 50% haemolytic complement (CH50) activity of serum. J. Vis. Exp. (37): 1923.

Dalal, I., Reid, B., Nisbet-Brown, E. and Roifman, C. M. 1998. The outcome of patients with hypogammaglobulinemia in infancy and early childhood. J. Pediatr 133(1): 144–146.

Davies, E. G., Cheung, M., Gilmour, K., Maimaris, J., Curry, J., Furmanski, A. et al. 2017. Thymus transplantation for complete DiGeorge syndrome: European experience. J. Allergy Clin. Immunol. 140(6): 1660–1670 e1616.

Davis, A. E., 3rd. 1988. C1 inhibitor and hereditary angioneurotic edema. Annu Rev. Immunol. 6: 595–628.

Demirdag, Y. Y. and Gupta, S. 2021. Update on Infections in Primary Antibody Deficiencies. Front Immunol. 12: 634181.

Dinauer, M. C. 2020. Neutrophil defects and diagnosis disorders of neutrophil function: an overview. Methods Mol. Biol. 2087: 11–29.

Donadieu, J., Beaupain, B., Fenneteau, O. and Bellanne-Chantelot, C. 2017. Congenital neutropenia in the era of genomics: classification, diagnosis, and natural history. Br J. Haematol. 179(4): 557–574.

Etzioni, A. 2009. Genetic etiologies of leukocyte adhesion defects. Curr. Opin. Immunol. 21(5): 481–486.

Feske, S., Picard, C. and Fischer, A. 2010. Immunodeficiency due to mutations in ORAI1 and STIM1. Clin. Immunol. 135(2): 169–182.

Fodil, N., Langlais, D. and Gros, P. 2016. Primary immunodeficiencies and inflammatory disease: a growing genetic intersection. Trends Immunol. 37(2): 126–140.

Frauwirth, K. A. and Thompson, C. B. 2002. Activation and inhibition of lymphocytes by costimulation. J. Clin. Invest. 109(3): 295–299.

Ghannam, A., Sellier, P., Defendi, F., Favier, B., Charignon, D., Lopez-Lera, A. et al. 2015. C1 inhibitor function using contact-phase proteases as target: evaluation of an innovative assay. Allergy 70(9): 1103–1111.

Gompels, M. M., Lock, R. J., Morgan, J. E., Osborne, J., Brown, A. and Virgo, P. F. 2002. A multicentre evaluation of the diagnostic efficiency of serological investigations for C1 inhibitor deficiency. J. Clin. Pathol. 55(2): 145–147.

Goronzy, J. J., Gustafson, C. E and Weyand, C. M. 2019. Immune deficiencies at the extremes of age. Clinical Immunology 535–543.e531.

Haddad, E. and Hoenig, M. 2019. Hematopoietic stem cell transplantation for severe combined immunodeficiency (SCID). Front Pediatr. 7: 481.

Henrickson, S. E., Ruffner, M. A. and Kwan, M. 2016. Unintended immunological consequences of biologic therapy. Curr. Allergy Asthma Rep. 16(6): 46.

Joseph, K., Bains, S., Tholanikunnel, B. G., Bygum, A., Aabom, A., Koch, C. et al. 2015. A novel assay to diagnose hereditary angioedema utilizing inhibition of bradykinin-forming enzymes. Allergy 70(1): 115–119.

Knight, V., Heimall, J. R., Wright, N., Dutmer, C. M., Boyce, T. G., Torgerson, T. R. et al. 2020. Follow-up for an abnormal newborn screen for severe combined immunodeficiencies (NBS SCID): A Clinical Immunology Society (CIS) survey of current practices. Int. J. Neonatal. Screen 6(3).

Li, H. H., Busse, P., Lumry, W. R., Frazer-Abel, A., Levy, H., Steele, T. et al. 2015. Comparison of chromogenic and ELISA functional C1 inhibitor tests in diagnosing hereditary angioedema. J. Allergy Clin. Immunol. Pract. 3(2): 200–205.

Lumniczky, K., Impens, N., Armengol, G., Candeias, S., Georgakilas, A. G., Hornhardt, S. et al. 2021. Low dose ionizing radiation effects on the immune system. Environ. Int. 149: 106212.

McDonald-McGinn, D. M., Sullivan, K. E., Marino, B., Philip, N., Swillen, A., Vorstman, J. A. et al. 2015. 22q11.2 deletion syndrome. Nat. Rev. Dis. Primers 1: 15071.

Moins-Teisserenc, H., Cordeiro, D. J., Audigier, V., Ressaire, Q., Benyamina, M., Lambert, J. et al. 2021. Severe altered immune status after burn injury is associated with bacterial infection and septic shock. Front Immunol. 12: 586195.

Notarangelo, L. D., Duse, M. and Ugazio, A. G. 1992. Immunodeficiency with hyper-IgM (HIM). Immunodefic Rev. 3(2): 101–121.

Pai, S. Y., Lurain, K. and Yarchoan, R. 2021. How immunodeficiency can lead to malignancy. Hematology Am. Soc. Hematol. Educ. Program 2021(1): 287–295.

Puck, J. M. 2012. Laboratory technology for population-based screening for severe combined immunodeficiency in neonates: the winner is T-cell receptor excision circles. J. Allergy Clin. Immunol. 129(3): 607–616.

Reith, W. and Mach, B. 2001. The bare lymphocyte syndrome and the regulation of MHC expression. Annu. Rev. Immunol. 19: 331–373.

Schmidt, R. E., Grimbacher, B. and Witte, T. 2017. Autoimmunity and primary immunodeficiency: two sides of the same coin? Nat. Rev. Rheumatol. 14(1): 7–18.

Schroder-Braunstein, J. and Kirschfink, M. 2019. Complement deficiencies and dysregulation: Pathophysiological consequences, modern analysis, and clinical management. Mol. Immunol. 114: 299–311.

Shearer, W. T., Dunn, E., Notarangelo, L. D., Dvorak, C. C., Puck, J. M., Logan, B. R. et al. 2014. Establishing diagnostic criteria for severe combined immunodeficiency disease (SCID), leaky SCID, and Omenn syndrome: the Primary Immune Deficiency Treatment Consortium experience. J. Allergy Clin. Immunol. 133(4): 1092–1098.

Shih, A. R. and Murali, M. R. 2015. Laboratory tests for disorders of complement and complement regulatory proteins. Am. J. Hematol. 90(12): 1180–1186.

Steiger, S., Rossaint, J., Zarbock, A. and Anders, H. J. 2022. Secondary immunodeficiency related to kidney disease (SIDKD)-definition, unmet need, and mechanisms. J. Am. Soc. Nephrol. 33(2): 259–278.

Stone, K. D., Feldman, H. A., Huisman, C., Howlett, C., Jabara, H. H. and Bonilla, F. A. 2009. Analysis of *in vitro* lymphocyte proliferation as a screening tool for cellular immunodeficiency. Clin. Immunol. 131(1): 41–49.

Tangye, S. G., Al-Herz, W., Bousfiha, A., Cunningham-Rundles, C., Franco, J. L., Holland, S. M. et al. 2022. Human inborn errors of immunity: 2022 update on the classification from the international union of immunological societies expert committee. J. Clin. Immunol.

Tarzi, M. D., Hickey, A., Forster, T., Mohammadi, M. and Longhurst, H. J. 2007. An evaluation of tests used for the diagnosis and monitoring of C1 inhibitor deficiency: normal serum C4 does not exclude hereditary angio-oedema. Clin. Exp. Immunol. 149(3): 513–516.

Toma, A., Fenaux, P., Dreyfus, F. and Cordonnier, C. 2012. Infections in myelodysplastic syndromes. Haematologica 97(10): 1459–1470.

Walkovich, K. and Vander Lugt, M. 2009. ZAP70-related combined immunodeficiency. 2009 Oct 20 [Updated 2021 Sep 23]. *In*: Adam, M. P., Everman, D. B., Mirzaa, G. M. et al. (eds.). GeneReviews® [Internet]. Seattle (WA): University of Washington, Seattle; 1993–2022. Available from: https://www.ncbi.nlm.nih.gov/books/NBK20221/.

Yamamoto, S., Kubotsu, K., Kida, M., Kondo, K., Matsuura, S., Uchiyama, S. et al. 1995. Automated homogeneous liposome-based assay system for total complement activity. Clin. Chem. 41(4): 586–590.

Yel, L. 2010. Selective IgA deficiency. J. Clin. Immunol. 30(1): 10–16.

Yu, H. H., Yang, Y. H. and Chiang, B. L. 2021. Chronic granulomatous disease: a comprehensive review. Clin. Rev. Allergy Immunol. 61(2): 101–113.

Chapter 9

Allergy Immunotherapy for Inhalant Allergens

Harold S. Nelson

Introduction

Allergy immunotherapy (AIT) is a form of treatment for allergic diseases whose aim is to induce tolerance to the causative allergens (Burks 2013). In most cases, this involves the administration of allergens or derivatives of allergens with an initial build-up of doses, followed by the administration of the highest achieved dose as a maintenance treatment for several years. The allergen is conventionally administered either as subcutaneous injections (subcutaneous immunotherapy or SCIT) or by placing a tablet or liquid preparation of the allergen under the tongue (sublingual immunotherapy or SLIT). In the case of SLIT tablets, treatment is often initiated with the maintenance dose, omitting the initial build-up. There are many alternatives to traditional SCIT and SLIT that are under study (Table 1), typically they promise fewer administrations of the agent, but as none are currently approved in the United States; they will only be briefly mentioned at the end of this chapter.

Table 1. Future approaches to SCIT.[1]

1. Alternative routes of administration
a. Intralymphatic
b. Epicutaneous
2. Adjuvants
a. Vitamin D
b. Probiotics
c. Ligands for the innate immune system
d. Nanoparticles
3. Modified allergens
a. Allergoids
b. Modified recombinant allergens
c. Non-IgE binding peptides

[1] Data from (Nelson 2022).

Professor of Medicine, Department of Medicine, Division of Allergy and Immunology, National Jewish Health, 1500 Jackson St. Denver, Colorado, USA 80206, University of Colorado Denver School of Medicine.
Email: nelsonh@njhealth.org

Indications for AIT

Many randomized, controlled studies have examined the effectiveness of AIT administered by both SCIT and SLIT in the treatment of allergic rhinoconjunctivitis and asthma. Studies have been positive with both approaches for reducing symptoms and medication use while inducing favorable changes in quality of life and specific immunologic markers (Calderon 2011). However, a Cochran systematic review in 2020, still found that the support for the treatment of asthma with SLIT was inadequate to recommend its use (Fulmali 2021).

AIT has also been used with non-inhalant allergens. SCIT with Hymenoptera venom and whole-body extract of fire ants has proven to reduce systemic reactions to the stings of these insects (Boyle 2012). There are a few studies reporting successful treatment of atopic dermatitis with house dust mite extracts by both SCIT and SLIT in patients sensitized to these allergens (Bae 2013; Pajno 2007). Finally, both oral and sublingual administration of several foods in patients with IgE-mediated food allergy has shown promising results.

Comparison of Efficacy of SCIT and SLIT

There are only a few studies that compared directly the efficacy of SCIT vs. SLIT using accepted dosing regimens for each. Two studies compared the response in subjects with seasonal allergic rhinitis caused by grass pollen, treating subjects with the recommended doses of timothy pollen extract by SLIT-tablet (75,000 SQ-U daily) or injection (100,000 SQ-U every one or two months) and including placebo or untreated controls (Aasbjerg 2014; Scadding 2017). In both studies the response to nasal challenge with timothy extract was the primary outcome and in both the timothy SCIT was significantly more effective than the timothy SLIT-tablets early (3 months and 1st GPS, respectively); later (15 months or 2nd GPS respectively) although the same trend in favor of SCIT continued, the differences were no longer statistically significant. The advantage of SLIT over SCIT is its greater safety. Unlike SCIT, no fatal reactions have been reported with SLIT; therefore, after the first administration of SLIT that should be done under medical observation, the approved SLIT tablets can be administered at home. Despite this apparent advantage, adherence to SLIT is considerably poorer than to SCIT (Kiel 2013).

Selection of Patients With Respiratory Allergies for AIT

The first consideration in evaluating a patient for AIT with inhalant allergens is understanding if their symptoms are due to allergy. The questions here are: is there evidence by skin or *in vitro* testing of IgE sensitization to the allergen in question?; is the patient significantly exposed to that allergen?; and, finally, does the occurrence of symptoms in the patient correspond to their pattern of exposure to that allergen(s)?

The next consideration is, does the severity of symptoms warrant embarking on a fairly expensive and somewhat inconvenient course of treatment. The most effective form of treatment would be avoidance; however, this is almost impossible for seasonal allergens, is difficult for most allergens causing perennial symptoms and is usually unacceptable to patients who have indoor pets to which they are sensitive. Fairly effective and reasonably priced pharmacologic treatments, including systemic and topical antihistamines and topical corticosteroids, provide variable relief for symptoms of allergic rhinitis.

Should AIT be then limited to those failing symptomatic treatment? Here is a place for discussion between the physician and the patient. The advantages of selecting AIT as an adjunct to symptomatic treatment, in addition to more complete symptoms relief, are the disease-modifying effects of AIT, such as reduction in the development of asthma in patients only experiencing rhinoconjunctivitis and persisting clinical improvement after discontinuation of a successful course of AIT. For patients with asthma, considerations are the greater seriousness of the disease, but also the greater danger of the treatment, especially if the asthma is not well controlled.

Contraindications for AIT

There are several contraindications to placing a patient on AIT. Perhaps the foremost is the presence of severe or poorly controlled bronchial asthma (Epstein 2021). European Academy of Allergy and Clinical Immunology (EAACI) guidelines list as absolute contraindications for SCIT: uncontrolled or severe asthma, active systemic autoimmune disorders, active malignant neoplasm and pregnancy; as relative contraindications: partially controlled asthma, beta-adrenergic blocker therapy, severe cardiovascular disease, systemic autoimmune disorders in remission, severe psychiatric disorders, poor adherence, primary and secondary immunodeficiency and a history of serious systemic reaction to AIT (Roberts 2018). The 3rd update of the U.S. immunotherapy practice parameters considers active autoimmune conditions as only a relative contraindication and states that AIT should be initiated only if the patient's asthma is stable with pharmacotherapy (Cox 2011).

Treatment of the Polyallergic Patient With AIT

The majority of patients in both the U.S. and Europe presenting to an allergy clinic for evaluation of an allergic respiratory condition are sensitized to multiple aeroallergens. (Nelson 2016). There is no difference in the response to AIT with a single allergen, whether they are sensitive to only the allergen being used for treatment or to multiple unrelated allergens (Nelson 2013). There is, however, a major disagreement between the majority of European and American allergists regarding the appropriate treatment of patients presenting with multiple allergies, as opposed to multiple positive skin tests most of which may not be clinically important. The US practice parameters recommend that patients be treated with a mixture(s) containing all clinically relevant allergen extracts (Cox 2011). European guidelines, however, do not recommend the use of mixtures of unrelated allergens (Demoly 2016; Roberts 2018). Instead, they recommend that only the most clinically important allergen extract be administered or if two extracts containing unrelated allergens are of equal importance, they are to be given on alternate days or during the same visit in the left and right arm with at least a 30-minute interval between injections. Support for the US practice is primarily provided by the studies of Lowell and Franklin who demonstrated, in two randomized placebo-controlled trials, that reduction or elimination of ragweed extract in a mixture of unrelated allergen extracts caused loss of protection against symptoms of allergic rhinitis during the ragweed pollen season, thus proving that ragweed pollen extract was clinically effective when administered in a mixture of unrelated pollen extracts.

The Immunologic Response to AIT

In general, the immunologic responses to SCIT and SLIT are the same and represent an allergen-specific shift from the abnormalities found in allergic patients toward the immune response found in non-allergic individuals (Jutel 2004). Early after initiation of AIT, there is suppression of mast cell and basophil responsiveness and an increase in allergen-specific regulatory cells secreting the cytokine interleukin-10 (IL-10), these include not only regulatory T-lymphocytes, but also regulatory B cells, Treg follicular cells and regulatory innate lymphoid cells (Shamji 2021). In addition, there is induction of iTr35 cells secreting IL-35 which are potential immune regulators (Shamji 2021). These cellular changes are accompanied by suppression of specific Immunoglobulin E (IgE) and enhanced production of specific IgG4 and IgA (Jutel 2004). Later, there is an allergen-specific immune deviation from Type-2 to Type-1 cytokine response (Hamid 1997).

Prescribing a Therapeutic Extract for AIT

The physician prescribing immunotherapy should be trained and experienced in prescribing and administering immunotherapy (Cox 2011). They must select the appropriate allergen extracts based on that patient's clinical history, allergen exposure and the results of tests for specific IgE antibodies

Figure 1. Allergy treatment extract prescription form.

Patient name	Prescribing physician
Date of birth	Address
Patient number	Telephone number
Telephone number	Fax

Extract Designation:

Trees (T); Grasses (G); Weeds (W); Molds (M); House Dust Mites (HDM); Cockroach (Cr); Cat (C); Dog (D)

New vials		Date prepared		Expiration date			
Vial From vial		/ /		/ /			
Vial From vial		/ /		/ /			
Vial From vial		/ /		/ /			
Allergen Number	Allergen Name[2]	Concentration Potency units[3]	Volume Added	Manufacturer	Lot #	Expiration Date[4]	
1							
2							
3							
4							
5							
6							
7							
8							
9							
10.							
Diluent							
Total Volume							
Treatment Schedule							
		Standard Schedule		Begin with Vial #4			
				Begin with Vial $5			
		Conservative Schedule		See attached			

(1) Modified From Cox (2011). (2) Name May be Botanical or Common (If Unique). (3) Examples: Weight by Volume (w/v), Protein Nitrogen Units (PNU), Allergy Units (AU), Bioequivalent Allergy Units (BAU), 50% Glycerin (50% G), Aqueous (AQ), Aluminum Precipitated (AP). (4) Expiration Date for the mixture is the Earliest of Any Component.

and ensure that effective doses of each unrelated allergen will be delivered with the maintenance injections. An example of a form for prescribing an AIT treatment extract is found in Figure 1.

If a patient is deemed to be a suitable candidate for immunotherapy, the prescribing physician must first decide whether to follow the European model, that AIT is administered for only one, or occasionally two unrelated allergen extracts, or follow the US practice of treating all clinically important allergies employing one or several vials containing mixtures of unrelated allergen extracts. If the European model is employed, the only decisions are the type of extract and the dose of the extract to be administered. If the US model is employed there are four considerations: selection of the allergen extracts to be included (i.e., aqueous or normal saline, 50% glycerinated saline or aluminum precipitated), adequate dosing of each allergen, attention to botanically related and hence often cross-acting allergens and avoidance of mixing extracts with strong proteolytic activity with other extracts which they may degrade.

Allergen Extracts

Potency and Standardization

In the US, there are a limited number of standardized extracts of inhalant allergens, namely cat hair and dander or pelt, the HDM *Dermatophagoides pteronyssinus* and *D. farinae*, short ragweed, the cross-reactive northern pasture grasses (NPG) timothy, June, meadow fescue, orchard, red top, rye, and sweet vernal. Also, Bermuda grass; that does not cross-react with the NPG. For these standardized extracts the U.S. Food and Drug Administration (FDA) has established a standard of potency, expressed in one of several units (e.g., Allergy Units; Bioequivalent Allergy Units) that must be met for the allergen extract to be released by the manufacturer.

The potencies of non-standardize products are generally expressed by the weight of crude material and the volume of extracting fluid (weight/volume) or the protein nitrogen content per unit volume (PNU/mL); neither of these expressions of potency bears a strong relation to allergenic potency. However, randomized, double-blind, placebo-controlled trials (RDBPC) trials have been conducted with non-standardized birch, dog dander and *Alternaria alternata* with the effective doses expressed as the content of major allergen in the maintenance dose. In Europe, extracts are more often standardized, but there are no agencies setting standards; instead, each manufacturer maintains its own within house standards.

Diluents, Adjuvants and Modifications in Dose

In the U.S. extracts are available in saline solution with 0.4% phenol as a preservative or they may contain 50% glycerin. For diluting the extracts saline may be used but far preferable is saline containing 0.03% human serum albumin (HSA). The HSA helps maintain potency, particularly of dilute extracts. In the US, there is one line of pollen extracts precipitated by aluminum, creating a deport product. In Europe, aluminum-precipitated extracts are much more commonly used and allergoids, created by mixing an allergen extract with an aldehyde resulting in some denaturation and clumping of the proteins are available for several allergens. Both of these modifications reduce reactivity with IgE and reduce systemic reactions.

Selection of Doses

The response to AIT is dose-dependent. RDBPC trials have been conducted with a limited number of allergen extracts and the effects as well as suboptimal doses have been expressed by the major allergen content of the maintenance dose. Some extract manufacturers have performed analyses on US allergen extracts to determine their content of major allergens. This information was employed to develop recommendations for dosing with U.S. allergy extracts that appeared in the 3rd update of the Immunotherapy: Practice Parameters (Table 2). In Table 2, a range of doses is given for the standardized extracts, this reflects the range of major allergen content in the US commercial extracts of these allergens.

Since the prescriber will not know the major allergen content of the extract he/she is employing, it is recommended that the middle of the recommended dose range be used. The major allergen content of the non-standardized pollen extracts has been in the same range as the standardized pollens, therefore approximately the same doses of non-standardized pollen extracts should be employed as is recommended for standardized pollens. Non-standardized dog dander extracts, with the exception of one acetone-precipitated product (Meiser 2001), are probably too weak to achieve the optimal dose. Most extracts of *Alternaria,* the only fungus for which a major allergen target dose is established, are too weak to deliver the proven effective dose, but the strongest available, given as 1 mL, undiluted, could come close to achieving this dose. There are no RDBPC trials performed with a cockroach or fungi other than *Alternaria* that report the major allergen content of the extract employed, nor is there information on the major allergen content of most of these

Table 2. Recommended dosing with US standardized extracts.[1]

Allergen	Extracts Available in the US	Dosing Recommended in Practice Parameter Mean (Range)
Short ragweed	1/10 w/v (100,000 AU/mL)	2,500 AU (1,000 to 4,000 AU)
Timothy grass	100,000 BAU/mL	2,500 BAU (1,000 to 4,000 BAU)
Bermuda grass	10,000 BAU/mL	900 BAU (300 to 1,500 BAU)
Cat hair and dander	5,000, 10,000 BAU/mL	2,500 BAU (1,000 to 4,000 BAU)
Dermatophagoides pteronyssinus	3,000, 5,000, 10,000 and 30,000 AU/mL	1,250 AU (500 to 2,000 AU)
Dermatophagoides farinae	3,000, 5,000, 10,000, and 30,000 AU/mL	1,250 AU (500 to 2,000 AU)

[1] Modified from Cox 2011.

extracts; accordingly, it is not known if effective AIT can be delivered with the presently available US commercial extracts. It is not customary to adjust the targeted dose for age or weight.

Attention to Cross-Allergenicity

It is important that cross-reacting allergen extracts be approached differently from non-cross-reacting extracts. To prevent overloading the treatment extract with a group of cross-reacting allergens, either the locally predominating species should be used to represent the group or a mixture of locally important members of the group should be prepared and treated as if they were a single pollen extract. Clinically important cross-reacting groups are listed in Table 3.

Table 3. Patterns of cross-reactivity of allergens.[1]

Trees	
Birch; Alder; Hazelnut; Hornbeam (strongly cross-reactive); Beech; Oak (moderately cross-reactive)	Use locally most important species
European Olive; Ash; Privet; Russian Olive	Use locally most important species
Cedar; Cypress; Juniper; Arborvitae	Use locally most important species
Pecan; Hickory	Use locally most important species
Poplar; Aspen; Cottonwood	Use locally most important species
Grasses	
NPG (Timothy; June; Orchard; Redtop; Meadow Fescue; Perennial Rye; Sweet Vernal	Use Timothy or a mixture of locally important members
Bermuda Grass	Not cross-reactive with NPG
Bahia, Johnson Grass	Use if locally important
Weeds	
Short; Giant; False and Western Ragweed	Use locally most important species
Southern and Slender Ragweed; Cocklebur, Burweed Marsh Elder	Use if locally important
Sages; Mugwort	Use locally most important species
Pigweed; Palmer's Amaranth; Western Water Hemp	Use locally most important species
Russian Thistle; *Kochia*; Lamb's Quarters	If both Russian Thistle and *Kochia* are locally important, use a mixture
Insects	
Dermatophagoides pteronyssinus and farinae	If both are locally important, use a mixture
Cockroach; German and American	Use a mixture

[1] From: Weber 2007 and Weber 2008.

Compatibility of Allergy Extracts for Mixing

Allergen extracts of cockroaches and fungi have strong proteolytic activities that have been shown to degrade the allergens contained in each other (Grier 2012) as well as extracts of pollens, animal danders and house dust mites (Nelson 1996). The proper procedure is that cockroach and fungal extracts are given separately and neither is mixed with pollen, dander or house dust mite extracts.

Preparing an Allergen Extract for AIT

A physician with training and expertise in allergen immunotherapy should be responsible for ensuring that compounding personnel are instructed and trained in the preparation of extracts for AIT (Cox 2011).

Single extracts or mixtures of allergen extracts suitable for AIT can be obtained from most commercial providers of allergen extracts. These will contain the proper concentration of the extract(s) that have been prepared under sterile conditions and will contain multiple vials of increasing concentration of the treatment extract to be used to build up to the maintenance dose unless this represents a refill of the maintenance concentration.

If, on the other hand, the extract for AIT is to be prepared in the clinic of the prescribing physician, there are conditions that should be met (Cox 2011). The compounding person must:

1. Be an appropriately trained health professional
2. Be trained in the preparation of allergenic products
3. Pass a written test on aseptic technique and extract preparation
4. Be able to correctly identify, measure and mix ingredients
5. Be able to demonstrate an understanding of antiseptic hand cleaning and disinfection of mixing surfaces
6. Annually pass a media-fill test

Competency can be assessed using quizzes prepared by the Advocacy Council of the American College of Allergy, Asthma and Immunology at (https://education.acaai.org, then under "Free courses for College members", highlight "allergen extract mixing quiz" (accessed June 7, 2023). Non-college members should go to (https://education.acaai.org/allergenextractquiznm) (ACAAI 2023b). The following additional resources are available with the quizzes: The ACAAI's Allergen Immunotherapy Extract Preparation: Physician Instruction Guide; An Allergen Extract Preparation-competency Check List to use in preparation for taking the Extract Preparation Quiz; the Allergen Extract Preparation Guidelines; and the portion of U.S. Pharmacopoeia Convention (USP) Chapter 797 that relates to allergen extract preparation.

Several commercial tests are available to assess sterile technique (i.e., media-fill tests). Information is available through the American College of Allergy, Asthma and Immunology at (hppts://education.acaai.org) (ACAAI 2023b) accessed June 7, 2023.

Management of AIT

Build-up Schedule

SCIT treatment must be started with a diluted extract, usually 1:1,000 v/v of the maintenance concentration in patients with no special risk (Table 4).

A somewhat more conservative build-up is recommended for patients with many strongly positive skin prick tests, controlled asthma or a history of systemic reactions to previous AIT. The build-up may be accomplished with injection visits once or twice a week or even daily, by cluster build-up with several injections per day on non-consecutive days by rush build-up with multiple injections on consecutive days (https://college.acaai.org/toolkits/allergen-extract-mixing-toolkit/)

Table 4. Representative conventional schedule for subcutaneous immunotherapy.[1] Patients with asthma or previous systemic reactions to AIT may require a more conservative schedule.

1:10,000 v/v Vial #5[2] Silver Cap	1:1,000 v/v Vial #4 Blue Cap	1:100 v/v Vial #3 Green Cap	1:10 v/v Vial #2 Gold Cap	1:1 v/v Maintenance Vial Red Cap
0.05 mL	0.05 mL	0.05 mL	0.05 mL	0.05 mL
0.10 mL	0.10 mL	0.10 mL	0.07 mL	0.07 mL
0.20 mL	0.20 mL	0.20 mL	0.10 mL	0.10 mL
0.40 mL	0.40 mL	0.40 mL	0.15 mL	0.15 mL
			0.25 mL	0.20 mL
			0.35 mL	0.30 mL
			0.50 mL	0.40 mL
				0.50 mL

From (Nelson 2021)
Vial #5 is used for highly sensitive patients (multiple large skin test reactions). Less sensitive patients begin with vial #4.

(ACAAI 2023a). The advantage of cluster and rush regimens is more rapidly reaching maintenance doses. The disadvantage of rush is more frequent systemic reactions. There is disagreement about whether cluster build up is associated with an increased incidence of systemic reactions (Epstein 2013; Winslow 2016). Whatever schedule is used, it is important to keep the extract at 4 degrees centigrade when the patient is not actually receiving their injection to avoid accelerated loss of potency. Loss of potency is more rapid in more dilute solutions, making it important to complete treatment with the first 1–2 vials as quickly as possible.

Although build-up schedules have been employed with SLIT, treatment with the currently approved SLIT tablets is initiated with the maintenance dose tablet.

Safety Precautions

No matter which build-up schedule is used, certain precautions are employed by some or all physicians in administering AIT. For SCIT, the treatment should be administered in a medical facility with trained personnel and equipment to manage systemic reactions (Cox 2011), use of two means of identification (such as name and birth date) should be used to ensure the administration of the correct extract to the patient, and the patient should remain under observation in the facility for 30 minutes following the injection (Cox 2011). If the patient has asthma, special care is indicated including determining that the asthma is well controlled because, if not, the injection should not be given (Cox 2011). The occurrence of large local or systemic reactions with SCIT can be reduced by the pre-administration of an antihistamine (Ohashi 2006).

Two safety concerns are quite controversial, prescribing an epinephrine autoinjector for all or most patients receiving SCIT (Epstein 2019) (the FDA mandates this for patients receiving SLIT tablets since administration occurs at home) and reduction in the dose of SCIT during the season of pollen contained in their treatment extract (Bernstein 2020; Lin 1992; Wong 2017). US allergists are close to evenly divided on both issues.

With SLIT, where the occurrence of serious systemic reactions is very uncommon except with the initial dose, the first dose should be administered under observation in the clinic, but subsequent doses are administered by the patient at home.

Modification in Doses

The dose of the SCIT extract may require reduction under certain circumstances such as

1. replacement of the maintenance extract when the previous vial is exhausted or expired;
2. an excessive number of consecutively missed injection visits; or the occurrence of a systemic reaction.

Table 5. Adjustments for gaps in SCIT treatment.[1]

Build-up Phase	
Up to 7 days late	Continue build-up as scheduled
8–13 days	Repeat the last dose
14–21 days	Reduce dose by 25%
21–28 days	Reduce dose by 50%
Maintenance Phase	
2–4 weeks late	Reduce dose by 75%
> weeks late	Reduce by one or more dilutions depending on the length of time and the patient's sensitivity

[1] Modified from the US Practice Parameters (Cox 2011).

While it is clear that all these situations require some adjustment in dose, there are few prospective studies testing the safety of different degrees of modifications. Empiric suggestions for adjustment for new vials is that the dose is reduced by 1/3 to 1/2 if the same extracts from the same providers are used to compound the new extract. This drop-back should be greater (e.g., 90%) if there is a change in the supplier of allergen extracts and still greater (e.g., 99%) if fungal or cockroach extracts are included. Suggestions for adjusting for missed doses are given in Table 5.

If the patient experiences a systemic reaction during build up, common practice is to administer the last tolerated dose the next time. If the reaction is severe or the patient is on maintenance, some reduction in dose is common. Also, if the reaction is severe, the physician should assess, with input from the patient, the appropriateness of continuing AIT.

Large Local Reactions

Large local reactions are common during the course of SCIT. They have been shown not to be predictive of a systemic reaction with the next injection (Tankersley 2000; Jutel and Kelso 2004) but may persist for 24 hours or more and cause patients discomfort. Two studies have demonstrated that the occurrence of large local reactions can be reduced by rinsing the syringe with epinephrine 1:1,000 prior to filling it with extract (Mustafa 2020; Sapsaprang 2020).

Duration of AIT

Studies of 3 or 4 years of SCIT with grass pollen extract have shown good clinical responses and persistence of improvement during 3 years of follow-up after AIT was stopped (Ebner 1994; Durham 1999). Other SCIT studies have shown that in patients with residual symptoms after 3 years 2 further years of treatment produced significant further improvement (Tabar 2011) or produced no further improvement (Stelmach et al. 2012). Thus, the usual recommendation is 3–5 years of AIT depending on how quickly the patient responds but stopping AIT if the patient has not responded by one year after reaching maintenance dosing.

A study with house dust mite SLIT found a good response with 3-year treatment, but a somewhat more prolonged remission with 4 or 5 years of treatment (Marogna et al. 2010). On the other hand, a study of both SCIT and SLIT treatment for 2 years found that the improvement with both approaches versus placebo, was significant after 2 years, but the benefit was largely lost one year after treatment was discontinued (Scadding et al. 2017) suggesting 2 years of either SCIT or SLIT, even if clinically effective while being administered was, of insufficient duration to provide long-lasting relief.

Future Approaches to AIT

Despite the overall efficacy and disease-modifying potential of SCIT and SLIT, both are underutilized in treating the increasing number of patients with respiratory allergies. Both involve some expense for most patients. SCIT, although probably somewhat more effective than SLIT, is associated with an increased potential for systemic reactions; for that reason, it must be administered in a facility prepared to treat these reactions. SCIT, on the other hand, can be self-administered at home. A big drawback is that both SCIT and SLIT involve a 3- to 5-year commitment and a number of studies suggest that a relatively small percentage placed on AIT persist with the treatment for that length of time that is probably necessary to achieve persisting improvement. The mechanisms underlying the improvement with AIT are thought to be understood, which encourages investigators to pursue new ways to achieve these immunologic changes by methods that require many fewer treatments, hopefully over a shorter period. Table 1 lists the more promising approaches that are currently under investigation to achieve improvements in SCIT (Nelson 2022). Of these, the most likely to see introduction into clinical use is the alternative routes of administration, the adjuvants vitamin D and probiotics and the allergoids. The other approaches will require extensive investigations and even if they succeed, they are a number of years away from approval.

Glossary of Abbreviations

ACAAI – American College of Allergy, Asthma and Immunology
AIT – Allergy Immunotherapy
AU – Allergy Units
AQ – Aqueous
AP – Aluminum Precipitated
BAU – Bioequivalent Allergy Units
EAACI – European Academy of Allergy and Clinical Immunology
GPS – Grass Pollen Season
HAS – Human Serum Albumin
50% G – 50% Glycerin
NPG – Northern Pasture Grasses
OIT – Oral Immunotherapy
PNU – Protein Nitrogen Units
RDBPC – Randomized, Double-Blind, Placebo-Controlled Trials
SCIT – Subcutaneous Immunotherapy
SLIT – Sublingual Immunotherapy
w/v – Weight by Volume

References

Aasbjerg, K., Backer, V., Lund, G., Holm, J., Nielsen, N. C., Holse, M. et al. 2014. Immunological comparison of allergen immunotherapy tablet treatment and subcutaneous immunotherapy against grass allergy. Clin. Exp. Allergy 44: 417–28.

ACAAI. 2023a. (https://college.acaai.org/toolkits/allergen-extract-mixing-toolkit/).

ACAAI. 2023b. (hppts://education.acaai.org).

Bae, J. M., Choi, Y. Y., Park, C. O., Chung, K. Y. and Lee, K. H. 2013. Efficacy of allergen-specific immunotherapy for atopic dermatitis: a systematic review and meta-analysis of randomized controlled trials. J. Allergy Clin. Immunol. 132: 110–7.

Bernstein, D. and Epstein, T. E. G. 2020. Safety of allergen immunotherapy in North America from 2008–2017: Lessons learned from the ACAAI/AAAAI National Surveillance Study of adverse reactions to allergen immunotherapy. Allergy Asthma Proc. 41: 108–111.

Boyle, R. J., Eiremeli, M., Hockenhull, J, Cherry, M. G., Bulsara, M. K., Daniels, M. and Oude Eiberink, J. N. G. 2012. Venom immunotherapy for preventing allergic reactions to insect stings. Cochrane Database Syst. Rev. 10: CD008838.

Burks, A. W., Calderon, M. A., Casale, T., Cox, L., Demoly, P., Jutel, M. et al. 2013. Update on allergy immunotherapy: American Academy of Allergy, Asthma & Immunology/European Academy of Allergy and Clinical Immunology/PRACTALL consensus report. J. Allergy Clin. Immunol. 131: 1288–96.

Calderon, M. A., Casale, T. B., Togias, A., Bousquet, J., Durham, S. R. and Demoly, P. 2011. Allergen-specific immunotherapy for respiratory allergies: from meta-analysis to registration and beyond. J. Allergy Clin. Immunol. 127: 30–38.

Cox, L., Nelson, H., Lockey, R, Calabria, C., Chacko, T., Finegold, I. et al. 2011. Allergen immunotherapy: a practice parameter third update. J. Allergy Clin. Immunol. 127: S1–S55.

Demoly, P., Passalacqua, G., Pfaar, O., Sastre, J. and Wahn, U. 2016. Management of the polyallergic patients with allergy immunotherapy: a practice-based approach. Allergy Asthma Clin. Immunol. 12: 2.

Durham, S. R., Walker, S. M., Varga, E. M., Jacobson, M. R., O'Brien, F. O., Noble, W. et al. 1999. Long-term clinical efficacy of grass-pollen immunotherapy. N Engl. J. Med. 341: 468–75.

Ebner, C., Kraft, D. and Ebner, H. 1994. Booster immunotherapy (BIT). Allergy 49: 38–42.

Epsein, T. G., Liss, G. M., Murphy-Berendts, K. and Bernstein, D. I. 2013. AAAAI and ACAAI surveillance study of subcutaneous immunotherapy, Year 3: what practices modify the risk of systemic reactions? Ann. Allergy Asthma Immunol. 110: 274–8.

Epstein, T. G., Liss, G. M., Berendts, K. M. and Bernstein, D. I. 2019. AAAAI/ACAAI Subcutaneous Immunotherapy Surveillance Study 2013–2017: fatalities, infections delayed reactions, and use of epinephrine autoinjectors. J. Allergy Clin. Immunol. Pract. 7: 1996–2003.

Epstein, T. G., Murphy-Berendts, K., Liss, G. M. and Bernstein, D. 2021. Risk factors for fatal and nonfatal reactions to immunotherapy (2008–2018): postinjection monitoring and severe asthma. Ann. Allergy Asthma Immunol. 127: 64–69.

Franklin, W. and Lowell, F. C. 1967. Comparison of two dosages of ragweed extract in the treatment of pollinosis. JAMA 201: 915–917.

Fulmali, A. and Kimkool, P. 2021. Is sublingual immunotherapy for asthma effective and safe? J. Allergy Clin. Immunol. 147: 1865–1872.

Grier, T. J., LeFevre, D. M., Duncan, E. A., Esch, R. E. and Coyne, T. C. 2012. Allergen stabilities and compatibilities in mixtures of high-protease fungal and insect extracts. Ann. Allergy Asthma Immunol. 108: 439–47.

Hamid, Q. A., Schotman, E., Jacobson, M. R., Walker, S. M. and Durham, S. R. 1997. Increases in IL-12 messenger RNA+ cells accompany inhibition of allergen-induced late skin responses after successful grass pollen immunotherapy. J. Allergy Clin. Immunol. 99: 254–60.

Jutel, M. and Kelso, J. M. 2004. The rate of systemic reactions to immunotherapy injections is the same whether or not the dose is reduced after a local reaction. Ann. Allergy Asthma Immunol. 92: 225–227.

Kiel, M. A., Röder, E., Gerth van Wijk, R., Al, M. J., Hop, W. C. and Rutten van Mölken, M. P. 2013. Real-life compliance and persistence among users of subcutaneous and sublingual allergen immunotherapy. J. Allergy Clin. Immunol. 132: 353–360.

Lin, M. S., Tanner, E., Lynn, J. and Friday, G. A. Jr. 1992. Nonfatal systemic allergic reactions induced by skin testing and immunotherapy. Ann. Allergy 71: 557–562.

Lowell, F. C. and Franklin, W. 1965. A double-blind study of the effectiveness and specificity of injection therapy in ragweed hay fever. N Engl. J. Med. 273: 675–679.

Marogna, M., Spadolini, I., Massolo, A., Canonica, G. W. and Passalacqua, G. 2010. Long-lasting effects of sublingual immunotherapy according to its duration: a 15-year prospective study. J. Allergy Clin. Immunol. 126: 969–75.

Meiser, J. B. and Nelson, H. S. 2001. Comparing conventional and acetone-precipitated dog allergen extract skin testing. J. Allergy Clin. Immunol. 107: 744–745.

Mustafa, S. S., Vadamalai, K., Bingemann, T. and Ramsey, A. 2020. Efficacy of epinephrine and diphenhydramine rinses in decreasing local reactions to subcutaneous aeroallergen immunotherapy. Allergy Asthma Proc. 41: 52–58.

Nelson, H. S., Iklé, D. and Buchmeier, A. 1996. Studies of allergen extract stability: the effects of dilution and mixing. J. Allergy Clin. Immunol. 98: 383–8.

Nelson, H., Blaiss, M., Nolte, H., Würtz, S. Ø., Andersen, J. S. and Durham, S. R. 2013. Efficacy and safety of the SQ-standardized grass allergy immunotherapy tablet in mono- and polysensitized subjects. Allergy 68: 252–5.

Nelson, H. S. 2016. Allergen immunotherapy (AIT) for the multiple-pollen sensitive patient. Expert Rev. Clin. Pharmacol. 9: 1443–1451.

Nelson, H. S. 2021. Chapter 15, Allergen Immunotherapy in Textbook of Allergy for the Clinician, 2nd Ed. Pudupakkam, K., Vedanthan Harold, S., Nelson, Shripad, N. Agashe, P. A. Mahest and Robit Katial (eds.). CRC Press, Taylor & Francis Group. Boca Raton, Florida and Abingdon, Oxon, England.

Nelson, H. S. 2022. Future directions in allergy immunotherapy. Allergy Asthma Proc. 43: xxx.

Ohashi, Y., Nakai, Y. and Murata, K. 2006. Effect of pretreatment with fexofenadine on the safety of immunotherapy in patients with allergic rhinitis. Ann. Allergy Asthma Immunol. 96: 600–605.

Pajno, G. B., Caminiti, L., Vita, D., Barbrerio, G., Salzano, G., Lombardo, F. et al. 2007. Sublingual immunotherapy in mite-sensitized children with atopic dermatitis: A randomized, double-blind placebo-controlled study. J. Allergy Clin. Immunol. 120: 164–170.

Roberts, G., Pfaar, O., Akdis, C. A., Ansotegui, I. J., Durham, S. R., Gerth van Wijk, R. et al. 2018. EAACI guidelines on allergen immunotherapy: allergic rhinoconjunctivitis. Allergy 73: 765–798.

Sapsaprang, S., Boonard, K., Pacharn, P., Srisuwatchari, W., Visisunthorn, N. and Jirapongsananuruk, O. 2020. Epinephrine-coated syringe for SCIT reduced local reactions: A randomized, double-blind, placebo-controlled trial. J. Allergy Clin. Immunol. Pract. 8: 1465–1467.

Scadding, G. W., Caldron, M. A., Shamji, M. H., Elfan, A. O., Penagos, M., Dumitru, F. et al. 2017. Effect of 2 years of treatment with sublingual grass pollen immunotherapy on nasal response to allergen challenge at 3 years among patients with moderate to severe seasonal allergic rhinitis: The GRASS randomized clinical trial. JAMA 317: 615–625.

Shamji, M. H., Layhadi, J. A., Sharif, H., Penagos, M. and Durham, S. R. 2021. Immunological responses and biomarkers for allergen-specific immunotherapy against inhaled allergens. JACI Pract. 9: 1769–78.

Stelmach, I., Sobocińska, A., Majak, P., Smejda, K., Jerzyńska, J. and Stelmach, W. 2012. Comparison of the long-term efficacy of 3- and 5-year house dust mite allergen immunotherapy. Ann. Allergy Asthma Immunol. 109: 274–278.

Tabar, A. I., Arroabarren, E., Echechipía, S., Garcia, B. E., Martin, S. and Alvarez-Puebla, M. J. 2011. Three years of specific immunotherapy may be sufficient in house dust mite respiratory allergy. J. Allergy Clin. Immunol. 127: 57–63.

Tankersley, M. S., Butler, K. K., Butler, W. K. and Goetz, D. W. 2000. Local reactions during allergen immunotherapy do not require dose adjustment. J. Allergy Clin. Immunol. 106: 840–3.

Weber, R. W. 2007. Cross-reactivity of pollen allergens: impact on allergen immunotherapy. Ann. Allergy Asthma Immunol. 99: 203–212.

Weber, R. W. 2008. Guidelines for using pollen cross-reactivity in formulating allergeíín immunotherapy. J. Allergy Clin. Immunol. 122: 219–221.

Winslow, A. W., Turbyville, J. C., Sublett, J. W., Sulett, J. L. and Polland, D. 2016. Comparison of systemic reactions in rush, cluster and standardized build aeroallergen immunotherapy. An. Allergy Asthma Immunol. 117: 542–545.

Wong, P. H., Quinn, J. M., Gomez, R. A. and Webb, C. N. 2017. Systemic reactions to immunotherapy during mountain cedar season: implications for seasonal dose adjustment. J. Allergy Clin. Immunol. Pract. 5: 1438–1439.

Chapter 10

Targeted and Biologic Therapeutics for Allergic and Immunologic Diseases

Bindon, Brittany,[1,#] *Zahid, Soombal,*[1,#] *Chapman, Nicholas*[2] *and Wang, Eileen*[1,*]

Introduction

Targeted and biologic therapeutics have rapidly expanded over the past few decades, revolutionizing the management and treatment of various disorders. Here, we discuss the targeted therapeutics approved for several allergic and immunologic disorders as well as promising agents under investigation. Efficacy, safety and logistical data is outlined to aid clinicians in precision medicine.

Asthma

Asthma is a chronic airway inflammatory disease affecting around 300 million people worldwide. Up to 10% of adult asthmatics have been reported to suffer from severe asthma, which is associated with increased morbidity and mortality (Manka and Wechsler 2018). Several biologic therapies have been approved for use in severe asthma, as seen in Table 1. These have dramatically changed the treatment landscape, providing patients with severe or refractory disease relief from exacerbations and symptoms as well as improved quality of life (QoL). However, important questions that remain are their cost-effectiveness, duration of use as well as predictors of response, thus warranting ongoing studies.

Anti-Immunoglobulin IgE

IgE is responsible for the initiation of Type 1 hypersensitivity reactions involved in the pathophysiology of many allergic disorders. Omalizumab is a recombinant humanized monoclonal antibody, which binds to the Cε3 domain of IgE, lowering free IgE levels and downregulating high-affinity IgE receptors (FcεRI) on basophils and mast cells (Kaplan et al. 2017).

Omalizumab

Efficacy Data

Omalizumab is approved for moderate-to-severe persistent asthma (6 years and older) with sensitization to perennial aeroallergens and symptoms inadequately controlled on inhaled

---
[1] National Jewish Health and the University of Colorado School of Medicine.
[2] St Joseph Hospital, Denver (Colorado).
[#] Co-First Authors.
[*] Corresponding author: wange@njhealth.org

Table 1. Biologics approved for treatment in asthma.

Mechanism of Action	Drug	Approved Indications in the US	Age Approved for Asthma (years)	Dosing and Frequency	Route	Phase 3 Clinical Trial Results		
						Exacerbation Reduction	Increased FEV1	Maintenance OCS Reduction
Anti-IgE	**Omalizumab**	2003 Asthma 2016 CSU 2020 CRSwNP	≥ 6	75–375 mg (based on weight, IgE level and age)	SC Office Home	✓	Minimal increase	
Anti-IL-5	**Mepolizumab**	2015 Asthma 2019 EGPA 2020 HES 2021 CRSwNP	≥ 6	100 mg 300 mg (EGPA and HES)	SC Office Home (for > 11 y.o.)	✓	✓	✓
	Reslizumab	2016 Asthma	≥ 18	3.0 mg/kg	IV Clinic/ Infusion center	✓	✓	✓ (Not done prospectively but post hoc analysis)
Anti-IL-5Rα	**Benralizumab**	2018 Asthma	≥ 12	30 mg	SC Office Home	✓	✓	✓
IL-4Rα (impacts IL-4 and IL-13)	**Dupilumab**	2017 A.D. 2018 Asthma 2019 CRSwNP 2022 EoE 2022 Prurigo Nodularis	≥ 6	200 mg or 300 mg 300 if OCS-dependent.	SC Home	✓	✓	✓
Anti-TSLP	**Tezepelumab**	2021 Asthma	≥ 12	210 mg	SC	✓	✓	*Not assessed in NAVIGATOR phase 3 RCT. However, not found to be significant in preliminary data from SOURCE phase 3 RCT

Table Adapted with permission from Wang, E. and Wechsler, M. E. 2022. A Rational Approach to Compare and Select Biologic Therapeutics in Asthma. Ann. Allergy Asthma Immunol. (Wang and Wechsler 2022).

Key: FDA: U.S. Food and Drug Administration; OCS: oral corticosteroid; CSU: chronic spontaneous urticaria; EGPA: eosinophilic granulomatosis polyangiitis; HES: hypereosinophilic syndrome; CRSwNP: chronic rhinosinusitis with nasal polyps; A.D.: Atopic dermatitis, OCS: oral corticosteroid; SC subcutaneous; FEV1: forced expiratory volume in one second; EoE: eosinophilic esophagitis.

corticosteroids (ICS). Omalizumab dosing is based on body weight and serum total IgE level as detailed in Table 1. In a pivotal phase 3 randomized control trial (RCT), adult and adolescent patients with allergic asthma treated with omalizumab had significantly fewer asthma exacerbations, greater reduction in daily inhaled corticosteroid (ICS) dose, symptoms and improved lung function, as measured by mean morning peak expiratory flow (PEF) and mean forced expiratory volume in 1 second (or FEV1) compared with placebo (Soler et al. 2001). These results were corroborated in children with allergic asthma as well (Milgrom et al. 2001). In a pooled analysis of various phase 3 RCTs, treatment with omalizumab led to lower incidences of serious asthma exacerbations requiring unscheduled outpatient visits, emergency room (ER) treatments and hospitalizations (Corren et al. 2003).

Special Populations

Asthma morbidity is known to be higher for the inner-city population, which is partly attributed to the prevalence of allergic sensitization as well as high exposure to indoor allergens. In the ICATA study, treatment with omalizumab significantly reduced the number of days with asthma symptoms in inner-city children and young adults as well as the proportion of patients who experienced exacerbations or who were hospitalized. Additionally, patients treated with omalizumab missed significantly fewer school days along with significant reductions in seasonal exacerbations compared with placebo (Busse et al. 2011). Building upon this, the PROSE study found that the odds of a fall season exacerbation were significantly lower with omalizumab treatment and patients had a lower risk of respiratory virus-associated exacerbation (Esquivel et al. 2017). Furthermore, omalizumab was found to decrease the frequency, duration and peak shedding of rhinovirus (RV) illnesses (Esquivel et al. 2017).

Real-World Studies

In a meta-analysis of 86 real-world observational studies, omalizumab significantly reduced the annual risk of asthma exacerbations as well as significantly reduced the proportion of patients receiving oral corticosteroid (OCS) (Bousquet et al. 2021). Omalizumab significantly improved lung function along with improvement in patient symptom control and QoL. Treatment also led to decreased health-care resource utilization including hospitalizations, ER visits and unscheduled physician visits.

Accessible biomarkers to assess responses are clinically pertinent. In the PROSPERO real-world study, clinical response to omalizumab was not impacted by baseline biomarkers, including blood eosinophil count (BEC) or fractional exhaled nitric oxide (FeNO) (Casale et al. 2019a). In contrast, RCT found that omalizumab's efficacy was deemed greatest in high baseline Type 2 (T2) biomarker subgroups (FeNO, BEC and serum periostin) when compared with the low-biomarker subgroups (Hanania et al. 2013). Given mixed results, further studies are warranted.

Other Disease Considerations

In addition to United States Food and Drug Administration (FDA) approval for allergic asthma, chronic spontaneous urticaria (CSU) and chronic sinusitis with nasal polyps, various case studies and small RCTs have demonstrated omalizumab's efficacy in off-label use for the treatment of non-allergic asthma (Garcia et al. 2013) and asthma with chronic obstructive pulmonary disease (COPD) overlap (Hanania et al. 2019). Additionally, omalizumab has proven beneficial in the off-label treatment of allergic bronchopulmonary aspergillosis (ABPA) (Li et al. 2017). Multiple case reports note the use of omalizumab off-label for idiopathic anaphylaxis (Kaminsky et al. 2021) and it has been used to prevent anaphylaxis as well as other associated symptoms in systemic mastocytosis (Jendoubi et al. 2020). These results, however, were not replicated in a more recent small RCT (Carter et al. 2021). Additionally, a rapidly expanding area of research is the use of off-label omalizumab as an add-on therapy for food oral immunotherapy (OIT), though additional studies are needed (Andorf et al. 2018).

Safety Data

In a systematic review, there were no significant differences in the frequency of adverse events (AE) between omalizumab and placebo, with most as mild to moderate in severity (Rodrigo et al. 2011). The most commonly reported AEs included nasopharyngitis, upper respiratory tract infection (URTI) and headache. Anaphylaxis, although a rare AE, has been reported in premarketing trials as well as post-marketing reports, with rates of 0.1–0.2% (Lieberman et al. 2017). Initial reports from RCTs prompted concern for malignancy associated with omalizumab use, the phase 4 EXCELS trial refuted this claim (Long et al. 2014). However, omalizumab was found to have a higher incidence rate of cardiovascular (CV)/cerebrovascular (CBV) serious AEs, though authors postulated this may be due to an imbalance in baseline asthma severity. This requires further investigation (Iribarren et al. 2017).

Uncontrolled asthma during pregnancy can increase the risk for adverse outcomes, including perinatal mortality, congenital anomalies, preterm birth as well as adverse maternal outcomes. Unfortunately, for many asthma medications, particularly biologics, pregnancy safety data is lacking. The omalizumab pregnancy registry, EXPECT, evaluated maternal, pregnancy and infant outcomes after exposure to omalizumab (Namazy et al. 2015). When compared to a disease-matched population of pregnant women not treated with omalizumab, there were similar rates of live births with no apparent increase in miscarriage or major congenital anomalies among women in both cohorts (Namazy et al. 2020). There was a slightly increased rate of low birth weight among infants exposed to omalizumab, although the investigators postulated this may have been driven by differences in underlying disease severity along with the increased prevalence of baseline comorbidities, like obesity.

Omalizumab Key Points

- Omalizumab is effective in adults and children with allergic asthma. It reduces seasonal asthma exacerbations along with respiratory virus exacerbations, particularly rhinovirus.

- Based on available data, there are no reliable biomarkers for predicting the response of omalizumab.

- Omalizumab has a favorable safety profile with a rare risk of anaphylaxis. There is no increased risk of malignancy, although there is a higher incidence rate of CV/CBV events in patients treated with omalizumab compared with the disease-matched cohort.

- Pregnancy safety data for omalizumab demonstrated no maternal deaths and no apparent increase in miscarriage and/or major congenital malformations, although there was a slight increased rate of low birthweight among infants exposed to omalizumab. As such, the decision to continue omalizumab during pregnancy should be individualized and based upon shared decision-making with the patient after a thorough discussion of risks and benefits.

Anti-Interleukin (IL)-5/5 Receptor (R)

IL-5 is the primary cytokine responsible for eosinophil production, activation and survival. Thus, disruption of the IL-5 receptor decreases eosinophils throughout the body (Kolbeck et al. 2010).

Reslizumab

Reslizumab is a humanized anti-IL-5 antibody (IgG4 kappa), FDA approved in 2016 for add-on maintenance therapy of severe eosinophilic asthma (SEA) in patients ages 18 years and older. Reslizumab is currently the only weight-based and IV anti-IL-5 asthma biologic therapy.

Efficacy Data

In duplicate, multicenter phase 3 RCTs, patients with uncontrolled eosinophilic asthma treated with reslizumab had significant reductions in the frequency of asthma exacerbations compared to placebo

(Castro et al. 2015). These findings were accompanied by significant improvements in lung function (FEV1), BEC and in patient-reported outcomes (PROs), including the asthma control questionnaire (ACQ) and asthma quality of life questionnaire. In various posthoc analyses, reslizumab also demonstrated efficacy in specific asthma cohorts; those with chronic rhinosinusitis with nasal polyps (CRSwNP) with or without aspirin sensitivity (Weinstein et al. 2019), late-onset asthma (Brusselle et al. 2017), OCS dependency (Nair et al. 2020) as well as multiple prior exacerbations within the past year (Wechsler et al. 2020). Notably, reslizumab was not found to be effective when administered to asthma patients unselected for eosinophil count (Corren et al. 2016).

The efficacy of reslizumab for the treatment of uncontrolled SEA has been confirmed in an open-label extension (OLE) and several real-world studies following FDA approval. In an OLE study of several phase 3 trials, reslizumab maintained improved lung function and asthma control in patients with moderate-to-SEA throughout the follow-up period of up to 3 years (Murphy et al. 2017). In a real-world study, patients sustained similar improvements along with a decreased frequency of asthma exacerbations throughout their treatment with reslizumab (Wechsler et al. 2021a).

Safety Data

In a pooled safety analysis, reslizumab demonstrated a favorable safety profile of long-term treatment, which was similar to the placebo. The most common AEs were asthma, nasopharyngitis and URTIs. There were three cases of anaphylaxis due to reslizumab infusion (Virchow et al. 2020).

Mepolizumab

Mepolizumab is an IL-5 receptor alpha monoclonal antibody (IgG1; kappa) FDA approved in 2015 for add-on maintenance therapy for patients 6 years of age or older with SEA.

Efficacy Data

In the MENSA phase 3 RCT, treatment with mepolizumab led to a significant reduction in exacerbations compared with placebo as well as significant improvements in lung function (FEV1), asthma symptoms and QoL (Ortega 2014). In the SIRIUS phase 3 RCT (Bel 2014), treatment with mepolizumab led to a significantly higher likelihood of OCS reduction as well as a reduction in asthma exacerbations despite OCS reduction. Mepolizumab's efficacy was sustained for up to 152 weeks, with improvements in exacerbations, asthma symptoms, lung function and OCS dose in the COSMEX OLE study (Khurana et al. 2019).

Real-World Studies

Various real-world studies further reinforce the efficacy of mepolizumab as an effective therapeutic agent in the treatment of SEA, which concluded that mepolizumab was associated with reduced exacerbations, including those requiring hospitalizations or ER presentations, decreased median daily OCS doses and improvement in lung function and QoL (Harrison et al. 2020).

Other Disease Considerations

In addition to various FDA-approved indications, mepolizumab is also being investigated as a treatment option for COPD, with promising results thus far although further studies are warranted to confirm its efficacy (Isoyama et al. 2021). Smaller case reports have been reported on the potential efficacy of mepolizumab, via off-label use, in the treatment of ABPA (Schleich et al. 2020) as well as Chronic Eosinophilic Pneumonia (CEP) (Bernard et al. 2020).

Safety Data

Mepolizumab demonstrated a favorable safety profile with the most frequently observed AEs reported as URTI, headache, worsening asthma and bronchitis. Serious AEs attributed to mepolizumab were rare with no episodes of anaphylaxis noted (Khatri et al. 2019). Rarely, mepolizumab therapy has been linked to opportunistic infections, including herpes zoster and helminth infections.

Benralizumab

Benralizumab is an anti-IL-5 receptor alpha monoclonal antibody (IgG1; kappa); FDA approved in 2017 for add-on maintenance therapy for patients 12 years or older with SEA.

Efficacy Data

In the CALIMA and SIROCCO phase 3 RCTs, benralizumab was associated with significantly lower annual exacerbation rates as well as improved lung function (pre-bronchodilator FEV1) (FitzGerald et al. 2016; Bleecker et al. 2016). In addition, treatment with benralizumab had significant improvement in all PROs, including rescue medication use, activity limitation and nighttime awakenings, with effects as early as day 1 (O'Quinn et al. 2019). Of importance, benralizumab's efficacy was maintained irrespective of baseline serum IgE level or atopy status (Chipps et al. 2018). Treatment with benralizumab led to a higher median reduction of OCS from baseline with higher odds of discontinuation as compared to placebo in the ZONDA trial (Nair et al. 2017). In a preliminary press release, treatment with benralizumab enabled 91% of patients to eliminate OCS or reduce their dose to ≤ 5 mg per day, with responses sustained for at least six months ("AstraZeneca, unpublished data"). The benefits of benralizumab were maintained throughout long-term use over 2 years with 50% of patients experiencing zero exacerbations during this period (FitzGerald et al. 2019).

Real-World Studies

Many real-world studies further demonstrate the efficacy and safety of benralizumab as an add-on therapy in SEA. In one study, benralizumab was associated with a significant depletion of BEC, reduction of asthma exacerbations, lung function (FEV_1), improvement in asthma symptoms and decrease in prednisone dose (from 25 to 0 mg) (Pelaia et al. 2020). These results were corroborated in a retrospective observational study with 95% of patients being able to suspend OCS use (Menzella et al. 2020).

Other Disease Considerations

Several case reports have reported the potential efficacy of off-label use of benralizumab in ABPA (Tomomatsu et al. 2020) and CEP (Isomoto et al. 2020).

Safety Data

Benralizumb has a favorable safety profile, with similar rates of AEs between treatment and placebo groups. Common AEs associated with benralizumab use include viral URTIs and worsening asthma, with rare reports of serious AEs (worsening asthma; pneumonia) (Busse et al. 2019).

Anti-IL5/5R Key Points

- There are currently three anti-IL5/5R biologics indicated for the treatment of SEA, reslizumab, mepolizumab and benralizumab. Mepolizumab is also FDA-approved for the treatment of CRSwNP, hypereosinophilic syndrome (HES) and eosinophilic granulomatosis polyangiitis (EGPA).

- The anti-IL5/5R biologics are efficacious, in terms of exacerbation reduction, FEV1 improvement, and OCS reduction with an acceptable safety profile in the treatment of SEA in children and adults.

- Long-term safety data for these medications are reassuring. While rare, there were reports of herpes zoster infections with mepolizumab and therefore if indicated, based upon risk factors and age, consider vaccination for herpes zoster prior to initiation of mepolizumab treatment.

Anti-IL-4/13

The IL-4 receptor axis interacts with IL-4 and IL-13 to promote T helper 2 (Th2) differentiation and inflammation, ultimately leading to downstream effects in various end organs and the pathogenesis of various allergic disorders (Harb and Chatila 2020).

Dupilumab

Dupilumab is a fully human monoclonal antibody to the IL-4 receptor alpha (α) subunit, which inhibits both IL-4 and IL-13 signaling. It is indicated as an add-on maintenance treatment for ages 6 years and older with moderate-to-severe eosinophilic or OCS-dependent asthma.

Efficacy Data

In phase 3, LIBERTY ASTHMA QUEST RCT (Castro et al. 2018), dupilumab led to a significant reduction in the rate of asthma exacerbations in adolescents and adults with uncontrolled asthma along with significant and rapid improvement in lung function (FEV1) with its greatest benefit among patients with baseline BEC of 300 cells/µL and FeNO 25 ppb.

In the LIBERTY ASTHMA VENTURE phase 3 RCT, dupilumab was found to be effective in children and adults with OCS-dependent severe asthma, leading to a significant decrease in OCS dose as well as increased likelihood of OCS discontinuation (Rabe et al. 2018), more pronounced in patients with baseline BEC 300 cells/µL. Dupilumab treatment also led to lower annualized rates of severe asthma exacerbations and higher FEV1 than placebo, both of which were more pronounced in patients with higher baseline BEC and FeNO levels. Similar to prior studies, dupilumab treatment led to a reduction in FeNO, as soon as by week two in this trial, which was sustained throughout treatment.

Real-World Studies

RCT findings have been corroborated with real-world evidence. In a retrospective, real-world cohort (Dupin et al. 2020), treatment of severe asthmatics with dupilumab led to significant improvement in clinical outcomes, including asthma symptoms and lung function. Notably, the daily prednisone dose significantly decreased from 20 to 5 mg and annual asthma exacerbations decreased from 4 to 1.

In another real-world, retrospective analysis (Mummler et al. 2021), switching to dupilumab in patients with prior insufficient response to anti-IL-5/5R or anti-IgE therapies was found to benefit most patients, with a significant increase in FEV1 and in Asthma Control Test (ACT) score. Half of the OCS-dependent patients were able to taper their OCS dose by more than 50%. Those with FeNO $\geq$ 25 ppb under prior therapy were more likely to be responders, although there were no other characteristics that differentiated responders. In another real-world, retrospective analysis (Bavaro et al. 2021), patients with aspirin-exacerbated respiratory disease (AERD) who previously received anti-IL-5/5R therapy were treated with dupilumab, after which sinonasal PROs (Sinonasal outcome test-22 (SNOT-22), smell/taste and congestion scores) significantly improved compared to baseline and after anti-IL-5/5R treatment. Although there were no differences in FEV1, annualized asthma exacerbation rate was significantly higher during treatment with anti-IL-5/5R compared with dupilumab treatment.

Other Disease Considerations

In addition to FDA-approved indications, case reports have demonstrated dupilumab's potential efficacy, via off-label use, in the treatment of refractory ABPA (Mikura et al. 2021).

Safety Data

Dupilumab's safety profile has been reported as acceptable and well-tolerated, with similar rates of AEs in both the dupilumab and placebo groups (Rabe et al. 2018). The most frequent AEs were

URTIs, bronchitis, sinusitis and influenza. Injection-site reactions were observed more frequently in the dupilumab group compared with the placebo. Notably, no AEs of conjunctivitis were observed.

During a phase 2b trial (Wenzel et al. 2016) transient elevation of BECs in patients treated with dupilumab was noted, particularly in those with higher baseline BECs. There was one report of the development of HES in a patient with a known high baseline BEC. This phenomenon has been repeatedly substantiated and has been attributed to dupilumab's inhibition of eosinophil migration into tissues via its interaction with IL-4 and IL-13. Fortunately, most cases are asymptomatic without clinical consequences (Rabe et al. 2018; Castro et al. 2018).

Dupilumab Key Points

- Dupilumab is currently indicated as an add-on maintenance treatment for adult and pediatric patients with moderate-to-severe eosinophilic or OCS-dependent asthma. It is currently only asthma biologic approved for an indication of OCS-dependent asthma.

- Dupilumab has proven efficacious in the treatment of asthma, which is based upon clinical trials and real-world studies, including in patients previously unresponsive to anti-IgE or anti-IL-5/5R biologics.

- With regards to biomarkers, the benefit of dupilumab is found to be greater among patients with baseline BEC of $\geq$ 300 cells/μL and FeNO $\geq$ 25 ppb as demonstrated in clinical trials.

- Dupilumab has an overall acceptable safety profile in the treatment of asthma. The increase in BEC has shown to often be transient and asymptomatic.

Tralokinumab and Lebrikizumab

Given dupilumab's efficacy in the treatment of asthma as well as IL-13's prominent role within the T2 pathway, anti-IL-13 monoclonal antibodies were of clinical interest in the treatment of uncontrolled asthma. However, RCTs did not demonstrate significant clinical benefits of these therapeutics, including tralokinumab (Panettieri et al. 2018) or lebrikizumab (Hanania et al. 2016).

Anti-Epithelial Cytokines

Tezepelumab

Thymic stromal lymphopoietin (TSLP) is a pleiotropic, epithelial cell-derived cytokine that is involved in the initiation of several inflammatory cascades. TSLP has been implicated in a variety of disorders, including allergic, autoimmune and chronic inflammatory disorders as well as several malignancies (Varricchi et al. 2018). Levels of human TSLP are increased in the airways of patients with asthma and correlate with disease severity (Li et al. 2018). Tezepelumab is an anti-TSLP human IgG2 monoclonal antibody, FDA-approved in December 2021 for add-on maintenance treatment of patients with severe asthma aged 12 years and older.

Efficacy Data

In the PATHWAY phase 2b trial, patients with severe, uncontrolled asthma treated with Tezepelumab had 71% lower rates of asthma exacerbations when compared with placebo, independent of baseline BEC. Additionally, Tezepelumab-reduced BEC, FeNO and total serum IgE levels across all groups (Corren et al. 2017). Treatment with Tezepelumab led to clinically meaningful improvements in asthma control, QoL and daily asthma symptoms (Corren et al. 2021b). Tezepelumb consistently reduced exacerbation rates irrespective of perennial allergy status (Corren et al. 2021a). Additionally, Tezepelumab reduced the rate of asthma exacerbations that required hospitalizations or ED visits. Of those who did require hospital admission, they spent fewer mean days in the hospital and/or ICU compared with those who received a placebo (Corren et al. 2020b). In the CASCADE exploratory phase 2 trial, (Emson et al. 2020) treatment with Tezepelumab resulted in a significantly greater reduction of airway submucosal eosinophils compared with placebo in patients with severe, uncontrolled asthma, irrespective of baseline BEC, with a corresponding reduction in T2 biomarkers such as BEC, serum T2 cytokines and FeNO.

In the NAVIGATOR phase 3 trial, adolescent and adult patients with severe, uncontrolled asthma treated with Tezepelumab experienced fewer exacerbations and had significantly improved lung function, asthma control, and health-related QoL than those who received a placebo (Menzies-Gow et al. 2021). Preliminary data from the ongoing SOURCE phase 3 trial, Tezepelumab did not significantly reduce OCS dose compared with placebo in adults with OCS-dependent asthma; however, full data has not yet been made publicly available ("AstraZeneca, unpublished data").

Other Disease Considerations

Given its promising role in multiple inflammatory disorders, Tezepelumab is currently under investigation for other disease considerations including severe CRSwNP, CSU, COPD as well as eosinophilic esophagitis (EoE) (Kemp 2021). However, Tezepelumab was not found to be efficacious in patients with severe atopic dermatitis (AD) (Simpson et al. 2019).

Safety Data

In phase 2 and phase 3 trials, the frequencies and types of AEs were similar between Tezepelumab and placebo groups (Corren et al. 2017; Menzies-Gow et al. 2021). The most commonly reported AEs were nasopharyngitis, URTI, headache, bronchitis and asthma.

Tezepelumab Key Points

- Tezepelumab is the most recently approved biologic for severe asthma and the only biologic approved for asthma without phenotype or biomarker limitations.
- Tezepelumab has an overall favorable safety profile.

Anti-IL-33 and Anti-ST2

IL-33 is an epithelial-derived alarmin released in response to tissue injury. When IL-33 binds to its receptor (ST2; IL-1 receptor-like 1), it initiates a downstream signaling cascade leading to T2 and non-T2 inflammation, which can contribute to airway disease. As such, it provides a potential therapeutic option in the management of airway disease and recent phase 3 studies have shown promising results.

Itepekimab is a new human IgG4P monoclonal antibody against IL-33. In a recent phase 2 trial, adults with moderate-to-severe asthma were randomized to receive SC itepekimab 300 mg, itepekimab plus dupilumab (referred to as combination therapy), dupilumab or placebo (Wechsler et al. 2021b). At the end of the trial, significantly fewer patients in the itepekimab and combination groups experienced an event indicating loss of asthma control. Lung function (FEV1) increased with itepekimab and dupilumab monotherapies but not with combination therapy. Although dupilumab efficacy was generally greater than that observed with itepekimab, the trial was not powered to compare these differences. The frequency of AEs was similar across treatment groups.

Astegolimab is a human IgG2 monoclonal antibody that blocks IL-33 signaling by selectively inhibiting ST2, the IL-33 receptor. In the ZENYATTA Phase 2b trial (Kelsen et al. 2021), asthma exacerbation rates were significantly improved relative to placebo in the astegolimab 70 mg and 490 mg groups, although not significant at the 210 mg dose. When adjusted for BEC < 300 cells/μL, results were comparable to the overall population. AEs were similar in astegolimab and placebo groups.

Asthma Key Points

- Although there are several biologics approved for the treatment of asthma, head-to-head comparator trials are lacking. See Table 1 for a comparison between available trial data.
- The decision to prescribe a biologic should be individualized with consideration of clinical characteristics and comorbidities, biomarkers, potential adverse effects as well as patient preferences.

Atopic Dermatitis

Atopic dermatitis (AD) is an inflammatory skin disease affecting both children and adults and is characterized by recurrent pruritus and eczematous lesions (Ratchataswan et al. 2021). Its treatment can often be challenging, although the recent development of various biologics as well as Janus Kinase (JAK) inhibitors has provided significant benefit in this population as seen in Tables 2 and 3.

Anti-IL 4/13 Therapeutics

Dupilumab

Dupilumab is indicated for the treatment of adult and pediatric patients ages 6 years and older with moderate-to-severe AD that is inadequately controlled with topical prescription therapies or when those therapies are not advisable.

Efficacy Data

In dual-phase 3 RCTs, SOLO 1 and SOLO 2, significantly more patients with moderate-to-severe AD treated with dupilumab monotherapy achieved an Investigator's Global Assessment score of 0/1 (IGA 0/1) and EASI75 (Eczema Area and Severity Index with $\geq$ 75% improvement) compared with placebo (Simpson et al. 2016). Dupilumab also significantly improved pruritus and QoL. These results were corroborated in the adolescent population in the LIBERTY AD ADOL phase 3 RCT (Simpson et al. 2020a). Additionally, dupilumab therapy with concomitant topical corticosteroids (TCS) was proven to be efficacious in the adult and pediatric populations in the phase 3 LIBERTY AD CHRONOS (Blauvelt et al. 2017) and LIBERTY AD PEDS RCTs (Paller et al. 2020), respectively, as well as in adults with inadequate response to, intolerance of, or for whom cyclosporine A (CsA) treatment was medically inadvisable in the LIBERTY AD CAFÉ RCT (de Bruin-Weller et al. 2018). Dupilumab's efficacy was sustained up to 76 weeks in adults (Deleuran et al. 2020) and 52 weeks in adolescents and children in various OLE studies (Cork et al. 2020; Cork et al. 2021).

Dupilumab leads to significant and rapid improvements in daily peak pruritus Numerical Rating scale (NRS) by day 2 in adults and day 5 in adolescents (Silverberg et al. 2020a). Dupilumab treatment showed rapid and sustained improvements in the magnitude of itch, starting with the first dose; responses progressively increased and were sustained through to the end of treatment up to 1 year. In addition to improving signs and symptoms of AD, dupilumab led to clinically significant improvement in comorbid asthma and/or sinonasal disease, if present (Boguniewicz et al. 2021).

Real-World Studies

Real-world studies, including a meta-analysis (Halling et al. 2021), supported dupilumab's efficacy in the treatment of AD, producing similar results to preceding clinical trials. In one particular real-world study (Ariens et al. 2020), dupilumab was efficacious in the treatment of difficult-to-treat AD, with over half of patients previously failing treatment on $\geq$ 2 immunosuppressive drugs, as evidenced by improvement in EASI score and PROs, such as pain, itch, anxiety/depression and QoL.

Table 2. Biologics for treatment in AD.

Biologic	Target	FDA Approval for AD	Age Approved for AD	Dosing and Frequency for AD		Route	Phase 3 Clinical Trial results		
							AD Severity (EASI; IGA)	Pruritus	S. Aureus Colonization
Dupilumab	IL-4Rα (impacts IL-4 and IL-13)	✓	≥ 6 years	Adults: 300 mg (after 600 mg LD)	Q2W	SC	✓	✓	✓ *Phase 2 results
				Pediatrics (Weight based) 15 to < 30 kg: 300 mg (600 mg LD)	Q4W				
				30 to < 60 kg: 200 mg (400 mg LD)	Q2W				
				≥ 60 kg: 300 (600 mg LD)	Q2W				
Tralokinumab	IL-13	✓	≥ 18 years	300 mg (after 600 mg LD)	Q2W *Can increase to Q4W if disease well controlled after 16 weeks	SC	✓	✓	✓
Lebrikizumab	IL-13			Not determined	Not determined	SC	✓ *Dose-Dependent	✓	(Not evaluated)
							*Only phase 2 Data available for lebrikizumab		
Nemolizumab	IL-31			60 mg	Q4W	SC	✓	✓	(Not evaluated)

Table 3. Janus Kinase (JAK) inhibitors being investigated in AD.

JAK inhibitor	JAK Selectivity	FDA Indications	Age Approved for AD	Dosing and Frequency for AD		Route of Administration	Phase 2 and 3 RCT results		Adverse Effects	Change in Lab Parameters in RCTs	Black Box Warning
							AD Severity (EASI/IGA)	Pruritus	Common AEs Reported in RCTs		
Ruxolitinib	JAK 1 JAK 2	**Mild-moderate AD** (2021) Oral: Myelofibrosis PV GVHD	≥ 12 years	1.5% cream	Twice daily (up to 20% BSA)	Topical	✓	✓ *As early as the first 12 hours	Nasopharyngitis URTI Headache Application site reactions AD	Transient platelet increase (~week 2)	✓ Serious infections, mortality, malignancy, MACE and thrombosis
Delgocitinib	JAK1 JAK2, JAK3 TYK 2	-- *Approved in Japan for AD	--	--	--	Topical	✓	✓ *As early as the first night	Nasopharyngitis Contact dermatitis Acne Application site folliculitis	--	--
Tofacitinib	JAK 1 JAK3	RA UC pcJIA PsA	--	2% ointment	Twice daily	Topical	✓ *Only phase 2 RCT	✓ *As early as day 2 of treatment	Nasopharyngitis Contact dermatitis Headache		✓ Serious infections, mortality, malignancy, MACE and thrombosis
Abrocitinib	JAK 1	**Moderate-severe AD** (2022)	≥ 18 years	100–200 mg	Once daily	Oral	✓	✓ *As early as day 2 of treatment	Nausea Headache Acne	CPK elevation increased LDL, HDL decreased platelets	✓ Serious infections, mortality, malignancy, MACE and thrombosis

Updacitinib	JAK 1	**Moderate-severe AD** (2022) RA PsA	≥ 12 years* and Less than 65 years * Must weigh at least 40 kg	15–30 mg	Once daily	Oral	✓	✓ *As early as day 2-3 of treatment	Acne URTI Nasopharyngitis AD Headache	CPK elevation increased LDL, HDL, Transaminitis Cytopenia (anemia; neutropenia)	✓ Serious infections, mortality, malignancy, MACE and thrombosis
Baricitinib	JAK 1 JAK 2	RA *Approved in the EU and Japan for AD	---	1, 2 or 4 mg *Doses used in phase 3 RCTs	Once daily	Oral	✓	✓	Nasopharyngitis, Headache Diarrhea	CPK elevation Increased LDL, HDL Creatinine elevation Hematologic changes (anemia, lymphopenia, neutropenia and thrombocytosis)	✓ Serious infections, malignancy and thrombosis

Key: PV: Polycythemia Vera; GVHD: Graft versus Host Disease; BSA: body surface area; RA: Rheumatoid Arthritis; UC: Ulcerative Colitis; pcJIA: polyarticular course juvenile idiopathic arthritis; PsA: psoriatic arthritis; CPK: creatine phosphokinase; LDL: Low-density lipoprotein; HDL: high-density lipoprotein

Safety Data

In terms of safety, dupilumab therapy for AD was found to have an acceptable safety profile in various phase 2, phase 3 and real-world studies. In the SOLO 1 and SOLO 2 phase 3 trials (Simpson et al. 2016), the overall incidence of AEs was similar in the dupilumab and placebo groups. Most AEs were mild. The most common AEs were exacerbations of AD, injection-site reactions and nasopharyngitis. Rates of conjunctivitis were higher in the dupilumab groups than in placebo groups (3–5% vs. 1%).

In a systematic review and meta-analysis of eight RCTs (Fleming and Drucker 2018), dupilumab was associated with decreased risk for skin infections, and eczema herpeticum infections with no increased risk of overall herpesvirus infections or overall infections compared to placebo.

Regarding conjunctivitis, a pooled analysis (Akinlade et al. 2019) analyzed 11 RCTs of dupilumab in AD, asthma, CRSwNP and EoE. The incidence of conjunctivitis was higher in dupilumab compared with placebo-treated patients in AD clinical trials (8.6 vs. 2.1%). Conjunctivitis was mostly mild to moderate, with most cases resolved during the treatment period. More severe AD at baseline, prior history of conjunctivitis and higher levels of serum T2 biomarkers (TARC, IgE, BEC) were associated with increased conjunctivitis risk. Dupilumab treatment was not associated with an increased incidence of conjunctivitis in asthma, CRSwNP and EoE trials. The pathogenesis of conjunctivitis during dupilumab treatment for AD is unknown, although patients may be at higher risk given the high prevalence of ocular disease in patients with AD. At this time, there is no consensus on treatment for conjunctivitis in dupilumab-treated patients, although ophthalmic preparations of corticosteroids, antibiotics, antihistamines and mast cell stabilizers were the most common treatments used in these trials.

Although dupilumab-associated facial erythema was not reported in phase 3 RCTs for AD, there have been reports in real-world studies (Waldman et al. 2020). The presence or absence of atopy or dupilumab-induced ocular disorder did not significantly impact the development of dupilumab facial redness (DFR). The majority of patients who developed this continued with their dupilumab therapy regardless, however, indicating that DFR was less symptomatically burdensome than their underlying skin condition.

Tralokinumab

Tralokinumab is an anti-IL-13, FDA-approved in late 2021 for the treatment of moderate-to-severe AD in adult patients whose disease is not adequately controlled with topical prescription therapies or when those therapies are not advisable.

Efficacy Data

In two dual phase 3 RCTs, ECZTRA 1 and ECZTRA 2 (Wollenberg et al. 2021a), significantly more adults with moderate-to-severe AD treated with tralokinumab monotherapy achieved an IGA 0/1 and EASI75 at week 16 compared with placebo. Treatment with tralokinumab also led to significant improvement compared with placebo in all key secondary endpoints, including pruritus, scoring atopic dermatitis (SCORAD) and Dermatology life quality index (DLQI) scores. Improvements in pruritus and sleep scores were rapid and sustained, with significant improvements compared with placebo as early as week 1. Additionally, treatment with tralokinumab led to a 10 times greater reduction in *S. aureus* colonization of lesional skin at week 16 compared with placebo. Tralokimumab response was maintained in both q2w and q4w groups through 52 weeks, though the response may be sustained as early as week 16. The subsequent ECZTRA 3 (Silverberg et al. 2021a) and ECZTRA 7 (Gutermuth et al. 2021) RCTs demonstrated that tralokinumab with concomitant TCS significantly improves AD signs and symptoms in adults with moderate-to-severe AD, including those with severe CSA-refractory AD.

Safety Data

In a pooled safety analysis (Simpson 2021), tralokinumab was found to be well tolerated with an acceptable safety profile for the treatment of moderate-to-severe AD. The frequency of AEs was similar for tralokinumab compared with placebo, with most AEs reported as mild to moderate in severity. The most common AEs included AD, URTIs and conjunctivitis. Similar to dupilumab, the incidence of conjunctivitis has been found to be significantly higher with tralokinumab compared with placebo, with most events characterized as mild to moderate and transient (Wollenberg et al. 2021b).

Lebrikizumab

Lebrikizumab, an anti-IL-13 monoclonal antibody, is currently under investigation for AD.

Efficacy Data

In phase 2 TREBLE RCT (Simpson et al. 2018), significantly more patients achieved EASI50 with lebrikizumab than with a placebo as well as an IGA 0/1 and SCORAD-50. In another phase 2 RCT (Guttman-Yassky et al. 2020), significantly more patients treated with lebrikizumab demonstrated dose-dependent improvements in EASI and pruritus NRS scores compared with placebo, with improvement seen as early as day 2. Notably, 5 of 12 lebrikizumab patients with prior dupilumab use (compared with 0/4 placebo patients) achieved EASI75 and 4 of 12 lebrikizumab patients achieved IGA 0/1.

Safety Data

Lebrikizumab was found to be well tolerated with an acceptable safety profile in the above trials. The frequencies of AEs were overall similar between lebrikizumab and placebo groups and mostly mild to moderate in severity (Simpson et al. 2018). Common AEs included URTI, nasopharyngitis and headaches (Guttman-Yassky et al. 2020). Of note, unlike in AD RCTs with dupilumab or tralokinumab, the frequencies of conjunctivitis in lebrikizimab groups were low.

Anti-IL 31

Nemolizumab

IL-31 is a proinflammatory cytokine implicated in the pathogenesis of AD, playing a key role in pruritus as well as dysregulation of the skin barrier (Kabashima et al. 2018). Nemolizumab is a humanized monoclonal antibody against the IL-31 receptor A subunit, which is currently under investigation for various dermatologic disorders, including AD, pruritus and prurigo nodularis.

Efficacy Data

In the phase 2 XCIMA trial (Ruzicka et al. 2017), nemolizumab treatment led to a significant, dose-dependent improvement in the pruritus visual-analog scale (VAS), as compared with placebo. Nemolizumab's clinical efficacy was sustained and/or progressively improved up to 64 weeks (Kabashima et al. 2018). In a subsequent phase 3 trial (Kabashima et al. 2020) of patients with moderate-to-severe AD, treatment with nemolizumab concomitantly with topical agents led to significantly greater improvement in pruritus compared with placebo as demonstrated by the LS mean percent change in VAS. Additionally, nemolizumab led to improvement in AD severity, QoL and sleep, although no inferences can be drawn from these measures as there was no adjustment for multiple comparisons in this study.

Safety Data

Nemolizumab was overall well tolerated with an acceptable safety profile in the treatment of AD as concluded by various phase 2 and 3 trials. Patients treated with nemolizumab or placebo had similar frequencies of AEs, with most reported as mild to moderate in severity (Kabashima et al. 2020). The most commonly reported AEs included AD and nasopharyngitis. Skin infections were overall similar between both groups. Although there was no AE related to asthma reported in the phase 3 trial, a dose-dependent increase in asthma events in patients with pre-existing asthma treated with nemolizumab compared with placebo (11.2% vs. 1.8%) has been noted (Silverberg et al. 2020b). These events were typically mild and reversible, with no de novo cases of asthma reported. Investigators postulated this may have been caused by improved QoL with an associated increase in activity levels and/or respiratory infections. In the above phase 2 and 3 trials, peripheral edema was reported in more patients compared with a placebo. With regards to laboratory parameters, treatment with nemolizumab compared with placebo led to increased CK levels, although unclear if this was clinically relevant.

Biologic Therapeutics and Atopic Dermatitis Key Points

- There are currently two biologics approved for moderate-to-severe AD, dupilumab and tralokinumab with several other agents under investigation in clinical trials.
- As with asthma, there are no head-to-head comparator trials and such an approach to treatment in AD must be individualized for each patient with consideration of comorbidities, available safety data and patient preferences. See Table 2 for a comparison between available trial data.
- Notably, dupilumab was found to have unique safety signals in the management of AD, such as conjunctivitis and facial erythema, though these were typically not treatment-limiting.

JAK Inhibitors

Janus Kinase (JAK) inhibitors represent a promising new therapy for the treatment of AD among other dermatologic conditions. In brief review, the JAK family consists of four receptor-associated kinases, JAK1, JAK2, JAK3, and tyrosine kinase 2 (TYK2), which are key components of the JAK-signal transducers and activators of transcription (JAK-STAT) pathway. This pathway is integral in signal transduction for many cytokines, including those implicated in the pathogenesis of AD, such as IL-4, IL-5, IL-13, IL-31, IL-22 and TSLP. As a result of this, JAK inhibition has been pursued as a novel treatment for AD (Chovatiya and Paller 2021). JAK inhibitors are synthetic small molecular compounds and therefore not biologics. At the time of this publication, three JAK inhibitors are currently FDA-approved for the treatment of AD. However, given the marked interest and development in oral and topical JAK inhibitors, the landscape of AD therapeutics will likely continue to expand. As such, we will review the current literature regarding JAK inhibitors for AD, see Table 3.

Topical JAK Inhibitors

Ruxolitinib

Ruxolitinib is a selective JAK 1 and JAK 2 inhibitor. Its topical formulation is indicated for the treatment of mild-to-moderate AD in adolescents (ages 12 years and older) and adults whose disease is not well controlled with topical prescription therapies or when those are not recommended.

Efficacy Data

In the dual phase 3 TRuE-AD1 and TRuE-AD2 studies (Papp et al. 2021), significantly more patients with mild-to-moderate AD treated with ruxolitinib achieved an IGA 0/1 and EASI75 compared with vehicle. Additionally, a significant reduction in itch was noted as early as 12 hours after initial application in the 1.5% ruxolitinib group.

Safety Data

In a pharmacokinetics analysis of the above RCTs, plasma concentrations of ruxolitinib were minimal following topical application of ruxolitinib cream and as such serious systemic AEs commonly associated with oral JAK inhibitors were infrequently observed (Gong et al. 2021). Ruxolitinib cream at all doses was overall well tolerated with an acceptable safety profile. The most common treatment emergent AEs (TEAEs) were similar between vehicle and treatment groups and included nasopharyngitis, URTIs, headache, application site reactions and AD. Application site reactions, such as stinging/burning, were infrequent (< 1%) and reported more in the vehicle group compared with treatment groups. Treatment with ruxolitinib did not lead to any clinically meaningful changes in hematologic parameters. Despite the above reassuring data, it is important to note that ruxolitinib cream currently possesses a black box warning for serious infections, mortality, malignancy, major adverse cardiovascular event (MACE) and thrombosis, based upon prior studies of oral JAK inhibitors to treat inflammatory conditions.

Delgocitinib

Delgocitinib is a novel topical pan-JAK inhibitor, which acts to inhibit all JAKs (JAK1, JAK2, JAK3 and tyrosine kinase 2). It is approved in Japan for the treatment of AD, though it remains under investigation for the treatment of AD in the US. It was granted Fast Track Designation by the FDA in 2020, to help expedite its development and review, for adults with moderate-to-severe chronic hand eczema.

Efficacy Data

In a phase 2 trial (Nakagawa et al. 2018), delgocitinib led to significant improvement in EASI score compared with the vehicle along with a percentage of body surface area (BSA) affected, nocturnal and daytime pruritus. Notably, a significant reduction in pruritus was noted as early as the first night of study treatment with JTE-052 at 0.5% and higher doses. IGA scores were improved at end of treatment with JTE ointment at doses of 0.5% and higher doses.

In a phase 3 trial, QBA4-1 (Nakagawa et al. 2020a), significantly more patients with moderate-to-severe AD treated with delgocitinib 0.5% ointment had clinically meaningful improvements in signs and symptoms of AD, as determined by mEASI, IGA and pruritus NRS scores with sustained improvements up to 28 weeks. These results were replicated in the pediatric population in a similar phase 3 trial (Nakagawa et al. 2021) and for up to 52 weeks in an open-label study, QBA4-2 (Nakagawa et al. 2020b).

Safety Data

Delgocitinib had a favorable safety profile in AD RCTs. In a pooled safety analysis (Nakagawa et al. 2020a), most AEs were mild with the most common AEs reported as nasopharyngitis, contact dermatitis, acne and application site folliculitis. Application site irritation symptoms were infrequent (< 2%) and mild, with no reports of skin atrophy or telangiectasia at the sites of application. Serious AEs were rarely attributed to the low systemic exposure to delgocitinib.

Tofacitinib

Tofacitinib is a potent JAK 1 and JAK 3 inhibitor.

Efficacy Data

In a phase 2a study (Bissonnette et al. 2016), treatment with 2% tofacitinib ointment BID showed significantly greater efficacy in patients with mild-to-moderate AD as measured by EASI, BSA, physician's global assessment (PGA) scores and pruritus as measured by Itch Severity Item (ISI). There was significant improvement in EASI and BSA by week 1 and improvement in pruritus by day 2.

Safety Data

With regards to its safety, tofacitinib ointment had comparable safety and tolerability effects when compared with a placebo (Bissonnette et al. 2016). The most frequently reported treatment-related AEs were mild and included nasopharyngitis, increased blood creatine phosphokinase (CPK), contact dermatitis and headache. Although oral tofacitinib carries an FDA black box warning for serious AEs, including serious infections, thrombosis and malignancies; none of these were reported in this limited trial.

Oral JAK Inhibitors

Abrocitinib

Abrocitinib is an oral, selective JAK 1 inhibitor approved by the FDA in January 2022 for the treatment of moderate-to-severe AD in adult patients whose disease is not controlled with other systemic drug products, including biologics or when the use of those therapies is inadvisable.

Efficacy Data

In the JADE MONO-1 phase 3 trial, adults and adolescents with moderate-to-severe AD treated with abrocitinib monotherapy had significant improvement in IGA and EASI75, with clinically meaningful responses noted as early as week 2 of treatment (Simpson et al. 2020b). These results were substantiated in a replicate phase 3 trials in adults, JADE MONO-2 (Silverberg et al. 2020c), and adolescents, JADE TEEN (Eichenfield et al. 2021). A pooled analysis of the above trials demonstrated abrocitinib's impact on itch, sleep disturbance, health-related QoL and work productivity (Silverberg et al. 2021b). In the JADE REGIMEN phase 3 trial, investigators found that reinitiation of abrocitinib effectively recaptured response after disease flare (Blauvelt et al. 2022).

In the JADE COMPARE phase 3 trial, adults with AD were randomized to receive, in addition to standard topical therapy, 100 mg or 200 mg abrocitinib once daily, 300 mg dupilumab SC Q2W or placebo (Bieber et al. 2021a). Compared with placebo, patients treated with either dose of abrocitinib had significant improvement in IGA and EASI75 responses at weeks 12 and 16. The 200 mg dose of abrocitinib had a superior itch response at week 2 compared with dupilumab. However, there were no significant differences in IGA and EASI75 responses between the groups at week 16.

Safety Data

In an integrated safety analysis, abrocitinib was deemed to have an acceptable safety and tolerability profile (Simpson et al. 2021). Most AEs reported were mild and self-limited. The most common dose-related, drug-related AEs were nausea, headache and acne. There was no dose-response relationship for serious infections, which was similar across placebo and treatment groups. The most frequent serious infections (0.2% or less for each type) in abrocitinib-treated patients included pneumonia, herpes simplex, and herpes zoster. There were three serious AEs determined as MACE as well as five events of venous thromboembolism (VTE) that occurred in the 200 mg group. There were three deaths due to gastric carcinoma (diagnosed on day 43), sudden death and COVID-19. With regards to lab evaluation, there was an asymptomatic, dose-dependent decrease in platelets, with nadir around week 4 with subsequent increase and plateau around week 12. Additionally, there was a dose-related, asymptomatic increase in CPK, which began at week 4 and plateaued at week 8, as well as a dose-dependent effect on low- or high-density lipoprotein (LDL; HDL) from baseline to week 16.

Updacitinib

Upadacitinib is an oral, reversible small-molecule JAK 1 inhibitor approved in January 2022 for the treatment of moderate-to-severe AD for ages 12 and older whose disease is not controlled with other systemic drug products, including biologics or when the use of those therapies is inadvisable.

Efficacy Data

In the dual Measure Up 1 and Measure Up 2 phase 3 RCTs (Guttman-Yassky et al. 2021), significantly more patients with moderate-to-severe AD treated with upadacitinib achieved an EASI75 and an IGA 0/1, with improvements noted as early as week 2. Additionally, significantly more patients had improvements in itch by day 2 and 3 with upadacitinib 30 and 15 mg, respectively, compared with placebo. These results were corroborated in the phase 3 AD Up trial, where adults and adolescents with moderate-to-severe AD were treated with upadacitinib in combination with TCS for 16 weeks (Reich et al. 2021). Upadacitinb's efficacy was sustained for up to 52 weeks with a clear dose response observed from week 2 onwards (Silverberg et al. 2021c).

In a head-to-head comparator phase 3 trial, Heads Up, investigators analyzed the efficacy of upadacitinib compared with dupilumab in adult patients with moderate-to-severe AD (Blauvelt et al. 2021). Significantly more patients receiving upadacitinib compared with dupilumab achieved an EASI75. Additionally, upadacitinib demonstrated superiority over dupilumab in all secondary endpoints analyzed, including significant improvement in the worst pruritus NRS as early as week 1, achievement of EASI75 as early as week 2 and achievement of EASI100.

Safety Data

Upadacitinib carries an FDA black box warning for treatment in RA including serious infections, malignancy and thrombosis. In the above RCTs, upadacitinib was overall well tolerated with an acceptable safety profile. Most AEs were reported as mild, with the most frequently reported AEs in the trials including acne, URTIs, nasopharyngitis, AD and headache. Acne was reported more frequently in the upadacitinib groups compared with placebo, as high as 17% in one trial (Guttman-Yassky et al. 2021). With regards to laboratory parameters, patients treated with upadacitinib infrequently developed abnormal liver function, cytopenias and/or elevated CPK. With regards to liver function, most were transaminitis elevations, which were mild to moderate and transient. Similarly, most cytopenias were transient in nature and mild to moderate in severity.

Baricitinib

Baricitinib is an oral, reversible, synthetic and selective JAK 1 and JAK 2 inhibitor. Although baricitinib has been approved for the treatment of moderate-to-severe AD in adult patients in the European Union (EU) and Japan, it remains under FDA review for this indication.

Efficacy Data

In dual-phase 3 monotherapy trails, BREEZE-AD1 and BREEZE-AD2 (Simpson et al. 2020c), significantly more patients with moderate-to-severe AD achieved the primary end point of a vIGA-AD 0/1 following treatment with baricitinib 4 mg or 2 mg groups compared with placebo. Additionally, improvements in sleep disturbance, skin pain and QoL measures were observed by week 1 in these groups. Baricitinib's efficacy was sustained over 68 weeks (Silverberg et al. 2021d). In the BREEZE-AD7 phase 3 trial, baricitinib 4 mg combination therapy with TCS significantly improved the signs and symptoms of moderate-to-severe AD (Reich et al. 2020). Additionally, baricitinib plus TCS led to significant improvement in PROs, including health-related QoL and work productivity (Wollenberg et al. 2021c). Notably, in posthoc analyses of the above trials, treatment with baricitinib produced significant and rapid improvements in symptoms of skin pain (Thyssen et al. 2021), itch and sleep disturbance, typically starting one day after taking the first dose of baricitinib (Buhl et al. 2021).

Safety Data

In a pooled safety analysis (Bieber et al. 2021b), baracitinib's safety profile was deemed acceptable, with the most common TEAEs reported as nasopharyngitis, headache, CPK elevations and diarrhea. The frequency of serious infections, opportunistic infections and conjunctival disorders was low and similar between treatment groups. The most common serious infections were eczema herpeticum, cellulitis and pneumonia. In this analysis, herpes zoster infections were infrequent, did not show dose-dependent increases and were lower than previously reported for RA patients treated with baricitinib. Alternatively, herpes simplex infections were reported more frequently in the AD trials compared to RA and were reported more frequently for baricitinib 4-mg as compared with 2-mg and placebo. The incidence rate of herpes simplex infections decreased with extended treatment, suggesting continued treatment with baricitinib does not lead to an increased incidence of herpes simplex infections.

Based on RA trials, baricitinib carries an FDA black box warning for serious infections, malignancy and thrombosis. However, in the AD trials, no malignancies, gastrointestinal perforations, CV events or tuberculosis were reported in the placebo-controlled period in baricitinib-treated patients, although in the extended data set, there were two positively adjudicated MACEs (2-mg group), two VTEs (4-mg group) and one death. With regards to laboratory changes, an increase in CPK was the most common laboratory change, which was mostly asymptomatic. Additionally, baricitinib was associated with increases in both LDL and HDL as well as small reversible increases in serum creatinine.

JAK Inhibitors Key Points

- There are currently three JAK inhibitors approved for the treatment of AD, including topical ruxolinitib, oral abrocitinib and upadacitinib, with several other JAK inhibitors under investigation.
- There are no head-to-head comparator trials between JAK inhibitors in the treatment of AD and as such, the approach to treatment must be individualized for each patient with consideration of comorbidities, available safety data and patient preferences. See Table 3 for a comparison of available trial data.
- Although approved JAK inhibitors have overall acceptable safety profiles, it is important to note they carry a black box warning, typically based upon prior outcomes in rheumatologic diseases. In the above trials, most AEs were mild and self-limited, although more serious AEs were reported in a few patients, including serious infections, MACE, VTE and death. Additionally, given derangements in laboratory parameters reported in trials, it is important to monitor while on treatment in these agents.

Chronic Rhinosinusitis With Nasal Polyps

Chronic rhinosinusitis with nasal polyps (CRSwNP) is characterized by chronic inflammation of nasal mucosa and paranasal sinuses. It is often associated with impaired QoL along with a substantial economic burden (Wu et al. 2021). Several biologics are currently indicated for the management of CRSwNP or nasal polyps (see Table 4).

Anti-IgE Therapy

Omalizumab

Omalizumab is indicated as an add-on maintenance treatment for nasal polyps in adult patients with inadequate response to intranasal corticosteroids (INCS). The recommended dosing is based on body weight and serum total IgE.

Efficacy Data

In dual-phase 3 studies, POLYP 1 and POLYP 2, omalizumab therapy in patients with severe CRSwNP with prior inadequate response to INCS led to significant improvement in endoscopic, clinical and PROs (Gevaert et al. 2020). Furthermore, patients with comorbid asthma and NSAID-exacerbated respiratory disease (NERD) had similar improvements compared to patients without NERD. In a subgroup analysis (Damask et al. 2021), omalizumab was consistently favored over placebo independent of underlying patient factors, including patients with BEC > 300 and ≤ 300 cells/μL with or without previous sinonasal surgery, asthma and aspirin sensitivity.

Table 4. Biologics for treatment in CRSwNP.

Biologic	Target	FDA Approval for CRSwNP	Age Approved for CRSwNP	Dosing and Frequency for CRSwNP	Route	Phase 3 Clinical Trial results			
						Nasal Polyp Burden	Nasal Congestion	Sense of Smell	Reduced Need for Surgery
Dupilumab	IL-4Rα (impacts IL-4 and IL-13)	✓	≥ 18 years	300 mg	SC	✓	✓	✓	✓
Omalizumab	IgE	✓	≥ 18 years	75–600 mg (Dosing based on serum total IgE and Bodyweight)	SC	✓	✓	✓	(Not Evaluated)
Mepolizumab	IL-5	✓	≥ 18 years	100 mg	SC	✓	✓	✓	✓
Benralizumab	IL-5Rα			30 mg	SC	✓	✓	✓	

Other Disease Considerations

Omalizumab has also been investigated in the management of AR as well as aeroallergen immunotherapy with promising results thus far; however, further studies are warranted (Verbruggen et al. 2009; Kopp et al. 2009).

Safety Data

Overall, omalizumab is well tolerated with an acceptable safety profile in the management of CRSwNP with no new or unexpected safety concerns identified compared with earlier trials in asthma and CSU. The most common AEs observed were similar to prior trials, including headache, nasopharyngitis, injection-site reactions and asthma exacerbation; all of which have been previously reported with omalizumab. There were no confirmed events of anaphylaxis in these trials.

Anti-IL 4/13 Therapeutics

Dupilumab

Dupilumab is FDA-approved as an add-on maintenance treatment in adult patients with inadequately controlled CRSwNP.

Efficacy Data

In dual-phase 3 trials, LIBERTY NP SINUS-24 and SINUS-52, adult patients with symptomatic CRSwNP, despite previous treatment with OCS, surgery or both, treated with dupilumab had significant improvement in Nasal Polyp Score (NPS), nasal congestion or obstruction and the sinus Lund-Mackay CT scores. Additionally, there was a significant improvement in the University of Pennsylvania Smell Identification Test (UPSIT), loss-of-smell and SNOT-22 total scores. In a prespecified pooled analysis, compared with the placebo, the dupilumab group had 74% fewer who needed treatment with OCS and 83% fewer who needed surgery. In patients with comorbid asthma, dupilumab significantly improved lung function and asthma control. In a subsequent analysis of the SINUS-24 and SINUS-52 (Mullol et al. 2021) dupilumab produced rapid, as soon as day 3, and sustained improvement in sense of smell, regardless of CRSwNP duration, prior sinonasal surgery, comorbid asthma or AERD.

In an analysis of patients with CRSwNP and comorbid AERD (Laidlaw et al. 2019), treatment with dupilumab led to a significant reduction in mean NPS compared with placebo. AERD and aspirin-tolerant patients both experienced significant improvements in the Lund-Mackay total, SNOT-22 total, UPSIT and ACQ scores compared with placebo.

Real-World Studies

As discussed previously in the asthma section, a real-world, retrospective analysis (Bavaro et al. 2021) evaluated the response to dupilumab in patients with AERD, who were previously treated with anti-IL-5 therapy for the management of asthma or CRSwNP. Following the transition to dupilumab, total SNOT-22, smell/taste and congestion scores significantly improved compared to baseline and after anti-IL-5 treatment with ACT score significantly improving from baseline.

Safety Data

Dupilumab was found to have a favorable safety profile in the treatment of CRSwNP, with no new or unexpected safety concerns identified in prior trials for asthma or AD. The most common AEs were nasopharyngitis, nasal polyps, headache, asthma, epistaxis and injection-site erythema.

Anti-IL-5/5R

Mepolizumab

Mepolizumab is also indicated in the treatment of CRSwNP.

Efficacy Data

In the phase 3 SYNAPSE trial, patients treated with mepolizumab had significant improvement in both total endoscopic NPS and nasal obstruction VAS compared to placebo (Han et al. 2021).

Real-World Studies

A 12-month real-world study (Detoraki et al. 2021) confirmed the above findings, noting the significant improvement of SNOT-22 scores in asthma patients receiving mepolizumab therapy with concomitant CRSwNP.

Safety Data

Mepolizumab's safety profile for the treatment of CRSwNP is favorable, echoing safety data from asthma RCTs. The most frequently reported AEs were nasopharyngitis, headache, epistaxis and sinusitis (Han et al. 2021).

Benralizumab

Benralizumab is being investigated for the treatment of CRSwNP, although it does not possess FDA approval for this indication currently.

Efficacy Data

In the phase 3 OSTRO study, patients with CRSwNP treated with benralizumab had a significant median reduction in NPS and patients reported Mean Nasal Blockage Score; however, no significant effect was seen in SNOT-22 scores, time to the first surgery, or need for OCS (Bachert et al. 2021).

Real-World Studies

In a real-world study (Bagnasco et al. 2020), treatment of patients with uncontrolled asthma and concomitant nasal polyps with benralizumab led to improvement in asthma-related outcomes as well as various sinonasal parameters, including resolution of anosmia. In another small real-world observational study, treatment benralizumab led to significant improvement in various clinical outcomes in patients with SEA and CRSwNP, including SNOT-22, subjective pain via the Numerical Rating Scale (NRS), Endoscopic NPS, Lund-Mackay CT score and BEC (Lombardo et al. 2020).

CRSwNP Key Points

- There are currently three biologics approved for CRSwNP, omalizumab, dupilumab and mepolizumab, with an overall acceptable safety profile and no new safety signals from earlier trials for alternative indications.
- There are no head-to-head comparator trials and as such, the approach to treatment in CRSwNP must be individualized for each patient with consideration of comorbidities, available safety data and patient preferences. See Table 4 for a comparison between available trial data.

Chronic Spontaneous Urticaria

Chronic Spontaneous Urticaria (CSU) is defined by the presence of recurrent hives and/or angioedema for greater than 6 weeks. It is estimated to affect up to 1% of the general population and is associated with a significant impact on QoL in affected patients. There is only one biologic currently approved for treatment in CSU (Johal et al. 2021).

Anti-IgE

Omalizumab

Omalizumab is indicated for CSU in adults and adolescents 12 years of age and older who remain symptomatic despite H1 antihistamine treatment. The recommended dosing is not dependent on serum IgE level or body weight, in contrast to dosing in asthma and CRSwNP. Although omalizumab has known efficacy in CSU, its mechanism of action is not fully understood in this disease.

Efficacy Data

In the ASTERIA I phase 3 RCT of patients with CSU who remained symptomatic despite treatment with approved dosages of H1 antihistamines, the mean weekly itch severity score (ISS) was significantly improved from baseline with omalizumab treatment (Saini et al. 2015). Treatment with omalizumab was found to be efficacious in adolescents and adults with persistent CSU despite treatment with H1 antihistamines up to four times the approved dose in the Glacial phase 3 RCT (Kaplan et al. 2013).

In a posthoc meta-analysis of the ASTERIA I/II and Glacial RCTs (Casale et al. 2015) omalizumab 300 mg was determined to have similar efficacy in patients with CSU regardless of the background therapy for urticaria. Omalizumab response patterns have been found to be dose-dependent and highest with omalizumab 300 mg, with some patients responding as early as week 4 after a single dose of omalizumab (Kaplan et al. 2016). In the phase 3b randomized, open-label OPTIMA RCT, omalizumab dosing increased from 150 mg to 300 mg helped more patients achieve symptom control and retreatment with omalizumab was as effective as initial therapy (Sussman et al. 2020).

In the X-ACT phase 3 RCT, omalizumab proved to be efficacious in the treatment of patients with CSU and angioedema refractory to high-dose antihistamines (Staubach et al. 2016). Omalizumab significantly improved QoL compared with the placebo. The mean number of angioedema days in the placebo group was three times higher than in the omalizumab group (mean 14.6 days vs. 49.5 days) during the 28-week treatment period.

In the XTEND-CIU study (Maurer et al. 2018), omalizumab was found to be efficacious with sustained control through 48 weeks of treatment along with retreatment upon flare. In a subsequent analysis of the XTEND-CIU study, treatment with omalizumab improved PROs regarding health-related QoL including sleep, anxiety, work productivity and activity, which occurred as early as week 12 and sustained up to the entire duration of the 48-week treatment period (Casale et al. 2019b).

Real-World Studies

A systematic review of 84 publications, including case reports/series and observational studies, evaluated the real-world efficacy of omalizumab in the treatment of CSU (Bernstein et al. 2018). The rate of treatment response to omalizumab was reported to be over 80% with complete response in over half of the patients. QoL outcomes, as measured by DLQI and CU-Q2oL improved by over 70%. Following omalizumab initiation, patients were able to discontinue routine medications, including antihistamines (60%), OCS (75.3%), leukotriene receptor antagonists (LTRA) (72.3%) as well as immunomodulatory agents (71.7%). In addition to CSU, omalizumab has been reported as efficacious in inducible urticarias as well, especially in those with high IgE (Yu et al. 2021).

Although many CSU patients respond to omalizumab at the licensed doses, some patients have refractory disease. Real-world studies have shown that some of these patients benefit from updosing of omalizumab. In a review article of nine observational real-world studies (Metz et al. 2020), omalizumab updosing to 450 or 600 mg Q4W resulted in improved disease control as well as QoL in CSU patients who did not previously respond to licensed doses, with complete response rates reported in up to 60% patients. There were no new safety signals reported at these higher doses.

Several biomarkers have been identified to help physicians predict response to omalizumab. In a systematic review (Fok et al. 2021), neither weak nor strong evidence for any parameters in predicting a good response to omalizumab was found. However, there was strong evidence that low total IgE at baseline was a predictor for poor or nonresponse to omalizumab. Particularly, in one chart review (Straesser et al. 2018), the adjusted OR for response to omalizumab was 13.81 for CSU patients with baseline serum IgE $\geq$ 168.0 IU/mL compared to those with baseline serum IgE $\leq$ 15.2 IU/mL. More recently, basophils have taken a prominent role in understanding disease pathophysiology and response to treatment in CSU. Omalizumab non-responders in CSU have been shown to have significantly lower baseline levels of FcεRI on basophils than responders (Deza et al. 2017). Higher baseline basophil count and basophil functional phenotype, as determined by response to anti-IgE stimulation, may be predictive of response to omalizumab as well (Johal et al. 2021). In addition to the above, other potential biomarkers that have been associated with poor response to omalizumab include eosinopenia (< 50 cells/μL), basopenia (< 10 cells/μL), high sensitivity C-Reactive Protein (> 3 mg/mL), obesity as well as worsening of CSU after initiation of omalizumab (Maurer et al. 2021a).

Safety Data

In phase 2 and 3 RCTs, omalizumab in the treatment of CSU was found to be well tolerated with an acceptable safety profile, with similar rates of AEs to placebo, with most reported as mild to moderate in severity. The most commonly reported AEs included URTIs, headaches, nasopharyngitis, skin and subcutaneous disorders and gastrointestinal disorders.

Ligelizumab

Ligelizumab is a next-generation, humanized IgG1 monoclonal antibody directed against IgE, which has shown to be promising in early studies regarding the treatment of CSU. Ligelizumab binds with high affinity to the Ce3 domain of IgE and leads to increased suppression of free IgE in atopic subjects compared with omalizumab (Arm et al. 2014).

In an early phase 2b trial, ligelizumab was found to have a clear dose response relationship and higher rates of complete response compared with omalizumab and placebo in patients with CSU that was inadequately controlled with standard-of-care therapy, such as H1-antihistamines (Maurer et al. 2019). In a follow-up OLE study, ligelizumab was found to be efficacious, with up to 75.8% of patients reporting cumulative complete responses following 52 weeks of treatment (Maurer et al. 2021b). In both trials, ligelizumab was reported to be well tolerated with a low overall incidence of treatment-related serious AEs, with the most frequently reported AEs characterized as non-serious nasopharyngitis, headache, URTI and urticaria. Ligelizumab's safety and efficacy in refractory CSU are currently being investigated in dual phase 3 trials, PEARL 1 and PEARL 2. At the time of this publication, preliminary data from these trials demonstrated the superiority of ligelizumab versus placebo at week 12 but not when compared with omalizumab ("Novartis, unpublished data"). Ligelizumab has been granted breakthrough designation status by FDA as of January 2021; however, it has yet to be approved for any indications.

In addition to the above studies, there are several ongoing clinical trials investigating ligelizumab's efficacy and safety profile in the treatment of peanut allergy (NCT04984876) as well as chronic inducible urticaria (NCT05024058).

Anti-IL-4/13

Dupilumab

Although not FDA indicated in CSU, preliminary data from the phase 3 LIBERTY CUPID trial has shown promising evidence for dupilumab's role in the treatment of moderate-to-severe CSU (Sanofi 2021). According to a press release in 2021, the study met its primary end points as assessed by change in ISS7 and Urticaria Activity Score over 7 days (UAS7) at 24 weeks in children and adults with refractory CSU. Dupilumab demonstrated an acceptable safety profile, similar to prior safety reports for approved indications.

CSU Key Points

* Omalizumab is the only biologic therapy currently approved for treatment in CSU, although additional agents are under investigation.
* Several biomarkers have been identified to help predict response to omalizumab in CSU, including but not limited to total IgE, baseline levels of FcεRI on basophils, baseline basophil count and basophil functional phenotype.

Other Eosinophilic Disorders

Eosinophilic Granulomatosis Polyangiitis

Eosinophilic granulomatosis with polyangiitis (EGPA) is a small vessel vasculitis characterized by eosinophilic infiltrate (Wechsler et al. 2017).

Anti-IL-5/5R

Mepolizumab

Mepolizumab is the only approved biologic agent for the treatment of EGPA. In pivotal RCTs, treatment with mepolizumab in EGPA led to significantly higher rates of remission (Wechsler et al. 2017) as well as a higher likelihood of OCS dose reduction by 50% or more (Steinfeld et al. 2019).

Real-world studies further confirm the efficacy of mepolizumab in the treatment of EGPA. In a six-month prospective, observational study of patients with EGPA and concomitant asthma (Caminati et al. 2021), patients had significant improvement in ACT, BEC, FEV1 and exacerbation rates following treatment with mepolizumab. Additionally, over 50% of patients were able to completely discontinue OCS. Another real-world study followed 16 relapsing or refractory EGPA patients receiving mepolizumab, which demonstrated a remission rate of 75% and a significantly decreased immunosuppressive requirement following mepolizumab therapy (Ueno et al. 2021). Although the approved dose of mepolizumab in the treatment of EGPA is 300 mg Q4W, this dosing regimen has recently been a topic of debate. Several real-world studies have demonstrated the efficacy of mepolizumab in EGPA when initiated for the treatment of asthma, even with this lower asthma-based dose of 100 mg Q4W (Bettiol et al. 2021). However, to confirm these findings, RCTs are necessary.

The safety profile for mepolizumab in the treatment of EGPA is similar to that seen in previous studies, with no new safety signals (Wechsler et al. 2017).

Other Anti-IL-5/5R

Several publications, including open-label studies and case reports, have demonstrated both reslizumab's and benralizumab's potential efficacy, via off-label use in EGPA (Manka et al. 2021; Guntur et al. 2021). Further studies are warranted.

Hypereosinophilic Syndrome

Hypereosinophilic syndrome (HES) is a rare group of disorders characterized by eosinophil-mediated organ damage or dysfunction.

Anti-IL-5/5R

Mepolizumab

Mepolizumab is currently the only FDA-approved biologic for the treatment of HES in patients aged 12 and older. In a pivotal RCT, significantly fewer patients with HES treated with mepolizumab compared to placebo experienced one or more flares or withdrew from the study compared to placebo (Roufosse et al. 2020). Its efficacy was sustained for up to 52 weeks in an OLE study (Gleich et al. 2021). The safety profile for mepolizumab in the treatment of HES was similar to that seen in prior studies.

Other Anti-IL5/5R

Smaller RCTs and case reports have documented the potential efficacy of reslizumab and benralizumab, via off-label use, in the treatment of HES (Kuruvilla 2018; Kuang et al. 2019).

Eosinophilic Esophagitis

Eosinophilic Esophagitis (EoE) is a chronic inflammatory T2 inflammatory disease of the esophagus characterized by esophageal dysfunction and eosinophilic infiltration of the esophageal mucosa (Hirano et al. 2020).

Anti-IL-4/13

Dupilumab

Recently, dupilumab has shown to be promising in the treatment of EoE. In a phase 2 RCT (Hirano et al. 2020), dupilumab significantly improved histologic features of EoE, including a reduction of peak esophageal intraepithelial eosinophil count by a mean of 86.8 eosinophils per high power field (hpf), EoE histologic scoring system (HSS) severity score by 68.3% and the endoscopic reference score by 1.6. Additionally, dupilumab significantly reduced dysphagia and even increased esophageal distensibility. Dupilumab is currently being investigated in an ongoing three-part phase 3 RCT, with preliminary data published as part of a press release for parts A & B. In part A, patients treated with dupilumab had a significant reduction in disease symptoms along with a 60% reduction in their esophageal eosinophilic count to a normal range. Patients also had a significant reduction in abnormal endoscopic findings ("Sanofi, unpublished data"). In Part B, patients treated with dupilumab had a significant reduction in disease symptoms and significantly more patients achieved histological remission. As a result of these promising results, the FDA granted breakthrough therapy designation to dupilumab for the treatment of patients 12 and older with EoE in September 2020.

Anti-IL-5/5R

Smaller RCTs have reported the efficacy of various anti-IL-5/5RA agents in EoE, including reslizumab, benralizumab and mepolizumab, via off-label use (Markowitz et al. 2018; Schneider and Rubinstein 2018; Assa'ad et al. 2011). However, further studies are warranted.

Immunodeficiencies

Humoral Immunodeficiencies and Immunoglobulin Replacement Therapy (IgRT)

Gamma globulin, also known as immunoglobulin replacement therapy (IgRT), has been used for decades in the treatment of inborn errors of immunity as well as secondary immunodeficiencies, including impaired specific antibody production with and without hypogammaglobulinemia. In addition to its ability to restore IgG, gamma globulin has several immunosuppressive and anti-inflammatory properties that can vary in different diseases and depend on dosing. At high dosing levels, IgRT can modulate lymphocyte levels, cytokine production, complement regulation and apoptosis (Ballow 2014).

We will focus this section on the use of gamma globulin in managing immune defects. IgRT primarily helps patients with clinically significant hypogammaglobulinemia and deficient antibody production by providing passive immunity, where bacteria and viruses can be neutralized, and phagocytosis and destruction of relevant pathogens are enhanced (Roifman et al. 1985).

IgRT is a pooled blood product collected from 1,000–100,000 screened donors per batch, depending on the manufacturer, allowing for significant antibody diversity and protection against a broad range of pathogens (Barahona Afonso and João 2016). This process, including fractionation, chromatography, viral inactivation and removal takes place over several months. There are additional quality control measures in place to ensure stable and safe solutions are produced ("FDA 2021").

IgRT Formulations

IgRT is available in intramuscular (IM), subcutaneous (SCIG) and intravenous (IVIG) forms. Dosing with IM has fallen out of favor given the limited quantity that could be administered, slow absorption, local degradation as well as associated pain and inconvenience (Lieberman and Berger 2013). Currently, FDA-approved SCIG and IVIG formulations in the United States and their select differences are summarized in Table 5. Commercial IgG products contain mainly IgG (> 95%), with small amounts of IgM and IgA. It should be noted that IgA content is lowest in Gammagard 5% solvent detergent and highest in Cutaquig. Choosing among products depends on several factors including insurance coverage, availability, dosing and frequency as well as comorbidities.

SCIG vs. IVIG

Potential selection factors for SCIG versus IVIG are outlined in Figure 1. On review of the US national survey for patients with PID, each treatment modality was reported to have appealing features and patients switched between SCIG and IVIG for a variety of reasons, including side effects and dosing frequency ("Immune Deficiency Foundation 2013"). More patients were found to have switched over to SCIG (n = 509), but there were still some who preferred IVIG (n = 134). As such, individual factors that drive satisfaction with therapy need to be considered to promote adherence.

There is no doubt, however, that the introduction of SCIG in 2006 changed the landscape for immunodeficiency diseases. Although PID patients appear to report little Ig treatment burden and are agreeable to either IVIG or SCIG, particularly when treatment is provided at home, SCIG is associated with higher satisfaction and patient preference (Jones et al. 2018). SCIG has also been found to be a more cost-effective option and less labor-intensive than IVIG for immunodeficient patients (Windegger et al. 2019). SCIG administration has consistently shown strong improvements in health-related QoL (Zuizewind et al. 2018; Lingman-Framme and Fasth 2013). Patients have felt more energetic, with increased emotional and social well-being with fewer restrictions on daily activities such as work and school (Samaan et al. 2014). In addition to the increased convenience, flexibility and independence, SCIG has the potential for higher as well as more steady mean serum IgG levels (Gustafson et al. 2008).

The serum half-life of gamma globulin is typically 3–4 weeks, but this can be shortened by states of hypermetabolism such as fever and infection (Alyanakian et al. 2003). Dosing in different disorders, the interval between doses, use of premedication and infusion rates can depend on patients and their disease factors. The starting dose of IVIG replacement therapy in PID management is typically 400–600 mg/kg every 3–4 weeks and for SCIG, typically around 100 mg/kg/week ("American Academy of Allergy Asthma and Immunology" 2011). Although most studies of SCIG have employed a design in which subjects were given IVIG therapy before being switched to SCIG (Berger et al. 2013), SCIG therapy is expected to be equally effective without the prior administration of IVIG (Misbah et al. 2009; Koterba and Stein 2015). Only SC HyQvia has initial

Table 5. IVIG and SCIG products that are available for use in humoral immunodeficiency disorders.

Products †	FDA Approved Ages for PID	IgA content (mcg/mL)	Stabilizer/regulator and related considerations
IVIG			
Asceniv 10%	≥ 12 years old	≤ 200	Glycine and polysorbate 80
Bivigam 10%	≥ 6 years old	≤ 200	Glycine
Flebogamma 5%, 10% DIF	5%: ≥ 2 years old 10%: ≥ 18 years old	5%: < 50 10%: < 100	D-sorbitol and polyethylene glycol Cannot be used in patients with hereditary fructose intolerance
Gammagard S/D (lyophilized)	≥ 2 years old	< 2.2	2% glucose, glycine, and polyethylene glycol Caution in diabetics
Gammaplex 5%, 10%	≥ 2 years old	5%: < 10 10%: < 20	5% sorbitol and glycine and polysorbate 80 Cannot be used in patients with hereditary fructose intolerance 10%: Glycine and polysorbate 80
Octagam 5%	6 to 16 years old and adults	< 200	Maltose Falsely elevates glucose readings in certain blood glucose monitoring systems May contain trace corn protein
Panzyga 10%	≥ 2 years old	100	Glycine
Privigen 10%	≥ 3 years old	< 25	L-proline Cannot be used in patients with hyperprolinemia
IVIG/SCIG			
Gammagard Liquid 10%	≥ 2 years old	37	Glycine
Gammaked 10%	≥ 2 years old	46	Glycine
Gamunex-C 10%	≥ 2 years old	46	Glycine
SCIG			
Cutaquig 16.5%	≥ 2 years old	≤ 600	Maltose
Cuvitru 20%	≥ 2 years old	80	Glycine
Hizentra 20%	≥ 2 years old	≤ 50	Proline and polysorbate 80 Cannot be used in patients with hyperprolinemia
HyQvia* 10% with recombinant human hyaluronidase	≥ 18 years old	37	Glycine
Xembify 20%	≥ 2 years old	Not specified	Glycine and polysorbate 80

PID: primary immunodeficiency, IVIG: intravenous immunoglobulin, S/D: solvent detergent, SCIG: subcutaneous immunoglobulin

† The description of these products, including brand name, are of therapies in the United States. Package inserts should be reviewed for dosing. In general, IVIG is every 3–4 weeks, SCIG can be weekly, every other week or daily with dose adjustments.

* Only subcutaneous formulation with monthly dosing and manufacturer instructions on starting therapy for patients naïve to immunoglobulin replacement

IVIG

SCIG

Advantages

* Less frequent dosing (i.e. every 3-4 weeks)
* Clinical monitoring with healthcare professionals

Advantages

* Self-administration at home for those able
* No IV access requirement
* Independence, flexibility
* Steady-state IgG levels
* Often reduced premedication

Disadvantages

* Intravenous access
* More systemic adverse effects
* Often requires premedication
* Infusion clinic or home nurse visits, cost consideration

Disadvantages

* More frequent infusions (e.g. weekly except for HyQvia)
* Multiple sites of infusion and localized site reactions; consider subcutaneous volume

Figure 1. Features of intravenous immunoglobulin (IVIG) versus subcutaneous immunoglobulin (SCIG).

dosing instructions outlined in its prescribing information for patients naïve to immune globulin treatment. HyQvia is also different from other SCIG products in that it is facilitated with recombinant human hyaluronidase, allowing for increased dispersion and absorption of IgG. HyQvia can thus be given in large volumes and at longer intervals such as every 3–4 weeks, similar to IVIG with favorable safety and efficacy data in PID patients (Hustad et al. 2021).

Monitoring

There has been debate over the years about the recommended IgG target. "Trough level" is relevant for IVIG whereas SCIG achieves a steady-state IgG level because the immunoglobulin molecules enter the circulation more gradually. Accumulated clinical evidence supports target levels of between 650–1,000 mg/dL and this has been reflected in US, European and Canadian guidelines (Shehata et al. 2010; Orange et al. 2010). A 2017 meta-analysis reinforced the efficacy of higher IgG levels while on replacement therapy and found that the incidence of pneumonia associated with 500 mg/dL trough levels was 5-fold that with 1,000 mg/dL (Perez et al. 2017). In agammaglobulinemia patients who are receiving IgRT, IgG levels greater than 800 mg/dL correlate with the minimization of severe infections (Albin and Cunningham-Rundles 2014). This higher trough level has also been suggested to be of value in patients with bronchiectasis to help prevent additional structural damage to the lung from infections. Objective parameters such as FEV1 have been shown to improve linearly with IgG trough levels of 800–1,100 mg/dL (Rich et al. 2008). Higher dosing does need to be carefully balanced with increased adverse effects. When changing a dose, several infusions may be needed to equilibrate to a new IgG level. While balancing risks and benefits, clinicians should approach dosing based on clinical outcomes rather than a specific level. Along with monitoring IgG levels, a complete blood count, hepatic transaminases and metabolic panel including glucose and serum creatinine are checked in patients on IgRT over time.

Safety Data

In counseling patients about risks and AEs, a few points should be covered. Gamma globulin is a pooled product from human donors. Even though there are numerous screening and preventive measures in place, there is a potential risk of pathogen transmission such as Hepatitis B, C and/or HIV. However, there has not been any transmission of the infectious disease reported from US-licensed IgRT products since mid-1994 (Guo et al. 2018).

Based on a patient's comorbidities, stabilizers or regulators used to prevent the polymerization of IgG molecules should be taken into consideration. For example, there are products that use glucose, and this should be avoided by diabetics. Similarly, sodium content is relevant for patients with certain cardiac conditions. The incidence of renal toxicity has decreased significantly after sucrose was removed from IgRT products, but rare incidents have still been reported (Dantal 2013).

Systemic adverse reactions are associated with IVIG likely due to the rapid dispersion of immunoglobulin. Reported percentages of common symptoms include headache (28%), fever (19%), nausea (14%), urticaria or nonspecific maculopapular rash (8–10%), flushing and myalgias (7%) and fatigue (5%) ("Immune Deficiency Foundation" 2002). These symptoms can occur during or after treatment and are usually self-limited. Aseptic meningitis is also a risk, particularly in patients with a history of migraines and those who have co-existing autoimmune and inflammatory diseases. Many side effects can be attenuated with premedication including acetaminophen, diphenhydramine, IV pre-hydration and/or slowing the infusion rate.

More serious complications include thromboembolic events, typically at higher doses (Brown and Ballas 2003) and rare but life-threatening anaphylaxis related to anti-IgA antibodies (Gharib 2016). The use of low IgA-containing preparations for IVIG or transition to SCIG should be considered in patients who are having difficulty tolerating IgRT related to the donor IgA. SCIG has been safely administered in patients who have had anti-IgA-antibody-related anaphylaxis (Horn et al. 2007). In addition to identifying patients with IgA deficiency and risk-stratifying hypercoagulable states, IgRT should always be started at the minimum effective dose and infusion rate to minimize a patient's risk of AEs. There is an associated boxed warning for IgRT products that includes thrombosis, renal dysfunction and/or acute renal failure. Individual patients may tolerate some products better than others as evidenced by AEs reported after a product change ("Immune Deficiency Foundation" 2002).

The occurrence of systemic AEs with SCIG is much lower in comparison with IVIG. SCIG can be associated with mild-to-moderate local injection-site erythema, swelling and tenderness. Although it has not been well studied, aseptic meningitis and renal and hematologic effects discussed above are considered to be less common with SCIG (Bonilla 2008). There are now more targeted therapies available for immunodeficient patients with specific genetic mutations, such as CTLA-4 defects, which are further discussed in the following section.

IgRT Key Points

- The choice between available IgRT products often hinges on insurance coverage, availability, dosing frequency as well as patient comorbidities. Currently, FDA-approved SCIG and IVIG formulations in the United States and their select differences are summarized in Table 5.

- The trough level is relevant for IVIG whereas SCIG achieves a steady-state IgG level. Target levels of between 650–1,000 mg/dL have been widely supported in the literature, with levels on the higher end being more effective at minimizing severe infections.

- Systemic adverse reactions are associated more frequently with IVIG rather than SCIG likely due to the more rapid dispersion of immunoglobulin with IVIG.

Cytotoxic T Lymphocyte–Associated Protein 4 (CTLA-4) Fusion Proteins

Abatacept and belatacept are recombinant CTLA-4 fusion proteins containing an extracellular domain of CTLA-4 and the Fc portion of a human immunoglobulin. The FDA has approved abatacept for adult RA, psoriatic arthritis, juvenile idiopathic arthritis and prophylaxis of acute graft versus host disease. Belatacept has an FDA indication for kidney transplant rejection prophylaxis.

Mechanism of Action

Given that these medications can replenish CTLA-4, they have been used off-label for two monogenic causes of immunodeficiency: CTLA-4 haploinsufficiency and LRBA deficiency. CTLA-4 helps limit immune responses by preventing the delivery of costimulatory signals needed for T cell activation, see Figure 2 (Walker 2013). LPS-responsive beige-like anchor protein (LRBA) works to maintain CTLA-4 expression on the cell surface (Khailaie et al. 2018). As such, deficiencies in either LRBA or CTLA-4 lead to excessive T cell activity. Both diseases share features of recurrent infection and hypogammaglobulinemia, interstitial lung disease (ILD), autoimmune manifestations including cytopenia, arthritis, enteropathy and lymphoproliferation as well as increased risk for lymphomas.

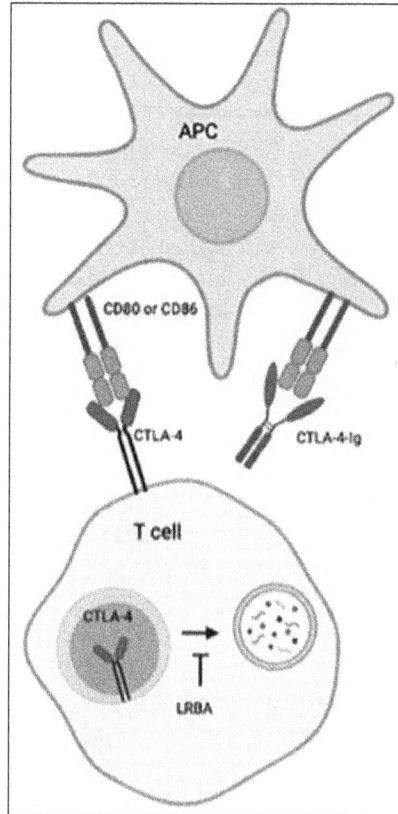

Figure 2. CTLA4-Ig binds to CD80/86 effectively replacing the non-functional CTLA-4 protein. LRBA controls the intracellular trafficking and degradation of CTLA4. In LRBA deficiency, there is increased CTLA4 turnover which is why CTLA4-Ig can play a role in replacement. (Reprinted with permission from Arnold, Chellapandian and Leiding. 2021. The Use of Biologic Modifiers as a Bridge to Hematopoietic Cell Transplantation in Primary Immune Regulatory Disorders. Front.Immunol).

Efficacy Data

CTLA-4-Ig has been shown to help control immune dysregulation caused by reduced CTLA-4 expression, resulting in improvements in autoimmune cytopenias, choroidopathy, enteropathy, hepatitis, lymphoproliferation, as well as a reduction in the use of other immunosuppressants (Tesch et al. 2020; Schwab et al. 2018). Furthermore, CTLA-4-Ig has had efficacy in the treatment of lymphoid infiltrations in the lung and central nervous system (van Leeuwen et al. 2018). Specifically, with regards to objective immune parameters, abatacept has led to improvement in naïve: effector

T cell ratios as well as functional antibody responses to polysaccharide vaccines, suggesting a rebalancing of the immune system (Arnold et al. 2021). In terms of QoL, one small, nonrandomized phase 2 trial demonstrated an 87.5% improvement in QoL and 57% improvement in fatigue in patients with common variable immunodeficiency (CVID) and ILD treated with abatacept, as compared with their baseline (von Spee-Mayer et al. 2021). In addition to reduced symptoms, 5 out of 8 patients had improvement in objective lung function and radiographic findings.

Safety Data

While both are CTLA-4-Ig, there are important differences between abatacept and belatacept of which clinicians should be informed. Unlike abatacept, belatacept carries an FDA Boxed Warning for post-transplant lymphoproliferative disorder and serious infections. Belatacept is indicated for IV administration with concomitant use of other immunosuppressants, such as mycophenolate mofetil or systemic corticosteroids. In contrast, abatacept can be administered IV or SC and the dosing has varied in off-label use with some CTLA-4 deficient patients receiving IV loading doses prior to SC administration. Abatacept carries a relatively safe AE profile with no significant increase in serious or overall infections reported with its use. However, it cannot be combined with TNF antagonists and anakinra, given an increase in serious AEs including malignancy and infections (Weinblatt et al. 2006). In addition, blood levels of Epstein-Barr Virus (EBV) and cytomegalovirus (CMV) should be monitored during CTLA4-Ig use, as severe viremia and neoplasms in patients have been described (Egg et al. 2018).

CTLA-4 fusion proteins have demonstrated the potential to downregulate severe autoimmunity and lymphocytic organ infiltration, mollifying the disease trajectory in patients with LRBA and CTLA-4 deficiencies. These medications can be added to the clinician's toolbox along with other therapies such as IVIG and sirolimus when bridging patients to the only known long-term cure for CTLA-4 insufficiency—hematopoietic stem cell transplant (Egg et al. 2021). Appropriate timing, dosing and duration of CTLA-4-Ig therapy are all areas that require further exploration in addition to conducting larger, controlled trials for CTLA4-Ig treatment in this patient population.

CTLA-4-Ig Key Points

- Abatacept and belatacept have been used off-label for two monogenic causes of immunodeficiency: CTLA-4 haploinsufficiency and LRBA deficiency.

- CTLA-4-Ig has been shown to help control immune dysregulation including improvement of autoimmune cytopenias, lymphoproliferation, and reduction in the use of other immunosuppressants.

- Belatacept carries an FDA Boxed Warning for post-transplant lymphoproliferative disorder and serious infections while abatacept does not. Abatacept cannot be combined with TNF antagonists and anakinra given a reported increase in serious AEs including malignancy and infections.

Autoinflammatory Syndromes

We will specifically examine periodic fever syndromes in this section and how interleukin-1 (IL-1) blockade can be used for the treatment of these disorders.

Although there are varying genetic mutations found in periodic fever syndromes, the defects often result in uncontrolled IL-1 production or uninhibited activity of IL-1 (Chae 2009). The overall failure in limiting the damage during inflammation leads to systemic manifestations such as fever and arthralgias in these patients. For mechanistic understanding, it should be noted that NLRP3 (nucleotide-binding domain, leucine-rich family, pyrin domain containing 3) produces cryopyrin. Cryopyrin is involved in proinflammatory cytokine release by regulating the protease caspase-1, which plays a role in activating interleukin-1 beta (IL-1β) (see Figure 3).

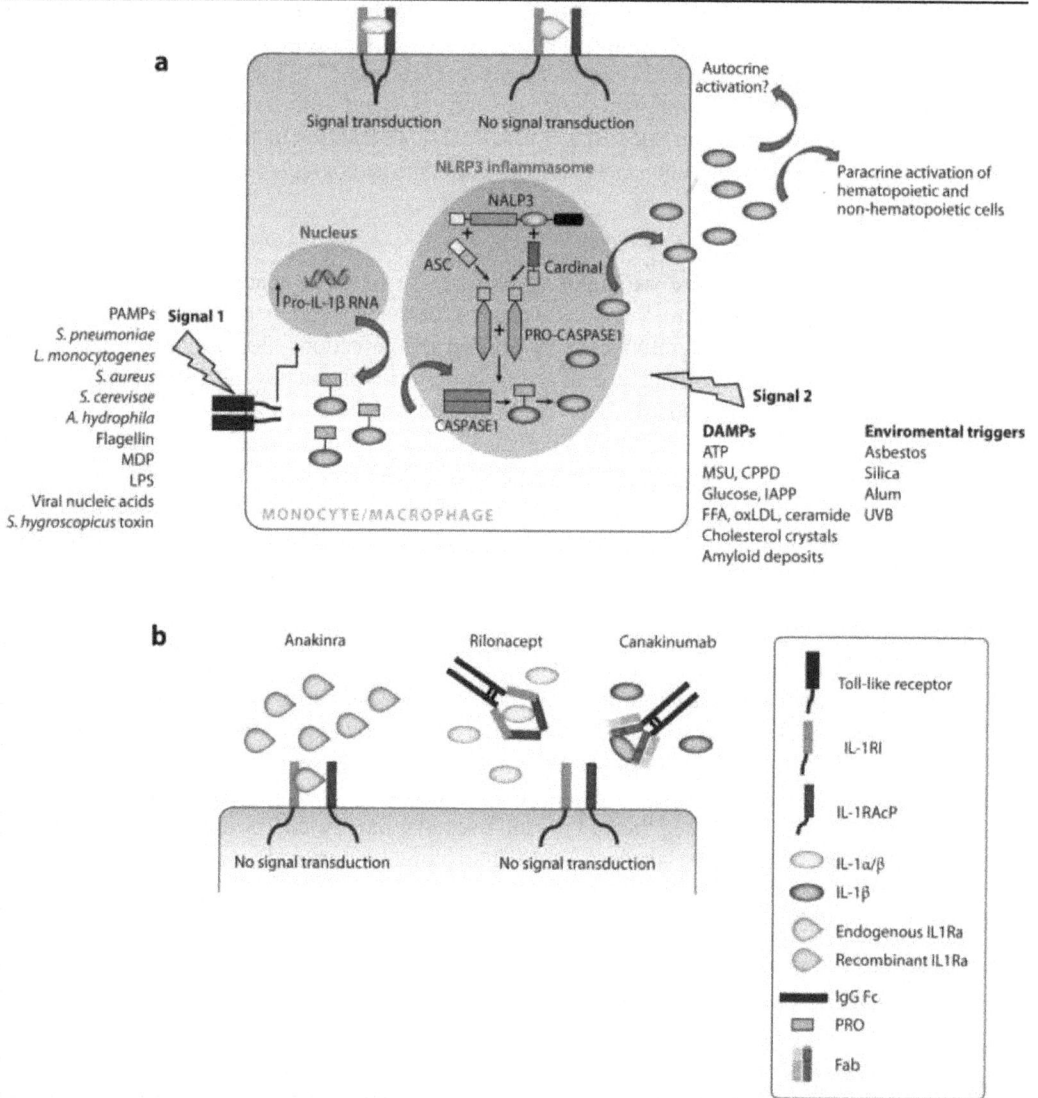

Figure 3. (a) Mechanism of IL-1 secretion and signaling. IL-1α and IL-1β are proinflammatory cytokines that activate cells by binding and signaling through the IL-1 receptor type I. IL-1β must be proteolytically cleaved into its active form by caspase-1. Mutations in NLRP-3 result in an overactive inflammasome resulting in increased activated IL-1β that drives inflammation. (b) Mechanism of IL-1 inhibition with the three currently approved treatments. (Reprinted with permission from Jesus and Goldbach-Mansky. 2014. IL-1 blockade in autoinflammatory syndromes. Annu. Rev. Med. 223–44).

CPPD: calcium pyrophosphate dehydrate crystals, DAMPs: danger-associated molecular patterns, FFA: free fatty acids; IAPP: islet amyloid polypeptide, LPS: lipopolysaccharide, MDP: muramyl dipeptide, MSU: monosodium urate, oxLDL: oxidized low-density lipoprotein, PAMPs: pathogen associated molecular patterns, ASC: adaptor molecule apoptosis-associated speck-like protein containing a CARD, NLRP-3: Nucleotide-binding domain, leucine rich family, pyrin domain containing 3, NALP3: NAcht Leucine-rich repeat Protein 3.

Three different therapies are available for IL-1 blockade in the US. Anakinra is an analog of the IL-1 receptor antagonist that can target IL-1 alpha (α) or IL-1 beta (β) and binds to the IL-1 receptor, neutralizing its biological effects. Rilonacept is a fusion protein that contains the extracellular portions of the IL-1 receptor and IL-1 receptor accessory protein and can neutralize IL-1α and IL-1β in blood circulation. Canakinumab is a monoclonal antibody that directly binds to only IL-1β. The mechanism of action for these drugs is outlined in Figure 3. Each of these medications is

Table 6. Available anti-IL-1 therapies in the US.

Therapy	Immunologic Target	Warnings and Precautions
Anakinra	Binds IL-1 receptor, affecting IL-1α and IL-1β activity levels	Bacterial and viral infections Use in combination with Tumor Necrosis Factor (TNF) blocking agents is not recommended Live vaccines should not be given concurrently Neutropenia has been reported with therapy
Canakinumab	Binds IL-1β	Bacterial and viral infections Live vaccines should not be given concurrently Neutropenia has been reported with therapy
Rilonacept	Binds IL-1β, IL-1α and IL-1 receptor antagonist	Bacterial and viral infections Live vaccines should not be given concurrently

self-administered but the frequency of administration varies. Further details about each medication are outlined in Tables 6 and 7.

Periodic Fever Syndromes

Cryopyrin-associated periodic syndromes (CAPS), TNF receptor-associated periodic syndrome (TRAPS), mevalonate kinase deficiency (also known as hyperimmunoglobulin D syndrome [HIDS]) and familial Mediterranean fever (FMF), have overlapping features in terms of the clinical phenotype. All three of the above medications are approved for CAPS in the US, but canakinumab is the only anti-IL-1 therapy that has FDA approval for other periodic fever syndromes (Dinarello et al. 2012).

Disease States

CAPS is a continuum of diseases, from most to least severe: chronic infantile neurological cutaneous and articular/neonatal onset multisystem inflammatory disease (CINCA/NOMID), Muckle-Wells syndrome (MWS) and familial cold-induced autoinflammatory syndrome (FCAS). These diseases are inherited in an autosomal dominant pattern and involve mutations of the NLRP3 (CIAS1) gene encoding cryopyrin. Each of these can present with fever, urticaria, arthralgias and conjunctivitis but only CINCA/NOMID is associated with facial dysmorphisms and developmental delay. Sensorineural, progressive hearing loss can be seen with MWS and CINCA/NOMID but not FCAS. IL-1 blockade is the recommended first-line therapy for patients with CAPS given that mutations in NLRP-3 result in an overactive inflammasome and increased IL-1β that perpetuates inflammation (Goldbach-Mansky 2011; Kuemmerle et al. 2011a). This relationship is depicted in Figure 3.

TRAPS is a disorder resulting from mutations in the tumor necrosis factor (TNF) receptor superfamily member one-A (TNFRSF1A or TNFR1) gene that leads to misfolding of the receptor (Gattorno et al. 2017). FMF involves mutations in the gene MEFV (Mediterranean fever) encoding protein pyrin. Both FMF and TRAPS are characterized by episodic attacks of severe inflammation associated with fever, malaise, serositis, myalgias and skin rashes.

HIDS is caused by a mutation in the mevalonate kinase gene (MVK). Presentation is in infancy with fevers lasting 3–7 days, painful lymphadenopathy, aphthous ulcers, abdominal pain, arthritis and skin with erythematous macules or urticaria-like lesions (Lainka et al. 2012).

Table 7. Targeted therapies for periodic fever syndromes with FDA approval.

Treatment	Level of Evidence	Age	Route of Administration	Dosing and Frequency	Relevant US FDA Approval
CAPS (mutation: NLRP3 [CIAS1])					
Canakinumab[1]	1B	≥ 4 years old	SC	Weight-based every 8 weeks	FCAS and MWS
Rilonacept[2]	1B	≥ 12 years old	SC	Weight-based for pediatric patients once weekly Adults: Loading dose: 320 mg, followed by 160 mg once weekly	FCAS and MWS
Anakinra[3]	2A	Any age	SC	Weight-based daily	NOMID/CINCA only
TRAPS (mutation: TNFRSF1A)					
Canakinumab	1B	≥ 2 years old	SC	Weight-based every 4 weeks	TRAPS
Rilonacept		Not FDA approved for this condition			
Anakinra	2B	Not FDA approved for this condition			
HIDS (MKD) (mutation: MVK)					
Canakinumab	1B	≥ 2 years old	SC	Weight-based every 4 weeks	HIDS
Rilonacept	NA	Not FDA approved for this condition			
Anakinra	2B	Not FDA approved for this condition			
FMF (mutation: MEFV)					
Canakinumab	1B	≥ 2 years old	SC	Weight-based every 4 weeks	FMF
Rilonacept	1B	Not FDA approved for this condition			
Anakinra	2B	Not FDA approved for this condition			

[1] Cankinumab is also FDA approved for SJIA and Still's disease (AOSD).

[2] Rilonacept is also FDA approved for DIRA and recurrent pericarditis.

[3] Anakinra is also FDA approved for RA and DIRA.

This table compiles data from the respective medication package inserts which can be reviewed for further information.

Centre for Evidence-based Medicine levels and grades of recommendation: 1B individual randomized controlled trial; 2A systematic review of cohort studies; 2B individual cohort study; 3B, individual case-control study; 4 case series.

SC: subcutaneous, CAPS: Cryopyrin-associated periodic syndromes, FCAS: familial cold-induced autoinflammatory syndrome, MWS: Muckle-Wells syndrome, CINCA/NOMID: chronic infantile neurological cutaneous and articular/neonatal-onset multisystem inflammatory disease, NLRP-3: Nucleotide-binding domain, leucine-rich family, pyrin domain containing 3, CIAS1: Cold-Induced Auto-inflammatory Syndrome-1, TNF receptor-associated periodic syndrome (TRAPS), TNFRSF1A: receptor superfamily member one-A, HIDS: hyperimmunoglobulin D syndrome, MKD: mevalonate kinase deficiency, MVK: mevalonate kinase gene, FMF: familial Mediterranean fever, MEFV: familial Mediterranean fever, NA: not applicable, FDA: United States Food and Drug Administration.

Anti-IL-1 Therapies

Canakinumab

Canakinumab has been approved for CAPS, TRAPS, HIDS and FMF. Up to a 97% response to canakinumab has been shown based on disease-activity scores, analysis of inflammatory markers and physician assessment in a placebo-controlled trial (Lachmann et al. 2009). In terms of AEs in this study, canakinumab was significantly different from placebo for an increased rate of suspected infections, with 67% in canakinumab group experiencing an infection vs. 25% in the placebo. Sustained remission, improved QoL and an excellent safety profile have been found with canakinumab use in pediatric and adult populations with open-label studies (Kuemmerle et al. 2011b; Yokota et al. 2017).

The efficacy of canakinumab for the treatment of TRAPS, HIDS and colchicine-resistant FMF was demonstrated in the CLUSTER RCT where significantly more patients receiving canakinumab had a complete response than those receiving placebo: 61% vs. 6% of patients with colchicine-resistant FMF, 35% vs. 6% of those with MVK deficiency and 45% versus 8% of those with TRAPS (De Benedetti et al. 2018). Increased dosing of canakinumab from 150 mg to 300 mg Q4W resulted in further improvements in disease control, particularly for HIDS. Infections, especially respiratory, were the most prevalent AEs. Patients should be informed about the increase in the rate of infections seen with canakinumab but otherwise, this therapy has been well tolerated and has consistently shown decreases in the frequency of attacks in patients with CAPS, TRAPS and HIDS (Kuemmerle et al. 2011c; Arostegui et al. 2017). There has also been substantial evidence to reinforce canakinumab use in FMF from RCT showing a reduction of flares and a decrease in inflammatory markers along with observational studies showing remission in most patients by 12 months with a high relapse rate upon treatment withdrawal (Gülez et al. 2020; van der Hilst et al. 2016).

Anakinra

Anakinra is FDA-approved for NOMID/CINCA. There have been observational studies for anakinra in CAPS showing reduced musculoskeletal symptoms and decreased inflammatory markers in the majority of patients (Goldbach-Mansky 2011). In a single-arm, open-label study, anakinra was given to 18 NOMID/CINCA patients with up to 5 years of follow-up showing rapid response with the disappearance of the rash. There was also improvement in hearing, resolution of headache, decrease in or disappearance of cochlear and leptomeningeal enhancement and reduced steroid use (Goldbach-Mansky et al. 2006). Global diary scores and inflammatory markers reduced significantly compared to the patient's own baseline. The most common AEs were headaches and arthralgia.

Treatment with anakinra in TRAPS has fewer data but has shown efficacy in an open-label trial and with on-demand therapy (Gattorno et al. 2008; Grimwood et al. 2015). In a registry-based study, anakinra induced a complete response in 26 of 33 patients (79%) and a partial response in 5 (ter Haar et al. 2013).

With HIDS, anakinra has been used to attenuate the severity and duration of acute events, ultimately improving disease control (van der Hilst et al. 2008). A prospective trial with 7 patients receiving on-demand anakinra showed that the attack duration was shorter and the maximum C-reactive protein level decreased. Additionally, a registry-based study of HIDS patients revealed that anakinra was effective in 24 (89%) of 27 patients, inducing complete remission in 6 (22%) (ter Haar et al. 2013).

A retrospective review of compiled FMF cases found that the use of anakinra resulted in a 77% complete response rate, with a partial response in an additional 19% of patients (van der Hilst et al. 2016). RCT by Ben-Zvi et al. has supported these positive findings, where 25 patients with colchicine-resistant FMF were given anakinra or placebo and the mean ± standard deviation (SD) number of attacks per patient per month was 1.7 ± 1.7 in those receiving anakinra and 3.5 ± 1.9 in those receiving placebo (Ben-Zvi et al. 2017). QoL was also improved. AEs included gastrointestinal and musculoskeletal symptoms as well as injection-site reactions as the most common, but these were comparable between anakinra and placebo. There were no severe AEs. Retrospective and registry-based reviews have also supported the reduction of flares, improvement in QoL and increased school attendance with anakinra use (Kurt et al. 2020; Sag et al. 2020).

More safety data is available for anakinra than canakinumab given its earlier release and approval. Five-year safety data for anakinra has shown that it is well tolerated in both pediatric and adult patients with CAPS. In this clinical cohort study, 43 patients with CAPS were monitored with a yearly rate of 7.7 AEs that decreased over time and were not dose-dependent (Ben-Zvi et al. 2017). The most frequent AEs were headaches and arthralgia.

A small open-label study in pediatric patients did reveal more noncompliance with anakinra than canakinumab presumably due to daily administration as opposed to every 4 or 8 weeks (Başaran et al. 2015). More frequent administration has also led to more injection-site reactions. A Cochrane review has demonstrated a statistically significant higher risk for serious infections associated with anakinra therapy in general (Singh et al. 2011). Like with canakinumab, patients should be informed of increased infection risk when being started on anakinra. Successful transitions from anakinra to canakinumab and vice versa have been documented (Cetin et al. 2015).

Rilonacept

Rilonacept is FDA-approved for CAPS, specifically FCAS and MWS. There is a single RCT that demonstrates the efficacy of rilonacept in CAPS. Hoffman et al. treated FCAS and MWS patients with rilonacept and reported a reduction in mean composite symptom score of 84% vs. 13% with placebo (Hoffman et al. 2008). Besides improvement in clinical findings, laboratory markers also improved. Rilonacept was generally well tolerated with the most common AEs being injection-site reactions, followed by URTIs. In an extended treatment duration of 72 weeks, rilonacept showed a favorable safety and tolerability profile in adult and pediatric patients with CAPS (Hoffman et al. 2012).

For FMF, RCT found that rilonacept reduced the number of attacks by greater than 50% of the baseline rate when compared to placebo, 75% vs. 35% respectively (Hashkes et al. 2012). There were no significant differences found between responders and non-responders in terms of baseline characteristics Most common AEs were injection-site reactions which were more often reported in patients receiving rilonacept than placebo (53 events vs. 13 events, respectively). At the present time, there is no published literature on rilonacept use in TRAPS and HIDS.

Additional Considerations

Each of the discussed periodic fever syndromes has distinct algorithms for management, including therapies separate from the anti-IL-1 blockade. These should be reviewed when caring for patients. Canakinumab, anakinra, and rilonacept have noticeable therapeutic effects in periodic fever syndromes with good tolerance but there are no controlled head-to-head trials between them.

There are new treatment approaches under development for periodic fever syndromes including small-molecule inhibitors of the NLRP3 inflammasome, such as MCC950 and therapies that lead to IL-1 inhibition through a different mechanism of action than previously discussed. Tranilast and dapansutrile are NLRP3 inhibitors that block the formation of inflammasomes, which are crucial for caspase 1 activation and thus IL-1β production (Huang et al. 2018; Klück et al. 2020). With ongoing research, we will obtain more data for existing therapies and potentially add new ones to our toolbox.

Anti-IL-1 Therapy Key Points

- Anakinra, canakinumab, and rilonacept are all approved for CAPS, but canakinumab is the only anti-IL-1 therapy that also has FDA approval for other periodic fever syndromes. Further details about each medication are outlined in Tables 6 and 7.

- In terms of AEs, anakinra and canakinumab have more frequently been associated with increased infection risk although they have also shown sustained remission of disease and an otherwise appreciable safety profile.

- The shared decision is of utmost importance when using these medications in an off-label manner to treat periodic fever syndromes. Patients should be informed that there are no controlled head-to-head trials between these drugs.

Hereditary Angioedema

Hereditary angioedema (HAE) is a rare, autosomal dominant disorder in which patients develop episodic swelling episodes of submucosal or subcutaneous tissues, without urticaria or pruritis. Different genetic mutations have been identified based on the subtype of HAE such as SERPING1 (Serpin Family G Member 1) in patients with deficient C1 esterase inhibitor (C1-INH) and Factor XII (FXII) gene mutations in HAE patients with normal C1-INH (Wilkerson and Moellman 2022). In most forms of HAE, enhanced generation of bradykinin, a potent mediator of vasodilation, leads to angioedema. C1 inhibitor replacement and drugs that act on the bradykinin pathway serve as an effective therapy. Existing HAE treatments target three areas in the pathway of bradykinin formation: replacement of C1-INH, inhibition of bradykinin formation through inhibition of kallikrein and antagonism of the bradykinin B2 receptor.

Management of acute attacks involves ensuring airway patency due to the life-threatening nature of laryngeal edema. Associated deaths from laryngeal edema range from 32.7–56% in a literature review of 23 HAE articles from September 2020 to April 2021 (Minafra et al. 2022). The United States Hereditary Angioedema Association Medical Advisory Board (US HAEA MAB) guidelines, updated in 2020, strongly recommend ecallantide, icatibant, plasma-derived C1-INH (pdC1-INH) or recombinant C1INH as first-line options for acute attacks (Busse et al. 2021). These therapies should be initiated as early as possible after the onset of swelling to shorten the duration and time to resolution (Craig et al. 2013).

Decisions about therapy should consider the burden of disease on an individual patient. Long-term prophylaxis is indicated for patients with frequent or severe attacks but is not limited to this population. Lanadelumab and pdC1-INH (specifically Cinryze and Haegarda) are listed as first-line prophylactic treatments per US HAEA MAB guidelines (Busse et al. 2021). We will review the eight most efficacious FDA-approved medications by their mechanism of action. The medications are also summarized in Table 8 with the distinction made between those used for acute versus prophylactic treatment. The treatment options below were studied in patients with absolute or functional deficiency of C1-INH. For HAE with normal C1-INH, treatments used are overall like those for HAE-C1-INH (Bork et al. 2020). However, there are no placebo-controlled clinical trials for the HAE with a normal C1-INH population and treatment experience is limited.

C1 Esterase Inhibitors

C1-INH therapies function to replace the missing or nonfunctional C1-INH in HAE patients. Brand names will be used to differentiate between the products. Berinert is a pdC1-INH indicated for acute attacks and was approved based on results from IMPACT-1. In this RCT, the 20-U/kg dose shortened duration of symptoms to 0.5 hours from 1.5 hours (Craig et al. 2009). With an OLE of this study, the median time for onset of symptom relief was 0.46 hours (Craig et al. 2011). There were

Table 8. Select FDA-approved treatments for hereditary angioedema.

Therapy	Indications	Route of Administration and Frequency	Mechanism of Action	Special Considerations
Plasma-derived C1 Inhibitor (Berinert)	Acute attacks All ages	IV on-demand can be self-administered	Inhibits plasma kallikrein and several coagulation factors	Risk of arterial and venous thromboembolic events, particularly at higher doses Derived from human plasma with a theoretical risk of infection transmission The most common adverse reaction is dysgeusia
Recombinant human C1 inhibitor (Ruconest)	Acute attacks ≥ 12 years old	IV on-demand can be self-administered	Inhibits plasma kallikrein and several coagulation factors	No more than 2 doses in 24 hours Rabbit-derived contraindicated in those with known or suspected allergy to rabbits Risk of arterial and venous thromboembolic events, particularly at higher doses Derived from human blood with a theoretical risk of infection transmission The common adverse reactions (≥ 2%) reported in clinical trials were headache, nausea, and diarrhea
Ecallantide (Kalbitor)	Acute attacks ≥ 12 years old	SC administered by HCP (to manage the risk of anaphylaxis)	Inhibits plasma kallikrein	Anaphylaxis has occurred in 3.5% of treated patients (Lunn and Banta 2011) Prolonged PTT The most common adverse reactions (≥ 3%) in treated patients are headache, nausea, diarrhea, pyrexia, injection site reactions, and nasopharyngitis
Icatibant (Firazyr)	Acute attacks ≥ 18 years old	SC on demand but with intervals of at least 6 hours, can be self-administered	Bradykinin B2 receptor antagonist	The most commonly reported adverse reactions are injection site reactions Other common adverse reactions (≥ 1%) include pyrexia, transaminase increase, dizziness, and rash
Plasma derived C1 inhibitor (Cinryze)	Prophylaxis ≥ 6 years old	IV, every 3–4 days, can be self-administered	Inhibits plasma kallikrein and several coagulation factors	Risk of arterial and venous thromboembolic events, particularly at higher doses Derived from human plasma with a theoretical risk of infection transmission The most common adverse reactions (≥ 5%) are headache, nausea, rash, vomiting, and fever

Plasma derived C1 inhibitor (Haegarda)	Prophylaxis ≥ 6 years old	SC, every 3–4 days, can be self-administered	Inhibits plasma kallikrein and several coagulation factors	Risk of arterial and venous thromboembolic events, particularly at higher doses Derived from human plasma leading to the theoretical risk of infection transmission The most common adverse reactions are injection site reactions, nasopharyngitis, and dizziness
Lanadelumab (Takhzyro)	Prophylaxis ≥ 12 years old	SC every 2 or 4 weeks can be self-administered	A monoclonal antibody that inhibits plasma kallikrein	The most common adverse reactions are injection site reactions, headache, rash, myalgia, dizziness, and diarrhea Prolonged PTT
Berotralstat (Orladeyo)	Prophylaxis ≥ 12 years old	Oral capsule daily with food	Plasma kallikrein inhibitor	The most common adverse reactions (≥ 10%) are abdominal pain, vomiting, diarrhea, back pain, and gastroesophageal reflux disease An increase in QT prolongation can occur at dosages higher than the recommended 150 mg once-daily dosage Note for drug-drug interaction with CYP2D6 and CYP3A4, P-gp and BCRP

Abbreviations: IV: intravenous; SC: subcutaneous; PTT: Partial thromboplastin time; P-gp: P-glycoprotein; BCRP: breast cancer resistance protein

This table compiles data from the respective medication package inserts which can be reviewed for further information.

no treatment-related safety concerns; however, 43.9% of patients experienced at least one mild or moderate AE. The most frequently reported AEs are listed in Table 8. Only dysgeusia was reported at a frequency higher than placebo (4.7% vs. 0%, respectively).

Ruconest, is a recombinant human C1-INH that has a mean plasma half-life of 3 hours, compared to the 33 hours of pdC1-INH (van Doorn et al. 2005). Ruconest nonetheless is effective in treating acute attacks of HAE. A sustained effect, despite the relatively short half-life, was shown in a posthoc analysis where relapse of symptoms did not occur in any patients at 24 hours and in 7.1% at 72 hours (Bernstein et al. 2017). Riedl et al. conducted a pooled analysis of three early trials, including 45 attacks with upper airway involvement, revealing a median time to onset of symptom relief of 67 minutes, with 91.1% of individuals with upper airway symptoms having relief onset by 4 hours (Riedl et al. 2017). All attacks resolved without the need for any additional medication, and no patients required intubation or tracheostomy. In these studies, Ruconest was deemed safe and well tolerated, with no thromboembolic events, anaphylaxis, or neutralizing antibodies observed. More specifically, in a North American phase 3 trial for Ruconest, no deaths and no discontinuations from treatment-related AEs were reported. Each treatment-related AE, such as headache or back pain was not reported in more than one patient (Riedl et al. 2014). The serious adverse reaction reported in clinical trials was the anaphylactic reaction in an otherwise healthy subject who had an undisclosed rabbit allergy. Ruconest is generated from the milk of transgenic rabbits so is contraindicated in patients with rabbit sensitization of clinical significance.

Cinryze is a pdC1-INH that can be used for prophylaxis against HAE attacks, as supported by randomized and open-label trials (Zuraw et al. 2010; Riedl et al. 2012). When treated with Cinryze, a 66% decrease in the number of attacks per study period has been noticed (6.26 attacks vs. 12.73 attacks) and there was also a decrease in the average severity and duration of attacks (Zuraw et al. 2010). Cinryze has been proven to be well tolerated and safe, with an AE profile no different from that of a placebo on a review of clinical trials performed so far (Farkas and Varga 2012).

Another pdC1-INH, Haegarda is also used for long-term prophylaxis. The COMPACT study was a phase 3, randomized, placebo-controlled study with patients who received Haegarda every 3 to 4 days versus placebo. For the group treated with 60 IU/kg, which is the currently approved dose, the attack rate was 0.52 per month versus 4.03 per month in the placebo group (Longhurst et al. 2017). Also, 83% of this population was attack-free during months 25 to 30 of treatment, showing sustained efficacy (Craig et al. 2019). A posthoc analysis of the data from the COMPACT study found greater improvement for multiple HAE-related QoL impairments, including a 42.9% improvement in anxiety and considerable improvement in work productivity compared with placebo who were using on-demand treatment alone (Lumry et al. 2018). Safety data has been positive and consistent among the different trials, with injection-site reactions being the most frequently reported.

Plasma Kallikrein Inhibitors

These medications inhibit the conversion of high molecular weight kininogen to bradykinin by selectively and reversibly inhibiting plasma kallikrein (Hofman et al. 2017). Reducing bradykinin helps to control the increased vascular permeability and resultant angioedema in HAE patients.

Ecallantide is a kallikrein inhibitor used for acute attacks that were evaluated in the EDEMA study series (Cicardi, Levy, et al. 2010). Patients reported treatment outcomes using a score of +100 to −100, with +100 being the most improvement that could be achieved. The median treatment outcome score at 4 hours was 50.0 in the ecallantide group and 0.0 in the placebo group. The primary safety concern is related to hypersensitivity reactions, with an anaphylaxis rate of 3.5% ('FDA Center for Drug Evaluation and Research 2022'). Therefore, patients must receive ecallantide with a health-care provider present.

Lanadelumab is a monoclonal antibody used for long-term prophylaxis that inhibits plasma kallikrein, with a half-life of around 2 weeks. The HELP trial supported the efficacy of lanadelumab by finding that both 300 mg Q2W and Q4W significantly decreased the number of HAE attacks

(Banerji et al. 2018). The 125 patients included in the trial had a baseline mean attack rate ranging from 3.2 to 4.0 attacks per month. During the treatment period with lanadelumab for 26 weeks, the mean number of attacks per month for the placebo group was 1.97; 0.53 for the Q4W group; and 0.26 for the Q2W group. Patients also experienced a 63.0% QOL improvement in the Q4W group, 80.8% in the Q2W group and 36.8% in the placebo group. The most commonly occurring AEs with greater frequency in the lanadelumab treatment groups were injection-site reactions (52.4% lanadelumab; 34.1% placebo) and dizziness (6.0% lanadelumab; 0% placebo). A 2021 real-life study reported these side effects with less frequency and no safety concerns or treatment discontinuation in 34 patients (Buttgereit et al. 2021).

Berotralstat is the most recent addition to medications available for HAE treatment, approved in 2020. It is an oral medication used to prevent attacks of HAE. APeX-2, a 3-part phase 3 trial, includes patients with HAE who experienced ≥ 2 investigator-confirmed attacks requiring treatment. In part 1, berotralstat was found to significantly reduce attacks relative to the placebo with 1.31 attacks in the treatment group per month versus 2.35 attacks in the placebo per month over 24 weeks (Zuraw et al. 2021). When studied over 48 weeks of treatment in part 2, mean attack rates among patients receiving berotralstat 150 mg/day declined by 67% from baseline; reductions in attack rates either continued or declined further from Part 1 to Part 2 of the study (Wedner et al. 2021). The durability of the treatment was supported by these findings. Drug-related AEs were reported in 13 of 39 (33%) and 11 of 34 (32%) participants in treatment and placebo groups, respectively. AEs were mild or moderate, with no serious drug-related events. Most commonly, gastrointestinal symptoms were reported including abdominal pain, diarrhea and vomiting but these were self-limited (Hwang et al. 2019). QoL analysis revealed improved daily functions of life, mood, emotional health and food intake (Aygören-Pürsün et al. 2018).

Inhibition of Bradykinin B2 Receptor

Icatibant blocks the effects of bradykinin by selectively inhibiting the bradykinin B2 receptor. The placebo-controlled FAST-3 study assessed a median time to 50% reduction in symptom severity. For the group of patients with cutaneous and abdominal attacks, the primary outcome was significantly shorter in the icatibant group (n = 43) compared with the placebo (2.0 hours vs. 19.8 hours) (Lumry et al. 2011). Similarly, in a posthoc analysis of laryngeal involvement (n = 21) median time to 50% reduction in symptom severity was 2.0 hours. The incidence of AEs was similar in icatibant- and placebo-treated subjects (41% and 52%, respectively). No drug-related serious AEs or deaths were reported.

Second-Line Therapies

Attenuated androgens, antifibrinolytics, and fresh frozen plasma (FFP) are considered second-line therapies in light of the newer medications outlined above. Orally administered 17α-alkylated androgens including danazol and stanozolol have an FDA indication for short- and long-term prophylaxis but not acute attacks (Busse et al. 2021). One way these medications improve HAE is by increasing the amount of C1-INH produced by the liver. If androgens are used, the dosage must be titrated to the lowest dose that provides effective control of attacks. Common side effects from the 17α-alkylated androgens include virilization in women along with menstrual irregularities, acne, changes in libido, increased aggression, weight gain, and increased blood pressure (Zuraw et al. 2016). These drugs can also cause hepatotoxicity, including the development of hepatic adenomas and hepatic carcinoma. The 17α-alkylated androgens cannot be used in certain groups because of these risks, including children and pregnant women (Busse et al. 2021).

Treatment with an antifibrinolytic agent, TXA, has been used for long-term HAE prophylaxis but is generally less effective than androgen regimens and is now rarely used (Banerji et al. 2020). The proposed mechanism of action is the inhibition of plasminogen conversion to plasmin leading to decreased activation of FXII (Wahn et al. 2020). There is no FDA indication for TXA use in HAE.

Common side effects of the antifibrinolytic drugs include nausea and diarrhea, vertigo, postural hypotension, fatigue, and muscle cramps or weakness. Because of the possible prothrombotic effect of antifibrinolytics, these should be avoided in patients at increased risk of venous thromboembolism. Neither 17α-alkylated androgens nor antifibrinolytic drugs are effective for the management of acute attacks.

Although fresh frozen plasma (FFP) has historically been used for acute attacks and short-term prophylaxis, it has also been reported to lead to paradoxical worsening as plasma contains factors that may generate more bradykinin (Prematta et al. 2007). There is no FDA indication for use of FFP in HAE. The efficacy of FFP has not been studied in RCTs. If another effective acute therapy is not available, FFP remains an off-label option with solvent detergent treated plasma being preferred as this would have reduced viral transmission risk (Wentzel et al. 2019).

Additional Considerations

Short-term prophylaxis has been particularly helpful in the context of surgeries given that trauma and stress are triggers for angioedema episodes (Williams and Craig 2015). The goal is to reduce the likelihood of swelling during a situation that may precipitate an attack. Plasma-derived C1-INH can be infused 1–12 hours prior (preferred treatment), but FFP and high-dose androgens 5 days prior and 3 days after the procedure have been used for short-term prophylaxis (Busse et al. 2021).

In general, C1-INH replacement is preferred for acute treatment and short-term and long-term prophylaxis in pregnancy and lactating women (Maurer et al. 2022; Busse et al. 2021). None of the HAE drugs have been rigorously studied during pregnancy. However, given that pdC1INH is a normal protein found in the plasma of all people, it has been used in pregnancy with good results per anecdotal reports (Hermans 2007; González-Quevedo et al. 2016; Caballero et al. 2012).

Future Directions

There has been incredible development in the field of HAE treatment, and much more is in the pipeline. PHA-022121 is a novel, small-molecule bradykinin B2 receptor antagonist progressing to phase 2 trials for the treatment and prevention of HAE attacks. It has shown about 20-fold more potency than icatibant at the human bradykinin B_2 receptor (Lesage et al. 2022). Oral plasma kallikrein inhibitor BCX7353 is now in phase 3 after showing that 50% of patients in the 150 mg group had a 70% or higher reduction in the number of attacks per month compared to their baseline (Hwang et al. 2019).

HAE Key Points

- Ecallantide, icatibant, plasma-derived C1-INH (pdC1-INH), and recombinant C1INH are considered first-line options for acute attacks. HAE-specific therapies should be initiated as early as possible after the onset of swelling to shorten the duration and time to resolution.
- Lanadelumab and pdC1-INH (specifically Cinryze and Haegarda) are considered first-line prophylactic treatments.
- These medications can be self-administered with exception of ecallantide given the increased risk of anaphylaxis in trials. These medications are summarized in Table 8 with the distinction made between those used for acute treatment versus those used for prophylaxis.

Glossary of Abbreviations

ABPA – Allergic Bronchopulmonary Aspergillosis
AR – Allergic Rhinitis
AERD – Aspirin Exacerbated Respiratory Disease
AD – Atopic Dermatitis

BSA – Body Surface Area
C1-INH – C1 Esterase Inhibitor
CV – Cardiovascular
CBV – Cerebrovascular
CEP – Chronic Eosinophilic Pneumonia
CIndU – Chronic Inducible Urticaria
CINCA/NOMID – Chronic Infantile Neurological Cutaneous and Articular/Neonatal Onset
                    Multisystem Inflammatory Disease
COPD – Chronic Obstructive Pulmonary Disease
CRSwNP – Chronic Rhinosinusitis With Nasal Polyps
CSU – Chronic Spontaneous Urticaria
CVID – Common Variable Immunodeficiency
CPK – Creatine Phosphokinase
CAPS – Cryopyrin-Associated Periodic Syndromes
CsA – Cyclosporine A
EoE – Eosinophilic Esophagitis
EGPA – Eosinophilic Granulomatosis Polyangiitis
Q2W – Every Two Weeks
Q4W – Every Four Weeks
FXII – Factor XII
FCAS – Familial Cold-Induced Autoinflammatory Syndrome
FMF – Familial Mediterranean Fever
FFP – Fresh Frozen Plasma
HAE – Hereditary Angioedema
FcεRI – High-Affinity Receptor For Ige
HES – Hypereosinophilic Syndrome
IgG – Immunoglobulin G
IgA – Immunoglobulin A
IgRT – Immunoglobulin Replacement Therapy
IT – Immunotherapy
ICS – Inhaled Corticosteroids
ILD – Interstitial Lung Disease
INCS – Intranasal Corticosteroids
IV – Intravenous
IVIG – Intravenous
JAK – Janus Kinase
LTRA – Leukotriene Receptor Antagonists
LDL, HDL – Low Or High-Density Lipoprotein
HIDS – Mevalonate Kinase Deficiency (Also Known As Hyperimmunoglobulin D Syndrome)
MWS – Muckle-Wells Syndrome
US HAEA MAB – The United States Hereditary Angioedema Association Medical Advisory Board
NPS – Nasal Polyp Score
NERD – NSAID Exacerbated Respiratory Disease
OCS – Oral Corticosteroid
OIT – Oral Immunotherapy
RV – Rhinovirus
TARC or CCL17 – Serum Thymus and Activation-Regulated Chemokine
SNOT-22 – Sinonasal Outcome Test-22
S. aureus – *Staphylococcus aureus*
SC – Subcutaneous
TSLP – Thymic Stromal Lymphopoietin

TRAPS – TNF Receptor-Associated Periodic Syndrome
TCS – Topical Corticosteroids
TXA – Tranexamic Acid
T2 – Type 2
FDA – United States Food and Drug Administration
UPSIT – University of Pennsylvania Smell Identification Test
URTI – Upper Respiratory Tract Infection
VTE – Venous Thromboembolism

Research Trial Glossary of Abbreviations

AE – Adverse Event
ACQ – Asthma Control Questionnaire
ACT – Asthma Control Test
BEC – Blood Eosinophil Count
CI – Confidence Interval
DLQI – Dermatology Life Quality Index
DFR – Dupilumab Facial Redness
EASI – Eczema Area and Severity Index
FEV1 – Forced Expiratory Volume in 1 Second
FeNO – Fractional Exhaled Nitric Oxide
HR – Hazard Ratio
hpf – High Power Field
IGA – Investigator's Global Assessment Score
ISS – Itch Severity Score
MACE – Major Adverse Cardiovascular Event
mEASI – Modified EASI
NRS – Numerical Rating Scale
OR – Odds Ratio
OLE – Open-Label Extension
PROs – Patient Reported Outcomes
PEF – Peak Expiratory Flow
QoL – Quality Of Life
RCT – Randomized Control Trial
RR – Relative Risk
SCORAD – Scoring Atopic Dermatitis Calculator
SD – Standard Deviation
TEAEs – Treatment Emergent AEs
UAS7 – Urticaria Activity Score Over 7 Days
VAS – Visual-Analog Scale

References

Akinlade, B., Guttman-Yassky, E., de Bruin-Weller, M., Simpson, E. L., Blauvelt, A., Cork, M. J. et al. 2019. Conjunctivitis in dupilumab clinical trials. Br J. Dermatol. 181: 459–73.

Albin, S. and Cunningham-Rundles, C. 2014. An update on the use of immunoglobulin for the treatment of immunodeficiency disorders. Immunotherapy 6: 1113–26.

Alyanakian, M. A., Bernatowska, E., Scherrmann, J. M., Aucouturier, P. and Poplavsky, J. L. 2003. Pharmacokinetics of total immunoglobulin G and immunoglobulin G subclasses in patients undergoing replacement therapy for primary immunodeficiency syndromes. Vox Sang 84: 188–92.

American Academy of Allergy Asthma and Immunology. 2011. Eight guiding principles for effective use of IVIG for patients with primary immunodeficiency.

Andorf, S., Purington, N., Block, W. M., Long, A. J., Tupa, D., Brittain, E. et al. 2018. Anti-IgE treatment with oral immunotherapy in multifood allergic participants: a double-blind, randomised, controlled trial. Lancet Gastroenterol. Hepatol. 3: 85–94.

Ariens, L. F. M., van der Schaft, J., Bakker, D. S., Balak, D., Romeijn, M. L. E., Kouwenhoven, T. et al. 2020. Dupilumab is very effective in a large cohort of difficult-to-treat adult atopic dermatitis patients: First clinical and biomarker results from the BioDay registry. Allergy 75: 116–26.

Arm, J. P., Bottoli, I., Skerjanec, A., Floch, D., Groenewegen, A., Maahs, S. et al. 2014. Pharmacokinetics, pharmacodynamics and safety of QGE031 (ligelizumab), a novel high-affinity anti-IgE antibody, in atopic subjects. Clin. Exp. Allergy 44: 1371–85.

Arnold, D. E., Chellapandian, D. and Leiding, J. W. 2021. The use of biologic modifiers as a bridge to hematopoietic cell transplantation in primary immune regulatory disorders. Front Immunol. 12: 692219.

Arostegui, J. I., Anton, J., Calvo, I., Robles, A., Iglesias, E., López-Montesinos, B. et al. 2017. Open-label, Phase II study to assess the efficacy and safety of canakinumab treatment in active hyperimmunoglobulinemia D with periodic fever syndrome. Arthritis Rheumatol. 69: 1679–88.

Assa'ad, A. H., Gupta, S. K., Collins, M. H., Thomson, M., Heath, A. T., Smith, D. A. et al. 2011. An antibody against IL-5 reduces numbers of esophageal intraepithelial eosinophils in children with eosinophilic esophagitis. Gastroenterology 141: 1593–604.

"AstraZeneca, unpublished data." In. 2020. Update on SOURCE Phase III trial for tezepelumab in patients with severe, oral corticosteroid-dependent asthma.

"AstraZeneca, unpublished data." In. 2021. New Fasenra data from the PONENTE trial show sustained, robust oral corticosteroid reductions in largest ever steroid-sparing trial in severe asthma.

Aygören-Pürsün, E., Bygum, A., Grivčheva-Panovska, V., Magerl, M., Graff, J., Steiner, U. C. et al. 2018. Oral plasma kallikrein inhibitor for prophylaxis in hereditary angioedema. N Engl. J. Med. 379: 352–62.

Bachert, C., Han, J. K., Desrosiers, M., Hellings, P. W., Amin, N., Lee, S. E. et al. 2019. Efficacy and safety of dupilumab in patients with severe chronic rhinosinusitis with nasal polyps (LIBERTY NP SINUS-24 and LIBERTY NP SINUS-52): results from two multicentre, randomised, double-blind, placebo-controlled, parallel-group phase 3 trials. Lancet 394: 1638–50.

Bachert, C., Han, J. K., Desrosiers, M. Y., Gevaert, P., Heffler, E., Hopkins, C. et al. 2021. Efficacy and safety of benralizumab in chronic rhinosinusitis with nasal polyps: A randomized, placebo-controlled trial. J. Allergy Clin. Immunol.

Bagnasco, D., Brussino, L., Bonavia, M., Calzolari, E., Caminati, M., Caruso, C. et al. 2020. Efficacy of Benralizumab in severe asthma in real life and focus on nasal polyposis. Respir. Med. 171: 106080.

Ballow, M. 2014. Mechanisms of immune regulation by IVIG. Curr. Opin. Allergy Clin. Immunol. 14: 509–15.

Banerji, A., Riedl, M. A., Bernstein, J. A., Cicardi, M., Longhurst, H. J., Zuraw, B. L. et al. 2018. Effect of Lanadelumab compared with placebo on prevention of hereditary angioedema attacks: a randomized clinical trial. JAMA 320: 2108–21.

Banerji, A., Davis, K. H., Brown, T. M., Hollis, K., Hunter, S. M., Long, J. et al. 2020. Patient-reported burden of hereditary angioedema: findings from a patient survey in the United States. Ann. Allergy Asthma Immunol. 124: 600–07.

Banerji, A., Hao, J., Ming, Y. et al. 2020. Long-term efficacy and safety of lanadelumab: final results from the HELP Open-Label Extension Study. Ann. Allergy, Asthma and Immunol. 125: S21.

Barahona Afonso, A. F. and João, C. M. 2016. The production processes and biological effects of intravenous immunoglobulin. Biomolecules 6: 15.

Başaran, Ö., Uncu, N., Çelikel, B. A., Taktak, A., Gür, G. and Cakar, N. 2015. Interleukin-1 targeting treatment in familial Mediterranean fever: an experience of pediatric patients. Mod. Rheumatol. 25: 621–4.

Bavaro, N., Gakpo, D., Mittal, A., Bensko, J. C., Laidlaw, T. M. and Buchheit, K. M. 2021. Efficacy of dupilumab in patients with aspirin-exacerbated respiratory disease and previous inadequate response to anti-IL-5 or anti-IL-5Ralpha in a real-world setting. J. Allergy Clin. Immunol. Pract. 9: 2910–12 e1.

Bel, E. H. 2014. Oral glucocorticoid-sparing effect of mepolizumab in eosinophilic asthma. N Engl. J. Med.

Ben-Zvi, I., Kukuy, O., Giat, E., Pras, E., Feld, O., Kivity, S. et al. 2017. Anakinra for colchicine-resistant familial mediterranean fever: a randomized, double-blind, placebo-controlled trial. Arthritis Rheumatol, 69: 854–62.

Berger, M., Jolles, S., Orange, J. S. and Sleasman, J. W. 2013. Bioavailability of IgG administered by the subcutaneous route. J. Clin. Immunol. 33: 984–90.

Bernstein, J. A., Relan, A., Harper, J. R. and Riedl, M. 2017. Sustained response of recombinant human C1 esterase inhibitor for acute treatment of hereditary angioedema attacks. Ann. Allergy Asthma Immunol. 118: 452–55.

Bernstein, J. A., Kavati, A., Tharp, M. D., Ortiz, B., MacDonald, K., Denhaerynck, K. et al. 2018. Effectiveness of omalizumab in adolescent and adult patients with chronic idiopathic/spontaneous urticaria: a systematic review of 'real-world' evidence. Expert Opin. Biol. Ther. 18: 425–48.

Bettiol, A., Urban, M. L., Dagna, L., Cottin, V., Franceschini, F., Del Giacco, S. et al. 2021. Mepolizumab for Eosinophilic Granulomatosis with Polyangiitis (EGPA): a European multicenter observational study. Arthritis Rheumatol.

Bieber, T., Simpson, E. L., Silverberg, J. I., Thaci, D., Paul, C., Pink, A. E. et al. 2021a. Abrocitinib versus placebo or dupilumab for atopic dermatitis. N Engl. J. Med. 384: 1101–12.

Bieber, T., Thyssen, J. P., Reich, K., Simpson, E. L., Katoh, N., Torrelo, A. et al. 2021b. Pooled safety analysis of baricitinib in adult patients with atopic dermatitis from 8 randomized clinical trials. J. Eur. Acad. Dermatol. Venereol. 35: 476–85.

Bissonnette, R., Papp, K. A., Poulin, Y., Gooderham, M., Raman, M., Mallbris, L. et al. 2016. Topical tofacitinib for atopic dermatitis: a phase IIa randomized trial. Br J. Dermatol. 175: 902–11.

Blauvelt, A., de Bruin-Weller, M., Gooderham, M., Cather, J. C., Weisman, J., Pariser, D. et al. 2017. Long-term management of moderate-to-severe atopic dermatitis with dupilumab and concomitant topical corticosteroids (LIBERTY AD CHRONOS): a 1-year, randomised, double-blinded, placebo-controlled, phase 3 trial. Lancet 389: 2287–303.

Blauvelt, A., Teixeira, H. D., Simpson, E. L., Costanzo, A., De Bruin-Weller, M., Barbarot, S. et al. 2021. Efficacy and safety of upadacitinib vs dupilumab in adults with moderate-to-severe atopic dermatitis: a randomized clinical trial. JAMA Dermatol. 157: 1047–55.

Blauvelt, A., Silverberg, J. I., Lynde, C. W., Bieber, T., Eisman, S., Zdybski, J. et al. 2022. Abrocitinib induction, randomized withdrawal, and retreatment in patients with moderate-to-severe atopic dermatitis: Results from the JAK1 Atopic Dermatitis Efficacy and Safety (JADE) REGIMEN phase 3 trial. J. Am. Acad. Dermatol. 86: 104–12.

Bleecker, E. R., FitzGerald, J. M., Chanez, P., Papi, A., Weinstein, S. F., Barker, P. et al. 2016. Efficacy and safety of benralizumab for patients with severe asthma uncontrolled with high-dosage inhaled corticosteroids and long-acting beta2-agonists (SIROCCO): a randomised, multicentre, placebo-controlled phase 3 trial. Lancet 388: 2115–27.

Boguniewicz, M., Beck, L. A., Sher, L., Guttman-Yassky, E., Thaci, D., Blauvelt, A. et al. 2021. Dupilumab improves asthma and sinonasal outcomes in adults with moderate to severe atopic dermatitis. J. Allergy Clin. Immunol. Pract. 9: 1212–23 e6.

Bonagura, V. R., Marchlewski, R., Cox, A. and Rosenthal, D. W. 2008. Biologic IgG level in primary immunodeficiency disease: the IgG level that protects against recurrent infection. J. Allergy Clin. Immunol. 122: 210–2.

Bonilla, F. A. 2008. Intravenous immunoglobulin: adverse reactions and management. J. Allergy Clin. Immunol. 122: 1238–9.

Bordone, L., Nanavati, C., Newman, K., Alexander, V., Wang, Y., Zuraw, B. et al. 2022. Pharmacodynamics and pharmacokinetics of PKK-LRx in patients with hereditary angioedema. Journal of Allergy and Clinical Immunology 149: AB165.

Bork, K., Machnig, T., Wulff, K., Witzke, G., Prusty, S. and Hardt, J. 2020. Clinical features of genetically characterized types of hereditary angioedema with normal C1 inhibitor: a systematic review of qualitative evidence. Orphanet J. Rare Dis. 15: 289.

Bousquet, J., Humbert, M., Gibson, P. G., Kostikas, K., Jaumont, X., Pfister, P. et al. 2021. Real-world effectiveness of omalizumab in severe allergic asthma: a meta-analysis of observational studies. J. Allergy Clin. Immunol. Pract. 9: 2702–14.

Brenard, E., Pilette, C., Dahlqvist, C., Colinet, B., Schleich, F., Roufosse, F. et al. 2020. Real-life study of mepolizumab in idiopathic chronic eosinophilic pneumonia. Lung 198: 355–60.

Brown, H. C. and Ballas, Z. K. 2003. Acute thromboembolic events associated with intravenous immunoglobulin infusion in antibody-deficient patients. J. Allergy Clin. Immunol. 112: 797–9.

Brusselle, G., Germinaro, M., Weiss, S. and Zangrilli, J. 2017. Reslizumab in patients with inadequately controlled late-onset asthma and elevated blood eosinophils. Pulm Pharmacol. Ther. 43: 39–45.

Buhl, T., Rosmarin, D., Serra-Baldrich, E., Fernandez-Penas, P., Igarashi, A., Konstantinou, M. P. et al. 2021. Itch and sleep improvements with baricitinib in patients with atopic dermatitis: a post hoc analysis of 3 phase 3 studies. Dermatol. Ther. (Heidelb) 11: 971–82.

Busse, P. J., Christiansen, S. C., Riedl, M. A., Banerji, A., Bernstein, J. A., Castaldo, A. J. et al. 2021. US HAEA Medical Advisory Board 2020 Guidelines for the Management of Hereditary Angioedema. J. Allergy Clin. Immunol. Pract. 9: 132–50.e3.

Busse, W. W., Morgan, W. J., Gergen, P. J., Mitchell, H. E., Gern, J. E., Liu, A. H. et al. 2011. Randomized trial of omalizumab (anti-IgE) for asthma in inner-city children. N Engl. J. Med. 364: 1005–15.

Busse, W. W., Bleecker, E. R., FitzGerald, J. M., Ferguson, G. T., Barker, P., Sproule, S. et al. 2019. Long-term safety and efficacy of benralizumab in patients with severe, uncontrolled asthma: 1-year results from the BORA phase 3 extension trial. Lancet Respir. Med. 7: 46–59.

Buttgereit, T., Vera, C., Weller, K., Gutsche, A., Grekowitz, E. M., Aykanat, S. et al. 2021. Lanadelumab efficacy, safety, and injection interval extension in HAE: A real-life study. J. Allergy Clin. Immunol. Pract. 9: 3744–51.

Caballero, T., Farkas, H., Bouillet, L., Bowen, T., Gompel, A., Fagerberg, C. et al. 2012. International consensus and practical guidelines on the gynecologic and obstetric management of female patients with hereditary angioedema caused by C1 inhibitor deficiency. J. Allergy Clin. Immunol. 129: 308–20.

Callewaert, C., Nakatsuji, T., Knight, R., Kosciolek, T., Vrbanac, A., Kotol, P. et al. 2020. IL-4Ralpha blockade by dupilumab decreases *Staphylococcus aureus* colonization and increases microbial diversity in atopic dermatitis. J. Invest Dermatol. 140: 191–202 e7.

Caminati, M., Crisafulli, E., Lunardi, C., Micheletto, C., Festi, G., Maule, M. et al. 2021. Mepolizumab 100 mg in severe asthmatic patients with EGPA in remission phase. J. Allergy Clin. Immunol. Pract. 9: 1386–88.

Carter, M. C., Maric, I., Brittain, E. H., Bai, Y., Lumbard, K., Bolan, H. et al. 2021. A randomized double-blind, placebo-controlled study of omalizumab for idiopathic anaphylaxis. J. Allergy Clin. Immunol. 147: 1004–10 e2.

Casale, T. B., Bernstein, J. A., Maurer, M., Saini, S. S., Trzaskoma, B., Chen, H. et al. 2015. Similar efficacy with omalizumab in chronic idiopathic/spontaneous urticaria despite different background therapy. J. Allergy Clin. Immunol. Pract. 3: 743–50 e1.

Casale, T. B., Luskin, A. T., Busse, W., Zeiger, R. S., Trzaskoma, B., Yang, M. et al. 2019a. Omalizumab effectiveness by biomarker status in patients with asthma: evidence from PROSPERO, a prospective real-world study. J. Allergy Clin. Immunol. Pract. 7: 156–64 e1.

Casale, T. B., Murphy, T. R., Holden, M., Rajput, Y., Yoo, B. and Bernstein, J. A. 2019b. Impact of omalizumab on patient-reported outcomes in chronic idiopathic urticaria: Results from a randomized study (XTEND-CIU). J. Allergy Clin. Immunol. Pract. 7: 2487–90 e1.

Castro, M., Zangrilli, J., Wechsler, M. E., Bateman, E. D., Brusselle, G. G., Bardin, P. et al. 2015. Reslizumab for inadequately controlled asthma with elevated blood eosinophil counts: results from two multicentre, parallel, double-blind, randomised, placebo-controlled, phase 3 trials. Lancet Respir. Med. 3: 355–66.

Castro, M., Corren, J., Pavord, I. D., Maspero, J., Wenzel, S., Rabe, K. F. et al. 2018. Dupilumab efficacy and safety in moderate-to-severe uncontrolled asthma. N Engl. J. Med. 378: 2486–96.

Cetin, P., Sari, I., Sozeri, B., Cam, O., Birlik, M., Akkoc, N. et al. 2015. Efficacy of interleukin-1 targeting treatments in patients with familial mediterranean Fever. Inflammation 38: 27–31.

Chae, J. J., Aksentijevich, I. and Kastner, D. L. 2009. Advances in the understanding of familial Mediterranean fever and possibilities for targeted therapy. Br J. Haematol. 146: 467–78.

Chipps, B. E., Newbold, P., Hirsch, I., Trudo, F. and Goldman, M. 2018. Benralizumab efficacy by atopy status and serum immunoglobulin E for patients with severe, uncontrolled asthma. Ann. Allergy Asthma Immunol. 120: 504–11 e4.

Chovatiya, R. and Paller, A. S. 2021. JAK inhibitors in the treatment of atopic dermatitis. J. Allergy Clin. Immunol. 148: 927–40.

Cicardi, M., Banerji, A., Bracho, F., Malbrán, A., Rosenkranz, B., Riedl, M. et al. 2010. Icatibant, a new bradykinin-receptor antagonist, in hereditary angioedema. N Engl. J. Med. 363: 532–41.

Cicardi, M., Levy, R. J., McNeil, D. L., Li, H. H., Sheffer, A. L., Campion, M. et al. 2010. Ecallantide for the treatment of acute attacks in hereditary angioedema. N Engl. J. Med. 363: 523–31.

Cork, M. J., Thaci, D., Eichenfield, L. F., Arkwright, P. D., Hultsch, T., Davis, J. D. et al. 2020. Dupilumab in adolescents with uncontrolled moderate-to-severe atopic dermatitis: results from a phase IIa open-label trial and subsequent phase III open-label extension. Br J. Dermatol. 182: 85–96.

Cork, M. J., Thaci, D., Eichenfield, L. F., Arkwright, P. D., Sun, X., Chen, Z. et al. 2021. Dupilumab provides favourable long-term safety and efficacy in children aged >/= 6 to < 12 years with uncontrolled severe atopic dermatitis: results from an open-label phase IIa study and subsequent phase III open-label extension study. Br J. Dermatol. 184: 857–70.

Corren, J., Casale, T., Deniz, Y. and Ashby, M. 2003. Omalizumab, a recombinant humanized anti-IgE antibody, reduces asthma-related emergency room visits and hospitalizations in patients with allergic asthma. J. Allergy Clin. Immunol. 111: 87–90.

Corren, J., Weinstein, S., Janka, L., Zangrilli, J. and Garin, M. 2016. Phase 3 study of reslizumab in patients with poorly controlled asthma: effects across a broad range of eosinophil counts. Chest 150: 799–810.

Corren, J., Parnes, J. R., Wang, L., Mo, M., Roseti, S. L., Griffiths, J. M. et al. 2017. Tezepelumab in adults with uncontrolled asthma. N Engl. J. Med. 377: 936–46.

Corren, J., Chen, S., Callan, L. and Gil, E. G. 2020. The effect of tezepelumab on hospitalizations and emergency department visits in patients with severe asthma. Ann. Allergy Asthma Immunol. 125: 211–14.

Corren, J., Castro, M., O'Riordan, T., Hanania, N. A., Pavord, I. D., Quirce, S., Chipps, B. E. et al. 2020. Dupilumab efficacy in patients with uncontrolled, moderate-to-severe allergic asthma. J. Allergy Clin. Immunol. Pract. 8: 516–26.

Corren, J., Ambrose, C. S., Salapa, K., Roseti, S. L., Griffiths, J. M., Parnes, J. R. et al. 2021a. Efficacy of tezepelumab in patients with severe, uncontrolled asthma and perennial allergy. J. Allergy Clin. Immunol. Pract. 9: 4334–42 e6.

Corren, J., Garcia Gil, E., Griffiths, J. M., Parnes, J. R., van der Merwe, R., Salapa, K. et al. 2021b. Tezepelumab improves patient-reported outcomes in patients with severe, uncontrolled asthma in PATHWAY. Ann. Allergy Asthma Immunol. 126: 187–93.

Craig, Timothy J., Robyn J. Levy, Richard L. Wasserman, Againdra K. Bewtra, David Hurewitz, Krystyna Obtułowicz et al. 2009. Efficacy of human C1 esterase inhibitor concentrate compared with placebo in acute hereditary angioedema attacks. Journal of Allergy and Clinical Immunology 124: 801–08.

Craig, T. J., Bewtra, A. K., Bahna, S. L., Hurewitz, D., Schneider, L. C., Levy, R. J. et al. 2011. C1 esterase inhibitor concentrate in 1085 Hereditary Angioedema attacks—final results of the I.M.P.A.C.T.2 study. Allergy 66: 1604–11.

Craig, T. J., Rojavin, M. A., Machnig, T., Keinecke, H. O. and Bernstein, J. A. 2013. Effect of time to treatment on response to C1 esterase inhibitor concentrate for hereditary angioedema attacks. Ann. Allergy Asthma Immunol. 111: 211–5.

Craig, T., Zuraw, B., Longhurst, H., Cicardi, M., Bork, K., Grattan, C. et al. 2019. Long-term outcomes with subcutaneous C1-inhibitor replacement therapy for prevention of hereditary angioedema attacks. J. Allergy Clin. Immunol. Pract. 7: 1793–802.e2.

Damask, C., Chen, M., Holweg, C. T. J., Yoo, B., Millette, L. A. and Franzese, C. 2021. Defining the efficacy of omalizumab in nasal polyposis: A POLYP 1 and POLYP 2 subgroup analysis. Am. J. Rhinol. Allergy: 19458924211030486.

Dantal, J. 2013. Intravenous immunoglobulins: in-depth review of excipients and acute kidney injury risk. Am. J. Nephrol. 38: 275–84.

De Benedetti, F., Gattorno, M., Anton, J., Ben-Chetrit, E., Frenkel, J., Hoffman, H. M. et al. 2018. Canakinumab for the treatment of autoinflammatory recurrent fever syndromes. N Engl. J. Med. 378: 1908–19.

de Bruin-Weller, M., Thaci, D., Smith, C. H., Reich, K., Cork, M. J., Radin, A. et al. 2018. Dupilumab with concomitant topical corticosteroid treatment in adults with atopic dermatitis with an inadequate response or intolerance to ciclosporin A or when this treatment is medically inadvisable: a placebo-controlled, randomized phase III clinical trial (LIBERTY AD CAFE). Br J. Dermatol. 178: 1083–101.

Deleuran, M., Thaci, D., Beck, L. A., de Bruin-Weller, M., Blauvelt, A., Forman, S. et al. 2020. Dupilumab shows long-term safety and efficacy in patients with moderate to severe atopic dermatitis enrolled in a phase 3 open-label extension study. J. Am. Acad. Dermatol. 82: 377–88.

Detoraki, A., Tremante, E., D'Amato, M., Calabrese, C., Casella, C., Maniscalco, M. et al. 2021. Mepolizumab improves sino-nasal symptoms and asthma control in severe eosinophilic asthma patients with chronic rhinosinusitis and nasal polyps: a 12-month real-life study. Ther. Adv. Respir. Dis. 15: 17534666211009398.

Deza, G., Bertolin-Colilla, M., Pujol, R. M., Curto-Barredo, L., Soto, D., Garcia, M., Hernandez, P. R. et al. 2017. Basophil FcepsilonRI expression in chronic spontaneous urticaria: a potential immunological predictor of response to omalizumab therapy. Acta Derm. Venereol. 97: 698–704.

Dinarello, Charles A., Anna Simon and Jos W. M. van der Meer. 2012. Treating inflammation by blocking interleukin-1 in a broad spectrum of diseases. Nature Reviews Drug Discovery 11: 633–52.

Diver, S., Khalfaoui, L., Emson, C., Wenzel, S. E., Menzies-Gow, A., Wechsler, M. E. et al. 2021. Effect of tezepelumab on airway inflammatory cells, remodelling, and hyperresponsiveness in patients with moderate-to-severe uncontrolled asthma (CASCADE): a double-blind, randomised, placebo-controlled, phase 2 trial. Lancet Respir. Med. 9: 1299–312.

Dupin, C., Belhadi, D., Guilleminault, L., Gamez, A. S., Berger, P., De Blay, F. et al. 2020. Effectiveness and safety of dupilumab for the treatment of severe asthma in a real-life French multi-centre adult cohort. Clin. Exp. Allergy 50: 789–98.

Egg, D., Schwab, C., Gabrysch, A., Arkwright, P. D., Cheesman, E., Giulino-Roth, L. et al. 2018. Increased risk for malignancies in 131 affected CTLA4 mutation carriers. Front Immunol. 9: 2012.

Egg, D., Rump, I. C., Mitsuiki, N., Rojas-Restrepo, J., Maccari, M. E., Schwab, C. et al. 2021. Therapeutic options for CTLA-4 insufficiency. J. Allergy Clin. Immunol.

Eichenfield, L. F., Flohr, C., Sidbury, R., Siegfried, E., Szalai, Z., Galus, R. et al. 2021. Efficacy and safety of abrocitinib in combination with topical therapy in adolescents with moderate-to-severe atopic dermatitis: The JADE TEEN randomized clinical trial. JAMA Dermatol. 157: 1165–73.

Emson, C., Diver, S., Chachi, L., Megally, A., Small, C., Downie, J. et al. 2020. CASCADE: a phase 2, randomized, double-blind, placebo-controlled, parallel-group trial to evaluate the effect of tezepelumab on airway inflammation in patients with uncontrolled asthma. Respir. Res. 21: 265.

Esquivel, A., Busse, W. W., Calatroni, A., Togias, A. G., Grindle, K. G., Bochkov, Y. A. et al. 2017. Effects of omalizumab on rhinovirus infections, illnesses, and exacerbations of asthma. Am. J. Respir. Crit. Care Med. 196: 985–92.

Farkas, H. and Varga, L. 2012. Human plasma-derived, nanofiltered, C1-inhibitor concentrate (Cinryze®), a novel therapeutic alternative for the management of hereditary angioedema resulting from C1-inhibitor deficiency. Biol. Ther. 2: 2.

FDA Center for Drug Evaluation and Research (CDER) application number 125277 summary review. Accessed February 6, 2022.

FitzGerald, J. M., Bleecker, E. R., Nair, P., Korn, S., Ohta, K., Lommatzsch, M. et al. 2016. Benralizumab, an anti-interleukin-5 receptor alpha monoclonal antibody, as add-on treatment for patients with severe, uncontrolled, eosinophilic asthma (CALIMA): a randomised, double-blind, placebo-controlled phase 3 trial. Lancet 388: 2128–41.

FitzGerald, J. M., Bleecker, E. R., Bourdin, A., Busse, W. W., Ferguson, G. T., Brooks, L. et al. 2019. Two-year integrated efficacy and safety analysis of benralizumab in severe asthma. J. Asthma Allergy 12: 401–13.

Fleming, P. and Drucker, A. M. 2018. Risk of infection in patients with atopic dermatitis treated with dupilumab: A meta-analysis of randomized controlled trials. J. Am. Acad. Dermatol. 78: 62–69 e1.

Fok, J. S., Kolkhir, P., Church, M. K. and Maurer, M. 2021. Predictors of treatment response in chronic spontaneous urticaria. Allergy 76: 2965–81.

Food and Drug Administration, 2021. In. Department of Health and Human Services. Code of Federal Regulations, Chapter I, Subchapter, F. Biologics. 21(7): Part 640, Subpart J. Immune Globulin (Human).

Garcia, G., Magnan, A., Chiron, R., Contin-Bordes, C., Berger, P., Taille, C. et al. 2013. A proof-of-concept, randomized, controlled trial of omalizumab in patients with severe, difficult-to-control, nonatopic asthma. Chest 144: 411–19.

Gattorno, M., Pelagatti, M. A., Meini, A., Obici, L., Barcellona, R., Federici, S. et al. 2008. Persistent efficacy of anakinra in patients with tumor necrosis factor receptor-associated periodic syndrome. Arthritis Rheum. 58: 1516–20.

Gattorno, M., Obici, L., Cattalini, M., Tormey, V., Abrams, K., Davis, N. et al. 2017. Canakinumab treatment for patients with active recurrent or chronic TNF receptor-associated periodic syndrome (TRAPS): an open-label, phase II study. Ann. Rheum Dis. 76: 173–78.

Gauvreau, G. M., Arm, J. P., Boulet, L. P., Leigh, R., Cockcroft, D. W., Davis, B. E., Mayers, I. et al. 2016. Efficacy and safety of multiple doses of QGE031 (ligelizumab) versus omalizumab and placebo in inhibiting allergen-induced early asthmatic responses. J. Allergy Clin. Immunol. 138: 1051–59.

Gevaert, P., Omachi, T. A., Corren, J., Mullol, J., Han, J., Lee, S. E. et al. 2020. Efficacy and safety of omalizumab in nasal polyposis: 2 randomized phase 3 trials. J. Allergy Clin. Immunol. 146: 595–605.

Gharib, A., Caperton, C. and Gupta, S. 2016. Anaphylaxis to IGIV in immunoglobulin-naïve common variable immunodeficiency patient in the absence of IgG anti-IgA antibodies: successful administration of low IgA-containing immunoglobulin. Allergy Asthma Clin. Immunol. 12: 23.

Gleich, G. J., Roufosse, F., Chupp, G., Faguer, S., Walz, B., Reiter, A. et al. 2021. Safety and efficacy of mepolizumab in hypereosinophilic syndrome: an open-label extension study. J. Allergy Clin. Immunol. Pract.

Goldbach-Mansky, R., Dailey, N. J., Canna, S. W., Gelabert, A., Jones, J., Rubin, B. I. et al. 2006. Neonatal-onset multisystem inflammatory disease responsive to interleukin-1beta inhibition. N Engl. J. Med. 355: 581–92.

Goldbach-Mansky, R. 2011. Current status of understanding the pathogenesis and management of patients with NOMID/CINCA. Curr. Rheumatol. Rep. 13: 123–31.

Gong, X., Chen, X., Kuligowski, M. E., Liu, X., Liu, X., Cimino, E. et al. 2021. Pharmacokinetics of Ruxolitinib in patients with atopic dermatitis treated with ruxolitinib cream: data from phase II and III studies. Am. J. Clin. Dermatol. 22: 555–66.

González-Quevedo, T., Larco, J. I., Marcos, C., Guilarte, M., Baeza, M. L., Cimbollek, S. et al. 2016. Management of pregnancy and delivery in patients with hereditary angioedema due to C1 inhibitor deficiency. J. Investig. Allergol. Clin. Immunol. 26: 161–7.

Grimwood, C., Despert, V., Jeru, I. and Hentgen, V. 2015. On-demand treatment with anakinra: a treatment option for selected TRAPS patients. Rheumatology (Oxford) 54: 1749–51.

Gülez, N., Makay, B. and Sözeri, B. 2020. Long-term effectiveness and safety of canakinumab in pediatric familial Mediterranean fever patients. Mod. Rheumatol. 30: 166–71.

Guntur, V. P., Manka, L. A., Denson, J. L., Dunn, R. M., Dollin, Y. T., Gill, M. et al. 2021. Benralizumab as a steroid-sparing treatment option in eosinophilic granulomatosis with polyangiitis. J. Allergy Clin. Immunol. Pract. 9: 1186–93 e1.

Guo, Y., Tian, X., Wang, X. and Xiao, Z. 2018. Adverse effects of immunoglobulin therapy. Front Immunol. 9: 1299.

Gustafson, R., Gardulf, A., Hansen, S., Leibl, H., Engl, W., Lindén, M. et al. 2008. Rapid subcutaneous immunoglobulin administration every second week results in high and stable serum immunoglobulin G levels in patients with primary antibody deficiencies. Clin. Exp. Immunol, 152: 274–9.

Gutermuth, J., Pink, A. E., Worm, M., Soldbro, L., Bjerregard Oland, C. and Weidinger, S. 2021. Tralokinumab plus topical corticosteroids in adults with severe atopic dermatitis and inadequate response to or intolerance of ciclosporin A: a placebo-controlled, randomized, phase III clinical trial (ECZTRA 7). Br J. Dermatol.

Guttman-Yassky, E., Bissonnette, R., Ungar, B., Suarez-Farinas, M., Ardeleanu, M., Esaki, H. et al. 2019. Dupilumab progressively improves systemic and cutaneous abnormalities in patients with atopic dermatitis. J. Allergy Clin. Immunol. 143: 155–72.

Guttman-Yassky, E., Blauvelt, A., Eichenfield, L. F., Paller, A. S., Armstrong, A. W., Drew, J. et al. 2020. Efficacy and safety of lebrikizumab, a high-affinity interleukin 13 inhibitor, in adults with moderate to severe atopic dermatitis: a phase 2b randomized clinical trial. JAMA Dermatol. 156: 411–20.

Guttman-Yassky, E., Teixeira, H. D., Simpson, E. L., Papp, K. A., Pangan, A. L., Blauvelt, A. et al. 2021. Once-daily upadacitinib versus placebo in adolescents and adults with moderate-to-severe atopic dermatitis (Measure Up 1 and Measure Up 2): results from two replicate double-blind, randomised controlled phase 3 trials. Lancet 397: 2151–68.

Halling, A. S., Loft, N., Silverberg, J. I., Guttman-Yassky, E. and Thyssen, J. P. 2021. Real-world evidence of dupilumab efficacy and risk of adverse events: A systematic review and meta-analysis. J. Am. Acad. Dermatol. 84: 139–47.

Han, J. K., Bachert, C., Fokkens, W., Desrosiers, M., Wagenmann, M., Lee, S. E. et al. 2021. Mepolizumab for chronic rhinosinusitis with nasal polyps (SYNAPSE): a randomised, double-blind, placebo-controlled, phase 3 trial. Lancet Respir. Med. 9: 1141–53.

Hanania, N. A., Wenzel, S., Rosen, K., Hsieh, H. J., Mosesova, S., Choy, D. F. et al. 2013. Exploring the effects of omalizumab in allergic asthma: an analysis of biomarkers in the EXTRA study. Am. J. Respir. Crit. Care Med. 187: 804–11.

Hanania, N. A., Korenblat, P., Chapman, K. R., Bateman, E. D., Kopecky, P., Paggiaro, P. et al. 2016. Efficacy and safety of lebrikizumab in patients with uncontrolled asthma (LAVOLTA I and LAVOLTA II): replicate, phase 3, randomised, double-blind, placebo-controlled trials. Lancet Respir. Med. 4: 781–96.

Hanania, N. A., Chipps, B. E., Griffin, N. M., Yoo, B., Iqbal, A. and Casale, T. B. 2019. Omalizumab effectiveness in asthma-COPD overlap: Post hoc analysis of PROSPERO. J. Allergy Clin. Immunol. 143: 1629–33 e2.

Harb, H. and Chatila, T. A. 2020. Mechanisms of dupilumab. Clin. Exp. Allergy 50: 5–14.

Harrison, T., Canonica, G. W., Chupp, G., Lee, J., Schleich, F., Welte, T. et al. 2020. Real-world mepolizumab in the prospective severe asthma REALITI-A study: initial analysis. Eur. Respir. J. 56.

Hashkes, P. J., Spalding, S. J., Giannini, E. H., Huang, B., Johnson, A., Park, G. et al. 2012. Rilonacept for colchicine-resistant or -intolerant familial Mediterranean fever: a randomized trial. Ann. Intern. Med. 157: 533–41.

Hermans, C. 2007. Successful management with C1-inhibitor concentrate of hereditary angioedema attacks during two successive pregnancies: a case report. Arch. Gynecol. Obstet. 276: 271–6.

Hirano, I., Dellon, E. S., Hamilton, J. D., Collins, M. H., Peterson, K., Chehade, M. et al. 2020. Efficacy of dupilumab in a phase 2 randomized trial of adults with active eosinophilic esophagitis. Gastroenterology 158: 111–22 e10.

Hoffman, H. M., Throne, M. L., Amar, N. J., Sebai, M., Kivitz, A. J., Kavanaugh, A. et al. 2008. Efficacy and safety of rilonacept (interleukin-1 Trap) in patients with cryopyrin-associated periodic syndromes: results from two sequential placebo-controlled studies. Arthritis Rheum. 58: 2443–52.

Hoffman, H. M., Throne, M. L., Amar, N. J., Cartwright, R. C., Kivitz, A. J., Soo, Y. et al. 2012. Long-term efficacy and safety profile of rilonacept in the treatment of cryopryin-associated periodic syndromes: results of a 72-week open-label extension study. Clin. Ther. 34: 2091–103.

Hofman, Z. L. M., de Maat, S., Suffritti, C., Zanichelli, A., van Doorn, C., Sebastian, S. A. E. et al. 2017. Cleaved kininogen as a biomarker for bradykinin release in hereditary angioedema. J. Allergy Clin. Immunol. 140: 1700–03.e8.

Horn, J., Thon, V., Bartonkova, D., Salzer, U., Warnatz, K., Schlesier, M. et al. 2007. Anti-IgA antibodies in common variable immunodeficiency (CVID): diagnostic workup and therapeutic strategy. Clin. Immunol. 122: 156–62.

Huang, Y., Jiang, H., Chen, Y., Wang, X., Yang, Y., Tao, J. et al. 2018. Tranilast directly targets NLRP3 to treat inflammasome-driven diseases. EMBO Mol. Med. 10.

Humbert, M., Beasley, R., Ayres, J., Slavin, R., Hebert, J., Bousquet, J. et al. 2005. Benefits of omalizumab as add-on therapy in patients with severe persistent asthma who are inadequately controlled despite best available therapy (GINA 2002 step 4 treatment): INNOVATE. Allergy 60: 309–16.

Hustad, N. B., Degerud, H. M., Hjelmerud, I., Fraz, M. S. A., Nordøy, I., Trøseid, M. et al. 2021. Real-world experiences with facilitated subcutaneous immunoglobulin substitution in patients with hypogammaglobulinemia, using a three-step ramp-up schedule. Frontiers in Immunology 12.

Hwang, J. R., Hwang, G., Johri, A. and Craig, T. 2019. Oral plasma kallikrein inhibitor BCX7353 for treatment of hereditary angioedema. Immunotherapy 11: 1439–44.

Immune Deficiency Foundation. 2002. *In*: Primary Immune Deficiency Diseases in America: The Second National Survey of Patients, Towson, Maryland.

Immune Deficiency Foundation. 2013. *In*: National Immunoglobulin Treatment Survey Report. Towson, Maryland.

Iribarren, C., Rahmaoui, A., Long, A. A., Szefler, S. J., Bradley, M. S., Carrigan, G. et al. 2017. Cardiovascular and cerebrovascular events among patients receiving omalizumab: Results from EXCELS, a prospective cohort study in moderate to severe asthma. J. Allergy Clin. Immunol. 139: 1489–95 e5.

Isomoto, K., Baba, T., Sekine, A., Aiko, N. and Ogura, T. 2020. Promising effects of benralizumab on chronic eosinophilic pneumonia. Intern. Med. 59: 1195–98.

Isoyama, S., Ishikawa, N., Hamai, K., Matsumura, M., Kobayashi, H., Nomura, A. et al. 2021. Efficacy of mepolizumab in elderly patients with severe asthma and overlapping COPD in real-world settings: A retrospective observational study. Respir. Investig. 59: 478–86.

Jendoubi, F., Gaudenzio, N., Gallini, A., Negretto, M., Paul, C. and Bulai Livideanu, C. 2020. Omalizumab in the treatment of adult patients with mastocytosis: A systematic review. Clin. Exp. Allergy 50: 654–61.

Johal, K. J., Chichester, K. L., Oliver, E. T., Devine, K. C., Bieneman, A. P., Schroeder, J. T. et al. 2021. The efficacy of omalizumab treatment in chronic spontaneous urticaria is associated with basophil phenotypes. J. Allergy Clin. Immunol. 147: 2271–80 e8.

Jones, G. L., Vogt, K. S., Chambers, D., Clowes, M. and Shrimpton, A. 2018. What is the burden of immunoglobulin replacement therapy in adult patients with primary immunodeficiencies? A systematic review. Front Immunol. 9: 1308.

Kabashima, K., Furue, M., Hanifin, J. M., Pulka, G., Wollenberg, A., Galus, R. et al. 2018. Nemolizumab in patients with moderate-to-severe atopic dermatitis: Randomized, phase II, long-term extension study. J. Allergy Clin. Immunol. 142: 1121–30 e7.

Kabashima, K., Matsumura, T., Komazaki, H., Kawashima, M. and Study Group Nemolizumab, J. P. 2020. Trial of nemolizumab and topical agents for atopic dermatitis with pruritus. N Engl. J. Med. 383: 141–50.

Kaminsky, L. W., Aukstuolis, K., Petroni, D. H. and Al-Shaikhly, T. 2021. Use of omalizumab for management of idiopathic anaphylaxis: A systematic review and retrospective case series. Ann. Allergy Asthma Immunol. 127: 481–87.

Kaplan, A., Ledford, D., Ashby, M., Canvin, J., Zazzali, J. L., Conner, E. et al. 2013. Omalizumab in patients with symptomatic chronic idiopathic/spontaneous urticaria despite standard combination therapy. J. Allergy Clin. Immunol. 132: 101–9.

Kaplan, A., Ferrer, M., Bernstein, J. A., Antonova, E., Trzaskoma, B., Raimundo, K. et al. 2016. Timing and duration of omalizumab response in patients with chronic idiopathic/spontaneous urticaria. J. Allergy Clin. Immunol. 137: 474–81.

Kaplan, A. P., Gimenez-Arnau, A. M. and Saini, S. S. 2017. Mechanisms of action that contribute to efficacy of omalizumab in chronic spontaneous urticaria. Allergy 72: 519–33.

Kelsen, S. G., Agache, I. O., Soong, W., Israel, E., Chupp, G. L., Cheung, D. S. et al. 2021. Astegolimab (anti-ST2) efficacy and safety in adults with severe asthma: A randomized clinical trial. J. Allergy Clin. Immunol. 148: 790–98.

Kemp, Adrian. 2021. Tezspire (tezepelumab) approved in the US for severe asthma. *In*: AstraZeneca.

Khailaie, S., Rowshanravan, B., Robert, P. A., Waters, E., Halliday, N., Badillo Herrera, J. D. et al. 2018. Characterization of CTLA4 trafficking and implications for its function. Biophys J. 115: 1330–43.

Khatri, S., Moore, W., Gibson, P. G., Leigh, R., Bourdin, A., Maspero, J. et al. 2019. Assessment of the long-term safety of mepolizumab and durability of clinical response in patients with severe eosinophilic asthma. J. Allergy Clin. Immunol. 143: 1742–51 e7.

Khurana, S., Brusselle, G. G., Bel, E. H., FitzGerald, J. M., Masoli, M., Korn, S. et al. 2019. Long-term safety and clinical benefit of mepolizumab in patients with the most severe eosinophilic asthma: The COSMEX study. Clin. Ther. 41: 2041–56 e5.

Klück, V., Tlta Jansen, Janssen, M., Comarniceanu, A., Efdé, M., Tengesdal, I. W. et al. 2020. Dapansutrile, an oral selective NLRP3 inflammasome inhibitor, for treatment of gout flares: an open-label, dose-adaptive, proof-of-concept, phase 2a trial. Lancet Rheumatol. 2: e270–e80.

Kolbeck, R., Kozhich, A., Koike, M., Peng, L., Andersson, C. K., Damschroder, M. M. et al. 2010. MEDI-563, a humanized anti-IL-5 receptor alpha mAb with enhanced antibody-dependent cell-mediated cytotoxicity function. J. Allergy Clin. Immunol. 125: 1344–53 e2.

Kopp, M. V., Hamelmann, E., Zielen, S., Kamin, W., Bergmann, K. C., Sieder, C. et al. 2009. Combination of omalizumab and specific immunotherapy is superior to immunotherapy in patients with seasonal allergic rhinoconjunctivitis and co-morbid seasonal allergic asthma. Clin. Exp. Allergy 39: 271–9.

Koterba, A. P. and Stein, M. R. 2015. Initiation of immunoglobulin therapy by subcutaneous administration in immunodeficiency patients naive to replacement therapy. Allergy Asthma Clin. Immunol. 11: 63.

Kuang, F. L., Legrand, F., Makiya, M., Ware, J., Wetzler, L., Brown, T. et al. 2019. Benralizumab for PDGFRA-negative hypereosinophilic syndrome. N Engl. J. Med. 380: 1336–46.

Kuemmerle-Deschner, J. B., Ramos, E., Blank, N., Roesler, J., Felix, S. D., Jung, T., Stricker, K. A. et al. 2011a. Canakinumab (ACZ885, a fully human IgG1 anti-IL-1β mAb) induces sustained remission in pediatric patients with cryopyrin-associated periodic syndrome (CAPS). Arthritis Res. Ther. 13: R34.

Kuemmerle-Deschner, J. B., Tyrrell, P. N., Koetter, I., Wittkowski, H., Bialkowski, A., Tzaribachev, N. P. et al. 2011b. Efficacy and safety of anakinra therapy in pediatric and adult patients with the autoinflammatory Muckle-Wells syndrome. Arthritis Rheum. 63: 840–9.

Kuemmerle-Deschner, Jasmin B., Hachulla, E., Cartwright, R., Hawkins, P. N., Tran, T. A., Bader-Meunier, B. et al. 2011c. Two-year results from an open-label, multicentre, phase III study evaluating the safety and efficacy of canakinumab in patients with cryopyrin-associated periodic syndrome across different severity phenotypes. Annals of the Rheumatic Diseases 70: 2095–102.

Kurt, T., Aydın, F., Nilüfer Tekgöz, P., Sezer, M., Uncu, N. and Çelikel Acar, B. 2020. Effect of anti-interleukin-1 treatment on quality of life in children with colchicine-resistant familial Mediterranean fever: A single-center experience. Int. J. Rheum. Dis. 23: 977–81.

Kuruvilla, M. 2018. Treatment of hypereosinophilic syndrome and eosinophilic dermatitis with reslizumab. Ann. Allergy Asthma Immunol. 120: 670–71.

Lachmann, H. J., Kone-Paut, I., Kuemmerle-Deschner, J. B., Leslie, K. S., Hachulla, E., Quartier, P. X. et al. 2009. Use of canakinumab in the cryopyrin-associated periodic syndrome. N Engl. J. Med. 360: 2416–25.

Laidlaw, T. M., Mullol, J., Fan, C., Zhang, D., Amin, N., Khan, A., Chao, J. et al. 2019. Dupilumab improves nasal polyp burden and asthma control in patients with CRSwNP and AERD. J. Allergy Clin. Immunol. Pract. 7: 2462–65 e1.

Lainka, E., Neudorf, U., Lohse, P., Timmann, C., Bielak, M., Stojanov, S. K. et al. 2012. Incidence and clinical features of hyperimmunoglobulinemia D and periodic fever syndrome (HIDS) and spectrum of mevalonate kinase (MVK) mutations in German children. Rheumatol. Int. 32: 3253–60.

Lesage, A., Marceau, F., Gibson, C., Loenders, B., Katzer, W., Ambrosi, H. D., Saupe, J. A. et al. 2022. *In vitro* pharmacological profile of PHA-022121, a small molecule bradykinin B(2) receptor antagonist in clinical development. Int. Immunopharmacol. 105: 108523.

Levy, R. J., Lumry, W. R., McNeil, D. L., Li, H. H., Campion, M., Horn, P. T. and Pullman, W. E. 2010. EDEMA4: a phase 3, double-blind study of subcutaneous ecallantide treatment for acute attacks of hereditary angioedema. Ann. Allergy Asthma Immunol. 104: 523–9.

Li, J. X., Fan, L. C., Li, M. H., Cao, W. J. and Xu, J. F. 2017. Beneficial effects of Omalizumab therapy in allergic bronchopulmonary aspergillosis: A synthesis review of published literature. Respir. Med. 122: 33–42.

Li, Y., Wang, W., Lv, Z., Li, Y., Chen, Y., Huang, K. C. J. et al. 2018. Elevated expression of IL-33 and TSLP in the airways of human asthmatics *in vivo*: a potential biomarker of severe refractory disease. J. Immunol. 200: 2253–62.

Lieberman, P. and Berger, M. 2013. Intramuscular versus intravenous immunoglobulin replacement therapy and measurement of immunoglobulin levels during immunoglobulin replacement therapy. J. Allergy Clin. Immunol. Pract. 1: 705–6.

Lieberman, P. L., Jones, I., Rajwanshi, R., Rosen, K. and Umetsu, D. T. 2017. Anaphylaxis associated with omalizumab administration: Risk factors and patient characteristics. J. Allergy Clin. Immunol. 140: 1734–36 e4.

Lingman-Framme, J. and Fasth, A. 2013. Subcutaneous immunoglobulin for primary and secondary immunodeficiencies: an evidence-based review. Drugs 73: 1307–19.

Lombardo, N., Pelaia, C., Ciriolo, M., Della Corte, M., Piazzetta, G., Lobello, N. P. et al. 2020. Real-life effects of benralizumab on allergic chronic rhinosinusitis and nasal polyposis associated with severe asthma. Int. J. Immunopathol. Pharmacol. 34: 2058738420950851.

Long, A., Rahmaoui, A., Rothman, K. J., Guinan, E., Eisner, M., Bradley, M. S. et al. 2014. Incidence of malignancy in patients with moderate-to-severe asthma treated with or without omalizumab. J. Allergy Clin. Immunol. 134: 560–67 e4.

Longhurst, H., Cicardi, M., Craig, T., Bork, K., Grattan, C., Baker, J. H. H. et al. 2017. Prevention of hereditary angioedema attacks with a subcutaneous C1 inhibitor. N Engl. J. Med. 376: 1131–40.

Lumry, W. R., Li, H. H., Levy, R. J., Potter, P. C., Farkas, H., Moldovan, D., Riedl, M., Li, H., Craig, T., Bloom, B. J. and Reshef, A. 2011. Randomized placebo-controlled trial of the bradykinin B$_2$ receptor antagonist icatibant for the treatment of acute attacks of hereditary angioedema: the FAST-3 trial. Ann. Allergy Asthma Immunol. 107: 529–37.

Lumry, William R., Timothy Craig, Bruce Zuraw, Hilary Longhurst, James Baker, Henry Li, H. et al. 2018. Health-related quality of life with subcutaneous C1-inhibitor for prevention of attacks of hereditary angioedema. The Journal of Allergy and Clinical Immunology: In Practice 6: 1733–41.e3.

Maetzel, A., Smith, M. D., Duckworth, E. J., Hampton, S. L., De Donatis, G. M., Murugesan, N. et al. 2022. KVD900, an oral on-demand treatment for hereditary angioedema: Phase 1 study results. J. Allergy Clin. Immunol.

Manka, L. A. and Wechsler, M. E. 2018. Selecting the right biologic for your patients with severe asthma. Ann. Allergy Asthma Immunol. 121: 406–13.

Manka, L. A., Guntur, V. P., Denson, J. L., Dunn, R. M., Dollin, Y. T., Strand, M. J. et al. 2021. Efficacy and safety of reslizumab in the treatment of eosinophilic granulomatosis with polyangiitis. Ann. Allergy Asthma Immunol. 126: 696–701 e1.

Markowitz, J. E., Jobe, L., Miller, M., Frost, C., Laney, Z. and Eke, R. 2018. Safety and efficacy of reslizumab for children and adolescents with eosinophilic esophagitis treated for 9 years. J. Pediatr. Gastroenterol. Nutr. 66: 893–97.

Maspero, J. F., FitzGerald, J. M., Pavord, I. D., Rice, M. S., Maroni, J., Rowe, P. J. G. et al. 2021. Dupilumab efficacy in adolescents with uncontrolled, moderate-to-severe asthma: LIBERTY ASTHMA QUEST. Allergy 76: 2621–24.

Maurer, M., Kaplan, A., Rosen, K., Holden, M., Iqbal, A., Trzaskoma, B. L. et al. 2018. The XTEND-CIU study: Long-term use of omalizumab in chronic idiopathic urticaria. J. Allergy Clin. Immunol. 141: 1138–39 e7.

Maurer, M., Gimenez-Arnau, A. M., Sussman, G., Metz, M., Baker, D. R., Bauer, A. et al. 2019. Ligelizumab for chronic spontaneous urticaria. N Engl. J. Med. 381: 1321–32.

Maurer, M., Gimenez-Arnau, A., Bernstein, J. A., Chu, C. Y., Danilycheva, I., Hide, M. M. et al. 2021a. Sustained safety and efficacy of ligelizumab in patients with chronic spontaneous urticaria: A one-year extension study. Allergy.

Maurer, M., Khan, D. A., Elieh Ali Komi, D. and Kaplan, A. P. 2021b. Biologics for the use in chronic spontaneous urticaria: when and which. J. Allergy Clin. Immunol. Pract. 9: 1067–78.

Maurer, M., Magerl, M., Betschel, S., Aberer, W., Ansotegui, I. J., Aygören-Pürsün, E. A. et al. 2022. The international WAO/EAACI guideline for the management of hereditary angioedema-The 2021 revision and update. Allergy.

McKenzie, A., Roberts, A., Malandkar, S., Feuersenger, H., Panousis, C. and Pawaskar, D. 2021. A phase I, first-in-human, randomized dose-escalation study of anti-activated factor XII monoclonal antibody garadacimab. Clin. Transl. Sci.

Menzella, F., Ruggiero, P., Galeone, C., Scelfo, C., Bagnasco, D. and Facciolongo, N. 2020. Significant improvement in lung function and asthma control after benralizumab treatment for severe refractory eosinophilic asthma. Pulm. Pharmacol. Ther. 64: 101966.

Menzies-Gow, A., Corren, J., Bourdin, A., Chupp, G., Israel, E., Wechsler, M. E. et al. 2021. Tezepelumab in adults and adolescents with severe, uncontrolled asthma. N Engl. J. Med. 384: 1800–09.

Metz, M., Vadasz, Z., Kocaturk, E. and Gimenez-Arnau, A. M. 2020. Omalizumab updosing in chronic spontaneous urticaria: an overview of real-world evidence. Clin. Rev. Allergy Immunol. 59: 38–45.

Mikura, S., Saraya, T., Yoshida, Y., Oda, M., Ishida, M., Honda, K. et al. 2021. Successful treatment of mepolizumab- and prednisolone-resistant allergic bronchopulmonary aspergillosis with dupilumab. Intern. Med. 60: 2839–42.

Milgrom, H., Berger, W., Nayak, A., Gupta, N., Pollard, S., McAlary, M. et al. 2001. Treatment of childhood asthma with anti-immunoglobulin E antibody (omalizumab). Pediatrics 108: E36.

Minafra, F. G., Gonçalves, T. R., Alves, T. M. and Pinto, J. A. 2022. The mortality from hereditary angioedema worldwide: a review of the real-world data literature. Clin. Rev. Allergy Immunol. 62: 232–39.

Misbah, S., Sturzenegger, M. H., Borte, M., Shapiro, R. S., Wasserman, R. L., Berger, M. et al. 2009. Subcutaneous immunoglobulin: opportunities and outlook. Clin. Exp. Immunol. 158 Suppl 1: 51–9.

Mitroulis, I., Skendros, P. and Ritis, K. 2010. Targeting IL-1beta in disease; the expanding role of NLRP3 inflammasome. Eur. J. Intern. Med. 21: 157–63.

Mullol, J., Bachert, C., Amin, N., Desrosiers, M., Hellings, P. W., Han, J. K. et al. 2021. Olfactory outcomes with dupilumab in chronic rhinosinusitis with nasal polyps. J. Allergy Clin. Immunol. Pract.

Mummler, C., Munker, D., Barnikel, M., Veit, T., Kayser, M. Z., Welte, T. et al. 2021. Dupilumab improves asthma control and lung function in patients with insufficient outcome during previous antibody therapy. J. Allergy Clin. Immunol. Pract. 9: 1177–85 e4.

Murphy, K., Jacobs, J., Bjermer, L., Fahrenholz, J. M., Shalit, Y., Garin, M. et al. 2017. Long-term safety and efficacy of reslizumab in patients with eosinophilic asthma. J. Allergy Clin. Immunol. Pract. 5: 1572–81 e3.

Nair, P., Wenzel, S., Rabe, K. F., Bourdin, A., Lugogo, N. L., Kuna, P. et al. 2017. Oral glucocorticoid-sparing effect of benralizumab in severe asthma. N Engl. J. Med. 376: 2448–58.

Nair, P., Bardin, P., Humbert, M., Murphy, K. R., Hickey, L., Garin, M. R. et al. 2020. Efficacy of intravenous reslizumab in oral corticosteroid-dependent asthma. J. Allergy Clin. Immunol. Pract. 8: 555–64.

Nakagawa, H., Nemoto, O., Igarashi, A. and Nagata, T. 2018. Efficacy and safety of topical JTE-052, a Janus kinase inhibitor, in Japanese adult patients with moderate-to-severe atopic dermatitis: a phase II, multicentre, randomized, vehicle-controlled clinical study. Br J. Dermatol. 178: 424–32.

Nakagawa, H., Nemoto, O., Igarashi, A., Saeki, H., Kaino, H. and Nagata, T. 2020a. Delgocitinib ointment, a topical Janus kinase inhibitor, in adult patients with moderate to severe atopic dermatitis: A phase 3, randomized, double-blind, vehicle-controlled study and an open-label, long-term extension study. J. Am. Acad. Dermatol. 82: 823–31.

Nakagawa, H., Nemoto, O., Igarashi, A., Saeki, H., Murata, R., Kaino, H. et al. 2020b. Long-term safety and efficacy of delgocitinib ointment, a topical Janus kinase inhibitor, in adult patients with atopic dermatitis. J. Dermatol. 47: 114–20.

Nakagawa, H., Nemoto, O., Igarashi, A., Saeki, H., Kabashima, K., Oda, M. et al. 2021. Delgocitinib ointment in pediatric patients with atopic dermatitis: A phase 3, randomized, double-blind, vehicle-controlled study and a subsequent open-label, long-term study. J. Am. Acad. Dermatol. 85: 854–62.

Namazy, J., Cabana, M. D., Scheuerle, A. E., Thorp, Jr., J. M., Chen, H., Carrigan, G. et al. 2015. The Xolair Pregnancy Registry (EXPECT): the safety of omalizumab use during pregnancy. J. Allergy Clin. Immunol. 135: 407–12.

Namazy, J. A., Blais, L., Andrews, E. B., Scheuerle, A. E., Cabana, M. D., Thorp, J. M. et al. 2020. Pregnancy outcomes in the omalizumab pregnancy registry and a disease-matched comparator cohort. J. Allergy Clin. Immunol. 145: 528–36 e1.

Novartis, unpublished data. 2021. *In*: Novartis provides an update on Phase III ligelizumab (QGE031) studies in chronic spontaneous urticaria (CSU).

O'Quinn, S., Xu, X. and Hirsch, I. 2019. Daily patient-reported health status assessment improvements with benralizumab for patients with severe, uncontrolled eosinophilic asthma. J. Asthma Allergy 12: 21–33.

Orange, J. S., Grossman, W. J., Navickis, R. J. and Wilkes, M. M. 2010. Impact of trough IgG on pneumonia incidence in primary immunodeficiency: A meta-analysis of clinical studies. Clin. Immunol. 137: 21–30.

Ortega. 2014. Mepolizumab treatment in patients with severe eosinophilic asthma. N Engl. J. Med.

Paller, A. S., Siegfried, E. C., Thaci, D., Wollenberg, A., Cork, M. J., Arkwright, P. D. et al. 2020. Efficacy and safety of dupilumab with concomitant topical corticosteroids in children 6 to 11 years old with severe atopic dermatitis: A randomized, double-blinded, placebo-controlled phase 3 trial. J. Am. Acad. Dermatol. 83: 1282–93.

Panettieri, R. A., Jr., Sjobring, U., Peterffy, A., Wessman, P., Bowen, K., Piper, E. et al. 2018. Tralokinumab for severe, uncontrolled asthma (STRATOS 1 and STRATOS 2): two randomised, double-blind, placebo-controlled, phase 3 clinical trials. Lancet Respir. Med. 6: 511–25.

Papp, K., Szepietowski, J. C., Kircik, L., Toth, D., Eichenfield, L. F., Leung, D. Y. M. et al. 2021. Efficacy and safety of ruxolitinib cream for the treatment of atopic dermatitis: Results from 2 phase 3, randomized, double-blind studies. J. Am. Acad. Dermatol. 85: 863–72.

Pelaia, C., Busceti, M. T., Crimi, C., Carpagnano, G. E., Lombardo, N., Terracciano, R. et al. 2020. Real-Life effects of benralizumab on exacerbation number and lung hyperinflation in atopic patients with severe eosinophilic asthma. Biomed. Pharmacother. 129: 110444.

Perez, E. E., Orange, J. S., Bonilla, F., Chinen, J., Chinn, I. K., Dorsey, M. et al. 2017. Update on the use of immunoglobulin in human disease: A review of evidence. J. Allergy Clin. Immunol. 139: S1–s46.

Prematta, M., Gibbs, J. G., Pratt, E. L., Stoughton, T. R. and Craig, T. J. 2007. Fresh frozen plasma for the treatment of hereditary angioedema. Ann. Allergy Asthma Immunol. 98: 383–8.

Rabe, K. F., Nair, P., Brusselle, G., Maspero, J. F., Castro, M., Sher, L. H. et al. 2018. Efficacy and safety of dupilumab in glucocorticoid-dependent severe asthma. N Engl. J. Med. 378: 2475–85.

Ratchataswan, T., Banzon, T. M., Thyssen, J. P., Weidinger, S., Guttman-Yassky, E. and Phipatanakul, W. 2021. Biologics for treatment of atopic dermatitis: current status and future prospect. J. Allergy Clin. Immunol. Pract. 9: 1053–65.

Reich, K., Kabashima, K., Peris, K., Silverberg, J. I., Eichenfield, L. F., Bieber, T., Kaszuba, A. et al. 2020. Efficacy and safety of baricitinib combined with topical corticosteroids for treatment of moderate to severe atopic dermatitis: a randomized clinical trial. JAMA Dermatol. 156: 1333–43.

Reich, K., Teixeira, H. D., de Bruin-Weller, M., Bieber, T., Soong, W., Kabashima, K. T. et al. 2021. Safety and efficacy of upadacitinib in combination with topical corticosteroids in adolescents and adults with moderate-to-severe atopic dermatitis (AD Up): results from a randomised, double-blind, placebo-controlled, phase 3 trial. Lancet 397: 2169–81.

Rich, A. L., Le Jeune, I. R., McDermott, L. and Kinnear, W. J. M. 2008. Serial lung function tests in primary immune deficiency. Clinical & Experimental Immunology 151: 110–13.

Riedl, M. A., Hurewitz, D. S., Levy, R., Busse, P. J., Fitts, D. and Kalfus, I. 2012. Nanofiltered C1 esterase inhibitor (human) for the treatment of acute attacks of hereditary angioedema: an open-label trial. Ann. Allergy Asthma Immunol. 108: 49–53.

Riedl, M. A., Bernstein, J. A., Li, H., Reshef, A., Lumry, W., Moldovan, D. H. et al. 2014. Recombinant human C1-esterase inhibitor relieves symptoms of hereditary angioedema attacks: phase 3, randomized, placebo-controlled trial. Ann. Allergy Asthma Immunol. 112: 163–69.e1.

Riedl, M. A., Li, H. H., Cicardi, M., Harper, J. R. and Relan, A. 2017. Recombinant human C1 esterase inhibitor for acute hereditary angioedema attacks with upper airway involvement. Allergy Asthma Proc. 38: 462–66.

Riedl, Marc A., Aleena Banerji and Richard Gower. 2021. Current medical management of hereditary angioedema: Follow-up survey of US physicians. Annals of Allergy, Asthma & Immunology 126: 264–72.

Rodrigo, G. J., Neffen, H. and Castro-Rodriguez, J. A. 2011. Efficacy and safety of subcutaneous omalizumab vs placebo as add-on therapy to corticosteroids for children and adults with asthma: a systematic review. Chest 139: 28–35.

Roifman, C. M., Lederman, H. M., Lavi, S., Stein, L. D., Levison, H. and Gelfand, E. W. 1985. Benefit of intravenous IgG replacement in hypogammaglobulinemic patients with chronic sinopulmonary disease. Am. J. Med. 79: 171–4.

Roufosse, F., Kahn, J. E., Rothenberg, M. E., Wardlaw, A. J., Klion, A. D., Kirby, S. Y. M. J. et al. 2020. Efficacy and safety of mepolizumab in hypereosinophilic syndrome: A phase III, randomized, placebo-controlled trial. J. Allergy Clin. Immunol. 146: 1397–405.

Ruzicka, T., Hanifin, J. M., Furue, M., Pulka, G., Mlynarczyk, I., Wollenberg, A. et al. 2017. Anti-Interleukin-31 receptor a antibody for atopic dermatitis. N Engl. J. Med. 376: 826–35.

Sag, E., Akal, F., Atalay, E., Akca, U. K., Demir, S., Demirel, D. et al. 2020. Anti-IL1 treatment in colchicine-resistant paediatric FMF patients: real life data from the HELIOS registry. Rheumatology (Oxford) 59: 3324–29.

Saini, S. S., Bindslev-Jensen, C., Maurer, M., Grob, J. J., Bulbul Baskan, E., Bradley, M. S. et al. 2015. Efficacy and safety of omalizumab in patients with chronic idiopathic/spontaneous urticaria who remain symptomatic on H1 antihistamines: A randomized, placebo-controlled study. J. Invest. Dermatol. 135: 925.

Samaan, K., Levasseur, M. C., Decaluwe, H., St-Cyr, C., Chapdelaine, H., Des Roches, A. and Haddad, E. 2014. SCIg vs. IVIg: let's give patients the choice! J. Clin. Immunol. 34: 611–4.

Sanofi, unpublished data. 2020. *In*: Dupixent (dupilumab) eosinophilic esophagitis trial meets both co-primary endpoints.

Sanofi. 2021. Dupixent® (dupilumab) significantly improved itch and hives in patients with chronic spontaneous urticaria, a step forward in demonstrating the role of type 2 inflammation in these patients.

Schleich, F., Vaia, E. S., Pilette, C., Vandenplas, O., Halloy, J. L., Michils, A. R. et al. 2020. Mepolizumab for allergic bronchopulmonary aspergillosis: Report of 20 cases from the Belgian Severe Asthma Registry and review of the literature. J. Allergy Clin. Immunol. Pract. 8: 2412–13 e2.

Schneider, A. and Rubinstein, A. 2018. Benralizumab intended for eosinophilic asthma leads to complete resolution of eosinophilic esophagitis. Annals of Allergy, Asthma and Immunology 121: S127.

Schwab, C., Gabrysch, A., Olbrich, P., Patiño, V., Warnatz, K., Wolff, D. et al. 2018. Phenotype, penetrance, and treatment of 133 cytotoxic T-lymphocyte antigen 4-insufficient subjects. J. Allergy Clin. Immunol. 142: 1932–46.

Shehata, Nadine, Valerie Palda, Tom Bowen, Elie Haddad, Thomas B. Issekutz, Bruce Mazer et al. 2010. The use of immunoglobulin therapy for patients with primary immune deficiency: an evidence-based practice guideline. Transfusion Medicine Reviews 24: S28–S50.

Silverberg, J. I., Pinter, A., Pulka, G., Poulin, Y., Bouaziz, J. D., Wollenberg, A. et al. 2020a. Phase 2B randomized study of nemolizumab in adults with moderate-to-severe atopic dermatitis and severe pruritus. J. Allergy Clin. Immunol. 145: 173–82.

Silverberg, J. I., Simpson, E. L., Thyssen, J. P., Gooderham, M., Chan, G., Feeney, C. et al. 2020b. Efficacy and safety of abrocitinib in patients with moderate-to-severe atopic dermatitis: a randomized clinical trial. JAMA Dermatol. 156: 863–73.

Silverberg, J. I., Yosipovitch, G., Simpson, E. L., Kim, B. S., Wu, J. J., Eckert, L. I. et al. 2020c. Dupilumab treatment results in early and sustained improvements in itch in adolescents and adults with moderate to severe atopic dermatitis: Analysis of the randomized phase 3 studies SOLO 1 and SOLO 2, AD ADOL, and CHRONOS. J. Am. Acad. Dermatol, 82: 1328–36.

Silverberg, J. I., de Bruin-Weller, M., Bieber, T., Soong, W., Kabashima, K., Costanzo, A. et al. 2021a. Upadacitinib plus topical corticosteroids in atopic dermatitis: Week 52 AD Up study results. J. Allergy Clin. Immunol.

Silverberg, J. I., Simpson, E. L., Wollenberg, A., Bissonnette, R., Kabashima, K., DeLozier, A. M. et al. 2021b. Long-term efficacy of baricitinib in adults with moderate to severe atopic dermatitis who were treatment responders or partial responders: an extension study of 2 randomized clinical trials. JAMA Dermatol. 157: 691–99.

Silverberg, J. I., Thyssen, J. P., Simpson, E. L., Yosipovitch, G., Stander, S., Valdez, H. et al. 2021c. Impact of oral abrocitinib monotherapy on patient-reported symptoms and quality of life in adolescents and adults with moderate-to-severe atopic dermatitis: a pooled analysis of patient-reported outcomes. Am. J. Clin. Dermatol. 22: 541–54.

Silverberg, J. I., Toth, D., Bieber, T., Alexis, A. F., Elewski, B. E., Pink, A. E. et al. 2021d. Tralokinumab plus topical corticosteroids for the treatment of moderate-to-severe atopic dermatitis: results from the double-blind, randomized, multicentre, placebo-controlled phase III ECZTRA 3 trial. Br J. Dermatol. 184: 450–63.

Simpson, E. L., Bieber, T., Guttman-Yassky, E., Beck, L. A., Blauvelt, A., Cork, M. J. et al. 2016. Two phase 3 trials of dupilumab versus placebo in atopic dermatitis. N Engl. J. Med. 375: 2335–48.

Simpson, E. L., Flohr, C., Eichenfield, L. F., Bieber, T., Sofen, H., Taieb, A. et al. 2018. Efficacy and safety of lebrikizumab (an anti-IL-13 monoclonal antibody) in adults with moderate-to-severe atopic dermatitis inadequately controlled by topical corticosteroids: A randomized, placebo-controlled phase II trial (TREBLE). J. Am. Acad. Dermatol. 78: 863–71 e11.

Simpson, E. L., Parnes, J. R., She, D., Crouch, S., Rees, W., Mo, M. et al. 2019. Tezepelumab, an anti-thymic stromal lymphopoietin monoclonal antibody, in the treatment of moderate to severe atopic dermatitis: A randomized phase 2a clinical trial. J. Am. Acad. Dermatol. 80: 1013–21.

Simpson, E. L., Lacour, J. P., Spelman, L., Galimberti, R., Eichenfield, L. F., Bissonnette, R. et al. 2020a. Baricitinib in patients with moderate-to-severe atopic dermatitis and inadequate response to topical corticosteroids: results from two randomized monotherapy phase III trials. Br J. Dermatol. 183: 242–55.

Simpson, E. L., Paller, A. S., Siegfried, E. C., Boguniewicz, M., Sher, L., Gooderham, M. J. et al. 2020b. Efficacy and safety of dupilumab in adolescents with uncontrolled moderate to severe atopic dermatitis: a phase 3 randomized clinical trial. JAMA Dermatol. 156: 44–56.

Simpson, E. L., Sinclair, R., Forman, S., Wollenberg, A., Aschoff, R., Cork, M. T. et al. 2020c. Efficacy and safety of abrocitinib in adults and adolescents with moderate-to-severe atopic dermatitis (JADE MONO-1): a multicentre, double-blind, randomised, placebo-controlled, phase 3 trial. Lancet 396: 255–66.

Simpson, E. L. 2021. Safety of specifically targeting interleukin 13 with tralokinumab in adult patients with moderate-to-severe atopic dermatitis: pooled analysis of five randomized, double-blind, placebo-controlled phase 3 and phase 2 trials. https://jofskin.org/index.php/skin/article/view/1164.

Simpson, E. L., Silverberg, J. I., Nosbaum, A., Winthrop, K. L., Guttman-Yassky, E., Hoffmeister, K. M. et al. 2021. Integrated safety analysis of abrocitinib for the treatment of moderate-to-severe atopic dermatitis from the phase II and phase iii clinical trial program. Am. J. Clin. Dermatol. 22: 693–707.

Singh, J. A., Wells, G. A., Christensen, R., Tanjong Ghogomu, E., Maxwell, L., Macdonald, J. K. G. et al. 2011. Adverse effects of biologics: a network meta-analysis and Cochrane overview. Cochrane Database Syst. Rev. 2011: Cd008794.

Soler, M., Matz, J., Townley, R., Buhl, R., O'Brien, J., Fox, H. J. et al. 2001. The anti-IgE antibody omalizumab reduces exacerbations and steroid requirement in allergic asthmatics. Eur .Respir. J. 18: 254–61.

Staubach, P., Metz, M., Chapman-Rothe, N., Sieder, C., Brautigam, M., Canvin, J. et al. 2016. Effect of omalizumab on angioedema in H1-antihistamine-resistant chronic spontaneous urticaria patients: results from X-ACT, a randomized controlled trial. Allergy 71: 1135–44.

Steinfeld, J., Bradford, E. S., Brown, J., Mallett, S., Yancey, S. W., Akuthota, P. et al. 2019. Evaluation of clinical benefit from treatment with mepolizumab for patients with eosinophilic granulomatosis with polyangiitis. J. Allergy Clin. Immunol. 143: 2170–77.

Straesser, M. D., Oliver, E., Palacios, T., Kyin, T., Patrie, J., Borish, L. S. et al. 2018. Serum IgE as an immunological marker to predict response to omalizumab treatment in symptomatic chronic urticaria. J. Allergy Clin. Immunol. Pract. 6: 1386–88 e1.

Sussman, G., Hebert, J., Gulliver, W., Lynde, C., Yang, W. H., Papp, K. et al. 2020. Omalizumab re-treatment and step-up in patients with chronic spontaneous urticaria: OPTIMA trial. J. Allergy Clin. Immunol. Pract. 8: 2372–78 e5.

Tapia-Abellán, A., Angosto-Bazarra, D., Martínez-Banaclocha, H., de Torre-Minguela, C., Cerón-Carrasco, J. P., Pérez-Sánchez, H. et al. 2019. MCC950 closes the active conformation of NLRP3 to an inactive state. Nat. Chem. Biol. 15: 560–64.

ter Haar, Nienke, Helen Lachmann, Seza Özen, Pat Woo, Yosef Uziel et al. 2013. Treatment of autoinflammatory diseases: results from the Eurofever Registry and a literature review. Annals of the Rheumatic Diseases 72: 678–85.

Tesch, V. K., Abolhassani, H., Shadur, B., Zobel, J., Mareika, Y., Sharapova, S. et al. 2020. Long-term outcome of LRBA deficiency in 76 patients after various treatment modalities as evaluated by the immune deficiency and dysregulation activity (IDDA) score. J. Allergy Clin. Immunol. 145: 1452–63.

Thyssen, J. P., Buhl, T., Fernandez-Penas, P., Kabashima, K., Chen, S., Lu, N. et al. 2021. Baricitinib rapidly improves skin pain resulting in improved quality of life for patients with atopic dermatitis: analyses from BREEZE-AD1, 2, and 7. Dermatol. Ther. (Heidelb) 11: 1599–611.

Tomomatsu, K., Sugino, Y., Okada, N., Tanaka, J., Oguma, T. and Asano, K. 2020. Rapid clearance of mepolizumab-resistant bronchial mucus plugs in allergic bronchopulmonary aspergillosis with benralizumab treatment. Allergol. Int. 69: 636–38.

Trischler, J., Bottoli, I., Janocha, R., Heusser, C., Jaumont, X., Lowe, P. et al. 2021. Ligelizumab treatment for severe asthma: learnings from the clinical development programme. Clin. Transl. Immunology 10: e1255.

Ueno, M., Miyagawa, I., Nakano, K., Iwata, S., Hanami, K., Fukuyo, S. et al. 2021. Effectiveness and safety of mepolizumab in combination with corticosteroids in patients with eosinophilic granulomatosis with polyangiitis. Arthritis Res. Ther. 23: 86.

van der Hilst, J. C. H., Bodar, E. J., Barron, K. S., Frenkel, J., Drenth, J. P. H., van der Meer, J. W. M. et al. 2008. Long-term follow-up, clinical features, and quality of life in a series of 103 patients with hyperimmunoglobulinemia D syndrome. Medicine (Baltimore) 87: 301–10.

van der Hilst, J. C. H., Moutschen, M., Messiaen, P. E., Lauwerys, B. R. and Vanderschueren, S. 2016. Efficacy of anti-IL-1 treatment in familial Mediterranean fever: a systematic review of the literature. Biologics 10: 75–80.

van Doorn, Martijn B. A., Jacobus Burggraaf, Tijtje van Dam, Anke Eerenberg, Marcel Levi, Cornelis E. Hack et al. 2005. A phase I study of recombinant human C1 inhibitor in asymptomatic patients with hereditary angioedema. Journal of Allergy and Clinical Immunology. 116: 876–83.

van Leeuwen, E. M., Cuadrado, E., Gerrits, A. M., Witteveen, E. and de Bree, G. J. 2018. Treatment of intracerebral lesions with abatacept in a CTLA4-haploinsufficient patient. J. Clin. Immunol. 38: 464–67.

Varricchi, G., Pecoraro, A., Marone, G., Criscuolo, G., Spadaro, G., Genovese, A. et al. 2018. Thymic stromal lymphopoietin isoforms, inflammatory disorders, and cancer. Front Immunol. 9: 1595.

Verbruggen, K., Van Cauwenberge, P. and Bachert, C. 2009. Anti-IgE for the treatment of allergic rhinitis--and eventually nasal polyps? Int. Arch. Allergy Immunol. 148: 87–98.

Virchow, J. C., Katial, R., Brusselle, G. G., Shalit, Y., Garin, M., McDonald, M. et al. 2020. Safety of reslizumab in uncontrolled asthma with eosinophilia: a pooled analysis from 6 trials. J. Allergy Clin. Immunol. Pract. 8: 540–48 e1.

von Spee-Mayer, C., Echternach, C., Agarwal, P., Gutenberger, S., Soetedjo, V., Goldacker, S. et al. 2021. Abatacept use is associated with steroid dose reduction and improvement in fatigue and CD4-dysregulation in CVID patients with interstitial lung disease. J. Allergy Clin. Immunol. Pract. 9: 760–70.e10.

Wahn, V., Aberer, W., Aygören-Pürsün, E., Bork, K., Eberl, W., Faßhauer, M. et al. 2020. Hereditary angioedema in children and adolescents—A consensus update on therapeutic strategies for German-speaking countries. Pediatr. Allergy Immunol. 31: 974–89.

Waldman, R. A., DeWane, M. E., Sloan, B. and Grant-Kels, J. M. 2020. Characterizing dupilumab facial redness: A multi-institution retrospective medical record review. J. Am. Acad. Dermatol. 82: 230–32.

Walker, L. S. 2013. Treg and CTLA-4: two intertwining pathways to immune tolerance. J. Autoimmun 45: 49–57.

Wechsler, M. E., Akuthota, P., Jayne, D., Khoury, P., Klion, A., Langford, C. A. P et al. 2017. Mepolizumab or placebo for eosinophilic granulomatosis with polyangiitis. N Engl. J. Med. 376: 1921–32.

Wechsler, M. E., Hickey, L., Garin, M. and Chauhan, A. 2020. Efficacy of reslizumab treatment in exacerbation-prone patients with severe eosinophilic asthma. J. Allergy Clin. Immunol. Pract. 8: 3434–42 e4.

Wechsler, M. E., Ford, L. B., Maspero, J. F., Pavord, I. D., Papi, A., Bourdin, A. et al. 2021a. Long-term safety and efficacy of dupilumab in patients with moderate-to-severe asthma (TRAVERSE): an open-label extension study. Lancet Respir. Med.

Wechsler, M. E., Peters, S. P., Hill, T. D., Ariely, R., DePietro, M. R., Driessen, M. T. et al. 2021b. Clinical outcomes and health-care resource use associated with reslizumab treatment in adults with severe eosinophilic asthma in real-world practice. Chest 159: 1734–46.

Wechsler, M. E., Ruddy, M. K., Pavord, I. D., Israel, E., Rabe, K. F., Ford, L. B. et al. 2021c. Efficacy and safety of itepekimab in patients with moderate-to-severe asthma. N Engl. J. Med. 385: 1656–68.

Wedner, H. J., Aygören-Pürsün, E., Bernstein, J., Craig, T., Gower, R., Jacobs, J. S. et al. 2021. Randomized trial of the efficacy and safety of berotralstat (BCX7353) as an oral prophylactic therapy for hereditary angioedema: results of APeX-2 through 48 weeks (Part 2). J. Allergy Clin. Immunol. Pract. 9: 2305–14.e4.

Weinblatt, M., Combe, B., Covucci, A., Aranda, R., Becker, J. C. and Keystone, E. 2006. Safety of the selective costimulation modulator abatacept in rheumatoid arthritis patients receiving background biologic and nonbiologic disease-modifying antirheumatic drugs: A one-year randomized, placebo-controlled study. Arthritis Rheum. 54: 2807–16.

Weinstein, S. F., Katial, R. K., Bardin, P., Korn, S., McDonald, M., Garin, M. et al. 2019. Effects of reslizumab on asthma outcomes in a subgroup of eosinophilic asthma patients with self-reported chronic rhinosinusitis with nasal polyps. J. Allergy Clin. Immunol. Pract. 7: 589–96 e3.

Wentzel, N., Panieri, A., Ayazi, M., Ntshalintshali, S. D., Pourpak, Z., Hawarden, D., Potter, P. et al. 2019. Fresh frozen plasma for on-demand hereditary angioedema treatment in South Africa and Iran. World Allergy Organ J. 12: 100049.

Wenzel, S., Ford, L., Pearlman, D., Spector, S., Sher, L., Skobieranda, F. et al. 2013. Dupilumab in persistent asthma with elevated eosinophil levels. N Engl. J. Med. 368: 2455–66.

Wenzel, S., Castro, M., Corren, J., Maspero, J., Wang, L., Zhang, B. et al. 2016. Dupilumab efficacy and safety in adults with uncontrolled persistent asthma despite use of medium-to-high-dose inhaled corticosteroids plus a long-acting beta2 agonist: a randomised double-blind placebo-controlled pivotal phase 2b dose-ranging trial. Lancet 388: 31–44.

Wilkerson, R. G. and Moellman, J. J. 2022. Hereditary Angioedema. Emerg. Med. Clin. North Am. 40: 99–118.

Williams, Anesu H. and Timothy J. Craig. 2015. Perioperative management for patients with hereditary angioedema. Allergy & Rhinology (Providence, R.I.) 6: 50–55.

Windegger, Tanja M., Son Nghiem, Kim-Huong Nguyen, Yoke-Lin Fung and Paul A. Scuffham. 2019. Cost–utility analysis comparing hospital-based intravenous immunoglobulin with home-based subcutaneous immunoglobulin in patients with secondary immunodeficiency. Vox Sanguinis 114: 237–46.

Wollenberg, A., Beck, L. A., de Bruin Weller, M., Simpson, E. L., Imafuku, S., Boguniewicz, M. et al. 2021a. Conjunctivitis in adult patients with moderate-to-severe atopic dermatitis: results from five tralokinumab clinical trials. Br J. Dermatol.

Wollenberg, A., Blauvelt, A., Guttman-Yassky, E., Worm, M., Lynde, C., Lacour, J. P. et al. 2021b. Tralokinumab for moderate-to-severe atopic dermatitis: results from two 52-week, randomized, double-blind, multicentre, placebo-controlled phase III trials (ECZTRA 1 and ECZTRA 2). Br J. Dermatol. 184: 437–49.

Wollenberg, A., Nakahara, T., Maari, C., Peris, K., Lio, P., Augustin, M. et al. 2021c. Impact of baricitinib in combination with topical steroids on atopic dermatitis symptoms, quality of life and functioning in adult patients with moderate-to-severe atopic dermatitis from the BREEZE-AD7 Phase 3 randomized trial. J. Eur. Acad. Dermatol. Venereol. 35: 1543–52.

Wu, Q., Yuan, L., Qiu, H., Wang, X., Huang, X. and Zheng Yang, R. 2021. Efficacy and safety of omalizumab in chronic rhinosinusitis with nasal polyps: a systematic review and meta-analysis of randomised controlled trials. BMJ Open 11: e047344.

Xiong, X. F., Zhu, M., Wu, H. X., Fan, L. L. and Cheng, D. Y. 2019. Efficacy and safety of dupilumab for the treatment of uncontrolled asthma: a meta-analysis of randomized clinical trials. Respir. Res. 20: 108.

Yokota, S., Imagawa, T., Nishikomori, R., Takada, H., Abrams, K., Lheritier, K. et al. 2017. Long-term safety and efficacy of canakinumab in cryopyrin-associated periodic syndrome: results from an open-label, phase III pivotal study in Japanese patients. Clin. Exp. Rheumatol. 35 Suppl 108: 19–26.

Yu, M., Terhorst-Molawi, D., Altrichter, S., Hawro, T., Chen, Y. D., Liu, B. X. T. et al. 2021. Omalizumab in chronic inducible urticaria: A real-life study of efficacy, safety, predictors of treatment outcome and time to response. Clin. Exp. Allergy 51: 730–34.

Zhao, Z. T., Ji, C. M., Yu, W. J., Meng, L., Hawro, T., Wei, J. F. et al. 2016. Omalizumab for the treatment of chronic spontaneous urticaria: A meta-analysis of randomized clinical trials. J. Allergy Clin. Immunol. 137: 1742–50 e4.

Zuizewind, C. A., van Kessel, P., Kramer, C. M., Muijs, M. M., Zwiers, J. C. and Triemstra, M. 2018. Home-based treatment with immunoglobulins: an evaluation from the perspective of patients and healthcare professionals. J. Clin. Immunol. 38: 876–85.

Zuraw, B. L., Busse, P. J., White, M., Jacobs, J., Lumry, W., Baker, J. et al. 2010. Nanofiltered C1 inhibitor concentrate for treatment of hereditary angioedema. N Engl. J. Med. 363: 513–22.

Zuraw, B. L., Davis, D. K., Castaldo, A. J. and Christiansen, S. C. 2016. Tolerability and effectiveness of 17-α-alkylated androgen therapy for hereditary angioedema: a re-examination. J. Allergy Clin. Immunol. Pract. 4: 948–55.e15.

Zuraw, B., Lumry, W. R., Johnston, D. T., Aygören-Pürsün, E., Banerji, A., Bernstein, J. A. et al. 2021. Oral once daily berotralstat for the prevention of hereditary angioedema attacks: A randomized, double-blind, placebo-controlled phase 3 trial. J. Allergy Clin. Immunol. 148: 164–72.e9.

Chapter 11

Environmental Control in Allergic Diseases

Sitesh Roy[1],* and *Thomas Platts-Mills*[2]

Introduction

Inhaled allergens are well known to trigger immediate hypersensitivity reactions among children and young adults with asthma and rhinitis. With sensitization to one or more of the major indoor allergens (such as dust mites, cats, dogs or cockroaches) if a significant accumulation of those relevant allergens is present in the house, it has been consistently found to be one of the strongest risk factors for asthma in population, case-control and prospective studies (Platts-Mills et al. 1997; Peat et al. 1996; Sporik et al. 1990; Sears et al. 1989; Squillace et al. 1997). Similarly many harmful, toxic or potentially noxious indoor air pollutants/irritants are known to induce inflammation in the airways of both allergic and non-allergic individuals. Indoor air is laden with both of the above and hence presents a unique opportunity to intervene for susceptible individuals.

This chapter reviews the specific environmental control measures for reducing exposure to such indoor allergens and other relevant harmful exposures. Also, where possible the measures with the most clinical evidence for their positive impact are delineated from the less proven or unproven techniques.

Core Principles

A causal relationship between allergen exposure and asthma has been evidenced from bronchoprovocation experiments demonstrating that these allergens can induce bronchospasm, eosinophilic airway inflammation and prolonged increases in bronchial hyper-reactivity (Cockcroft et al. 1979; Calhoun et al. 1994). The stronger proof is evidenced by moving some asthmatic children or adults from their homes to a different low-allergen residential setting resulting in major improvements in their clinical symptoms and bronchial hyper-reactivity (Platts-Mills et al. 1997; Platt-Mills et al. 1982; Kerrebijn 1970). This background provides a powerful rationale for recommending that allergic patients should reduce allergen exposure in their houses as part of the management of asthma and allergic rhinitis (Sharma et al. 2007).

[1] Founder-Director Dr Roy Health Solutions Clinics, Mumbai, India.
[2] Professor of Medicine, Division of Allergy, Asthma and Immunology, University of Virginia, Charlottesville, Virginia USA.
* Corresponding author: siteshroy@gmail.com

Dominant allergens vary based on region, climate, housekeeping practices and pet ownership. In particular, there are now well-defined geographic areas where dust mites or cockroaches or pet dander are the strongest contributors to asthma risk. It is also possible that certain indoor allergens, such as house dust mites/storage mites, are more important in the pathogenesis of allergic airway disease than others, and this is an area of active investigation (Erwin et al. 2005a, Erwin et al. 2005b; Erwin et al. 2007; Platts-Mills et al. 2007).

Specific monoclonal antibody-based assays have been developed to monitor allergen levels during controlled trials and to test the specific measures recommended to control exposure to dust mites, cat, dog and cockroach antigens (Erwin and Platts-Mills 2005; Luczynska et al. 1989; Chapman et al. 1988). These techniques have facilitated detailed studies of specific allergens and have helped to define effective control measures, but due to the exquisite specificity of these measurements, some forms of the specific allergen (e.g., some isoforms of Der p 1) may escape detection (van Ree 2007).

Why Is Allergen Avoidance Important?

Allergen avoidance is appropriate for symptomatic patients with clinically relevant allergic responses documented either via positive skin tests (*in vivo*) or serum assays (*in vitro*) for specific immunoglobulin E (IgE) antibodies (Cloutier et al. 2020; Matsui and Peng 2020). It is important to implement a comprehensive environmental control plan for all, or as many as possible, of the allergens that are identified as clinically relevant to that patient based on specific testing (Matsui and Peng 2020).

Patient Education and Cost

Patient/parent education is essential for the successful modification of the home environment and for influencing the natural history of allergies. Simply handing a sheet of recommendations to a patient without providing detailed education about the proposed measures considering the practicality of implementation for that patient or specific follow-up is unlikely to be effective.

Several studies have examined the use of allergy testing and specific advice about the avoidance of relevant allergens in the primary care (family physicians/general practitioners) setting (Bobb and Ritz 2003; Sibbald et al. 1997; Brydon 1993; Smith et al. 2015). Indeed, some interventions can be both effective and practical, such as removal of old carpeting from the home of dust mite-allergic patients, overall results have been mixed. It still makes good sense for the primary care physician to provide such education on the basis of skin test or specific IgE blood test results, which can play a major role in educating the patient about the relevance of allergen exposure and in encouraging compliance with measures proposed following evaluation by an allergy specialist. Perhaps the primary hurdle is lack of sufficient time to explain the proposed interventions. Often times, the primary educational role falls on the technician, nurse, nurse practitioner or nurse assistant, who can spend time with patients, discussing allergen avoidance, asthma therapy and smoking cessation.

The clinician should be mindful that major environmental modifications, such as removing carpeting, modifying heating systems, professional pest management or replacing old upholstered furniture, are expensive and may not be affordable to many families. Recognition of this and an initial emphasis on low-cost interventions would greatly enhance patient cooperation and outcomes.

Importance of Addressing All Allergens Relevant to That Patient

Studies showing that environmental control was effective were those in which the specific measures taken were tailored to the patient and addressed all of the major allergens to which each patient was sensitized (Morgan et al. 2004; van Schayck et al. 2007). The literature contains many studies that addressed single interventions, which often fail to demonstrate efficacy (Leas et al. 2018). It is imperative for future environmental control studies to use validated outcome measurements and adequate sample sizes to show clinically meaningful benefits.

Urban children with moderate-to-severe asthma represent a population that has been studied with regard to the impact of environmental allergen control on asthma. Comprehensive environmental modification in these children is effective in reducing asthma symptoms and appears to be cost-effective if carefully performed (Morgan et al. 2004; Kattan et al. 2005).

Assessing the Efficacy of Avoidance Measures

Improvement in the patient's symptoms is the most practical means of assessing the effectiveness of allergen control and avoidance measures in clinical practice. Repeating skin testing or *in vitro* testing is not recommended. Even when allergic individuals are able to avoid an allergen, the immunologic changes that result are not easily predicted despite changes in clinical manifestations of the allergy. A study on college students who experienced a prolonged decrease in exposure to cats showed a highly significant decrease in immunoglobulin G (IgG) to Fel d 1 but very little change in immunoglobulin E (IgE) antibody (Erwin et al. 2014).

Principles of Environmental Allergen Control

- Control potential sources of allergen (e.g., pets, rodents and cockroaches).
- Minimize sites in which mold or dust mites can grow.
- Minimize reservoirs of allergen (e.g., soft toys, upholstered sofas, carpets and uncovered pillows or bedding).
- Clinicians should know the cost of interventions and emphasize less expensive measures initially.
- Recognize that a minority of patients are primarily exposed outside their home, in environments they cannot directly control (e.g., work or school).
- For motivated patients who have adequate resources, we suggest the implementation of avoidance measures for all of the indoor allergens to which the patient is allergic/sensitized.

House Dust Mites

Dust mites (*Dermatophagoides pteronyssinus* and *D. farinae*) are arthropods of the class Arachnida that colonize bedding, sofas, carpets or any woven material. In tropical countries like India, other species like Blomia tropicalis, also have a great role to play in inciting allergies. Dust mites do not bite, and aside from causing allergic diseases, they are not known to pose any other harm to humans. Patients might have difficulty conceptualizing house dust mites because neither the dust mites, nor their debris, can be seen by the naked eye under normal circumstances. The first scientific proof of house dust mites as the main allergen contributor to house dust which had been documented to trigger asthma attacks since 1698 in medical literature, was in October 1964 in a landmark publication by Voorhorst and the Spieksma's from Germany (Voorhorst et al. 1964).

Dust mites absorb humidity from the atmosphere and feed on organic matter (including shed human and animal skin particles), usually with the aid of fungal degradation. They require nests to live in, a source of food (generally readily available in indoor environments with humans and pets) and sufficient humidity. Dust mite infestation is far less common in arid and high-altitude climates. In addition, in areas that have prolonged cold winters, indoor environments can be so dry that they are usually free of dust mites.

Dust mite fecal particles contain a complex mixture of allergenic dust mite-derived proteins, endotoxin, enzymes and dust mite and bacterial DNA, all of which can be immuno-stimulatory (Wan et al. 1999; Ghaemmaghami et al. 2001). These particles are relatively large and heavy and become transiently airborne after vigorous disturbance and settle rapidly with no allergen detectable in the air within 15 minutes (Tovey et al. 1981). Thus, air filtration only has a minor role in controlling exposure to dust mite allergens. Instead, exposure is believed to occur primarily by proximity to dust mite debris during time spent in bed, on the floor or upholstered furniture.

Dust mite avoidance has been shown both to decrease symptoms and decrease non-specific bronchial hyper-reactivity (Wilson and Platts-Mills 2018). Additionally, in a double-blind controlled trial on children with a history of repeated severe episodes of asthma, mite-proof encasings have been shown to decrease these acute episodes of asthma requiring treatment in a hospital setting (Murray et al. 2017; Platts-Mills et al. 2017).

The decision to recommend avoidance of mite allergens as a treatment requires evidence that the patient is sensitized and that mite exposure is playing a significant role in the patient's symptoms (clinical relevance of exposure to the allergen). Given the widespread prevalence of these allergens in the home environment and the necessary education plus interventions needed to get successful results, some clinicians are not fully convinced that this should be a primary part of the treatment.

In tropical countries like India, severe mite allergy is often seen in tertiary care clinics and up to 60–70% of patients with allergic rhinitis and asthma are sensitized to these allergens. Most patients have high exposure to mite allergens in their homes and hence dust mite avoidance measures are relevant and necessary. Given the lack of knowledge about dust mite allergies and the suboptimal use of moderate or high dose-inhaled/nasal steroids to manage these conditions allergen avoidance is still an effective first step along with pharmacotherapy for many allergic patients. Hence, it is inappropriate to ignore the dominant role of exposure to mite allergens as a cause of allergic disease and certainly, all mite-allergic patients should be advised to take steps to decrease exposure in the home.

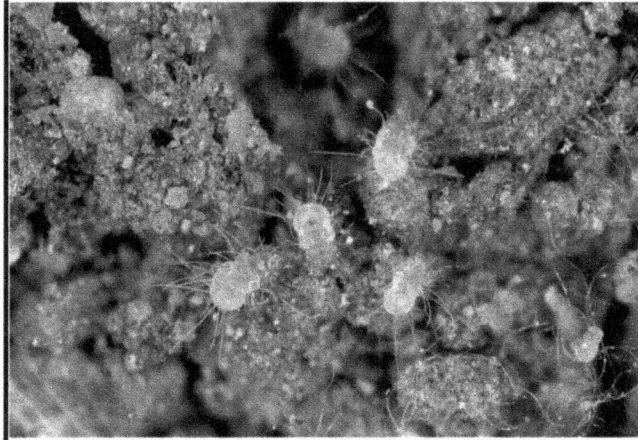

Figure 1. House Dust Mite.

Potential Options for Dust Mite Control

Effective avoidance measures include physical barriers, controlling humidity and removing areas, such as carpets and furniture that can harbor dust mite colonies. Other potential measures to reduce exposure to dust mite allergens include heat treatment, acaricides and allergen-denaturing agents.

Physical Barriers

Physical barriers used to control domestic allergen exposure include covers for pillows, mattresses, box springs, comforters and furniture cushions.

The simplest types of covers are plastic, which is uncomfortable for many patients due to non-breathability and hence sweating. Identifying a variety of alternative fabrics, including coated plastics, permeable synthetics that allow vapor and air movement, non-woven synthetics that allow airflow without passage of particles > 1 micron in diameter, and finely woven fabrics with pore sizes as small as 2 microns has required considerable effort (Vaughan et al. 1999). Woven fabrics with a designated pore size up to approximately 6 microns are preferable because these are very effective at controlling the passage of dust mite as well as cat allergens, while still permitting adequate air flow. These fabrics will also completely block the passage of immature and adult live dust mites. Woven fabrics are identifiable by their smooth texture, higher relative cost, and ability to be laundered repeatedly. In contrast, non-woven materials, which look and feel similar to heavyweight paper towels, can retain allergen on the surface and lose integrity with repeated washing (Miller et al. 2007).

The use of bedding covers as an isolated intervention is unlikely to reduce rhinitis or asthma symptoms to a clinically meaningful degree. Instead, bedding covers should be a component of a comprehensive plan to reduce exposure to dust mites, as well as any other allergens that are important to that patient.

- Over 1,100 adults with asthma and dust mite sensitivity, were randomly assigned to receive allergen-impermeable bed covers or placebo bed covers that allowed passage of dust mite allergen (Woodcock et al. 2003). Although applied without proper advice about washing bedding, the covers produced a significant decrease in dust mite allergen for three months. However, the changes in dust mite allergen were modest and were not associated with decreased asthma symptoms.

- A systematic review of just two trials led the reviewers to conclude that controlled trials of allergen avoidance for perennial allergic rhinitis were not convincing (Nurmatov et al. 2012). This was partly for technical reasons in assessing symptoms and also because only a limited number of subjects in these studies were selectively allergic to dust mite.

Even though the use of dust mite-impermeable bedding covers (as an isolated intervention) is probably not sufficient to produce clinical improvement, this intervention is an essential component of any strategy to reduce dust mite exposure (Morgan et al. 2004; Shedd et al. 2007). The key here is that effective allergen avoidance must target all of the allergens that are important for that patient (Woodcock et al. 2003; Terreehorst et al. 2003; Luczynska et al. 2003).

Minimizing Upholstery and Fabric Reservoirs

Efforts should be made to restrict the presence of carpets, upholstered furniture and drapes in the environment of the dust mite-allergic person in order to reduce the sites that can be colonized by dust mites or covered by their allergens. Wet wiping of surfaces as opposed to dusting and vacuuming of floors using a vacuum equipped with a high-efficiency particulate air (HEPA) filter or with double-thickness bags should be performed regularly. The number of stuffed toys in children's bedrooms should be minimized. Carpeting can be removed and replaced with finished floors (tiles, marble and wood) and washable area rugs.

These measures are particularly important in the rooms where the patient spends the greatest amount of time, such as the bedroom and living rooms where the television and computer are used.

Regulation of Humidity

Decreasing humidity can reduce dust mite replication and maintaining relative humidity below 50% is recommended. This can be accomplished by the regular opening of windows in a dry climate or air conditioning in a humid climate (Korsgaard 1983). Humidifiers should be generally avoided because they can easily become contaminated, and overuse will result in improved growth of mites and fungi. Dehumidifiers may be effective in reducing humidity in selective areas; e.g., bedroom, but not the whole house. Patients who report dry nasal passages should be encouraged to keep the temperature of their houses lower and to use saline nasal sprays before going to bed instead of humidifying the entire bedroom.

Upper floors usually have less humidity than lower floors. Carpets tend to become and remain damp in high-humidity areas, after which they can become a rich source of bacterial, fungal, and dust mite allergens (Platts-Mills et al. 1987). In some climates, apartments have dramatically less humidity than houses and commonly have up to 10-fold less dust mite allergen. In such situations, moving to an apartment on the second or higher floor may be an effective method of reducing dust mite exposure.

Heat Treatment

Both dry heat and steam treatments can eradicate dust mites and reduce exposure to dust mite allergens. One study demonstrated that commercial steam cleaning of carpets kills dust mites and reduces dust mite allergen levels (Colloff et al. 1995). In another study, asthmatic patients were randomized to receive treatment of mattresses and duvets with hot air (110°C/230°F) and steam, as well as steam cleaning of carpets vs. sham treatments (Htut et al. 2001). A single active environmental treatment resulted in a significant and sustained reduction in Der p 1 and 2 dust mite allergen concentrations and a reduction in bronchial reactivity as determined by bronchoprovocation testing that was maintained for 9 to 12 months.

Thus, washing sheets, pillow cases, mattress pads, and blankets weekly in hot water effectively reduces dust mite counts (McDonald and Tovey 1992). We recommend that bedding be washed in hot water (55°C or 120°F) with any detergent and when available dried in an electric clothes dryer on a hot setting (McDonald and Tovey 1992; Miller et al. 1996). The placing of mattresses and pillows in the hot sun for 4 hours in tropical countries, as a measure to kill house dust mites, while seemingly intuitive, actually ends up leaving a lot of dead mite body parts and feces in these and has not been scientifically proven to make a difference.

Insecticides and Allergen-Denaturing Agents

The use of chemicals to kill dust mites or denature allergens has also been investigated, but the data in favor of this approach are modest. Several chemicals have been tested, but only benzyl benzoate and tannic acid have been commonly used. Prolonged eradication of dust mites is not possible with commercially available chemicals.

- Benzyl benzoate is highly toxic to dust mites in the laboratory setting, but when applied to carpets, produces only a modest decrease in allergens ($< 60\%$) that is short-lived (Hayden et al. 1992).
- Tannic acid potently denatures proteins *in vitro*, but has a minimal effect when applied to carpets that harbor dust mites and other allergens (Woodfolk et al. 1994).

Impact on Asthma Control

A number of small controlled trials have successfully documented a decrease in dust mite allergen for six months or more following a range of interventions (Platts-Mills et al. 1997; Murray et al. 2017; Woodcock et al. 2003; Htut et al. 2001; Ehnert et al. 1992; Walshaw and Evans 1986; Gøtzsche et al. 1998). Each of these studies reported benefits, and four studies found a highly significant decrease in non-specific bronchial hyper-reactivity. It is important to note that over one-half of the reported trials of dust mite avoidance have failed because the measures proposed did not reduce allergen exposure for a significant period (Gøtzsche et al. 1998; Platts-Mills et al. 1999; Singh and Jaiswal 2013).

There are several conclusions from these studies:

- Successful controlled trials have used combinations of physical measures, including pillow covers, mattress covers, washing bedding in hot water and carpet removal, rather than chemical treatments.
- At least three to 6 months of sustained intervention was necessary to demonstrate clinical benefit.

Thus, patients should be encouraged to institute dust mite control measures that they can effectively sustain over time, and they should be advised to have patience as symptoms improve gradually and could lead to decreased medication requirements over time.

Summary of Avoidance Measures for House Dust Mites

1. Cover pillows and mattresses with zippered covers, which are impermeable to mites and mite allergens.
2. Wash bedsheets, pillowcases, and blankets in hot or warm water ($\approx 55°C$) with detergent or dry them in an electric dryer on the hot setting weekly.
3. When necessary, blankets should be replaced with those that can be washed.
4. Comforters (or duvets) should be removed or covered with fine zippered covers.
5. Use washable, vinyl or roll-type window covers instead of heavy curtains or drapery.
6. Remove clutter, soft toys and upholstered furniture.
7. Where possible, carpets should be removed or replaced with area rugs that can be cleaned/washed.
8. Replace carpets with polished flooring (tile, marble, wood, etc.) where possible.
9. Reduce upholstered furniture, particularly old sofas.
10. Vacuum weekly using a cleaner with a HEPA filtration system.
11. Control humidity to < 50% relative humidity at normal comfortable temperatures with air conditioning.
12. Allergy sufferers living in overtly damp housing might need to move to a new home and preferably live on the second or higher floor.

Practical Cost-Effective Dust Mites Control Measures

- Encase mattress, pillows and box springs in allergen-impermeable zippered covers. Finely woven zippered covers for pillows and duvets are preferable.
- Wash bedding weekly in warm water with detergent or use an electric dryer in the hot setting.
- Reduce indoor humidity to < 50% when practical; e.g., by using air conditioners in warmer climates.

Pets

Indoor pets are a common source of allergens, and the majority of pet-allergic patients are reactive to cats, dogs or both. However, a growing number of exotic animals are kept as pets, including reptiles, birds, insects, rodents, ferrets and monkeys, and allergic responses to these animals have also been reported (Phillips and Lockey 2009).

The most effective measure in controlling allergens derived from animals is to persuade the family or patient not to keep animals in the house. Scales shed from the animal's skin, i.e., pet dander (comparable with human dander) is the major source of animal allergens. Keeping a pet outdoors is effective, but restricting the animal to one part of the house is ineffective because animal allergens, particularly those from cats, are easily airborne & carried on clothing. Both cat and dog allergens can remain airborne for extended periods due to carriage on particles that, because of their small size, settle slowly. Many pets are regarded as "members of the family," hence aggressive efforts to persuade the patient to get rid of the animal (or animals) are unwise. Recognizing this, many efforts have been made to control cat allergens while the animal remains in the house (de Blay et al. 1991). The clinical effectiveness of these measures is not well-established, and patients must understand that the presence of a cat in the house represents such a large source of allergen that none of the proposed measures can consistently control allergen exposure (Wood et al. 1998).

Even when cats are removed from the house, allergens persist for many weeks or months (Wood et al. 1989). This phenomenon explains the increase in symptoms sometimes observed when a cat-allergic patient moves into a home in which cats were previously living. Aggressive cleaning measures can accelerate the removal of allergens. The quantity of cat allergen that accumulates in carpets, sofas and mattresses which are major reservoirs is difficult to remove without aggressive cleaning and removal of the old carpeting and upholstered furniture.

Cat allergen is transferred on clothing and can easily be detected in schools and in houses without a cat (Custovic et al. 1996; Gelber et al. 1993; Perzanowski et al. 1999). The quantities found in these sites are sometimes surprisingly high, such as 80 mcg per gram of dust of the antigen Fel d 1 (the major cat allergen) or Can f 1(the major dog allergen). In some cases, this is well within the range of allergen concentration found in homes with an animal. Furthermore, this passively transferred allergen can become airborne and cause symptoms (Almqvist et al. 2001; Bollinger et al. 2005; Platts-Mills et al. 2005). Patients who are highly allergic to cat or dog allergens should be informed about this potential source of ongoing exposure so that they can better understand their symptom patterns. Further research is needed on the effectiveness of avoidance measures for reducing cat allergen exposure in houses without a cat (Konradsen et al. 2015).

Specific Control Measures

In homes without a pet, levels of animal allergens may be effectively reduced through aggressive cleaning and the use of room air cleaners (Platts-Mills et al. 1997; de Blay et al. 1991). As mentioned previously, patients should be counseled that these measures are unlikely to be effective if the animal remains in the home.

Air Filters/Purifiers

In general, room air cleaners will only be effective if allergen reservoirs (including the pet itself as well as old carpets and upholstered furniture) are removed because otherwise, the air currents they create can increase the quantity of allergen becoming airborne. Air cleaners on an uncarpeted floor can reduce the concentration of airborne animal allergens, although studies have reported conflicting results regarding the impact of this reduction on symptoms of allergic rhinitis and asthma (Wood et al. 1998; van der Heide et al. 1999).

An expert panel organized by the American Academy of Allergy, Asthma and Immunology, conducted a systematic review concluding that there was evidence of benefit from the use of air filters in patients with allergic airway disease, but neither the magnitude of the effect nor the optimal techniques had been established (Sublett et al. 2010). In most positive studies, clinical benefit was demonstrated only after a prolonged period of use (e.g., a minimum of one year). Based on the available studies, that panel suggested that allergic patients choose one of the following options (Sublett et al. 2010):

- A room air purifier optimized for the room size it is placed in with a HEPA filter, particularly one that directs filtered air toward the individual's head during sleep (note: HEPA filters were developed in the early 1940s and used first by the Manhattan Project to contain the spread of airborne radioactive contaminants).

- If a central house air filtration system is present in the home, then disposable HEPA filters be used that are regularly changed (a relatively expensive option). HEPA filters have much higher air flow resistance and require more powerful air pumps and for this reason, are more expensive.

Aggressive Cleaning

Regular cleaning and the use of a vacuum cleaner with an effective filtration system are recommended. A controlled trial has reported lower allergen levels and clinical improvement in asthma measures in homes cleaned with vacuums equipped with HEPA filters, compared with vacuums without specialized filters (Popplewell et al. 2007). The homes in that study did not have pets, but the treatment was effective for cat-allergic subjects.

Bathing Pets

The effect of bathing pets regularly has been studied (de Blay et al. 1991; Avner et al. 1997; Nageotte et al. 2006). Washing cats, a challenging & unnatural task in itself, less often than weekly is unlikely to result in any meaningful improvement in symptoms, as some studies have shown that cat allergen in the air returns to pre-bath levels as quickly as one to three days later (Nageotte et al. 2006). The effect of washing dogs regularly has been less well studied. Twice weekly washing may be helpful.

"Hypoallergenic" Animals

There is no published scientific literature confirming the existence of "hypoallergenic" breeds of cats or dogs. However, there may be individual animals with lower or higher levels of allergen. In addition, there are ways of lowering the amount of allergen an animal produces, as described below.

Cats

The majority of people with cat allergy are sensitized to the protein Fel d 1. Efforts to decrease the amount of Fel d 1 produced or secreted by cats include the following:

- *Specialized food* — The addition of polyclonal antibodies specific for Fel d 1 to cat chow can reduce allergen shedding by pet cats (74). One technology, which is commercially available, involves the immunization of chickens with Fel d 1 to generate IgY antibodies (avian equivalent of human IgG), which can then be collected from egg yolks and used to supplement cat chow (Satyaraj et al. 2019a). This approach has been shown to reduce Fel d 1 levels in cat saliva and hair and be safe for the animals (Satyaraj et al. 2019a; Satyaraj et al. 2019b). A small pilot study of allergic patients in cat exposure chambers found some reduction in nasal symptoms, but larger studies are needed to determine if household levels of allergen are reduced by a clinically meaningful degree (Satyaraj et al. 2019c).

- *Genetic modification and breeding* — Several approaches to creating hypoallergenic cats have been suggested. These range from knocking out the gene for Fel d 1 to breeding cats that have lower Fel d 1 level, to simply encouraging breeding among select cats with lower allergen levels. Some Siberian cats have been monitored for Fel d1 levels to encourage lower allergen levels. However, companies that claim to have bred cats with lower levels have not provided objective evidence for their claims. Most importantly, no studies have been published to show that a so-called "hypoallergenic cat" results in lower levels of Fel d 1 in the house. Preliminary studies exposing cat-allergic subjects to the animals reported few symptoms, although no allergen measurements have been published (Spector S personal communication).

- *Vaccination (experimental)* — An experimental approach to reducing the amount of allergen secreted by cats involves immunizing the animals against their own endogenous Fel d 1. This was done using a vaccine based on the cucumber mosaic virus with both Fel d 1 and a tetanus toxoid-based peptide. Vaccination-induced high-affinity antibodies capable of neutralizing Fel d 1 and reducing its levels in the animals' secretions and appeared to be well tolerated by the cats, although larger and longer-term studies are needed (Thoms et al. 2019). It also remains to be seen whether levels are reduced enough to impact the symptoms of allergic patients. Reducing Fel d1 might have some deleterious health effects for that pet.

Dogs

There is no convincing evidence that certain breeds of dogs are less allergenic than others (Lockey 2012). The best study to date compared concentrations of the major dog allergen Can f 1 in samples from two groups of dogs and the homes they occupied (Vredegoor et al. 2012). The first group of 196 dogs consisted of breeds that are promoted on the Internet or by breeders as "hypoallergenic" (e.g., Labradoodle, Poodle, Spanish Waterdog, Airedale terrier), and the second group consisted of 160 dogs of breeds that carry no such claims (Labrador, Golden retriever and 46 other breeds, as well as various mixed breeds). Can f 1 concentrations in the animals' coats and in the settled and airborne dusts from their homes were compared. No differences were found in allergen levels in the homes of the two groups. Interestingly, concentrations of allergen in hair samples from the hypoallergenic group were significantly higher than those of the control group, although this was not reflected in home dust levels. Within each breed, there was marked variability among individual animals, a phenomenon also noted in earlier studies (Ramadour et al. 2005; Heutelbeck et al. 2008). This study confirmed the findings of an earlier, smaller study (Nicholas et al. 2011).

- *Other investigational approaches* — One study reported positive symptomatic benefits in cat-allergic subjects treated with injections of high-affinity monoclonal antibodies to Fel d 1 (Orengo et al. 2018).

Summary Practical Proven Animal Dander Control Measures

- Find the pet a new home, or at minimum, keep the animal out of the patient's bedroom
- Once the animal has been removed, the premises should be cleaned thoroughly
- Keep the pet in a room with a HEPA filter air cleaner/purifier, and replace the filter as recommended by the manufacturer
- Keep animals outside (e.g., in the garage or kennel)
- Cover air ducts of central air conditioning that lead to bedroom with filters or use air conditioners/air cleaners with HEPA filtration systems. Replace filters as recommended by the manufacturer
- Use air filters and vacuums with HEPA filters. Replace the filter as recommended by the manufacturer. Using an air filter can only reduce airborne allergens
- Washing cats does not reduce allergen levels significantly
- Washing dogs is a normal practice for outdoor dogs in hot climates and is well-accepted. Washing dogs twice a week may help
- Reduce reservoirs if the pet cannot be relocated to a new home: Remove carpets, reduce upholstered furniture to a minimum, replace drapes with blinds and/or vacuum weekly using a vacuum with good filtration (i.e., double thickness bags and/or HEPA filtration)

Rodents

Mice and rats produce urinary proteins that are allergenic in occupational (e.g., laboratory workers), school (Sheehan et al. 2009; Permaul et al. 2012) and domestic settings (Platts-Mills et al. 1990; Eggleston et al. 1990; Phipatanakul et al. 2000; Matsui et al. 2005). Mouse allergens are measurable in nearly all inner-city, multifamily homes and as many as 50 percent of suburban homes (Matsui et al. 2005; Chew et al. 2003). However, the levels in inner-city homes have been as much as 100-fold higher than those in suburban homes (Matsui et al. 2006), and levels in inner-city schools are often higher than in homes (Permaul et al. 2012).

Exposure of infants to mice allergens has been associated with the development of asthma, independent of other factors (Phipatanakul et al. 2005). Mouse exposure also correlates with poorer asthma control, increased acute care visits and increased health care utilization among inner-city children sensitized to mouse allergens (Matsui et al. 2004; Ahluwalia et al. 2013). In adults in the community (non-laboratory workers), sensitization to mouse allergens is significantly associated with asthma and asthma morbidity (Phipatanakul et al. 2007).

Exposure to rodents can be assessed by asking if mice or rats are ever sighted at home or if the family has seen evidence of their presence (droppings; nests) (Phipatanakul et al. 2012). However, mouse allergen can be high even if the answers to these questions are negative, as rodents may remain entirely hidden from sight.

- *Specific control measures* — Professional extermination (i.e., rodenticide application, traps) and integrated pest management (keeping food and trash in covered containers, sealing cracks in the walls, doors and floors, targeted cleaning and use of allergen-proof mattress and pillow encasements and portable air purifiers) are usually necessary to reduce rodent allergen levels significantly and maintain the improvements (Matsui et al. 2007; Sheehan et al. 2010; Phipatanakul et al. 2004). Mice can become resistant to rodenticides (Endepols et al. 2013). Evidence for the effectiveness of ultrasonic devices that deter the entry of mice into homes is lacking (Vantassel 2012). Even with effective use of these measures and lowering of mouse allergen levels, it can be difficult to demonstrate an impact on asthma symptoms, which may be due to the choice of control groups or the need to target all relevant allergens simultaneously (Matsui et al. 2017; Bacharier et al. 2017). Integrated Pest Management (IPM) involves removing facilitative factors including food, water and shelter leading to a reduced environmental carrying capacity for cockroaches and rodents along with blocking means of ingress and, when necessary, killing or trapping pests using either targeted application of chemicals or mechanical methods.

Practical Proven Rodent Control Measures

- Consult a professional exterminator.
- Periodically clean the home thoroughly and use baits if relevant.
- All food should be stored in sealed containers. Do not store garbage inside.
- Repair holes in walls, doors and floors and block other entry points.

Cockroaches

Evidence that allergens derived from the German cockroach, *Blattella germanica*, are important has come from case-control studies and provocation studies done in North America (Gelber et al. 1993; Call et al. 1992; Kang et al. 1979). As an example, one study of 476 children found that the combination of specific skin test positivity and exposure to cockroach allergen was associated with significantly higher rates of hospitalization, compared with when this combination was absent (0.37 vs. 0.11 hospitalizations per child per year) (Wang et al. 2009; Rosenstreich et al. 1997). Patients should be asked if they have seen cockroaches in the home, although roaches may be present even if they have not been sighted. Sticky traps may be placed near food or water sources to determine if there is an infestation and to evaluate if control measures are helping, as described in a 2013 practice parameter regarding assessment and exposure control measures for cockroaches (Portnoy et al. 2013).

- *Specific control measures* — The 2013 practice parameter recommends IPM to eliminate and prevent cockroach infestation. IPM includes removing reservoirs of accumulated cockroach debris, cleaning the area, reducing or eliminating cockroaches (placing multiple baited traps and poisons) and removing factors that facilitate infestation (e.g., standing water, access to refuse, papers or unwashed dishes) (Sheehan et al. 2010; Portnoy et al. 2013). Air filtration is not helpful in reducing cockroach allergen exposure, as the allergen settles quickly and does not

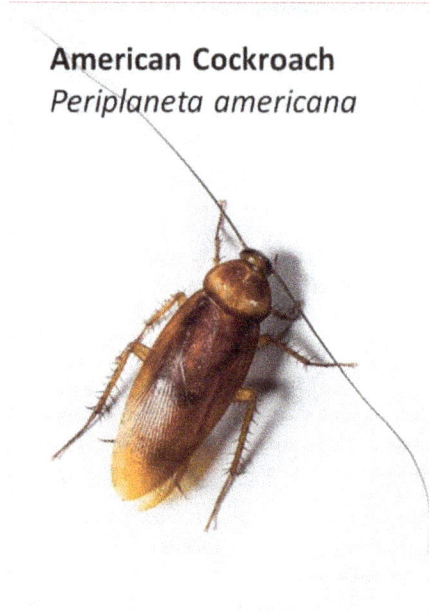

Figure 2. American Cockraoch.

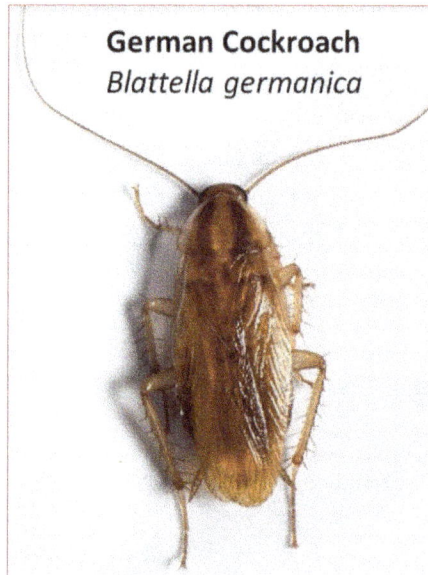

Figure 3. German Cockroach.

remain airborne. Professional extermination may be necessary, particularly if there is cockroach infestation in a multifamily building (Portnoy et al. 2013).

Despite the ability to measure cockroach allergen and a good understanding of the measures necessary to reduce exposure (Sever et al. 2007), initial interventional trials were unsuccessful (Gergen et al. 1999; Carter et al. 2001). It is likely that cockroach allergen reduction alone is not sufficient to impact symptoms, as was demonstrated in other studies targeting single allergens. This may be particularly true for patients living in poor conditions who may be exposed to high levels of multiple allergens. However, a subsequent trial that included a combined strategy to reduce exposure to cockroaches, dust mites and other indoor asthma triggers was successful in reducing symptoms and improving lung function in urban children with asthma (Morgan et al. 2004).

Practical Proven Cockroach Allergen Control Measures

- Use poison bait or traps to control.
- Consult a professional exterminator for severe infestation
- Periodically clean the home thoroughly.
- Encase all food fully and do not store garbage or papers inside the home.
- Fix water leaks and seal entry points of insects.

Other Insects

Moths (order Lepidoptera) and Asian ladybugs (ALBs) (*Harmonia axyridis*) which were imported to the United States from 1916 until 1990 as a biologic means of controlling aphids are examples of other insects that have been associated with allergic reactions in regularly exposed individuals (Yarbrough et al. 1999; Sharma et al. 2006; Nakazawa et al. 2006; Goetz 2008). Allergy to ALBs has been increasingly reported as a source of seasonal indoor respiratory symptoms, particularly chronic cough, rhinitis and asthma (Nakazawa et al. 2006). Most cases have been reported in rural areas of the central, mid-western and southern United States. They can also bite and cause local reactions.

ALBs enter homes through external cracks and crevices and then infest spaces within walls. They secrete a brown liquid that may stain walls and produce an unpleasant smell when handled. The source of the allergen(s) is not clear (112). Extracts for allergy skin testing and ALB-specific immunoglobulin E (IgE) immunoassays are not yet commercially available. Some allergy specialists in affected communities have produced extracts for skin testing using the beetles directly (Nakazawa et al. 2006).

Moths on the other hand have a layer of powdery scales on their wings, which sheds easily and can lead to direct contact allergic reactions as well as become airborne and give rise to inhaled allergies (Kausar 2018). Also the excrement of moths, their larvae and eggs can also elicit allergic reactions. The urticating scales on the underside of their abdomen also cause skin irritation due to their barbed nature, and if airborne can cause asthma or respiratory inflammation. Entomologists who work with moths are at the highest risk of allergies as are bakers exposed to the scales of flour moths (Makinen-Kiljunen et al. 2001).

Specific Control Measures

The primary protection is to have tight windows and walls to decrease access to these insects such as eliminating cracks around windows and doors and tears in window screens. The next most promising control measure for ALBs is the treatment of the outside of a house with pyrethroid chemicals prior to cold weather (Nakazawa et al. 2006). Other measures for ALBs, such as treating the already infested walls with chemicals, sound waves and traps have not been consistently helpful. In cases of severe allergy, it may be necessary for patients to move to a more tightly-built house or into a more urban area. Hot laundering of clothes as well as storing clothes in plastic bags so that the moths cannot feed on them have been successful interventions that seem to limit exposure in allergic individuals. A professional extermination might be necessary in some cases. Perimeter pesticide sprays may give temporary relief in preventing some insect infestations, but effective sprays kill all insects non-specifically, and the benefit is generally short-lived.

Indoor Molds

Indoor molds and fungi are most problematic in homes with high humidity, standing water or water damage. If the home of a mold-allergic patient contains visible mold or smells of mold, then remediation for this allergen is in order.

A randomized trial of indoor mold remediation in patients with asthma and visible mold growth in the home demonstrated benefit, regardless of whether patients were sensitized to four common allergenic molds by skin prick testing (Burr et al. 2007). In this study, which did not include a placebo/sham intervention, 164 homes housing 232 asthmatic patients were randomly assigned to undergo cleaning with detergent and fungicide and installation of an attic fan or to have this intervention performed one year later. There was a dramatic difference between the two groups at six months, with improvement in breathing symptoms in 52 and 0% of patients in the intervention and control groups, respectively, although some placebo effect was inevitable and some of the patients in the deferred intervention group performed mold remediation on their own. Medication use decreased 41% in the intervention group and increased 17% among control patients. The benefit in patients not sensitized to the four tested molds was posited to be secondary to the reduction in mycotoxins and volatile irritant substances emitted by molds. However, the effect could also reflect a failure to identify allergic patients when using only four molds and prick tests. Another similar randomized trial also found modest benefits (Kercsmar et al. 2006). The quality of mold extracts cannot be assumed and because of this, some investigators consider that intradermal tests for mold are more reliable. In addition, the situation with molds such as aspergillus, candida, or trichophyton is different because the allergen may be, or is growing on the patients. In that case, antifungal treatment may be necessary to reduce exposure.

Practical Proven Indoor Mold Control Measures

- Clean moldy surfaces with a dilute bleach solution.
- Fix water leaks.
- Reduce indoor humidity to < 50%.
- Avoid the use of humidifiers.
- Use air conditioners in warm climates.
- Evaporative (or swamp) coolers should be avoided or cleaned regularly.
- Avoid living in very poorly ventilated damp homes.

Outdoor Allergens

Outdoor allergens, especially pollens and molds, are difficult to avoid short of limiting contact with the outside world. However, patients with documented sensitivity to pollen and mold allergens

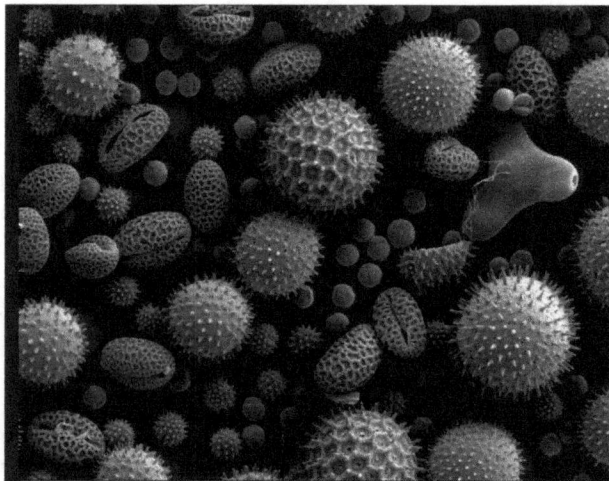

Figure 4. Tree, Grass, Weed Pollens.

can enact several measures during peak seasons when symptoms are most severe. These include closing the windows at home and in the car, using air conditioners to filter the air and staying indoors when possible. Showering before bed to remove allergens from hair and skin can help reduce contamination of the bedding. Over-the-counter saline sprays and rinses can be used to wash allergens from the nasal lining after outdoor exposure.

For patients motivated to do so, the removal of allergenic plants from their immediate surroundings can sometimes be helpful. Trees, shrubs and flowering plants that are pollinated by insects rather than by air are generally less allergenic, and a listing of such plants, as well as an approach to identifying other plants of low allergenic potential, has been published (Green et al. 2018).

Volatile Organic Compounds (VOCs)

VOCs are a large group of chemicals found in many products we use to build or maintain our homes. Once they are in our home they release or "off-gas" into the indoor air we breathe and can reach high levels in closed spaces. They are irritant by nature when inhaled. Common examples of VOCs in homes are benzene, ethylene glycol, formaldehyde, methylene chloride, tetracholo-ethylene, toluene, limonene, xylene and 1,3–butadiene. These are found in paints, varnishes, solvents, adhesives, caulks, carpets, vinyl flooring, composite wood products, upholstery, foam, cooking and cleaning products. Inhaling VOCs over prolonged periods have many harmful health effects but especially affects people with asthma, making their symptoms worse. Higher levels can lead to eye, nose and throat irritation, headaches, nausea/vomiting, dizziness as well as worsening of asthma symptoms. Young children and the elderly are more susceptible to VOC effects (Internet US EPA).

Specific Control Measures

Source control by removal or reduction of the number of products that could give off VOCs in the home is the key intervention. Discard unused paints, varnishes, adhesives and caulks after their household work is done. If these have to be stored then put them in a garage or outside the house. Choose low-VOC options for paints, wood and furnishing. Good ventilation by opening doors and windows helps keep VOC levels down. Use of exhaust fans when available can help too. Lowering the household ambient temperature and humidity levels leads to less off-gassing of VOCs (Internet). Air cleaners/purifiers have been studied for their ability to remove VOCs from homes and found to have suboptimal efficacy in doing so. The ones with activated carbon filters perform most efficiently within their recommended range of function. Some oxidation based air cleaners even emit VOC's like formaldehyde and acetone of their own by slow "outgassing" and should be avoided (Ye et al. 2021).

Changing Environment and Lifestyle Impact on Allergen Exposure and Disease

While many different forms of the disease have been influenced by changes in human diet and lifestyle, this is particularly true for allergic diseases (Platts-Mills 2015). Thus typically making houses warmer in the UK made it more comfortable to sit and watch TV and may have contributed to the growth of dust mites in homes. However, in the last 40 years, a series of changes have had the potential to lead to decreased accumulations of allergens in houses. The most obvious is the widespread adoption of whole house air conditioners in the USA. Equally, many houses removed fitted carpets and converted to wood or tile floors with area rugs. These changes were all accompanied by increased public awareness of the relevance of indoor allergens to asthma in children. More recently, the development of computers and the Internet has made it easy for patients and parents to access websites about allergen or particularly, dust mite avoidance.

In the Asia Pacific Region studies from Singapore, China, Taiwan and parts of urban/semiurban India have demonstrated rising house dust mites triggered allergies and asthma (Acevedo et al. 2019). The most likely explanation would be the urbanization of diet and lifestyle with longer times spent indoors on mobile phones, laptops/computers and/or TV leading to prolonged exposure to indoor allergens and greater chances of sensitization, hence allergy and asthma. Many house dust mite-allergic patients also report that they breathe better and have far less allergic symptoms, when they are outdoors in fresh air and sunlight or are away from their home on vacations. It is quite natural, that they are exposed to far less house dust mite allergens for hours and days at end in such situations. Thus, the myriad of undeniable benefits of regular outdoor activities and exercise would seem to work favorably for almost anyone who either has or is at risk for house dust mite triggered allergy/asthma.

Conclusion

Effective indoor allergen avoidance begins with the identification of those allergens that are relevant to a specific patient, through a careful history combined with specific allergy testing (*in vivo* or *in vitro*). Once the patient's sensitivities have been defined, specific practical, cost-effective measures for each allergen should be implemented. Encouraging safe, outdoor activity/exercise, a healthy diet rich in anti-oxidant, anti-inflammatory foods plus a healthy lifestyle that can benefit almost any chronic disease, certainly has its appeal for allergic individuals.

Environmental interventions can alter the natural history of allergic diseases and should be an integral part of the management of any allergic patients along with pharmacotherapy and also immunotherapy when appropriate. Future research and guidelines should focus on what makes a difference rather than trying to do too much and burdening the patient/family (Le Cann et al. 2017). As we continue to learn more about early life exposure to environmental allergens, molecular patterns of allergen sensitization, internal biodiversity and subsequent disease development, preventive approaches might evolve to reduce the burden of allergic diseases.

Glossary of Abbreviations

ALB – Asian Ladybug
HEPA – High-Efficiency Particulate Air
IPM – Integrated Pest Management
VOC – Volatile Organic Compounds

References

Acevedo, N., Zakzuk, J. and Caraballo, L. 2019. House dust mite allergy under changing environments. Allergy Asthma Immunol. Res. 11(4): 450.

Ahluwalia, S. K., Peng, R. D., Breysse, P. N. et al. 2013. Mouse allergen is the major allergen of public health relevance in Baltimore City. J. Allergy Clin. Immunol. 132: 830.

Almqvist, C., Wickman, M., Perfetti, L. et al. 2001. Worsening of asthma in children allergic to cats, after indirect exposure to cat at school. Am. J. Respir. Crit. Care Med. 163: 694.

Avner, D. B., Perzanowski, M. S., Platts-Mills, T. A. and Woodfolk, J. A. 1997. Evaluation of different techniques for washing cats: quantitation of allergen removed from the cat and the effect on airborne Fel d 1. J. Allergy Clin. Immunol. 100: 307.

Bacharier, L. B. 2017. Reducing exposure to mouse allergen among children and adolescents with asthma is achievable, but is it enough? JAMA 317: 1023.

Bobb, C. and Ritz, T. 2003. Do asthma patients in general practice profit from a structured allergy valuation and skin testing? A pilot study. Respir. Med. 97: 1180.

Bollinger, M. E., Eggleston, P. A., Flanagan, E. and Wood, R. A. 1996. Cat antigen in homes with and without cats may induce allergic symptoms. J. Allergy Clin. Immunol. 97: 907.

Brydon, M. 1993. The effectiveness of a peripatetic allergy nurse practitioner service in managing atopic allergy in general practice—a pilot study. Clin. Exp. Allergy 23: 1037.

Burr, M. L., Matthews, I. P., Arthur, R. A. et al. 2007. Effects on patients with asthma of eradicating visible indoor mould: a randomised controlled trial. Thorax 62: 767.

Calhoun, W. J., Dick, E. C., Schwartz, L. B. and Busse, W. W. 1994. A common cold virus, rhinovirus 16, potentiates airway inflammation after segmental antigen bronchoprovocation in allergic subjects. J. Clin. Invest 94: 2200.

Call, R. S., Smith, T. F., Morris, E. et al. 1992. Risk factors for asthma in inner city children. J. Pediatr. 121: 862.

Carter, M. C., Perzanowski, M. S., Raymond, A. and Platts-Mills, T. A. 2001. Home intervention in the treatment of asthma among inner-city children. J. Allergy Clin. Immunol. 108: 732.

Chapman, M. D., Aalberse, R. C., Brown, M. J. and Platts-Mills, T. A. 1988. Monoclonal antibodies to the major feline allergen Fel d I. II. Single step affinity purification of Fel d I, N-terminal sequence analysis, and development of a sensitive two-site immunoassay to assess Feld I exposure. J. Immunol. 140: 812.

Chew, G. L., Perzanowski, M. S., Miller, R. L. et al. 2003. Distribution and determinants of mouse allergen exposure in low-income New York City apartments. Environ. Health Perspect. 111: 1348.

Cockcroft, D. W., Ruffin, R. E., Frith, P. A. et al. 1979. Determinants of allergen-induced asthma: dose of allergen, circulating IgE antibody concentration, and bronchial responsiveness to inhaled histamine. Am. Rev. Respir. Dis. 120: 1053.

Colloff, M. J., Taylor, C. and Merrett, T. G. 1995. The use of domestic steam cleaning for the control of house dust mites. Clin. Exp. Allergy 25: 1061.

Custovic, A., Green, R., Taggart, S. C. et al. 1996. Domestic allergens in public places. II: Dog (Canf1) and cockroach (Bla g 2) allergens in dust and mite, cat, dog and cockroach allergensin the air in public buildings. Clin. Exp. Allergy 26: 1246.

de Blay, F., Chapman, M. D. and Platts-Mills, T. A. 1991. Airborne cat allergen (Fel d I). Environmental control with the cat *in situ*. Am. Rev. Respir. Dis. 143: 1334.

Eggleston, P. A., Ansari, A. A., Ziemann, B. et al. 1990. Occupational challenge studies with laboratory workers allergic to rats. J. Allergy Clin. Immunol. 86: 63.

Ehnert, B., Lau-Schadendorf, S., Weber, A. et al. 1992. Reducing domestic exposure to dust mite allergen reduces bronchial hyperreactivity in sensitive children with asthma. J. Allergy Clin. Immunol. 90: 135.

Endepols, S., Klemann, N., Song, Y. and Kohn, M. H. 2013. Vkorc L variation in house mice during warfarin and difenacoum field trials. Pest Manag. Sci. 69: 409.

Erwin, E. A. and Platts-Mills, T. A. 2005. Allergens. Immunol. Allergy Clin. North Am. 25: 1.

Erwin, E. A., Custis, N. J., Satinover, S. M. et al. 2005a. Quantitative measurement of IgE antibodies to purified allergens using streptavidin linked to a high-capacity solid phase. J. Allergy Clin. Immunol. 115: 1029.

Erwin, E. A., Wickens, K., Custis, N. J. et al. 2005b. Cat and dust mite sensitivity and tolerance in relation to wheezing among children raised with high exposure to both allergens. J. Allergy Clin. Immunol. 115: 74.

Erwin, E. A., Rönmark, E., Wickens, K. et al. 2007. Contribution of dust mite and cat specific IgE to total IgE: relevance to asthma prevalence. J. Allergy Clin. Immunol. 119: 359.

Erwin, E. A,, Woodfolk, J. A., James, H. R. et al. 2014. Changes in cat specific IgE and IgG antibodies with decreased cat exposure. Ann. Allergy Asthma Immunol. 112: 545.

Expert Panel Working Group of the National Heart, Lung, and Blood Institute (NHLBI) administered and coordinated National Asthma Education and Prevention Program Coordinating Committee (NAEPPCC), Cloutier, M. M., Baptist, A. P. et al. 2020. 2020 Focused Updates to the Asthma Management Guidelines: A Report from the National Asthma Education and Prevention Program Coordinating Committee Expert Panel Working Group. J. Allergy Clin. Immunol. 146: 1217.

Gelber, L. E., Seltzer, L. H., Bouzoukis, J. K. et al. 1993. Sensitization and exposure to indoor allergens as risk factors for asthma among patients presenting to hospital. Am. Rev. Respir Dis. 147: 573.

Gergen, P. J., Mortimer, K. M., Eggleston, P. A. et al. 1999. Results of the National Cooperative Inner-City Asthma Study (NCICAS) environmental intervention to reduce cockroach allergen exposure in inner-city homes. J. Allergy Clin. Immunol. 103: 501.

Ghaemmaghami, A. M., Robins, A., Gough, L. et al. 2001. Human T cell subset commitment determined by the intrinsic property of antigen: the proteolytic activity of the major mite allergen Der p 1 conditions T cells to produce more IL-4 and less IFN-gamma. Eur. J. Immunol. 31: 1211.

Goetz, D. W. 2008. Harmonia axyridis ladybug invasion and allergy. Allergy Asthma Proc. 29: 123.

Gøtzsche, P. C., Hammarquist, C. and Burr, M. 1998. House dust mite control measures in the management of asthma: meta-analysis. BMJ 317: 1105.

Green, B. J., Levetin, E., Horner, W. E. et al. 2018. Landscape plant selection criteria for the allergic patient. J. Allergy Clin. Immunol. Pract. 6: 1869.

Hayden, M. L., Rose, G., Diduch, K. B. et al. 1992. Benzyl benzoate moist powder: investigation of acaricidal (correction of acarical) activity in cultures and reduction of dust mite allergens in carpets. J. Allergy Clin. Immunol. 89: 536.

Heutelbeck, A. R., Schulz, T., Bergmann, K. C. and Hallier, E. 2008. Environmental exposure to allergens of different dog breeds and relevance in allergological diagnostics. J. Toxicol. Environ. Health A 71: 751.

Htut, T., Higenbottam, T. W., Gill, G. W. et al. 2001. Eradication of house dust mite from homes of atopic asthmatic subjects: a double-blind trial. J. Allergy Clin. Immunol. 107: 55.

Information about ladybug control measures is available through the Internet at: ipm.osu.edu/lady/lady.htm (Accessed on June 17, 2009).

Information about VOC's is available through the internet at: https://www.health.state.mn.us/communities/environment/air/toxins/voc.htm (Accessed June 10, 2022).

Kang, B., Vellody, D., Homburger, H. and Yunginger, J. W. 1979. Cockroach cause of allergic asthma. Its specificity and immunologic profile. J. Allergy Clin. Immunol. 63: 80.

Kattan, M., Stearns, S. C., Crain, E. F. et al. 2005. Cost-effectiveness of a home-based environmental intervention for inner-city children with asthma. J. Allergy Clin. Immunol. 116: 1058.

Kausar, M. A. 2018. A review of respiratory allergies caused by Insects. Bioinformation 14(9): 540.

Kercsmar, C. M., Dearborn, D. G., Schluchter, M. et al. 2006. Reduction in asthma morbidity in children as a result of home remediation aimed at moisture sources. Environ. Health Perspect. 114: 1574.

Kerrebijn, K. F. 1970. Endogenous factors in childhood CNSLD: Methodological aspects in population studies. p.38. *In*: Bronchitis III, Orie, N. G. M. and van der Lende, R. (eds.). Royal Vangorcum Assen, The Netherlands.

Konradsen, J. R., Fujisawa, T., van Hage, M. et al. 2015. Allergy to furry animals: New insights, diagnostic approaches, and challenges. J. Allergy Clin. Immunol. 135: 616.

Korsgaard, J. 1983. House-dust mites and absolute indoor humidity. Allergy 38: 85.

Le Cann, P., Paulus, H., Glorennec, P. et al. 2017. Home environmental interventions for the prevention or control of allergic and respiratory diseases: what really works. J. Allergy Clin. Immunol. Pract. 5(1): 66.

Leas, B. F., D'Anci, K. E., Apter, A. J. et al. 2018. Effectiveness of indoor allergen reduction in asthma management: A systematic review. J. Allergy Clin. Immunol. 141: 1854.

Lockey, R. F. 2012. The myth of hypoallergenic dogs (and cats). J. Allergy Clin. Immunol. 130: 910.

Luczynska, C., Tredwell, E., Smeeton, N. and Burney, P. 2003. A randomized controlled trial of mite allergen-impermeable bed covers in adult mite-sensitized asthmatics. Clin. Exp. Allergy 33: 1648.

Luczynska, C. M., Arruda, L. K., Platts-Mills, T. A. et al. 1989. A two-site monoclonal antibody ELISA for the quantification of the major Dermatophagoides spp. allergens, Der p I and Der f I. J. Immunol. Methods 118: 227.

Makinen-Kiljunen, S., Mussalo-Rauhamaa, H., Petman, L. et al. 2001. A baker's occupational allergy to flour moth (Ephestia kuehniella). Allergy 56: 696.

Matsui, E. C., Simons, E., Rand, C. et al. 2005. Airborne mouse allergen in the homes of inner-city children with asthma. J. Allergy Clin. Immunol. 115: 358.

Matsui, E. C. and Wood, R. A. 2006. Questions physicians often ask about allergens that trigger asthma. J. Respir. Dis. 27: 511.

Matsui, E. C., Eggleston, P. A., Buckley, T. J. et al. 2006. Household mouse allergen exposure and asthma morbidity in inner-city preschool children. Ann. Allergy Asthma Immunol. 97: 514.

Matsui, E. C., Perzanowski, M., Peng, R. D. et al. 2017. Effect of an integrated pest management intervention on asthma symptoms among mouse-sensitized children and adolescents with asthma: a randomized clinical trial. JAMA 317: 1027.

Matsui, E. C. and Peng, R. D. 2020. 2020 Updated Asthma Guidelines: Indoor allergen reduction. J. Allergy Clin. Immunol. 146: 1283.

McDonald, L. G. and Tovey, E. 1992. The role of water temperature and laundry procedures in reducing house dust mite populations and allergen content of bedding. J. Allergy Clin. Immunol. 90: 599.

Miller, J. D. and Miller, A. 1996. Ten minutes in a clothes dryer kills all mites in blankets. J. Allergy Clin. Immunol. 97: 423.

Miller, J. D., Naccara, L., Satinover, S. and Platts-Mills, T. A. 2007. Nonwoven in contrast to woven mattress encasings accumulate mite and cat allergen. J. Allergy Clin. Immunol. 120: 977.

Morgan, W. J., Crain, E. F., Gruchalla, R. S. et al. 2004. Results of a home-based environmental intervention among urban children with asthma. N Engl. J. Med. 351: 1068.

Murray, C. S., Foden, P., Sumner, H. et al. 2017. Preventing severe asthma exacerbations in children. A randomized trial of mite-impermeable bedcovers. Am. J. Respir. Crit. CareMed. 196: 150.

Nageotte, C., Park, M., Havstad, S. et al. 2006. Duration of airborne Fel d 1 reduction after cat washing. J. Allergy Clin. Immunol. 118: 521.

Nakazawa, T., Satinover, S. M., Naccara, L. et al. 2007. Asian ladybugs (Harmonia axyridis): a new seasonal indoor allergen. J. Allergy Clin. Immunol. 119: 421.

Nicholas, C. E., Wegienka, G. R., Havstad, S. L. et al. 2011. Dog allergen levels in homes with hypoallergenic compared with non hypoallergenic dogs. Am. J. Rhinol. Allergy 25: 252.

Nurmatov, U., van Schayck, C. P., Hurwitz, B. and Sheikh, A. 2012. House dust mite avoidance measures for perennial allergic rhinitis: an updated Cochrane systematic review. Allergy 67: 158.

Orengo, J. M., Radin, A. R., Kamat, V. et al. 2018. Treating cat allergy with monoclonal IgG antibodies that bind allergen and prevent IgE engagement. Nat. Commun. 9: 1421.

Peat, J. K., Tovey, E., Toelle, B. G. et al. 1996. House dust mite allergens. A major risk factor for childhood asthma in Australia. Am. J. Respir. Crit. Care Med. 153: 141.

Permaul, P., Hoffman, E., Fu, C. et al. 2012. Allergens in urban schools and homes of children with asthma. Pediatr Allergy Immunol. 23: 543.

Perzanowski, M. S., Rönmark, E., Nold, B. et al. 1999. Relevance of allergens from cats and dogs to asthma in the northernmost province of Sweden: schools as a major site of exposure. J. Allergy Clin. Immunol. 103: 1018.

Phillips, J. F. and Lockey, R. F. 2009. Exotic pet allergy. J. Allergy Clin. Immunol. 123: 513.

Phipatanakul, W., Eggleston, P. A., Wright, E. C. et al. 2000. Mouse allergen. II. The relationship of mouse allergen exposure to mouse sensitization and asthma morbidity in inner-city children with asthma. J. Allergy Clin. Immunol. 106: 1075.

Phipatanakul, W., Cronin, B., Wood, R. A. et al. 2004. Effect of environmental intervention on mouse allergen levels in homes of inner-city Boston children with asthma. Ann. Allergy Asthma Immunol. 92: 420.

Phipatanakul, W., Celedón, J. C., Sredl, D. L. et al. 2005. Mouse exposure and wheeze in the first year of life. Ann. Allergy Asthma Immunol. 94: 593.

Phipatanakul, W., Litonjua, A. A., Platts-Mills, T. A. et al. 2007. Sensitization to mouse allergen and asthma and asthma morbidity among women in Boston. J. Allergy Clin. Immunol. 120: 954.

Phipatanakul, W., Matsui, E., Portnoy, J. et al. 2012. Environmental assessment and exposure reduction of rodents: a practice parameter. Ann. Allergy Asthma Immunol. 109: 375.

Piacentini, G. L., Martinati, L., Mingoni, S. and Boner, A. L. 1996. Influence of allergen avoidance on the eosinophil phase of airway inflammation in children with allergic asthma. J. Allergy Clin. Immunol. 97: 1079.

Platts-Mills, J. A., Custis, N. J., Woodfolk, J. A. and Platts-Mills T. A. 2005. Airborne endotoxin in homes with domestic animals: implications for cat-specific tolerance. J. Allergy Clin. Immunol. 116: 384.

Platts-Mills, T. A., Tovey, E. R., Mitchell, E. B. et al. 1982. Reduction of bronchial hyperreactivity during prolonged allergen avoidance. Lancet 2: 675.

Platts-Mills, T. A., Hayden, M. L., Chapman, M. D. and Wilkins, S. R. 1987. Seasonal variation in dust mite and grass-pollen allergens in dust from the houses of patients with asthma. J. Allergy Clin. Immunol. 79: 781.

Platts-Mills, T. A., Longbottom, J., Edwards, J. et al. 1987. Occupational asthma and rhinitis related to laboratory rats: serum IgG and IgE antibodies to the rat urinary allergen. J. Allergy Clin. Immunol. 79: 505.

Platts-Mills, T. A., Vervloetmz, D., Thomas, W. R. et al. 1997. Indoor allergens and asthma: report of the Third International Workshop. J. Allergy Clin. Immunol. 100: S2.

Platts-Mills, T. A., Chapman, M. D. and Wheatly, L. M. 1999. Control of house dust mite in managing asthma. Conclusions of meta-analysis are wrong. BMJ 318: 870.

Platts-Mills, T. A. 2007. The role of indoor allergens in chronic allergic disease. J. Allergy Clin. Immunol. 119: 297.

Platts-Mills, T. A. 2015. The allergy epidemics: 1870–2010. J. of Allergy and Clin. Immunol. 136(1): 3.

Platts-Mills, T. A. E. and Woodfolk, J. A. 2017. Mite avoidance as a logical treatment for severe asthma in childhood. Why Not? Am. J. Respir. Crit. Care Med. 196: 119.

Popplewell, E. J., Innes, V. A., Lloyd-Hughes, S. et al. 2000. The effect of high-efficiency and standard vacuum-cleaners on mite, cat and dog allergen levels and clinical progress. Pediatr. Allergy Immunol. 11: 142.

Portnoy, J., Chew, G. L., Phipatanakul, W. et al. 2013. Environmental assessment and exposure reduction of cockroaches: a practice parameter. J. Allergy Clin. Immunol. 132: 802.

Ramadour, M., Guetat, M., Guetat, J. et al. 2005. Dog factor differences in Can f 1 allergen production. Allergy 60: 1060.

Rosenstreich, D. L., Eggleston, P., Kattan, M. et al. 1997. The role of cockroach allergy and exposure to cockroach allergen in causing morbidity among inner-city children with asthma. N Engl. J. Med. 336: 1356.

Satyaraj, E., Gardner, C., Filipi, I. et al. 2019a. Reduction of active Fel d1 from cats using an antiFeld1 egg IgY antibody. Immun. Inflamm. Dis. 7: 68.

Satyaraj, E., Li, Q., Sun, P. and Sherrill, S. 2019b. Anti-Fel d1 immunoglobulin Y antibody-containing egg ingredient lowers allergen levels in cat saliva. J. Feline Med. Surg. 21: 875.

Satyaraj, E., Wedner, H. J. and Bousquet, J. 2019c. Keep the cat, change the care pathway: A transformational approach to managing Fel d 1, the major cat allergen. Allergy 74Suppl 107: 5.

Sever, M. L., Arbes, S. J. Jr, Gore, J. C. et al. 2007. Cockroach allergen reduction by cockroach control alone in low-income urban homes: a randomized control trial. J. Allergy Clin. Immunol. 120: 849.

Sharma, H. P., Hansel, N. N., Matsui, E. et al. 2007. Indoor environmental influences on children's asthma. Pediatr Clin. North Am. 54: 103.

Sharma, K., Muldoon, S. B., Potter, M. F. and Pence, H. L. 2006. Ladybug hypersensitivity among residents of homes infested with ladybugs in Kentucky. Ann. Allergy Asthma Immunol. 97: 528.

Shedd, A. D., Peters, J. I., Wood, P. et al. 2007. Impact of home environment characteristics on asthma quality of life and symptom scores. J. Asthma 44: 183.

Sheehan, W. J., Rangsithienchai, P. A., Muilenberg, M. L. et al. 2009. Mouse allergens in urban elementary schools and homes of children with asthma. Ann. Allergy Asthma Immunol. 102: 125.

Sheehan, W. J., Rangsithienchai, P. A., Wood, R. A. et al. 2010. Pest and allergen exposure and abatement in inner-city asthma: a work group report of the American Academy of Allergy, Asthma & Immunology Indoor Allergy/Air Pollution Committee. J. Allergy Clin. Immunol. 125: 575.

Sibbald, B., Barnes, G. and Durham, S. R. 1997. Skin prick testing in general practice: a pilot study. J. Adv. Nurs. 26: 537.

Singh, M. and Jaiswal, N. 2013. Dehumidifiers for chronic asthma. Cochrane Database Syst. Rev. CD003563.

Smith, H., Horney, D., Goubet, S. et al. 2015. Pragmatic randomized controlled trial of a structured allergy intervention for adults with asthma and rhinitis in general practice. Allergy 70: 203.

Spector, S, personal communication.

Sporik, R., Holgate, S. T., Platts-Mills, T. A. and Cogswell, J. J. 1990. Exposure to house-dust mite allergen (Der p I) and the development of asthma in childhood. A prospective study. N Engl. J. Med. 323: 5024.

Sears, M. R., Herbison, G. P., Holdaway, M. D. et al. 1989. The relative risks of sensitivity to grass pollen, house dust mite and cat dander in the development of childhood asthma. Clin. Exp. Allergy 19: 419.

Squillace, S. P., Sporik, R. B., Rakes, G. et al. 1997. Sensitization to dust mites as a dominant risk factor for asthma among adolescents living in central Virginia. Multiple regression analysis of a population-based study. Am. J. Respir. Crit. Care Med. 156: 1760.

Sublett, J. L., Seltzer, J., Burkhead, R. et al. 2010. Air filters and air cleaners: rostrum by the American Academy of Allergy, Asthma & Immunology Indoor Allergen Committee. J. Allergy Clin. Immunol. 125: 32.

Terreehorst, I., Hak, E., Oosting, A. J. et al. 2003. Evaluation of impermeable covers for bedding in patients with allergic rhinitis. N Engl. J. Med. 349: 237.

Thoms, F., Jennings, G. T., Maudrich, M. et al. 2019. Immunization of cats to induce neutralizing antibodies against Fel d 1, the major feline allergen in human subjects. J. Allergy Clin. Immunol. 144: 193.

Tovey, E. R., Chapman, M. D., Wells, C. W. and Platts-Mills T. A. 1981. The distribution of dust mite allergen in the houses of patients with asthma. Am. Rev. Respir. Dis. 124: 630.

US EPA: https://www.epa.gov/indoor-air-quality-iaq/volatile-organic-compounds-impact-indoor-air-quality (Accessed June 10, 2022).

van der Heide, S., van Aalderen, W. M., Kauffman, H. F. et al. 1999. Clinical effects of air cleaners in homes of asthmatic children sensitized to pet allergens. J. Allergy Clin. Immunol. 104: 447.

van Ree, R. 2007. Indoor allergens: relevance of major allergen measurements and standardization. J. Allergy Clin. Immunol. 119: 270.

van Schayck, O. C., Maas, T., Kaper, J. et al. 2007. Is there any role for allergen avoidance in the primary prevention of childhood asthma? J. Allergy Clin. Immunol. 119: 1323.

Vantassel, S. M., Hygnstrom, S. E. and Ferraro, D. M. 2012. Controlling house mice. Revised March 2012. Lincoln (NE): University of Nebraska-Lincoln Extension. http://www.ianrpubs.unl.edu/live/g1105/build/g1105.pdf (Accessed on October 31, 2013).

Vaughan, J. W., McLaughlin, T. E., Perzanowski, M. S. and Platts-Mills, T. A. 1999. Evaluation of materials used for bedding encasement: effect of pore size in blocking cat and dust mite allergen. J. Allergy Clin. Immunol. 103: 227.

Voorhorst, R., Spieksma-Boezeman, M. I. and Spieksma, F. T. 1964. Is a mite (Dermatophagoides spp.) the producer of the house dust mite allergen? Allerg. Asthma (Leipz) 10: 329

Vredegoor, D. W., Willemse, T., Chapman, M. D. et al. 2012. Can f 1 levels in hair and homes of different dog breeds: lack of evidence to describe any dog breed as hypoallergenic. J. Allergy Clin. Immunol. 130: 904.

Walshaw, M. J. and Evans, C. C. 1986. Allergen avoidance in house dust mite sensitive adult asthma. QJ Med. 58: 199.

Wan, H., Winton, H. L., Soeller, C. et al. 1999. Der p 1 facilitates transepithelial allergen delivery by disruption of tight junctions. J. Clin. Invest 104: 123.

Wang, J., Visness, C. M., Calatroni, A. et al. 2009. Effect of environmental allergen sensitization on asthma morbidity in inner-city asthmatic children. Clin. Exp. Allergy 39: 1381.

Wilson, J. M. and Platts-Mills, T. A. E. 2018. Home environmental interventions for house dust mite. J. Allergy Clin. Immunol. Pract. 6: 1.

Wood, R. A., Chapman, M. D., Adkinson, N. F. Jr and Eggleston, P. A. 1989. The effect of cat removal on allergen content in household-dust samples. J. Allergy Clin. Immunol. 83: 730.

Wood, R. A., Johnson, E. F., Van Natta, M. L. et al. 1998. A placebo-controlled trial of a HEPA air cleaner in the treatment of cat allergy. Am. J. Respir. Crit. Care Med. 158: 115.

Woodcock, A., Forster, L., Matthews, E. et al. 2003. Control of exposure to mite allergen and allergen-impermeable bed covers for adults with asthma. N Engl. J. Med. 349: 225.

Woodfolk, J. A., Hayden, M. L., Miller, J. D. et al. 1994. Chemical treatment of carpets to reduce allergen: a detailed study of the effects of tannic acid on indoor allergens. J. Allergy Clin. Immunol. 94: 19.

Yarbrough, J. A., Armstrong, J. L., Blumberg, M. Z. et al. 1999. Allergic rhinoconjunctivitis caused by Harmonia axyridis (Asian lady beetle, Japanese lady beetle, or lady bug). J. Allergy Clin. Immunol. 104: 704.

Ye, Q., Krechmer, J. E., Shutter, J. D. et al. 2021. Real-Time laboratory measurements of VOC emissions, removal rates, and byproduct formation from consumer grade oxidation based air cleaners. Env. Sci. Technol. Lett. 12: 1020–1025.

Chapter 12

Insect Allergy

Diagnostic Procedures and Venom Immunotherapy

Karla E. Adams[1],* and *David B.K. Golden*[2]

◇◇

Introduction

Reactions to insect stings and bites are well characterized and range from localized cutaneous reactions to potentially life-threatening anaphylaxis. After a known or suspected allergic reaction to an insect sting, patients require counseling on the diagnosis, treatment and prognosis of the condition. In addition, patients must be advised on insect avoidance, possible emergency treatment of future sting reactions and the role of referral to an allergy specialist for further evaluation. When indicated, allergy testing should be done via skin testing or *in vitro* testing, with adjunct laboratory evaluation conducted if needed and available. Patients with insect-triggered severe allergic reactions who have a confirmatory diagnostic evaluation should be considered candidates for immunotherapy in order to decrease their risk of recurrent reactions with future stings. This chapter will review the characteristics of insect-triggered allergic reactions, the diagnostic evaluation tools that are available, treatment considerations and key factors that must be taken into account for all venom-allergic patients.

Insects

We begin with a review of the most common stinging insects known to trigger allergic reactions in humans. Important factors to understand when considering insect allergy include knowledge of entomology and the evolutionary relationship of insects. For example, one of the largest orders of insects is the Hymenoptera order, which consists of over 150,000 known species that have significant economic and ecological impact as pollinators and predators. One Hymenoptera sub-order is the Aprocrita, which is characterized by the presence of a petiole or narrow waist between the first two segments of the abdomen. In parasitoid species, this flexibility allows them to deposit eggs via an ovipositor. The monophyletic Aculeata clade has an evolved ovipositor that stings and delivers venom to prey for protection and defense. Within the Aculeata, common culprits for stinging insect reactions include members of the Apidae (honeybees), Vespidae (yellow jackets,

[1] Associate Professor of Pediatrics, Allergy & Immunology Division, Department of Medicine, Wilford Hall Ambulatory Surgical Center, 1100 Wilford Hall Loop, Bldg. 4554, Lackland AFB, San Antonio TX 78236.
[2] Associate Professor of Medicine, Johns Hopkins University, 25 Crossroads Drive #410, Owings Mills, MD 21117.
Email: dbkgolden@gmail.com
* Corresponding author: karla.e.adams2.mil@health.mil

Table 1. Common stinging and biting insects.

Order	Family	Subfamily	Genus	Common Name
Hymenoptera	Apidae	Apinae	*Apis*	Honeybee
			Bombus	Bumblebee
	Vespidae	Vespinae	*Vespula*	Yellow jacket
			Dolichovespula	Hornet
		Polistinae	*Polistes*	Wasp
	Formicidae	Myrmicinae	*Solenopsis*	Fire ant
			Pogonomyrmex	Harvester ant
		Myrmeciinae	*Myrmecia*	Jack jumper ant
		Ponerinae	*Pachycondyla*	Samsum ant
Diptera	Culicidae	Culicinae	*Aedes*	Mosquito
Coleoptera	Coccinellidae	Coccinellinae	*Harmonia*	Ladybug
Hemiptera	Reduviidae	Triatominae	*Triatoma*	Kissing bug

hornets and wasps) and Formicidae (ant) families. Table 1 shows common stinging and biting insects implicated in human allergic disease.

Flying Hymenoptera

Flying members of the Hymenoptera order are some of the most common human stinging insects. Survey data estimates a lifetime prevalence of a Hymenoptera sting ranging from 56.6% to 94.5% (Incorvaia et al. 1997; Kalyoncu et al. 1997). Stings can occur in any age group and are commonly seen in individuals whose occupations place them at higher risk for exposure, such as landscapers or honeybee keepers. In North America, common flying Hymenoptera stings are from *Vespula* species (yellow jackets), *Dolichovespula* (hornets), *Polistes* (wasps) and *Apis mellifera* (honeybee). Depending on geography, however, some locations may have a different distribution of individual species, which needs to be considered as it pertains to the specific allergens that need to be present in diagnostic and therapeutic extracts.

The characteristics or historical details of each sting event are important as the information may point to the trigger culprit. For example, aggressive Hymenoptera such as *Vespula* or *Polistes* species can sting with little to no provocation. Vespids are scavengers who are often present in outdoor settings where food is present (e.g., picnics, near trash receptacles). Although most yellow jackets can sting multiple times due to a retractable stinger, some species do tend to leave the stinger embedded in the skin. *Polistes* species are less aggressive though they can also sting multiple times with a retractable stinger if disturbed. The Apidae family, which includes honeybees and bumblebees, are typically docile species that will sting in defense if they feel threatened. Honeybees have a barbed stinger that may be retained in the skin, which offers clues as to the trigger of a reaction if present. Bumblebees are rare culprits of insect stings. The exception in the Apidae family is the Africanized honeybee (*Apis mellifera scutellata*), which was introduced to South America in the 1950s but has since interbred with the European honeybee and expanded its habitat to now include North America. Africanized honeybees are very aggressive, can chase prey over long distances and often swarm and sting in large numbers.

Stinging Ants

The Formicidae family includes over 14,000 species of ants. Of these, only a few species are known to trigger allergic reactions in humans. In the United States (U.S.), the two imported fire ant (IFA) species, *Solenopsis invicta* and *Solenopsis richteri* are the most common stinging ants in the south. Both are now endemic species in the southern U.S. after their inadvertent introduction through the port of Mobile, Alabama in the 1930s. *S. invicta* is present throughout the southern U.S., whereas

S. richteri is found in northwest Alabama and northeast Mississippi. Annually, the IFA sting rate is up to 58% (deShazo et al. 1984). The mechanism behind IFA stings is important to understand as it explains how IFA local reactions occur. The IFA bites down with its mandible then curves its abdomen in order to pierce the skin with its stinger. While anchored on its mandible, the IFA will pivot and reposition its abdomen to sting again and deliver a mixture of venom and piperidine alkaloids. The result is a circular rosette of stings that over 24 hours becomes a sterile pseudopustule. IFAs are very aggressive and will swarm with minimal disruption of their characteristic mound. Native fire ant species, *S. geminata*, *S. xiloni* and *S. aureus*, are widely distributed across the world though are only rarely implicated as causes of allergic reactions in humans.

Other stinging ants that are associated with allergic reactions include members of the *Myrmecia*, *Pachycondyla* and *Pogonomyrmex* genera. The distribution of these species determines their impact on human stinging reactions. For instance, most allergic stinging ant reactions in Australia are due to *Myrmecia pilosula* (Jack Jumper ant) and *Myrmecia pyriformis* (bull ant), which affect up to 2.7% of the population (Brown et al. 2003).

Biting Insects

Several other insect orders such as the Diptera (mosquitoes), Coleoptera (ladybugs) and Hemiptera (kissing bugs) are associated with adverse reactions when they come in contact with humans. While most reactions to these insects are self-limited cutaneous reactions, rare systemic allergic reactions have also been reported (Peng et al. 2004; Anderson and Belnap 2015). There are several commercial extracts to evaluate for reactions to mosquito in the U.S., though they are limited by a lack of standardization (Crisp and Johnson 2013). The lack of commercial extract availability for other biting insects limits routine evaluation and treatment of affected patients.

Epidemiology

The prevalence of Hymenoptera venom allergy (HVA) is estimated to be 3% in adults and 0.8% in children (Settipane et al. 1972; Golden et al. 1989). The exact prevalence of HVA is unclear and likely underreported with factors such as age, occupation and location all playing a role. For example, HVA was noted in 19% of children from the European Anaphylaxis Registry (Grabenhenrich et al. 2016). In a retrospective analysis of the epidemiology of anaphylaxis at a large tertiary center in the U.S., Hymenoptera stings were the second most common trigger for anaphylaxis seen in 24.6% of patients (Gonzalez-Estrada et al. 2017). Certain occupations are at increased exposure and thus presumably at increased risk for developing HVA. Bee keepers, for instance, have a prevalence of HVA of 14% to 32% (Muller 2005). Comparatively, firefighters in Spain have an HVA prevalence of 19.7%, which is 3-fold higher than the local general population in a recent study (Soriano-Gomis et al. 2021).

Insect-Triggered Fatalities

Fatal reactions due to stinging insects have occurred in patients with and without a history of previous insect reactions. Overall, the rate of fatal insect stings is estimated to be 0.1 cases per million annually (Turner et al. 2017). Despite recent data that shows an increase in venom-triggered anaphylaxis, the fatality case rate has remained stable or decreased over the same period (Liew et al. 2009; Motosue et al. 2017). In the U.S., Caucasian race, male sex and age over 60 were noted as risk factors for fatal insect reactions (Jerschow et al. 2014).

Clinical Features

As the diagnosis of HVA is clinical, the historical details that surround a stinging insect reaction such as the location of the sting, activity surrounding the event, visualization of the culprit insect or nearby nests, the timing of symptom onset and the characteristics of each symptom, as well as any treatments used are all key facts that need to be obtained in order to arrive at the diagnosis. Historical details such as the presence of a retained stinger may point to one species over another but may not be definitive. Similarly, the presence of a pseudopustule after an ant sting may indicate IFA as the culprit, though its absence may not completely rule out IFA as patients may not be on the lookout for these lesions. Identification of insects by patients or family is not reliable and thus should not drive the selection of which flying Hymenoptera species to test to evaluate for HVA (Baker et al. 2014).

Allergic symptoms after an insect sting range from localized cutaneous symptoms to systemic reactions or anaphylaxis. Local reactions are characterized by pruritus, erythema and edema that is contiguous to the site of the sting. Large local reactions (LLRs) are late-phase IgE-mediated cutaneous reactions that start within 24 to 48 hours after a sting and are associated with erythema and edema 10 cm in diameter and larger. LLRs can be debilitating as they can cross joints and affect daily activities (e.g., LLRs in the lower extremities can lead to difficulty ambulating). Systemic cutaneous reactions are characterized by the development of diffuse urticaria with or without angioedema not contiguous with the sting site. Finally, in some patients, an insect sting can lead to multi-system allergic symptoms that start within minutes of a sting and are better described as anaphylaxis. Anaphylaxis is characterized by the acute onset of symptoms that can be severe and life-threatening. Symptoms of anaphylaxis include cutaneous symptoms (flushing, urticaria with or without angioedema), respiratory symptoms (coughing, wheezing, shortness of breath), gastrointestinal symptoms (nausea, vomiting, diarrhea and abdominal pain), or cardiovascular symptoms (light-headedness, hypotension or shock and arrhythmias). Rarely, Kounis syndrome (a form of cardiac anaphylaxis) can occur after an insect sting (Jairam et al. 2010; Ridolo et al. 2012). Biphasic reactions, or the recurrence of allergic symptoms without re-exposure, can occur up to 72 hours after the initial symptoms and have been described in 5% to 25% of patients (Ellis and Day 2007; Lee et al. 2015). Table 2 summarizes the clinical features of insect-triggered reactions.

A large number of insect stings can sometimes cause toxic reactions that are non-immunologic. Acute kidney injury can occur in toxic envenomation due to arterial hypotension, hemolysis, rhabdomyolysis or a direct toxic effect on renal tubules (Silva et al. 2017). Other examples of atypical reactions after Hymenoptera stings include the development of serum sickness-like reactions, neurologic symptoms, acquired cold urticaria and chronic urticaria (Light et al. 1977; Jairam et al. 2010; Wong and Borici-Mazi 2012; Kutlu et al. 2013).

Table 2. Clinical features of insect-triggered reactions.

Reaction Type	Signs and Symptoms	Onset After a Sting
Large Local Reaction	• Pruritus • Edema • Erythema • Diameter $\geq$ 10 cm • May cross joints or affect entire extremity	• 24–48 hours
Systemic Cutaneous	• Urticaria ± angioedema non-contiguous with sting site • Flushing, sensation of warmth	• Immediate-hours
Anaphylaxis	• Cutaneous: urticaria, angioedema, flushing • Upper/Lower Respiratory: rhinitis, congestion, sneezing, cough, wheezing, shortness of breath, chest tightness, stridor • Cardiovascular: hypotension, shock, arrhythmia, tachycardia, loss of consciousness • Gastrointestinal: nausea, emesis, diarrhea, abdominal pain • Genitourinary: uterine cramps	• Immediate-hours • Biphasic symptoms in some

Natural History and Prognosis

The natural history of venom allergy is largely dependent on the specific clinical pattern being evaluated. For instance, asymptomatic venom sensitization, or the presence of venom-specific IgE (sIgE) without a correlating history of a sting-triggered reaction, can be seen in up to 15% of patients via skin testing (Golden et al. 1989). However, only 5% of asymptomatic though sensitized patients go on to have systemic symptoms with a deliberate sting (Sturm et al. 2014). LLRs tend to recur with future stings. In these patients, repeat stings are associated with systemic symptoms in 5% to 10% of adults and 2% to 7% of children (Graft et al. 1984; Mauriello et al. 1984; Golden et al. 2004). This risk may be dependent on the number of previous LLRs. In a small prospective study, patients with at least two LLRs had zero risk for systemic symptoms on re-sting (Pucci et al. 2015). In contrast, in patients who were followed prospectively after one LLR, 24% had systemic reactions on a subsequent sting (Bilo et al. 2019). Patients who experience systemic cutaneous symptoms have a 10% to 15% risk of recurrent systemic symptoms though less than a 3% chance of a more severe reaction with a future sting (van der Linden et al. 1994; Golden et al. 2004; Golden et al. 2006; Lange et al. 2016). Finally, patients at the highest risk of recurrence are those with insect-triggered anaphylaxis which is associated with a 30% to 70% risk of systemic symptoms with future stings (Reisman 1992; Golden et al. 2004; Lange et al. 2016).

Factors that affect the prognosis of HVA include the previous clinical history, knowledge of the natural history of the clinical pattern, the risk for future exposures and an assessment of patient-specific factors that may place them at risk. For example, patients with LLRs may experience significant morbidity and a decrement in their quality of life (QOL) if their occupation or hobbies place them at high risk of recurrent insect stings. In others, underlying medical problems such as respiratory or cardiovascular disease may place them at higher risk for severe insect-triggered symptoms or intolerance of immediate treatment for anaphylaxis. While the single best predictor for recurrent insect sting reactions is the history of a previous clinical reaction, understanding the variables that confer additional risk and impact HVA morbidity is key to providing personalized medical recommendations.

Diagnostics

Venoms

We begin our review of diagnostics with a discussion of venom extracts, procurement, cross-reactivity and availability, as extracts are central to both the diagnosis and the treatment of HVA. Honeybee venom is collected by electrical stimulation, whereas Vespid venom is obtained via direct dissection of the venom sacs followed by purification of the venom obtained. For IFA, whole ants are crushed to produce a whole-body extract (WBE). The difference in procurement is important as it allows for the standardization of venom extracts (flying Hymenoptera extracts), whereas IFA WBEs are not standardized. In the U.S., single venom lyophilized extracts exist for *Apis*, *Polistes* (*mixed species*), *Vespula* (*mixed species*) and two *Dolichovespula* species (yellow and white-faced hornet). A mixed Vespid extract that contains yellow jacket, yellow hornet and white-faced hornet venoms is also available. IFA WBE is available as a single species extract (*S. richteri*; *S. invicta*) or a mixture of both. Table 3 reviews the characteristics of venom extracts in the U.S.

Knowledge of the composition of venom extracts is key to understanding cross-reactivity patterns, which in turn aids in the interpretation of HVA diagnostic tests. Table 4 shows sample venom allergens, function if known and availability of recombinant allergens. Major allergens in honeybee venom include phospholipase A_2 (Api m 1) and hyaluronidase (Api m 2). Honeybee venom also has a unique allergen called melittin or Api m 4. Honeybee component allergens that are commercially available for clinical testing include Api m 1, 2, 3, 5 and 10. Major allergens in Vespid venom include Antigen 5 (e.g., Ves v 5, Dol a 5, etc.), phospholipase A_1 (Ves v 1, etc.)

Table 3. Hymenoptera extracts and practical aspects of venom immunotherapy in the United States.

	Flying Hymenoptera	Imported Fire Ant
Extracts	Standardized venom extracts	Non-standardized whole body extracts
Single Allergen	Honeybee Yellow jacket White-faced hornet Yellow hornet Wasp	*Solenopsis invicta* *Solenopsis richteri*
Mixtures	Mixed Vespid: Yellow jacket, White-faced hornet, Yellow hornet	Mixture *S. invicta* and *S. richteri*
Immunotherapy Starting Dose	0.001 to 0.01 μg for single venom extracts 0.003 to 0.03 μg for mixed Vespid extract	0.05 ml of 1:100,000 weight/volume extract
Immunotherapy Maintenance Dose	100 μg for single venom extracts 300 μg for mixed Vespid extract	0.5 ml of a 1:100 weight/volume extract

Table 4. Sample venom allergens and characteristics.

Insect	Allergen	Available Recombinant Allergen	Allergen Name/Function
Apis mellifera	Api m 1 Api m 2 Api m 3 Api m 4 Api m 5 Api m 10	rApi m 1 rApi m 2 rApi m 3 rApi m 5 rApi m 10	Phospholipase A2 Hyaluronidase Acid Phosphatase Melittin Dipeptidyl peptidase IV Icarapin
Vespula vulgaris	Ves v 1 Ves v 2 Ves v 3 Ves v 5	rVes v 1 rVes v 3 rVes v 5	Phospholipase A1 Hyaluronidase Dipeptidyl peptidase IV Antigen 5
Dolichovespula maculate	Dol m 1 Dol m 2 Dol m 5		Phospholipase A1 Hyaluronidase Antigen 5
Polistes dominula	Pol d 1 Pol d 4 Pol d 5	rPol d 1 rPol d 5	Phospholipase A1 Protease Antigen 5
Solenopsis invicta	Sol i 1 Sol i 2 Sol i 3 Sol i 4		Phospholipase A1 Function unknown Antigen 5 Homologous Sol i 2

and hyaluronidase (Ves v 2, etc.). The phospholipase found in Vespids is not related to honeybee phospholipase, however, hyaluronidase cross-reactivity can be seen due to the presence of cross-reactive carbohydrate determinants (CCDs) (Hemmer et al. 2001). The domestic Mediterranean wasp, *Polistes dominulus*, is now increasingly found in North America and poses a diagnostic dilemma due to only partial cross-reactivity with commercial extracts that include *P. annularis*, *P. fuscatus*, *P. exclamans* and *P. metricus* (Severino et al. 2006).

IFA extracts are composed of a mixture of piperidine alkaloids and several major allergenic proteins. There is extensive cross-reactivity between the two IFA species. Sol i 1 is a phospholipase that can cross-react with Vespid phospholipase (Hoffman et al. 1988). Sol i 3 is a member of the Antigen 5 family and is homologous with Vespid Antigen 5 though only limited cross-reactivity is seen. Sol r 1–3 are homologous to Sol i 1–3 though there is no analogous Sol i 4 antigen in *S. richteri*.

Additional limitations in regard to venom extract availability also need to be carefully considered. In the U.S., a venom shortage due to the loss of a commercial manufacturer in 2016 placed a significant strain on the ability to test for and treat HVA (Golden et al. 2017). A total lapse in the commercial supply of venom allergen extracts in Canada and Australia occurred for more than one year. In Europe, dialyzed venoms and depot venom extracts are available and provide additional options not presently available in the U.S. Finally, it is important to note that not all species endemic to a particular location will be represented in available commercial extracts, which poses a risk of underdiagnosis or under treatment in select populations.

Indications for Venom Testing

The decision to test for venom allergy is dependent on the clinical history of anaphylaxis after an insect sting. Conducting diagnostic testing for HVA without a correlating clinical history may reveal sensitization only and thus should be avoided. There is potential harm in recommending venom allergy testing, and thus it should be limited to patients who have a clear indication for venom immunotherapy (VIT). There are many people who have positive venom allergy tests but have a low risk of anaphylaxis to a future sting. A positive test can cause fear and may inhibit normal outdoor activities in some patients or families, and will usually also lead to a prescription of epinephrine auto-injectors which carry significant psychological and financial burdens. A positive test can also lead to administrative barriers (e.g., waiver request) for someone seeking to serve in the U.S. military and affiliated services even if they have never had a severe reaction to a sting. Therefore, venom testing should only be done in those with a clear history of anaphylaxis who are candidates for VIT. Venom testing and VIT are not generally recommended for patients with LLRs or systemic cutaneous reactions since their future risk of a more severe reaction is low. If, however, the patient is experiencing significant morbidity from recurrent LLRs or systemic cutaneous reactions, then testing and VIT can be considered in order to improve their QOL.

Testing for HVA is classically done via skin testing or serologic testing to assess the presence of sIgE of the venom in question. If testing to the first modality is negative, then testing should be repeated with the other available test. Timing is important as positive venom testing is more likely when done within 3 years of the last sting in patients with and without venom-triggered allergic reactions (Golden et al. 1989). Patients who test negative on skin testing and serologic testing should have testing repeated prior to determining that VIT is not indicated.

Table 5 provides a summary of available diagnostic tests that should be considered for patients undergoing workups for HVA.

Skin Tests

Synonyms

Prick skin test, skin test, scratch test, puncture test, intracutaneous testing and intradermal testing.

Test Explanation and Interpretation

Skin tests to evaluate for insect allergy can be conducted depending on the availability of commercial extracts. For flying Hymenoptera sting reactions, all five of the standardized venom extracts are utilized for testing. Protocols can vary and may include an initial prick test of each venom at a concentration of 100 µg/mL. Prick testing with venoms has poor sensitivity and is not utilized by most experts in the U.S. If the prick test is performed and is positive for some of the venoms, intradermal (ID) tests should be performed only for the venoms that were negative. Intradermal testing can be done starting at concentrations of 0.001 µg/mL to 0.01 µg/mL of each venom. If negative, a 10-fold higher venom concentration is placed intradermally until a positive test is noted or a maximum concentration of 1 µg/mL is reached. Utilizing venom concentrations higher than 1 µg/mL for ID testing increases the risk of a false positive test and thus should be avoided (Georgitis and Reisman 1985).

Table 5. Venom allergy diagnostic tests benefits and limitations.

Diagnostic Modality	Benefits	Limitations
Venom Skin Test		
	• Results within hours	• Requires specialized training to conduct • Small risk of adverse reaction • Dependent on availability of relevant allergens • Cannot conduct in some patients (e.g., dermatographism) • Concurrent medications may interfere with interpretation
***In Vitro* Tests**		
	• No need to stop routine medications • No risk for triggering allergic reaction • Underlying medical conditions typically not a factor	• Results may take days or weeks • Cost
Venom Specific IgE	• No specialized training needed to conduct	• Limited interpretation in patients with elevated total IgE levels • Results not interchangeable across testing platforms
Component Resolved Diagnostics	• Role in differentiating multiple sensitizations • Increased clinical sensitivity with multiple allergen panels	• Dependent on commercial availability of native and recombinant component allergens that are geographically relevant
Serum Basal Tryptase	• Role in evaluating for underlying condition associated with risk (e.g., mast cell disease, Hereditary α-tryptasemia), marker for increased reaction severity, adverse reactions to immunotherapy or relapse after immunotherapy	• Timing of test needs to be considered • No commercial test available to test α and β tryptase levels • Elevated total tryptase may be due to other medical conditions
Basophil Activation Test	• Role in differentiating multiple sensitizations • Predictor for adverse reactions with venom immunotherapy and risk for relapse	• Lack of commercial availability • Timing of collection and running the test • Lack of standardized reporting, validation and interpretation across labs
Sting Challenge Test		
	• Significant research application to determine factors that impact risk or protection in venom allergy • Prognostic information in patients who are receiving venom immunotherapy • Improved quality of life for some patients	• Significant risk for triggering anaphylaxis • Requires trained personnel to collect/identify insects, perform challenge, recognize/treat anaphylaxis • Patient factors may contraindicate this test • Concurrent medications may interfere with interpretation • Dependent on availability of relevant species

There are variable methods in regard to the technique of ID testing and interpretation. In the U.S., a volume of 0.02 to 0.03 mL of venom extract is placed intradermally to raise a 3 to 4 mm bleb (Bernstein et al. 2008). However, the product package insert for Hymenoptera venoms recommends placing the ID test with a 0.05 mL injection. A positive venom ID test is defined as a wheal of 3 to 5 mm above the negative control with surrounding erythema although some use the method of Norman to define a positive ID test (wheal of 5 to 10 mm with a flare of 11 mm to 20 mm) (Golden et al. 2017). A positive test at the prick step or any ID step is sufficient evidence of the presence of venom-IgE and thus no further testing needs to be done for that venom. Although the skin test result (i.e., size of the wheal) is not a reliable predictor of reaction severity, the concentration at which a venom skin test becomes positive may be indicative of a higher degree of sensitivity which in turn correlates with increased frequency of reactions.

Recent advances in skin testing have looked at faster protocols (e.g., single-step ID testing using at 1 μg/mL concentration) or simultaneous ID testing which show promising results regarding safety and cost reduction (Strohmeier et al. 2013; Quirt et al. 2016). This may also allow for the use of a much smaller number of ID tests, especially in young children.

Skin testing for IFA hypersensitivity uses a similar protocol as in flying Hymenoptera allergy. Selection of which WBE to use for testing is at the discretion of the allergist, though testing for single IFA species can be done based on geographic location or an IFA WBE mix can be utilized. A prick test at a concentration of 1×10^{-3} weight/volume (wt/vol) can be considered initially. If the prick test is negative, then ID testing at an initial concentration of 1×10^{-6} wt/vol can be done. Similar to flying Hymenoptera ID testing, increasing 10-fold concentrations of WBE is used until the test is positive or a maximum concentration of 1×10^{-3} wt/vol is reached.

Indications

Venom skin testing should be considered for any patient who presents with symptoms of anaphylaxis after a Hymenoptera sting, although it may be of more potential harm than benefit in individuals who do not require VIT (e.g., no history of anaphylaxis). All five flying Hymenoptera should be tested, as patient recollection and identification of what insect stung them is not sufficient. IFA alone may be tested in endemic areas if the history is typical and consistent with ant-triggered symptoms only. Select patients who have not experienced anaphylaxis (e.g., patients with LLRs) but have recurrent exposures or those who experience significant morbidity after a sting may undergo additional testing and consideration of VIT based on shared decision-making and patient values and preferences.

Clinical Co-Relationship and Limitations

Venom skin testing should be done as soon as feasible, though in some patients, a skin test done within days to weeks after an insect reaction may be negative due to a refractory period after mast cell degranulation. In these patients, skin tests should be repeated in a few months or alternatively *in vitro* testing can be considered as up to 10% of patients with a negative skin test will have evidence of sIgE via serologic testing. Negative venom skin testing does not eliminate all risks or rule out a diagnosis of HVA. Patients with convincing histories of HVA may still be at risk with subsequent stings despite negative skin testing and thus require repeat testing or additional diagnostics in order to optimally exclude HVA. Patients whose sting-triggered symptoms occurred remotely from testing may have negative testing due to a loss of sensitization. In a study of a general adult population (mostly asymptomatic), positive venom tests became negative at an estimated rate of 12% annually (Golden et al. 1997). Table 6 lists the possible reasons for negative skin test results that should be considered.

While a benefit of skin testing is that results are immediate, this implies that commercial venom extracts are available in order to conduct the testing. As noted previously, any shortage of venom

Table 6. Possible reasons for a negative venom skin test.

Improper test placement
Refractory period after a sting
Loss of sensitization (e.g., prolonged time between last sting and testing)
Lack of relevant allergens in extracts
Underlying mast cell disease

extracts in a region will have a direct impact on testing availability. Finally, the specific species sources used to create commercial extracts has profound influence on the sensitivity of diagnostic tests and the effectiveness of VIT.

Special Precautions

Conducting venom skin tests requires specific training on the management of venom extracts including reconstitution and dilution of extracts, proper technique for placement of prick and ID tests and interpretation of the test results. Data on risks for venom skin testing is limited. A survey study of practicing allergists from 1979 to 1982 noted adverse reactions in up to 1.4% of patients undergoing venom skin testing (Lockey et al. 1989). Currently, adverse reactions with skin testing are likely seen in less than 1% based on expert evidence. While special precaution needs to be taken for patients at higher risk for reactions or those who may not tolerate a systemic reaction or its treatment (e.g., patients with poorly controlled asthma may require that their asthma control be optimized prior to testing), venom skin testing remains a safe procedure and important diagnostic tool for the evaluation of HVA. A consideration for these special populations is to conduct *in vitro* testing first as it does not carry the same potential risks, then conduct skin testing if *in vitro* testing is negative.

Interfering Agents

Agents that interfere with venom skin testing are the same as for other allergen skin tests. First and second-generation antihistamines block the downstream effects of histamine release after mast cell activation and thus should be held by patients for 3 to 5 days prior to skin testing (Bernstein et al. 2008). Other medications with antihistamine properties (e.g., tricyclic antidepressants) may blunt skin test reactivity and should be held (if possible) for 1 to 2 weeks prior to skin testing. Newer medications such as mirtazapine or quetiapine have also been shown to suppress skin test responses so efforts should be made to hold these medications prior to skin testing (Kjaer et al. 2021). Omalizumab can decrease skin test reactivity by suppressing the late-phase skin response within 2 weeks of initiation though this effect reverses upon cessation of omalizumab (Ong et al. 2005; Corren et al. 2008). While beta-blockers (BB) are not known to interfere with skin test results, their use may be associated with increased severity or treatment-refractory anaphylaxis in patients who experience a systemic reaction to skin testing. The decision to skin test on or off a BB must be individualized after carefully weighing all the risks.

In Vitro Testing

Venom-Specific IgE Testing

Synonyms

Serology, RAST testing, ImmunoCAP™ testing and immunoassay.

Test Explanation and Interpretation

Serologic testing can be conducted to evaluate for the presence of free (unbound) venom sIgE. The first *in vitro* test for allergens was the Phadebas radioallergosorbent test (RAST) (Pharmacia, Uppsala, Sweden), which was a solid-phase radioimmunoassay. Since then, the term "RAST" continues to be used interchangeably with other serologic tests though currently available testing platforms are not radioimmunoassays. Available serologic tests are singleplex solid-phase or liquid-phase enzyme-linked immunosorbent assays (ELISA) that utilize fluorescence or chemiluminescence for antigen-antibody detection. Because each commercial testing platform utilizes different techniques to bind the allergen to its solid-phase matrix, the reported sIgE values are not interchangeable across testing platforms. ImmunoCAP™ is the most commonly used platform worldwide and has become the *de facto* standard for research and clinical reporting. The result of serologic testing is a quantitative sIgE value typically reported as kUa/L. While values > 0.35 kUa/L are considered to be positive and clinically relevant, laboratory technical improvements allow for the ability to report values between 0.10 and 0.35 kUa/L. The clinical utility of a lowered positive threshold is unknown though it may be beneficial in some patients. For example, the use of recombinant allergens and decreasing the diagnostic cut off to 0.10 kUa/L was associated with increased diagnostic sensitivity in a group of patients with undetectable venom-IgE (Michel et al. 2016).

Indications

Venom serology testing is indicated in patients with clinical histories of insect-triggered systemic or anaphylactic reactions. As with skin testing, serologic testing needs to be completed for all five flying Hymenoptera species for patients with a flying insect-triggered reaction. A serologic test for IFA is also commercially available and can be obtained for patients with IFA-triggered symptoms.

In vitro testing is particularly useful in patients who cannot undergo skin testing (e.g., patients unable to stop antihistamines, patients with dermatographism or those who are unlikely to tolerate skin testing). Serologic testing also becomes particularly helpful in patients who have a negative skin test for venoms.

Clinical Co-Relationship and Limitations

Evidence of venom sIgE obtained through serology in a patient with insect-triggered anaphylaxis is diagnostic of HVA. Similar to skin testing, serologic testing should only be done in patients with supporting clinical histories of HVA. Positive venom serology in a patient who has not had a systemic reaction to that insect is only indicative of sensitization and is associated with only a slightly increased future risk for that patient (and is not an indication for VIT). Furthermore, the absolute value of a serologic test does not offer any additional prognostic utility (i.e., no association with increased risk of a reaction or severity of a reaction). Another limitation to consider is the discordance between skin tests and serologic tests (e.g., skin tests may be positive in up to 20% of patients with negative venom serology) and thus they are best thought of as complementary testing modalities. Finally, additional limitations for serologic testing include the cost of the test and increased time to diagnosis since results of most *in vitro* tests are reported in days or weeks.

Special Precautions

There are no special precautions that need to be taken for serologic testing. Trained phlebotomists and available commercial platforms for *in vitro* testing are needed in order to run the tests. Patient factors that may place them at increased risk for systemic reactions are not a precaution for *in vitro* testing, hence this testing modality is a great option for patients who cannot stop medications that may interfere with skin testing or who have underlying risk factors that place them at higher risk with skin testing.

Interfering Agents

Special attention must be given to the interpretation of serologic tests in patients with elevated total serum IgE levels as non-specific binding may be seen. Similar precautions should be taken with respect to patients on omalizumab. Omalizumab is a biologic monoclonal antibody that binds free IgE and prevents its binding to mast cells. Commercial testing for total IgE does not discriminate between free and bound IgE, so total IgE values tend to increase upon initiation of omalizumab. Limited data on aeroallergen sIgE responses showed increased allergen-sIgE with omalizumab treatment that was dependent on pre-treatment sIgE levels (Mizuma et al. 2015). In a study evaluating the effects of omalizumab on the accuracy and reproducibility of total IgE and allergen-specific testing, total serum IgE levels were dependent on the diagnostic platform being utilized with ImmunoCAP™ showing the least reduction compared to five other assays (Hamilton 2006). Omalizumab decreased ImmunoCAP™ allergen-sIgE by 0.8% to 27.8% and showed a reduction of honeybee-IgE of 12.6% (Hamilton 2006).

Component Resolved Diagnostics

Synonyms

Component testing, component-specific testing, molecular allergy diagnostics and CRD.

Test Explanation and Interpretation

Component-resolved diagnostics (CRD) provides a more detailed immunologic sensitization profile for individual patients. Serologic testing using whole venom extracts measures sIgE against a complement of multiple venom proteins, whereas CRD tests for individual venom proteins. The result is a quantitative value of sIgE directed against the individually tested venom allergen component.

CRD can help differentiate between cross-reactivity and true clinical sensitization in patients who are polysensitized. Sensitization to multiple venoms can be due to the presence of sIgE directed against CCD moieties (found in plants and venoms) and homologous venom proteins or may be due to true clinically relevant sensitization to more than one insect. Extensive cross-reactivity is noted within the Vespinae subfamily (yellow jackets and hornets) and is less common between *Polistes* and Vespinae. European data shows frequent cross-reactivity between honeybees and Vespids (Muller et al. 2009). Testing to honeybee component allergens (Api m 1, Api m 2, Api m 3, Api m 5 and Api m 10) and Vespid allergens (Ves v 1 and Ves v 5) can differentiate honeybee and Vespid cross-reactivity from double sensitization. Resolving *Polistes* and yellow jacket double sensitization poses a problem due the to limited components available to distinguish between the two. A recent study showed promising results using Pol d 1 testing to improve the diagnostic accuracy of *Polistes* primary sensitization (Bilo et al. 2021). While CCDs are a common cause for multiple sensitizations, this may not be the case for *Polistes* species as their venom has been shown to be CCD-free (Blank et al. 2013).

The individualized venom sensitization profile that CRD provides is important for its diagnostic utility as well as its potential for risk stratification in venom-allergic patients. In the case of honeybee allergy, sensitization to Api m 10 was the best predictor for treatment failure with honeybee immunotherapy in a retrospective study of 115 patients (Frick et al. 2016). Furthermore, in immunotherapy responders, induction of tolerance as supported by the presence of Api m 10 specific-IgG4 was only seen in patients whose honeybee immunotherapy extracts contained detectable amounts of Api m 10. Subsequent studies have confirmed the finding of low to undetectable levels of Api m 10 in several commercial extracts (Blank et al. 2017). Adverse reactions to honeybee immunotherapy have also been associated with the presence and level of sIgE to Api m 4 (Ruiz et al. 2015; Ruiz et al. 2016). This data suggests a significant role for individualized venom sensitization profiles in venom-allergic patients for the diagnosis and management of HVA.

The use of species-specific recombinant components can add to the clinical sensitivity of venom testing. For example, yellow jacket venom spiked with recombinant rVes v 5 increased the sensitivity of *in vitro* testing from 83% to 94% (Vos et al. 2013). Initial data using recombinant honeybee allergen in a liquid-phase platform revealed positivity to rApi m 1 in 97% of honeybee allergic patients (Muller et al. 2009). Subsequent studies, however, have shown decreased sensitivity using rApi m 1 that ranges from 57% to 79% (Hofmann et al. 2011; Korosec et al. 2011). Reasons for this wide range may be the platform used (liquid-phase vs. solid-phase matrix), regional differences in sensitization patterns or the cell type in which the recombinant protein was expressed. Improvement in test sensitivity can also be achieved by testing with panels of venom components over single allergen testing. For example, testing single recombinant honeybee allergens was associated with test sensitivity ranging from 23% to 72%, which increased to 94% when evidence of sIgE to any one of multiple allergens was considered diagnostic for honeybee allergy (Kohler et al. 2014). Table 4 shows the currently available recombinant venom allergens in the U.S.

Indications

CRD can be considered in patients with evidence of multiple sensitizations without a correlating history of reactions to stings of multiple Hymenoptera genera. It can also be considered in patients who test negative with venom skin testing or with standard serologic testing using whole venom extracts as this provides an additional sensitive diagnostic tool. Finally, CRD testing should be considered in all honeybee allergic patients since the specific sensitization pattern that is elucidated through CRD has clinical implications for treatment (i.e., selection of therapeutic extracts that contain venom allergens relevant to the patient's sensitization pattern) and can assist with risk stratification for adverse events with immunotherapy and risk for relapse.

Clinical Co-Relationship and Limitations

Limitations for CRD testing include the commercial availability of venoms that are geographically relevant and the availability of the full range of known component allergens in each venom. Differences in the sensitivity of CRD commercial platforms must also be taken into account when interpreting CRD test results. Overall, CRD is less sensitive for initial diagnosis than whole venom serum IgE testing. This may be due to the limited number of allergen components available for testing and/or reduced binding by component allergens compared to natural allergen proteins.

Special Precautions

There are no special precautions that need to be taken for CRD testing.

Interfering Agents

There are no known interfering agents with CRD testing, however, interference from concurrent use of omalizumab is undefined though possible based on omalizumab's mechanism of action.

Serum Basal Tryptase

Synonyms

Tryptase, baseline tryptase, total tryptase and serum tryptase.

Test Explanation and Interpretation

While not a diagnostic test for HVA, serum basal tryptase (sBT) is an important adjunct test that should be considered in the context of insect-triggered reactions. Tryptase is a serine protease that exists in two major isoforms, α and β tryptase. Alpha tryptase is released constitutively from resting mast cells and reflects the overall mast cell burden. Beta tryptase is released from mast cells upon activation and degranulation. A total tryptase value represents the sum of α and β tryptase. After mast cell activation, peak elevations in total tryptase are seen at 1 to 2 hours then gradually return to normal after 24 to 48 hours. An elevated baseline tryptase level can be seen in patients who have underlying mast cell disease (MCD) due to increased mast cell burden or other mast cell disorders. Currently, there are no commercial tests available for α and β tryptase values. Commercial testing for total tryptase are ELISA-based assays that describe values ≤ 11.4 ng/mL to be in the normal range.

An elevated sBT may be associated with systemic mastocytosis, FIP1L1-PDGFRA+ neoplasms, myelodysplastic syndromes and hereditary α-tryptasemia (HαT). Clonal MCD was seen in up to 7.9% of HVA patients whereas up to 88% of patients with venom allergy and an elevated sBT were subsequently diagnosed with MCD (Bonadonna et al. 2009; Niedoszytko et al. 2014). Using an insurance claims database, a recent U.S. study showed an MCD prevalence of 0.097% in patients with HVA (Schuler et al. 2021). The differences in reported prevalence may be related to the population used for each study (general population vs. referral centers). Because venom allergy may be the presenting symptom for MCD, sBT levels should be considered in all HVA patients as a screening tool for MCD. The clinical history of venom reactions may also point to an underlying MCD. In a cohort of patients with normal sBT levels, hypotension and absence of cutaneous symptoms after an insect sting were the most relevant factors associated with an underlying MCD (Zanotti et al. 2015). Finally, patients with underlying MCD and HVA may have negative standard evaluations for venom allergy (i.e., venom skin testing) and thus should have a sBT level checked for further evaluation (Kranke et al. 2004; Bonadonna et al. 2009).

Even without underlying MCD, an elevated sBT is a marker for venom allergy severity and can assist with risk stratification. While sBT values > 11.4 ng/mL are generally considered to be elevated, data from venom-allergic patients has shown that even mild elevations of sBT are associated with increased reaction severity. Several investigators have shown an increased risk for severe sting anaphylaxis with sBT levels > 8 ng/mL (Borer-Reinhold et al. 2011; Francuzik et al. 2021). Farioli et al. utilized sBT levels to risk stratify venom reaction severity with levels < 4 ng/mL associated with low risk, levels between 4 ng/mL and 7.5 ng/mL considered medium risk and levels > 7.5 ng/mL associated with high risk (Farioli et al. 2019).

The clinical utility of the sBT level is also important as it relates to risks associated with VIT treatment and risks after immunotherapy is stopped. In patients receiving VIT, elevated sBT levels were associated with an increased risk of reactions during build-up, which was prominent in those on Vespid immunotherapy (Rueff et al. 2010). In a small prospective study of children with honeybee allergy, sBT levels of > 7.75 ng/mL were associated with an increased risk of anaphylaxis during VIT build-up (Cichocka-Jarosz et al. 2011). An elevated sBT level is also a marker for relapse after VIT and thus should be considered in all patients prior to stopping treatment (Golden et al. 2017).

Finally, the discovery of HαT and its association with venom allergy also poses a challenge in the interpretation of an elevated sBT. In a recent study of venom-allergic patients, increased germline copy number of α-tryptase sequences at *TPSAB1,* consistent with HαT, was the most common cause of an elevated sBT in 65% of patients (Selb et al. 2021). While HαT is seen in 5.6% of healthy individuals, an increased HαT prevalence of 9.2% was noted in a Slovenian cohort of venom-allergic patients with severe anaphylaxis (Lyons et al. 2021).

Indications

Consider obtaining a sBT level in all patients with HVA given its utility in evaluating for underlying MCD, as a biomarker for adverse side effects during VIT and as a risk factor for relapse after completion of immunotherapy. A sBT level should also be part of the diagnostic evaluation in patients with a convincing clinical history of insect-triggered anaphylaxis who test negative to routine venom skin tests or serologic tests.

Clinical Co-Relationship and Limitations

The optimal timing for obtaining a tryptase level depends on the goals of the evaluation. For instance, obtaining a tryptase level within 1 to 2 hours of the start of clinical symptoms will help confirm mast cell activation. Given the significant elevation in tryptase that some venom-allergic patients may experience during insect-triggered anaphylaxis, obtaining a tryptase level a week or more after the reaction is recommended to establish a baseline tryptase level.

A limitation of sBT testing includes the lack of availability of a commercial test for α and β tryptase levels. In addition, the current cut-off values for a normal sBT level may be insufficient for establishing potential risks of underlying MCD or risks with immunotherapy (Zanotti et al. 2015). To that end, routine testing for the *KIT* p.D816V mutation has been proposed as a potential biomarker for underlying MCD in venom-allergic patients with normal sBT levels (Selb et al. 2021).

Special Precautions

There are no special precautions that need to be taken for sBT testing.

Interfering Agents

There are no known interfering agents with sBT testing.

Basophil Activation Test

Synonyms

Cellular *in vitro* test.

Test Explanation and Interpretation

The basophil activation test (BAT) is designed to test basophil reactivity upon allergen exposure. Basophils that are sensitized with sIgE are stimulated *in vitro* with allergen leading to the expression of two basophil activation markers, CD 203c and CD63. BAT quantifies the expression of CD203c and CD63 on the basophil cell surface via flow cytometry. Aside from the quantified level of CD203c or CD63, basophil sensitivity can also be measured by the percentage ratio of basophil response at two venom dilutions, 0.1 µg/mL and 1 µg/mL, also known as the 0.1/1 ratio.

Test Rationale

BAT has been clinically useful in venom-allergic patients who have negative skin tests and serologic tests (Korosec et al. 2009; Korosec et al. 2013). In a small study of patients with systemic mastocytosis, however, the BAT did not add additional information to standard tests (Bonadonna et al. 2012). In patients with double sensitization, BAT testing was a helpful diagnostic tool to rule out irrelevant sensitization (Bokanovic et al. 2020). Increased basophil sensitivity or increased 0.1/1 ratios were noted in a cohort of HVA patients who experienced side effects during VIT build-up (Kosnik et al. 2005). Basophil sensitivity correlated with systemic side effects in children undergoing VIT build-up (Zitnik et al. 2012). Finally, BAT may be predictive of VIT effectiveness and risk for relapse. A positive BAT correlated with positive sting challenge results in 80% of patients who completed at least 3 years of honeybee VIT, whereas 87.5% of non-reactors had a negative BAT (Kucera et al. 2010).

Indications

Consider obtaining venom BAT testing in patients who have convincing clinical histories for HVA but who fail to show sIgE on standard tests or in patients who are polysensitized. Since BAT may be predictive of side effects during VIT, obtaining the test prior to VIT might assist with risk mitigation for patients on VIT. Furthermore, BAT could be considered in patients who are on VIT where there is a concern for ineffectiveness (e.g., systemic reaction to a field sting despite maintenance dose VIT) or in those where VIT is completed to gauge the potential for relapse.

Clinical Co-Relationship and Limitations

The lack of commercial availability of the BAT test is one of a few limitations hampering the routine use of this test in HVA. Additionally, the test must be run within 4 to 24 hours of collection so any delay in transit to specialty labs could lead to inadequate samples. There is also significant lab-to-lab variability in the way BAT results are reported as well as interpreted. Finally, various reports have noted that 10% to 20% of the patients tested with the BAT have basophils that do not respond to antigen stimulation (non-responders) which may be due to alterations of intracellular signaling (Santos et al. 2021). The clinical significance of the non-responder phenotype is unknown but needs to be elucidated prior to the mainstream application of BAT testing in HVA.

Special Precautions

There are no special precautions that need to be taken for BAT testing. The technical requirements of the test need to be taken into accounts such as the timing of the blood sample collection and transport to a specialized lab in order to obtain optimal results.

Interfering Agents

There are no known interfering agents with BAT testing. The impact of the concurrent use of biologics such as omalizumab is undefined.

Sting Challenge Test

Synonyms

Deliberate sting challenge and intentional sting challenge.

Test Explanation and Interpretation

Challenge testing is the gold standard tool to diagnose a clinical allergy, confirm the resolution of an allergy or demonstrate the efficacy of therapeutic interventions. In the case of venom allergy, the sting challenge has been used to determine the level of reactivity in patients prior to VIT, to establish the efficiency of VIT and to monitor the persistence of immunologic protection after completion of VIT. In research settings, sting challenge protocols allow for the comparison of factors that may influence risk or protection in venom allergy. Outside of research settings, performing a sting challenge in an untreated patient is generally not recommended due to its associated risks. For patients that are undergoing treatment with VIT, a sting challenge can be considered as it may provide treatment prognostic information that can guide treatment (Rueff et al. 2001).

Practical aspects of sting challenge testing must be considered prior to conducting the test. Patient selection must be deliberate in that patients at higher risk (i.e., patients with uncontrolled asthma or patients not being actively treated with VIT) would not be ideal candidates for sting challenges. The selection of the insects must also be deliberate and depends on the goal of the evaluation (e.g., in the case of suspected multiple sensitizations, challenge testing to multiple insects may clarify which insects need to be included in a VIT prescription). For flying Hymenoptera, mature insects should be selected as the amount and composition of venom depends on the developmental stage of the insect. The location of a sting challenge should take into account the inherent risks of anaphylaxis, so testing should be carried out in a hospital setting such as an intensive care unit. The patient should have intravenous access and medications needed to treat anaphylaxis should be immediately available.

Technical expertise is a requirement for sting challenges. Flying insects can be cooled prior to the challenge to avoid inadvertent agitation and venom loss. The insect is then placed on the patient's forearm using a syringe with wire mesh to decrease the risk of escape of the insect. The occurrence of the sting is confirmed via direct observation as well as patient confirmation of a burning sensation at the site. Objective measurement of the resulting wheal and flare at the sting site should occur as well as the measurement of vital signs before and after the sting. Patients who report symptoms should have confirmation via observation and quantification. Allergic symptoms after a sting challenge should be promptly treated with emergency medications with close monitoring for the resolution of symptoms. Interpretation of a positive sting challenge depends on the indications for why the test was done. For example, if the test is done to provide proof of VIT effectiveness and the patient subsequently has objective symptoms with the challenge, then their maintenance VIT dose should be increased to provide additional protection (Rueff et al. 2001). Protocols for IFA sting challenges are also available as described in a research setting (Tankersley et al. 2002).

Clinical Co-Relationship and Limitations

Sting challenge results are dependent on several factors such as the species of an insect used, the severity of the previous reaction and skin test reactivity (Golden et al. 2006). The severity of a sting challenge-triggered reaction is related to the age of the patient as well as the time interval from the sting to symptoms (van der Linden et al. 1994). As not all sting challenges will result in symptoms, a negative sting challenge may not necessarily preclude or inform future risk (Franken et al. 1994; van der Linden et al. 1994). Of sting-allergic patients who do not react to a single challenge sting, 20% will react to a repeat sting challenge at a later time. Due to the risk of anaphylaxis, the decision to perform a sting challenge must be carefully weighed for each patient. The risk of boosting sensitization should also be taken into account. On the other hand, the decision not to perform a sting challenge may also have detrimental effects. In a pilot study that assessed disease-specific health-related QOL, an improvement in QOL was noted after tolerance of a sting challenge in patients on VIT (Fischer et al. 2013).

Special Precautions

Due to the risk of inducing a systemic or anaphylactic reaction with a sting challenge, trained personnel that can identify and treat allergic reactions are required for sting challenge tests. Experienced staff that can procure and identify the species of an insect used for testing are also needed. Finally, patient selection must be deliberate in order to identify and exclude patients at high risk for reactions who should not be candidates for sting challenges.

Interfering Agents

Similar to skin tests, any medication that will blunt the allergic response should be held prior to sting challenge testing.

Others

Platelet-Activating Factor (PAF)

While not diagnostic for HVA, serum levels of platelet-activating factor (PAF) can be considered as an adjunct test. PAF plays a role in the allergic response by inducing inflammation and cellular signaling. PAF is produced by platelets, macrophages, neutrophils, monocytes and endothelial cells. It is rapidly degraded by platelet-activating factor-acetylhydrolase (PAF-AH), also known as lipoprotein-associated phospholipase A2 (Lp-PLA2). Serum PAF levels correlate directly and proportionally with allergic reaction severity (Vadas et al. 2013). Decreased levels of PAF-AH also correlate with reaction severity in HVA patients (Pravettoni et al. 2014). Lp-PLA2 is commercially available as a test and marker for vascular inflammation and cardiovascular risk in patients.

Therapeutics

Background

Treatment for insect-triggered reactions depends on the clinical symptoms experienced by the patient. For example, local reactions typically require minimal supportive treatment such as cool compresses, topical corticosteroids or oral antihistamines. IFA pseudopustules should be left undisturbed; lesions are sterile and will self-resolve but excoriation can lead to infection. Patients who experience LLRs after insect stings can receive supportive treatment such as cool compresses and elevation of the affected extremity if edema is present. Oral antihistamines and/or a short course of corticosteroids can also be considered for LLRs that affect QOL or for persistent symptoms. If a patient experiences systemic cutaneous symptoms that do not progress, treatment with an oral antihistamine can be considered with close monitoring. Insect-triggered anaphylaxis follows the same treatment algorithm as for other causes of anaphylaxis. The first line treatment for anaphylaxis is intramuscular epinephrine at a dose of 0.01 mg/kg for children and 0.3 mg to 0.5 mg in adults. Epinephrine can be repeated every 5 to 15 minutes if symptoms are progressing or worsening (Shaker et al. 2020). Adjunct treatments include placing the patient in a recumbent position or Trendelenburg, providing supplemental oxygen and placement of an intravenous line for fluids or medications. Additional medications that can be considered include antihistamines, H2-antagonists and corticosteroids, although the benefits of these medications have been questioned (Shaker et al. 2020).

After the initial treatment of insect-triggered allergic reactions is completed, patients need counseling on avoidance measures that are specific to the geographical location and the culprit insect in order to prevent future stings. Counseling needs to be patient-centered and should take patient occupation and hobbies into consideration. Patients who experience systemic reactions to insects need to be advised to carry epinephrine auto-injector kits and require education on the proper indication and use of the kits. Patients can also benefit from a detailed written allergy plan in case of future exposures. Finally, patients should be referred to an allergist to discuss further evaluation and treatment options.

Venom Immunotherapy

Synonyms

Venom subcutaneous immunotherapy, VIT, allergy shots, specific immunotherapy, allergen-specific immunotherapy and imported fire ant whole-body extract immunotherapy.

Explanation of Treatment Modality

VIT is the only disease-modifying treatment available for venom allergy. Previous protocols utilized whole-body flying Hymenoptera extracts to treat HVA. Despite a report in 1956 detailing the effectiveness of purified venom extracts for testing and treatment, it would take an additional 22 years for whole-body flying Hymenoptera extracts to fall out of favor (Fackler and Loveless 1956). Whole-body extracts were proven ineffective at preventing systemic reactions in the first controlled trial of VIT in 1978 (Hunt et al. 1978). In comparison, the risk of a systemic reaction to a sting was less than 5% in patients treated with VIT (Hunt et al. 1978).

Immunotherapy to treat ant allergy utilizes WBE in the case of IFA allergy (U.S.) and venom extracts to treat Jack Jumper ant hypersensitivity (Australia). Although placebo-controlled trials for the use of IFA WBE are not available, a retrospective study showed 98% efficacy in preventing recurrent anaphylaxis (Freeman et al. 1992). VIT to *M. pilosula* (Jack Jumper ant) was highly effective at preventing reactions compared to placebo (Brown et al. 2003).

Mechanism of Action

VIT induces both short-term protection and long-term sustained unresponsiveness by skewing the immune system away from a Th2 response. Immunologic changes seen with VIT include the induction of venom-specific $CD4^+CD25^+$ regulatory T cells and upregulation of IL-10 and TGF-β production which leads to peripheral T cell tolerance (Akdis and Akdis 2011). B cell responses are similarly affected by the switch from IgE-producing B cells to IgG4-producing B cells. Regulatory B cell production further suppresses venom-specific T cell proliferation and contributes to the tolerogenic immune response seen with immunotherapy. The function of IgG4 as a blocking antibody has been considered an important mechanism of immune tolerance though its presence alone has not been shown to be a consistent biomarker for VIT effectiveness (Muller et al. 1989; Ewan et al. 1993; Akdis and Akdis 2011). A better measure of the blocking activity of allergen-specific IgG has been elucidated through the measurement of inhibition of allergen presentation using the novel IgE-facilitated allergen binding (FAB) assay (Wachholz et al. 2003; Shamji et al. 2006). While VIT was associated with increased IgG4 and IgE-FAB inhibition in a group of honeybee-allergic children, it was the sustained and persistent decline in venom-specific IgE that was thought to be the underlying mechanism for prolonged clinical efficacy of VIT (Varga et al. 2009).

Indications

VIT is indicated for patients who experience anaphylaxis after an insect sting and who are shown to produce sIgE to the insect in question. It can also be considered for select cases, such as those experiencing debilitating or recurrent LLRs, as it has been shown to decrease the size and duration of LLRs (Golden et al. 2009). IFA WBE in a child with debilitating LLRs from IFA stings showed similar results (Hagan 2000). Children who experience systemic cutaneous reactions to IFA typically have similar cutaneous-only reactions with repeat stings (Nguyen and Napoli 2005). The current stinging insect practice parameter no longer recommends testing and immunotherapy treatment for patients of any age who experience systemic cutaneous reactions (Golden et al. 2017). In patients with cutaneous-only reactions, immunotherapy can be considered if they are recurrent and impact a patient's QOL or may be optional for IFA-triggered patients given that only limited data is available for these patients.

Venom Selection

VIT utilizes commercial venom extracts as single venom or a mixed Vespid extract. Single venoms (honeybee, yellow jacket, white-faced and yellow hornet, *Polistes* wasp) are available at a concentration of 100 µg/mL, whereas a mixed Vespid extract (yellow jacket, two hornet species) is available at a concentration of 300 µg/mL (100 µg/ml of each venom). For IFA allergy, immunotherapy utilizes a non-standardized WBE extract of *S. invicta* or *S. richteri* available in a 1:10 wt/vol concentration.

The selection of which venoms to include in a VIT prescription is dependent on the clinical history as well as the diagnostic results. The clinical history determines which patients should receive immunotherapy (i.e., patients with anaphylaxis after an insect sting), whereas the diagnostic results (i.e., skin testing or *in vitro* testing) determine what extracts are included in the prescription. For cases where the diagnostic results are not concordant with the history (e.g., evidence of sensitization to multiple venoms but only one reported insect-triggered reaction), additional diagnostic evaluation such as CRD or BAT testing can and should be considered to delineate true clinical allergy versus sensitization. If additional testing is not available or if the results are not clarified, then all venoms showing positive tests should be included in the VIT prescription. While there may be risks with this process in that patients may be treated with venoms that they are not clinically allergic too, the risk of missing a potentially relevant allergen outweighs any potentially negative effects.

Dosing and Protocols

Protocols for VIT and IFA WBE immunotherapy vary but follow a pattern similar to aeroallergen immunotherapy. The process can be divided into an up-dosing or build-up regimen and a maintenance regimen. The standard starting dose for VIT ranges between 0.001 to 0.01 µg for single venoms and 0.003 to 0.03 µg for the mixed Vespid extract. The target maintenance dose is 100 µg for single venoms or 300 µg for mixed Vespid extracts. The use of a 50 µg maintenance dose has been studied and appears to be protective in children, though data from adults is mixed (Golden et al. 1981; Reisman and Livingston 1992; Houliston et al. 2011; Konstantinou et al. 2011). Several studies have looked at different venom starting doses. In a cohort of HVA patients who underwent honeybee or Vespid build-up, there were zero systemic reactions using a 1 µg starting venom dose (Roumana et al. 2009). In a small, randomized pilot study, initial treatment with four monthly 100 µg VIT doses was tolerated without systemic reactions and was shown to be protective during a sting challenge (Vos et al. 2019). Table 3 summarizes practical considerations for VIT.

Up-dosing can be done via several different methods; conventional, modified rush, rush or ultra-rush protocols. Conventional schedules entail delivery of 1 to 2 weekly doses of venom extract over months until the maintenance dose is reached. Modified rush protocols involve the delivery of multiple extract doses over several hours, which is repeated weekly until the maintenance dose is reached, usually after 6 to 8 weeks. Rush and ultra-rush protocols complete the entire build-up process over the course of days to hours, respectively. While conventional build-up schedules are typically considered safe, they are also associated with a potential delay in achieving maintenance doses compared to accelerated schedules and thus take longer to provide protection. Compared to rush aeroallergen schedules, which are associated with an increased risk of local and systemic side effects, rush VIT protocols have not been shown to carry the same increased risk of side effects. On the other hand, ultra-rush VIT protocols have been identified as a risk factor for adverse effects during VIT (Rueff et al. 2010; Brown et al. 2012).

VIT can be spaced out to a conventional maintenance interval (CMI) of every 4 weeks once the maintenance dose has been reached and tolerated. After 12 to 18 months of CMI immunotherapy, extended maintenance intervals (EMI) of 6 to 8 weeks can be considered. EMIs, of up to 12 weeks, have been shown to be safe and effective in the treatment of HVA and may improve adherence (Cavallucci et al. 2010; Simioni et al. 2013). An EMI of 6 months was not protective in a cohort of honeybee-allergic patients (Goldberg and Confino-Cohen 2007). However, a recent study investigating the use of a progressively prolonged maintenance interval of up to 26 weeks was significant for no systemic reactions to 108 field stings sustained after an EMI of 20 weeks (Kontou-Fili et al. 2018).

Immunotherapy for IFA typically starts at a concentration of 0.05 mL of a 1:100,000 wt/vol concentration (Golden et al. 2017). Up-dosing can occur using a conventional build-up regimen, though safe and effective rush protocols have been reported for IFA in both children and adults (Judd et al. 2008; Arseneau et al. 2013). For IFA, the maintenance dose is typically 0.5 ml of a 1:100 wt/vol concentrate given monthly (Freeman et al. 1992).

Duration

The standard length of treatment for a VIT course is 3 to 5 years although longer treatment courses are superior (Keating et al. 1991; Lerch and Muller 1998). Longer treatment courses should be considered for patients at high risk for relapse. Risk factors for relapse include elevated baseline serum tryptase, underlying mast cell disorder, systemic reactions during VIT (to venom injection or insect sting), severe reactions to pre-VIT sting, honeybee sting anaphylaxis, frequent unavoidable insect exposure, age and underlying medical conditions (Golden et al. 2017). Lifelong VIT should be considered for patients with MCD as they are at high risk for life-threatening anaphylaxis if VIT is stopped (Oude Elberink et al. 1997). In fact, patients who relapse after VIT completion are at increased risk for an underlying clonal MCD and further evaluation should be considered (Bonadonna et al. 2018). A small survey study of patients who received IFA WBE immunotherapy showed no difference in field sting outcomes for patients who received less than 3 years versus those who received over 3 years of treatment (Forester et al. 2007). Because limited data exists on the natural history of IFA hypersensitivity, and because of the frequency of ant stings in endemic areas, prolonged treatment courses of longer than 5 years should be considered.

Limitations

There are several known limitations of VIT treatment. As VIT relies on the availability of venom extracts, any shortage in venom procurement or commercial availability will directly impact the ability to provide this service. Venom extracts also need to cover all endemic species in a region in order to effectively treat sensitized patients. The logistics of VIT must also be considered as it is a time-intensive program that has a high risk for non-adherence due to planned and non-planned events (Bilo et al. 2021).

Safety

Adverse reactions to VIT range from localized cutaneous symptoms to systemic reactions. Systemic symptoms themselves can range from mild symptoms (e.g., a few hives) to moderate or severe symptoms where multiple organ systems are involved. Systemic reactions occur in a small number of patients during the build-up phase of immunotherapy and are rare during the maintenance phase. Given the risks associated with untreated HVA, every effort must be made to adjust treatment regimens for patients who experience side effects with VIT. Modifications after a systemic reaction to VIT include a reduction of the next dose provided and consideration for premedication, if not already done. The use of antihistamine premedication can help decrease the risk of local and systemic adverse reactions to immunotherapy (Brockow et al. 1997). The addition of omalizumab is an effective treatment strategy in patients who experience recurrent systemic reactions to immunotherapy (Galera et al. 2009; Kontou-Fili and Filis 2009).

Reactions to immunotherapy may depend on the type of venom used. In a systematic review, honeybee immunotherapy was associated with a systemic reaction incidence of 25% whereas Vespid immunotherapy reactions were seen in up to 5.8% (Incorvaia et al. 2011). A different systematic review noted adverse systemic reactions in 14.2% of patients treated with honeybee VIT and 2.8% of patients treated with Vespid VIT (Boyle et al. 2012). An observational prospective study noted an increased risk of reactions during build-up VIT in patients with higher sBT levels, which was most prominent in those on Vespid immunotherapy (Rueff et al. 2010).

Cardiovascular Disease and Medications

The cardiovascular system is of particular importance in HVA patients. Venom-induced anaphylaxis more commonly involves cardiovascular symptoms (e.g., hypotension, loss of consciousness) compared to non-venom causes of anaphylaxis (Francuzik et al. 2021). Concurrent cardiovascular disease is also more commonly seen in venom-triggered anaphylaxis and is associated with a higher risk of severity (Francuzik et al. 2021). One reason for these findings includes possible impaired compensatory mechanisms from underlying cardiovascular disease. Another contributing factor may be the concurrent use of cardiovascular medications such as BB and angiotensin-converting enzyme inhibitors (ACE-I). These medications have long been considered risk factors for increased reaction severity in anaphylaxis due to their interruption of normal physiologic compensation during a systemic reaction. Data regarding the risks of these medications has been inconsistent, with studies showing both a positive and negative association (Rueff et al. 2009; Stoevesandt et al. 2012). Recent studies, however, have found that neither BB nor ACE-I use is associated with increased risks during VIT initiation or maintenance VIT (Stoevesandt et al. 2014; Stoevesandt et al. 2015). A recent large, prospective study concluded that cardiovascular medication use was not associated with increased risk or severity of systemic reactions to VIT (Sturm et al. 2021).

Differences in study results may be related to the study population utilized (e.g., underrepresentation of patients on cardiovascular medications), as well as an inability to separate risks associated with underlying cardiovascular disease from its treatment. A meta-analysis of anaphylaxis of all causes found that the risk of severe anaphylaxis was 3- to 5-fold higher with underlying cardiovascular disease compared to the pooled effect of both BB and ACE-I (Tejedor-Alonso et al. 2019). In most patients, the risk of untreated cardiovascular disease is substantial. This, in turn, makes the risk of stopping antihypertensive medications outweigh the risk of their continuation. Therefore, while the impact that underlying cardiovascular disease or medication use should be considered, it should not detract from offering VIT to these patients.

Mast Cell Disease

Patients with MCD are at increased risk of adverse reactions during immunotherapy and treatment failure with VIT. A systemic review in 2009 reported a risk of systemic side effects in MCD patients up to 20% although only 7.6% required the use of epinephrine or necessitated the discontinuation of treatment (Niedoszytko et al. 2009). Both conventional and rush protocols were tolerated in a case series of IFA allergic patients with underlying MCD (Nath et al. 2019). VIT effectiveness based on sting challenges or field stings is lower in MCD patients (76.1% and 66.7%, respectively) (Niedoszytko et al. 2009). Furthermore, as both severe and fatal reactions have occurred in MCD patients after the discontinuation of VIT, MCD patients with HVA should be considered candidates for lifelong treatment to ensure continued immunologic protection (Oude Elberink et al. 1997; Reimers and Müller 2005).

Treatment Failure

Patients who continue to experience reactions to field stings despite maintenance immunotherapy or those who relapse after completion of VIT require special attention and modifications. Patients who have field sting reactions despite maintenance dose VIT should be considered candidates for increased maintenance dosing (e.g., 200 µg for single venom extracts, 1 ml of a

1:100 wt/vol IFA WBE extract). Reasons for treatment failure include the use of venom extracts that may not cover the patient's sensitizations due to underrepresented allergens or missing species-specific allergens, underlying MCD, those with severe initial sting reactions, and patients with honeybee allergy (Golden et al. 2017). Mitigation strategies that can be considered include increasing the total maintenance dose of immunotherapy, provision of lifelong immunotherapy, consideration of additional diagnostic testing (in case of a new sensitization), and evaluation for an underlying MCD if not already done.

Special Precautions

Immunotherapy programs require specific training for technicians and nursing staff in order to ensure the safe delivery of allergen injections. Staff must be trained on the management of venom extracts (e.g., dilutions, mixing kits), dosage schedules and intervals. Given its inherent risks, staff must also be trained on the recognition and prompt treatment of adverse reactions to VIT. As noted, individualized risk stratification that takes a patient's venom clinical history, underlying medical conditions, medication use and future exposure risk must all be considered in order to mitigate the risks associated with VIT.

Conclusion

Allergy to stinging insects is a worldwide problem that is associated with significant morbidity and mortality for those affected. While much is known about insect allergy, diagnosis and treatment options, there still remain significant gaps and questions that need to be investigated in order to provide individualized diagnostics and treatments for patients. Recent laboratory advances are the right step in this direction as they have elucidated the reasons why differential responses are seen in the standard diagnostic tests and treatment options for HVA. Continued research and development using these new techniques is needed to provide standardized precise diagnostics and treatment options for HVA patients.

Glossary of Abbreviations

ACE-I – Angiotensin Converting Enzyme Inhibitor
BAT – Basophil Activation Test
CCD – Cross-Reactive Carbohydrate Determinants
CMI – Conventional Maintenance Interval
CRD – Component Resolved Diagnosis
ELISA – Enzyme-Linked Immunosorbent Assays
EMI – Extended Maintenance Intervals
FAB – Facilitated Allergen Binding
HVA – Hymenoptera Venom Allergy
ID – Intradermal
IFA – Imported Fire Ant
LLR – Large Local Reaction
MCD – Mast Cell Disease
PAF – Platelet-Activating Factor
PAF-AH – Platelet-Activating Factor Acetyl Hydrolase
QOL – Quality of Life
RAST – Radioallergosorbent Test
sBT – Serum Basal Tryptase
sIgE – Specific IgE
VIT – Venom Immunotherapy
WBE – Whole-Body Extracts

References

Akdis, C. A. and Akdis, M. 2011. Mechanisms of allergen-specific immunotherapy. J. Allergy Clin. Immunol. 127(1): 18–27.

Anderson, C. and Belnap, C. 2015. The kiss of death: a rare case of anaphylaxis to the bite of the red margined kissing bug. Hawaii J. Med. Public Health 74(9 Suppl 2): 33–35.

Arseneau, A. M., Nesselroad, T. D., Dietrich, J. J., Moore, L. M., Nguyen, S., Hagan, L. L. et al. 2013. A 1-day imported fire ant rush immunotherapy schedule with and without premedication. Ann. Allergy Asthma Immunol. 111(6): 562–566.

Baker, T. W., Forester, J. P., Johnson, M. L., Stolfi, A. and Stahl, M. C. 2014. The HIT study: Hymenoptera Identification Test—how accurate are people at identifying stinging insects? Ann. Allergy Asthma Immunol. 113(3): 267–270.

Bernstein, I. L., Li, J. T., Bernstein, D. I., Hamilton, R., Spector, S. L., Tan, R. et al. 2008. Allergy diagnostic testing: an updated practice parameter. Ann. Allergy Asthma Immunol. 100(3 Suppl 3): S1–148.

Bilo, M. B., Martini, M., Pravettoni, V., Bignardi, D., Bonadonna, P., Cortellini, G. et al. 2019. Large local reactions to Hymenoptera stings: Outcome of re-stings in real life. Allergy 74(10): 1969–1976.

Bilo, M. B., Braschi, M. C., Piga, M. A., Antonicelli, L. and Martini, M. 2021. Safety and adherence to venom immunotherapy during COVID-19 pandemic. J. Allergy Clin. Immunol. Pract. 9(2): 702–708.

Bilo, M. B., Martini, M., Bonadonna, P., Cinti, B., Da Re, M., Gabrielli, O. et al. 2021. Prevalence of Pol d 1 sensitization in polistes dominula allergy and its diagnostic role in vespid double-positivity. J. Allergy Clin. Immunol. Pract. 9(10): 3781–3787.

Blank, S., Neu, C., Hasche, D., Bantleon, F. I., Jakob, T. and Spillner, E. 2013. Polistes species venom is devoid of carbohydrate-based cross-reactivity and allows interference-free diagnostics. J. Allergy Clin. Immunol. 131(4): 1239–1242.

Blank, S., Etzold, S., Darsow, U., Schiener, M., Eberlein, B., Russkamp, D. et al. 2017. Component-resolved evaluation of the content of major allergens in therapeutic extracts for specific immunotherapy of honeybee venom allergy. Hum. Vaccin. Immunother. 13(10): 2482–2489.

Bokanovic, D., Arzt-Gradwohl, L., Schwarz, I., Schrautzer, C., Laipold, K., Aberer, W. et al. 2020. Possible utility of basophil activation test in dual honeybee and vespid sensitization. J. Allergy Clin. Immunol. Pract. 8(1): 392–394 e395.

Bonadonna, P., Perbellini, O., Passalacqua, G., Caruso, B., Colarossi, S., Dal Fior, D. et al. 2009. Clonal mast cell disorders in patients with systemic reactions to Hymenoptera stings and increased serum tryptase levels. J. Allergy Clin. Immunol. 123(3): 680–686.

Bonadonna, P., Zanotti, R., Melioli, G., Antonini, F., Romano, I., Lenzi, L. et al. 2012. The role of basophil activation test in special populations with mastocytosis and reactions to hymenoptera sting. Allergy 67(7): 962–965.

Bonadonna, P., Zanotti, R., Pagani, M., Bonifacio, M., Scaffidi, L., Olivieri, E. et al. 2018. Anaphylactic reactions after discontinuation of hymenoptera venom immunotherapy: a clonal mast cell disorder should be suspected. J. Allergy Clin. Immunol. Pract. 6(4): 1368–1372.

Borer-Reinhold, M., Haeberli, G., Bitzenhofer, M., Jandus, P., Hausmann, O., Fricker, M. et al. 2011. An increase in serum tryptase even below 11.4 ng/mL may indicate a mast cell-mediated hypersensitivity reaction: a prospective study in Hymenoptera venom allergic patients. Clin. Exp. Allergy 41(12): 1777–1783.

Boyle, R. J., Elremeli, M., Hockenhull, J., Cherry, M. G., Bulsara, M. K., Daniels, M. et al. 2012. Venom immunotherapy for preventing allergic reactions to insect stings. Cochrane Database Syst. Rev. 10: CD008838.

Brockow, K., Kiehn, M., Riethmuller, C., Vieluf, D., Berger, J. and Ring, J. 1997. Efficacy of antihistamine pretreatment in the prevention of adverse reactions to Hymenoptera immunotherapy: a prospective, randomized, placebo-controlled trial. J. Allergy Clin. Immunol. 100(4): 458–463.

Brown, S. G., Franks, R. W., Baldo, B. A. and Heddle, R. J. 2003. Prevalence, severity, and natural history of jack jumper ant venom allergy in Tasmania. J. Allergy Clin. Immunol. 111(1): 187–192.

Brown, S. G., Wiese, M. D., Blackman, K. E. and Heddle, R. J. 2003. Ant venom immunotherapy: a double-blind, placebo-controlled, crossover trial. Lancet 361(9362): 1001–1006.

Brown, S. G., Wiese, M. D., van Eeden, P., Stone, S. F., Chuter, C. L., Gunner, J. et al. 2012. Ultrarush versus semirush initiation of insect venom immunotherapy: a randomized controlled trial. J. Allergy Clin. Immunol. 130(1): 162–168.

Cavallucci, E., Ramondo, S., Renzetti, A., Turi, M. C., Di Claudio, F., Braga, M. et al. 2010. Maintenance venom immunotherapy administered at a 3-month interval preserves safety and efficacy and improves adherence. J. Investig. Allergol. Clin. Immunol. 20(1): 63–68.

Cichocka-Jarosz, E., Sanak, M., Szczeklik, A., Brzyski, P., Gielicz, A. and Pietrzyk, J. J. 2011. Serum tryptase level is a better predictor of systemic side effects than prostaglandin D2 metabolites during venom immunotherapy in children. J. Investig. Allergol. Clin. Immunol. 21(4): 260–269.

Corren, J., Shapiro, G., Reimann, J., Deniz, Y., Wong, D., Adelman, D. et al. 2008. Allergen skin tests and free IgE levels during reduction and cessation of omalizumab therapy. J. Allergy Clin. Immunol. 121(2): 506–511.

Crisp, H. C. and Johnson, K. S. 2013. Mosquito allergy. Ann. Allergy Asthma Immunol. 110(2): 65–69.

deShazo, R. D., Griffing, C., Kwan, T. H., Banks, W. A. and Dvorak, H. F. 1984. Dermal hypersensitivity reactions to imported fire ants. J. Allergy Clin. Immunol. 74(6): 841–847.

Ellis, A. K. and Day, J. H. 2007. Incidence and characteristics of biphasic anaphylaxis: a prospective evaluation of 103 patients. Ann. Allergy Asthma Immunol. 98(1): 64–69.

Ewan, P. W., Deighton, J., Wilson, A. B. and Lachmann, P. J. 1993. Venom-specific IgG antibodies in bee and wasp allergy: lack of correlation with protection from stings. Clin. Exp. Allergy 23(8): 647–660.

Fackler, W. R. and Loveless, M. H. 1956. Wasp venom allergy and immunity. Ann. Allergy 14(5): 347–366.

Farioli, L., Losappio, L. M., Schroeder, J. W., Preziosi, D., Scibilia, J., Caron, L. et al. 2019. Basal tryptase levels can predict clinical severity in hymenoptera venom anaphylaxis and ischemic cardiovascular disorders. J. Investig. Allergol. Clin. Immunol. 29(2): 162–164.

Fischer, J., Teufel, M., Feidt, A., Giel, K. E., Zipfel, S. and Biedermann, T. 2013. Tolerated wasp sting challenge improves health-related quality of life in patients allergic to wasp venom. J. Allergy Clin. Immunol. 132(2): 489–490.

Forester, J. P., Johnson, T. L., Arora, R. and Quinn, J. M. 2007. Systemic reaction rates to field stings among imported fire ant-sensitive patients receiving > 3 years of immunotherapy versus < 3 years of immunotherapy. Allergy Asthma Proc. 28(4): 485–488.

Francuzik, W., Rueff, F., Bauer, A., Bilo, M. B., Cardona, V., Christoff, G. et al. 2021. Phenotype and risk factors of venom-induced anaphylaxis: A case-control study of the European Anaphylaxis Registry. J. Allergy Clin. Immunol. 147(2): 653–662 e659.

Franken, H. H., Dubois, A. E., Minkema, H. J., van der Heide, S. and de Monchy, J. G. 1994. Lack of reproducibility of a single negative sting challenge response in the assessment of anaphylactic risk in patients with suspected yellow jacket hypersensitivity. J. Allergy Clin. Immunol. 93(2): 431–436.

Freeman, T. M., Hylander, R., Ortiz, A. and Martin, M. E. 1992. Imported fire ant immunotherapy: effectiveness of whole body extracts. J. Allergy Clin. Immunol. 90(2): 210–215.

Frick, M., Fischer, J., Helbling, A., Rueff, F., Wieczorek, D., Ollert, M. et al. 2016. Predominant Api m 10 sensitization as risk factor for treatment failure in honey bee venom immunotherapy. J. Allergy Clin. Immunol. 138(6): 1663–1671 e1669.

Galera, C., Soohun, N., Zankar, N., Caimmi, S., Gallen, C. and Demoly, P. 2009. Severe anaphylaxis to bee venom immunotherapy: efficacy of pretreatment and concurrent treatment with omalizumab. J. Investig. Allergol. Clin. Immunol. 19(3): 225–229.

Georgitis, J. W. and Reisman, R. E. 1985. Venom skin tests in insect-allergic and insect-nonallergic populations. J. Allergy Clin. Immunol. 76(6): 803–807.

Goldberg, A. and Confino-Cohen, R. 2007. Effectiveness of maintenance bee venom immunotherapy administered at 6-month intervals. Ann. Allergy Asthma Immunol. 99(4): 352–357.

Golden, D. B., Kagey-Sobotka, A., Valentine, M. D. and Lichtenstein, L. M. 1981. Dose dependence of Hymenoptera venom immunotherapy. J. Allergy Clin. Immunol. 67(5): 370–374.

Golden, D. B., Marsh, D. G., Kagey-Sobotka, A., Freidhoff, L., Szklo, M., Valentine, M. D. et al. 1989. Epidemiology of insect venom sensitivity. JAMA 262(2): 240–244.

Golden, D. B., Marsh, D. G., Freidhoff, L. R., Kwiterovich, K. A., Addison, B., Kagey-Sobotka, A. et al. 1997. Natural history of Hymenoptera venom sensitivity in adults. J. Allergy Clin. Immunol. 100(6 Pt 1): 760–766.

Golden, D. B., Kagey-Sobotka, A., Norman, P. S., Hamilton, R. G. and Lichtenstein, L. M. 2004. Outcomes of allergy to insect stings in children, with and without venom immunotherapy. N Engl. J. Med. 351(7): 668–674.

Golden, D. B., Breisch, N. L., Hamilton, R. G., Guralnick, M. W., Greene, A., Craig, T. J. et al. 2006. Clinical and entomological factors influence the outcome of sting challenge studies. J. Allergy Clin. Immunol. 117(3): 670–675.

Golden, D. B., Kelly, D., Hamilton, R. G. and Craig, T. J. 2009. Venom immunotherapy reduces large local reactions to insect stings. J. Allergy Clin. Immunol. 123(6): 1371–1375.

Golden, D. B., Bernstein, D. I., Freeman, T. M., Tracy, J. M., Lang, D. M. and Nicklas, R. A. 2017. AAAAI/ACAAI joint venom extract shortage task force report. Ann. Allergy Asthma Immunol. 118(3): 283–285.

Golden, D. B., Demain, J., Freeman, T., Graft, D., Tankersley, M., Tracy, J. et al. 2017. Stinging insect hypersensitivity: A practice parameter update 2016. Ann. Allergy Asthma Immunol. 118(1): 28–54.

Gonzalez-Estrada, A., Silvers, S. K., Klein, A., Zell, K., Wang, X. F. and Lang, D. M. 2017. Epidemiology of anaphylaxis at a tertiary care center: A report of 730 cases. Ann. Allergy Asthma Immunol. 118(1): 80–85.

Grabenhenrich, L. B., Dolle, S., Moneret-Vautrin, A., Kohli, A., Lange, L., Spindler, T. et al. 2016. Anaphylaxis in children and adolescents: The European anaphylaxis registry. J. Allergy Clin. Immunol. 137(4): 1128–1137 e1121.

Graft, D. F., Schuberth, K. C., Kagey-Sobotka, A., Kwiterovich, K. A., Niv, Y., Lichtenstein, L. M. et al. 1984. A prospective study of the natural history of large local reactions after Hymenoptera stings in children. J. Pediatr. 104(5): 664–668.

Hagan, L. L. 2000. Resolution of debilitating large local reaction from imported fire ant stings with rush immunotherapy: a case report. Pediatric Asthma, Allergy & Immunology 14(4): 333–338.

Hamilton, R. G. 2006. Accuracy of US Food and Drug Administration-cleared IgE antibody assays in the presence of anti-IgE (omalizumab). J. Allergy Clin. Immunol. 117(4): 759–766.

Hemmer, W., Focke, M., Kolarich, D., Wilson, I. B., Altmann, F., Wohrl, S. et al. 2001. Antibody binding to venom carbohydrates is a frequent cause for double positivity to honeybee and yellow jacket venom in patients with stinging-insect allergy. J. Allergy Clin. Immunol. 108(6): 1045–1052.

Hoffman, D. R., Dove, D. E., Moffitt, J. E. and Stafford, C. T. 1988. Allergens in Hymenoptera venom. XXI. Cross-reactivity and multiple reactivity between fire ant venom and bee and wasp venoms. J. Allergy Clin. Immunol. 82(5 Pt 1): 828–834.

Hofmann, S. C., Pfender, N., Weckesser, S., Huss-Marp, J. and Jakob, T. 2011. Added value of IgE detection to rApi m 1 and rVes v 5 in patients with Hymenoptera venom allergy. J. Allergy Clin. Immunol. 127(1): 265–267.

Houliston, L., Nolan, R., Noble, V., Pascoe, E., Hobday, J., Loh, R. et al. 2011. Honeybee venom immunotherapy in children using a 50-mug maintenance dose. J. Allergy Clin. Immunol. 127(1): 98–99.

Hunt, K. J., Valentine, M. D., Sobotka, A. K., Benton, A. W., Amodio, F. J. and Lichtenstein, L. M. 1978. A controlled trial of immunotherapy in insect hypersensitivity. N Engl. J. Med. 299(4): 157–161.

Incorvaia, C., Mauro, M. and Pastorello, E. A. 1997. Hymenoptera stings in conscripts. Allergy 52(6): 680–681.

Incorvaia, C., Frati, F., Dell'Albani, I., Robino, A., Cattaneo, E., Mauro, M. et al. 2011. Safety of hymenoptera venom immunotherapy: a systematic review. Expert Opin. Pharmacother. 12(16): 2527–2532.

Jairam, A., Kumar, R. S., Ghosh, A. K., Hasija, P. K., Singh, J. I., Mahapatra, D. et al. 2010. Delayed Kounis syndrome and acute renal failure after wasp sting. Int. J. Cardiol. 138(1): e12–14.

Jerschow, E., Lin, R. Y., Scaperotti, M. M. and McGinn, A. P. 2014. Fatal anaphylaxis in the United States, 1999–2010: temporal patterns and demographic associations. J. Allergy Clin. Immunol. 134(6): 1318–1328 e1317.

Judd, C. A., Parker, A. L., Meier, E. A. and Tankersley, M. S. 2008. Successful administration of a 1-day imported fire ant rush immunotherapy protocol. Ann. Allergy Asthma Immunol. 101(3): 311–315.

Kalyoncu, A. F., Demir, A. U., Ozcan, U., Ozkuyumcu, C., Sahin, A. A. and Baris, Y. I. 1997. Bee and wasp venom allergy in Turkey. Ann. Allergy Asthma Immunol. 78(4): 408–412.

Keating, M. U., Kagey-Sobotka, A., Hamilton, R. G. and Yunginger, J. W. 1991. Clinical and immunologic follow-up of patients who stop venom immunotherapy. J. Allergy Clin. Immunol. 88(3 Pt 1): 339–348.

Kjaer, H. F., Mortz, C. G. and Bindslev-Jensen, C. 2021. Does treatment with antidepressants, antipsychotics, or benzodiazepines hamper allergy skin testing? Clin. Transl. Allergy 11(7): e12060.

Kohler, J., Blank, S., Muller, S., Bantleon, F., Frick, M., Huss-Marp, J. et al. 2014. Component resolution reveals additional major allergens in patients with honeybee venom allergy. J. Allergy Clin. Immunol. 133(5): 1383–1389, 1389 e1381–1386.

Konstantinou, G. N., Manoussakis, E., Douladiris, N., Hatziioannou, A., Giavi, S., Saxoni-Papageorgiou, P. et al. 2011. A 5-year venom immunotherapy protocol with 50 mug maintenance dose: safety and efficacy in school children. Pediatr. Allergy Immunol. 22(4): 393–397.

Kontou-Fili, K. and Filis, C. I. 2009. Prolonged high-dose omalizumab is required to control reactions to venom immunotherapy in mastocytosis. Allergy 64(9): 1384–1385.

Kontou-Fili, K., Pitsios, C., Kompoti, E., Giannakopoulos, D. and Kouridakis, S. 2018. Safety and efficacy of a progressively prolonged maintenance interval of venom immunotherapy. Int. Arch. Allergy Immunol. 176(1): 39–43.

Korosec, P., Erzen, R., Silar, M., Bajrovic, N., Kopac, P. and Kosnik, M. 2009. Basophil responsiveness in patients with insect sting allergies and negative venom-specific immunoglobulin E and skin prick test results. Clin. Exp. Allergy 39(11): 1730–1737.

Korosec, P., Valenta, R., Mittermann, I., Celesnik, N., Erzen, R., Zidarn, M. et al. 2011. Low sensitivity of commercially available rApi m 1 for diagnosis of honeybee venom allergy. J. Allergy Clin. Immunol. 128(3): 671–673.

Korosec, P., Silar, M., Erzen, R., Celesnik, N., Bajrovic, N., Zidarn, M. et al. 2013. Clinical routine utility of basophil activation testing for diagnosis of hymenoptera-allergic patients with emphasis on individuals with negative venom-specific IgE antibodies. Int. Arch. Allergy Immunol. 161(4): 363–368.

Kosnik, M., Silar, M., Bajrovic, N., Music, E. and Korosec, P. 2005. High sensitivity of basophils predicts side-effects in venom immunotherapy. Allergy 60(11): 1401–1406.

Kranke, B., Sturm, G. and Aberer, W. 2004. Negative venom skin test results and mastocytosis. J. Allergy Clin. Immunol. 113(1): 180–181.

Kucera, P., Cvackova, M., Hulikova, K., Juzova, O. and Pachl, J. 2010. Basophil activation can predict clinical sensitivity in patients after venom immunotherapy. J. Investig. Allergol. Clin. Immunol. 20(2): 110–116.

Kutlu, A., Aydin, E., Goker, K., Karabacak, E. and Ozturk, S. 2013. Cold-induced urticaria with systemic reactions after hymenoptera sting lasting for 10 years. Allergol. Immunopathol. 41(4): 283–284.

Lange, J., Cichocka-Jarosz, E., Marczak, H., Krauze, A., Tarczon, I., Swiebocka, E. et al. 2016. Natural history of Hymenoptera venom allergy in children not treated with immunotherapy. Ann. Allergy Asthma Immunol. 116(3): 225–229.

Lee, S., Bellolio, M. F., Hess, E. P., Erwin, P., Murad, M. H. and Campbell, R. L. 2015. Time of onset and predictors of biphasic anaphylactic reactions: a systematic review and meta-analysis. J. Allergy Clin. Immunol. Pract. 3(3): 408–416 e401–402.

Lerch, E. and Muller, U. R. 1998. Long-term protection after stopping venom immunotherapy: results of re-stings in 200 patients. J. Allergy Clin. Immunol. 101(5): 606–612.

Liew, W. K., Williamson, E. and Tang, M. L. 2009. Anaphylaxis fatalities and admissions in Australia. J. Allergy Clin. Immunol. 123(2): 434–442.

Light, W. C., Reisman, R. E., Shimizu, M. and Arbesman, C. E. 1977. Unusual reactions following insect stings. Clinical features and immunologic analysis. J. Allergy Clin. Immunol. 59(5): 391–397.

Lockey, R. F., Turkeltaub, P. C., Olive, C. A., Baird-Warren, I. A., Olive, E. S. and Bukantz, S. C. 1989. The Hymenoptera venom study. II: Skin test results and safety of venom skin testing. J. Allergy Clin. Immunol. 84(6 Pt 1): 967–974.

Lyons, J. J., Chovanec, J., O'Connell, M. P., Liu, Y., Selb, J., Zanotti, R. et al. 2021. Heritable risk for severe anaphylaxis associated with increased alpha-tryptase-encoding germline copy number at TPSAB1. J. Allergy Clin. Immunol. 147(2): 622–632.

Mauriello, P. M., Barde, S. H., Georgitis, J. W. and Reisman, R. E. 1984. Natural history of large local reactions from stinging insects. J. Allergy Clin. Immunol. 74(4 Pt 1): 494–498.

Michel, J., Brockow, K., Darsow, U., Ring, J., Schmidt-Weber, C. B., Grunwald, T. et al. 2016. Added sensitivity of component-resolved diagnosis in hymenoptera venom-allergic patients with elevated serum tryptase and/or mastocytosis. Allergy 71(5): 651–660.

Mizuma, H., Tanaka, A., Uchida, Y., Fujiwara, A., Manabe, R., Furukawa, H. et al. 2015. Influence of Omalizumab on allergen-specific IgE in patients with adult asthma. Int. Arch. Allergy Immunol. 168(3): 165–172.

Motosue, M. S., Bellolio, M. F., Van Houten, H. K., Shah, N. D. and Campbell, R. L. 2017. Increasing emergency department visits for anaphylaxis, 2005–2014. J. Allergy Clin. Immunol. Pract. 5(1): 171–175 e173.

Muller, U., Helbling, A. and Bischof, M. 1989. Predictive value of venom-specific IgE, IgG and IgG subclass antibodies in patients on immunotherapy with honey bee venom. Allergy 44(6): 412–418.

Muller, U. R. 2005. Bee venom allergy in beekeepers and their family members. Curr. Opin. Allergy Clin. Immunol. 5(4): 343–347.

Muller, U. R., Johansen, N., Petersen, A. B., Fromberg-Nielsen, J. and Haeberli, G. 2009. Hymenoptera venom allergy: analysis of double positivity to honey bee and Vespula venom by estimation of IgE antibodies to species-specific major allergens Api m1 and Ves v5. Allergy 64(4): 543–548.

Nath, P., Adams, K., Schapira, R. and Edwards, K. 2019. Imported fire ant hypersensitivity and mastocytosis: A case series of successful venom immunotherapy. Ann. Allergy Asthma Immunol. 122(5): 541–542.

Nguyen, S. A. and Napoli, D. C. 2005. Natural history of large local and generalized cutaneous reactions to imported fire ant stings in children. Ann. Allergy Asthma Immunol. 94(3): 387–390.

Niedoszytko, M., de Monchy, J., van Doormaal, J. J., Jassem, E. and Oude Elberink, J. N. 2009. Mastocytosis and insect venom allergy: diagnosis, safety and efficacy of venom immunotherapy. Allergy 64(9): 1237–1245.

Niedoszytko, M., Bonadonna, P., Oude Elberink, J. N. and Golden, D. B. 2014. Epidemiology, diagnosis, and treatment of Hymenoptera venom allergy in mastocytosis patients. Immunol. Allergy Clin. North Am. 34(2): 365–381.

Ong, Y. E., Menzies-Gow, A., Barkans, J., Benyahia, F., Ou, T. T., Ying, S. et al. 2005. Anti-IgE (omalizumab) inhibits late-phase reactions and inflammatory cells after repeat skin allergen challenge. J. Allergy Clin. Immunol. 116(3): 558–564.

Oude Elberink, J. N., de Monchy, J. G., Kors, J. W., van Doormaal, J. J. and Dubois, A. E. 1997. Fatal anaphylaxis after a yellow jacket sting, despite venom immunotherapy, in two patients with mastocytosis. J. Allergy Clin. Immunol. 99(1 Pt 1): 153–154.

Peng, Z., Beckett, A. N., Engler, R. J., Hoffman, D. R., Ott, N. L. and Simons, F. E. 2004. Immune responses to mosquito saliva in 14 individuals with acute systemic allergic reactions to mosquito bites. J. Allergy Clin. Immunol. 114(5): 1189–1194.

Pravettoni, V., Piantanida, M., Primavesi, L., Forti, S. and Pastorello, E. A. 2014. Basal platelet-activating factor acetylhydrolase: prognostic marker of severe Hymenoptera venom anaphylaxis. J. Allergy Clin. Immunol. 133(4): 1218–1220.

Pucci, S., D'Alo, S., De Pasquale, T., Illuminati, I., Makri, E. and Incorvaia, C. 2015. Risk of anaphylaxis in patients with large local reactions to hymenoptera stings: a retrospective and prospective study. Clin. Mol. Allergy 13: 21.

Quirt, J. A., Wen, X., Kim, J., Herrero, A. J. and Kim, H. L. 2016. Venom allergy testing: is a graded approach necessary? Ann. Allergy Asthma Immunol. 116(1): 49–51.

Reimers, A. and Müller, U. 2005. Fatal outcome of a Vespula sting in a patient with mastocytosis after specific immunotherapy with honey bee venom. Allergy Clin. Immunol. Int. J. WAO Org. 17(Suppl 1): S69–S70.

Reisman, R. E. 1992. Natural history of insect sting allergy: relationship of severity of symptoms of initial sting anaphylaxis to re-sting reactions. J. Allergy Clin. Immunol. 90(3 Pt 1): 335–339.

Reisman, R. E. and Livingston, A. 1992. Venom immunotherapy: 10 years of experience with administration of single venoms and 50 micrograms maintenance doses. J. Allergy Clin. Immunol. 89(6): 1189–1195.

Ridolo, E., Olivieri, E., Montagni, M., Rolli, A. and Senna, G. E. 2012. Type I variant of Kounis syndrome secondary to wasp sting. Ann. Allergy Asthma Immunol. 109(1): 79–81.

Roumana, A., Pitsios, C., Vartholomaios, S., Kompoti, E. and Kontou-Fili, K. 2009. The safety of initiating Hymenoptera immunotherapy at 1 microg of venom extract. J. Allergy Clin. Immunol. 124(2): 379–381.

Rueff, F., Wenderoth, A. and Przybilla, B. 2001. Patients still reacting to a sting challenge while receiving conventional Hymenoptera venom immunotherapy are protected by increased venom doses. J. Allergy Clin. Immunol. 108(6): 1027–1032.

Rueff, F., Przybilla, B., Bilo, M. B., Muller, U., Scheipl, F., Aberer, W. et al. 2009. Predictors of severe systemic anaphylactic reactions in patients with Hymenoptera venom allergy: importance of baseline serum tryptase-a study of the European Academy of Allergology and Clinical Immunology Interest Group on Insect Venom Hypersensitivity. J. Allergy Clin. Immunol. 124(5): 1047–1054.

Rueff, F., Przybilla, B., Bilo, M. B., Muller, U., Scheipl, F., Aberer, W. et al. 2010. Predictors of side effects during the buildup phase of venom immunotherapy for Hymenoptera venom allergy: the importance of baseline serum tryptase. J. Allergy Clin. Immunol. 126(1): 105–111 e105.

Ruiz, B., Serrano, P., Verdu, M. and Moreno, C. 2015. Sensitization to Api m 1, Api m 2, and Api m 4: association with safety of bee venom immunotherapy. Ann. Allergy Asthma Immunol. 114(4): 350–352.

Ruiz, B., Serrano, P. and Moreno, C. 2016. IgE-Api m 4 is useful for identifying a particular phenotype of bee venom allergy. J. Investig. Allergol. Clin. Immunol. 26(6): 355–361.

Santos, A. F., Alpan, O. and Hoffmann, H. J. 2021. Basophil activation test: Mechanisms and considerations for use in clinical trials and clinical practice. Allergy 76(8): 2420–2432.

Schuler, C. F. 4th., Volertas, S., Khokhar, D., Yuce, H., Chen, L., Baser, O. et al. 2021. Prevalence of mastocytosis and Hymenoptera venom allergy in the United States. J. Allergy Clin. Immunol. 148(5): 1316–1323.

Selb, J., Rijavec, M., Erzen, R., Zidarn, M., Kopac, P., Skerget, M. et al. 2021. Routine KIT p.D816V screening identifies clonal mast cell disease in Hymenoptera allergic patients regularly missed using baseline tryptase levels alone. J. Allergy Clin. Immunol. 148(2): 621–626.

Settipane, G. A., Newstead, G. J. and Boyd, G. K. 1972. Frequency of Hymenoptera allergy in an atopic and normal population. J. Allergy Clin. Immunol. 50(3): 146–150.

Severino, M. G., Campi, P., Macchia, D., Manfredi, M., Turillazzi, S., Spadolini, I. et al. 2006. European Polistes venom allergy. Allergy 61(7): 860–863.

Shaker, M. S., Wallace, D. V., Golden, D. B. K., Oppenheimer, J., Bernstein, J. A., Campbell, R. L. et al. 2020. Anaphylaxis-a 2020 practice parameter update, systematic review, and Grading of Recommendations, Assessment, Development and Evaluation (GRADE) analysis. J. Allergy Clin. Immunol. 145(4): 1082–1123.

Shamji, M. H., Wilcock, L. K., Wachholz, P. A., Dearman, R. J., Kimber, I., Wurtzen, P. A. et al. 2006. The IgE-facilitated allergen binding (FAB) assay: validation of a novel flow-cytometric based method for the detection of inhibitory antibody responses. J. Immunol. Methods 317(1-2): 71–79.

Silva, G. B. D. J., Vasconcelos, A. G. J., Rocha, A. M. T., Vasconcelos, V. R., Barros, J. N., Fujishima, J. S. et al. 2017. Acute kidney injury complicating bee stings—a review. Rev. Inst. Med. Trop. Sao Paulo 59: e25.

Simioni, L., Vianello, A., Bonadonna, P., Marcer, G., Severino, M., Pagani, M. et al. 2013. Efficacy of venom immunotherapy given every 3 or 4 months: a prospective comparison with the conventional regimen. Ann. Allergy Asthma Immunol. 110(1): 51–54.

Soriano-Gomis, V., Cabrera-Beyrouti, R., Serrano-Delgado, P., Jimenez-Rodriguez, T. W., Gomez, M. B. and Fernandez-Sanchez, J. 2021. Epidemiology of Hymenoptera venom allergy in the Valencia Fire Brigade (Spain). J. Allergy Clin. Immunol. Pract. 9(2): 1037–1038 e1032.

Stoevesandt, J., Hain, J., Kerstan, A. and Trautmann, A. 2012. Over- and underestimated parameters in severe Hymenoptera venom-induced anaphylaxis: cardiovascular medication and absence of urticaria/angioedema. J. Allergy Clin. Immunol. 130(3): 698–704 e691.

Stoevesandt, J., Hain, J., Stolze, I., Kerstan, A. and Trautmann, A. 2014. Angiotensin-converting enzyme inhibitors do not impair the safety of Hymenoptera venom immunotherapy build-up phase. Clin. Exp. Allergy 44(5): 747–755.

Stoevesandt, J., Hosp, C., Kerstan, A. and Trautmann, A. 2015. Hymenoptera venom immunotherapy while maintaining cardiovascular medication: safe and effective. Ann. Allergy Asthma Immunol. 114(5): 411–416.

Strohmeier, B., Aberer, W., Bokanovic, D., Komericki, P. and Sturm, G. J. 2013. Simultaneous intradermal testing with hymenoptera venoms is safe and more efficient than sequential testing. Allergy 68(4): 542–544.

Sturm, G. J., Kranzelbinder, B., Schuster, C., Sturm, E. M., Bokanovic, D., Vollmann, J. et al. 2014. Sensitization to Hymenoptera venoms is common, but systemic sting reactions are rare. J. Allergy Clin. Immunol. 133(6): 1635–1643 e1631.

Sturm, G. J., Herzog, S. A., Aberer, W., Alfaya Arias, T., Antolin-Amerigo, D., Bonadonna, P. et al. 2021. beta-blockers and ACE inhibitors are not a risk factor for severe systemic sting reactions and adverse events during venom immunotherapy. Allergy 76(7): 2166–2176.

Tankersley, M. S., Walker, R. L., Butler, W. K., Hagan, L. L., Napoli, D. C. and Freeman, T. M. 2002. Safety and efficacy of an imported fire ant rush immunotherapy protocol with and without prophylactic treatment. J. Allergy Clin. Immunol. 109(3): 556–562.

Tejedor-Alonso, M. A., Farias-Aquino, E., Perez-Fernandez, E., Grifol-Clar, E., Moro-Moro, M. and Rosado-Ingelmo, A. 2019. Relationship between anaphylaxis and use of beta-blockers and angiotensin-converting enzyme inhibitors: a systematic review and meta-analysis of observational studies. J. Allergy Clin. Immunol. Pract. 7(3): 879–897 e875.

Turner, P. J., Jerschow, E., Umasunthar, T., Lin, R., Campbell, D. E. and Boyle, R. J. 2017. Fatal anaphylaxis: mortality rate and risk factors. J. Allergy Clin. Immunol. Pract. 5(5): 1169–1178.

Vadas, P., Perelman, B. and Liss, G. 2013. Platelet-activating factor, histamine, and tryptase levels in human anaphylaxis. J. Allergy Clin. Immunol. 131(1): 144–149.

van der Linden, P. W., Hack, C. E., Struyvenberg, A. and van der Zwan, J. K. 1994. Insect-sting challenge in 324 subjects with a previous anaphylactic reaction: current criteria for insect-venom hypersensitivity do not predict the occurrence and the severity of anaphylaxis. J. Allergy Clin. Immunol. 94(2 Pt 1): 151–159.

Varga, E. M., Francis, J. N., Zach, M. S., Klunker, S., Aberer, W. and Durham, S. R. 2009. Time course of serum inhibitory activity for facilitated allergen-IgE binding during bee venom immunotherapy in children. Clin. Exp. Allergy 39(9): 1353–1357.

Vos, B., Kohler, J., Muller, S., Stretz, E., Rueff, F. and Jakob, T. 2013. Spiking venom with rVes v 5 improves sensitivity of IgE detection in patients with allergy to Vespula venom. J. Allergy Clin. Immunol. 131(4): 1225–1227, 1227 e1221.

Vos, B., Dubois, A. E. J., Rauber, M. M., Pfutzner, W., Miehe, M., Bohle, B. et al. 2019. Initiating yellow jacket venom immunotherapy with a 100-mug dose: A challenge? J. Allergy Clin. Immunol. Pract. 7(4): 1332–1334 e1334.

Wachholz, P. A., Soni, N. K., Till, S. J. and Durham, S. R. 2003. Inhibition of allergen-IgE binding to B cells by IgG antibodies after grass pollen immunotherapy. J. Allergy Clin. Immunol. 112(5): 915–922.

Wong, C. G. and Borici-Mazi, R. 2012. Delayed-onset cold anaphylaxis after hymenoptera sting. Ann. Allergy Asthma Immunol. 109(1): 77–78.

Zanotti, R., Lombardo, C., Passalacqua, G., Caimmi, C., Bonifacio, M., De Matteis, G. et al. 2015. Clonal mast cell disorders in patients with severe Hymenoptera venom allergy and normal serum tryptase levels. J. Allergy Clin. Immunol. 136(1): 135–139.

Zitnik, S. E., Vesel, T., Avcin, T., Silar, M., Kosnik, M. and Korosec, P. 2012. Monitoring honeybee venom immunotherapy in children with the basophil activation test. Pediatr. Allergy Immunol. 23(2): 166–172.

Chapter 13A

Role of Yoga and Ayurveda in the Management of Allergic Disorders

Kashinath G. Metri[1,*] and *Pudupakkam K. Vedanthan*[2]

Introduction

Allergic disorders have become a common health issue worldwide in the last two decades (Zhang and Zhang 2019; Naha et al. 2012). Allergy is the body's hypersensitivity response after exposure to a specific harmless substance (Johansson et al. 2004). Abnormal immune response/hyperactivity is the hallmark of all allergic disorders (Maeda et al. 2019). It is essential to understand the factors involved in the development of hypersensitivity.

Strong heritability and a western lifestyle seem to contribute to the increasing prevalence of allergic diseases (Antonogeorgos et al. 2021). Changes in maternal and infant diets (Sicherer et al. 2008), exposure to antibiotics in infancy, indoor air pollutants (especially cigarette smoke) and aeroallergens have been suggested as environmental factors (Holgate 2000). Further, growing evidence suggests that stress is strongly involved in the cause and maintenance of many chronic non-communicable diseases, including allergic disorders (Liezmann et al. 2011; Misery et al. 2022). Chronic stress exacerbates existing allergies and could be an independent cause of chronic allergic diseases (Dave et al. 2011). Stress reaction causes dysregulation in neuroendocrine-immune function by exaggerating sympathetic tone and hypothalamic-pituitary-adrenal axis activity (Guilliams 2010; Rohleder 2004). Further, it leads to increased production of inflammatory cytokines and mast cell activity involved in allergic disorders (Liezmann et al. 2012).

Diet is an important determinant of health. Food also has immunological significance (López-Varela et al. 2002). Studies have shown that malnutrition significantly affects immune function (Woon et al. 2018). Similarly, excess fast food consumption is also associated with allergic disorders (Vo Ehrenstien et al. 2015; Ellwood et al. 2013). Fast foods are processed with added preservatives, coloured and refined. Such food is not a functional food and is highly unhealthy with a negligible quantity of fibre and antioxidants (Von Ehrenstein et al. 2015; Rutkowski et al. 2014). Evidence suggests that artificial colours in fast food cause allergies (Stevens et al. 2013). Fast food consumption may increase cytokine production and immune system dysregulation, contributing to allergic disorders (Myles 2014).

---

[1] Assistant Professor, Department of Yoga, Central University of Rajasthan.
[2] The University of Colorado at Anschutz Campus in Aurora, Colorado. USA.
Email: pkv1947@gmail.com
* Corresponding author: kgmhetre@gmail.com

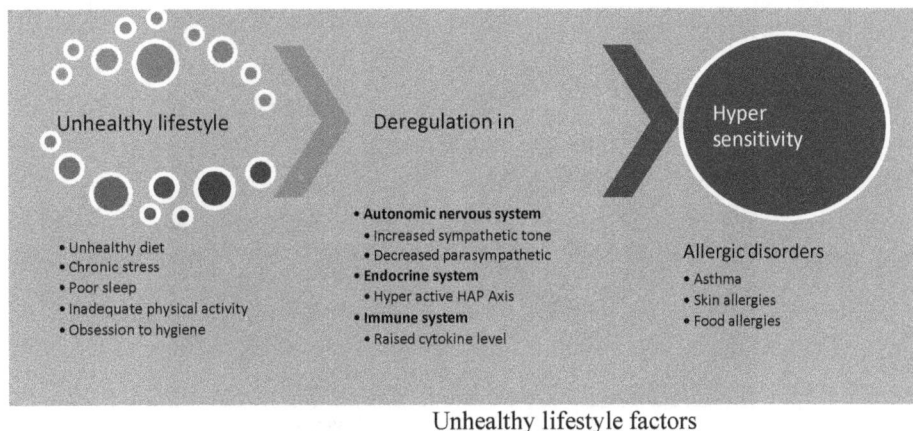

Unhealthy lifestyle factors

Figure 1. Pathophysiology of allergic disorders.

Good quality sleep is important for health (Wu and Yang 2020). Sleep strongly connects with immune functioning (Moldofsky et al. 1995). Sleep deprivation is associated with increased inflammatory cytokine production and dysregulation in neuroendocrine and immune functions (Rico-Rosillo and Vega-Robledo 2018; Briançon-Marjollet et al. 2015; Kim et al. 2022; Oztürk et al. 1999). Further, studies have found a strong association between sleep deprivation with allergic diseases such as asthma and allergic rhinitis (Koinis-Mitchell et al. 2012).

Physical activity is also an important determinant of health. Adequate physical activity has an appositive impact on the immune system (Nieman and Wentz 2019). A recent review by Kuder et al. offers promising evidence of the additional benefit of increased physical activity as a non-pharmacologic treatment for asthma (Kuder et al. 2021). Prossegger et al. demonstrated that recreational winter exercise at moderately cold temperatures reduces allergic airway inflammation measured as fractional oral exhaled nitric oxide, and nasal eosinophilic cell count and induces sustainable improvements in allergic symptoms (Prossegger et al. 2019).

Yoga

Yoga has gained popularity in the last two decades as the most commonly recommended complementary medicine due to its therapeutic benefits for various chronic disorders (Dutta et al. 2022). Yoga, a lifestyle intervention, involves several mind-body practices that help promote health and well-being (Shawn and Keytaz 2021).

The discipline of yoga was discovered, developed and practiced by ancient sages of the Indian continent (Basavareddi 2015). Yoga includes Yama (self-discipline), Niyama (social conduct), Āsana (yoga postures), Prāṇāyāma (yoga breathing techniques), Pratyāhāra (control over senses), Dhāraṇā (focusing meditation) and Dhyāna (defocusing meditation) and Samādhi (transcendence), which makes it a popular discipline (White 2019).

Allergic Disorders According to Yoga

According to yoga, every living being comprises five distinct aspects (Pancha Kosha) of existence. They are (a) *annamayakōśa*, the physical anatomical component, which is made of chemicals (pockets of particles, atoms, cells, tissues and organ systems); (b) *prāṇamayakōśa*, the vital body, the bio-magnetic field responsible for all physiological functions (movement and reproduction); (c) *Manōmayakōśa*, the mind (perception and emotions); (d) *vijñānamayakōśa*, the intellectual discriminating component of the mind; (e) *ānandamayakōśa*, the causal bliss field, (stable, rested and thoughtless state) (Bhagat 2018). According to yoga, allergy is a peripheral manifestation

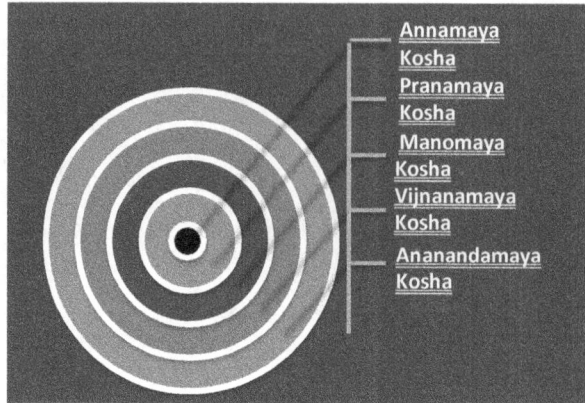

Depicts the five aspects of human existence.

Figure 2. Five layers of human consciousness (Pancha Kosha).

of *Ādhi* (emotional imbalances in the Manōmayakōśa) that begins in the mind and shows up as immune hyper-reactivity in *annamayakōśa*. *Ādhi* also diverts the person from a healthy lifestyle (Bhavanani 2011).

Techniques of Yoga-Based Lifestyle Change for Allergic Disorders

Diet Modification

Yoga's uniqueness lies in studying the influence of food on the mental state (Rosen 2011) and classifies them under three categories: those that make the mind calm and stable (Satvika), those which excite negative emotions (Rajasic) and those that cause drowsiness/laziness (Tamasic) (Khanna et al. 2013). Thus, the recommended Satvika food for health is nutritious, simple, wholesome, freshly cooked and saatmya (suitable) foods consumed in moderate quantities (Bhagavat Gita). Avoid processed, deep-fried, refined, heavily spiced foods considered rajasic and fermented, preserved or stale foods as tamasic. Yoga and Ayurveda also suggest that persons with allergic diseases should follow the Satvika diet and avoid food that aggravates the allergy symptoms. Identify the allergens in the food and prevent them initially but develop tolerance to use healthy food items later as the system becomes more stable through regular yoga practices (Arya et al. 2021).

Yoga Kriyas (Cleansing Techniques)

Kriyas refer to techniques of cleansing the internal passages. The recommended cleaning techniques (Kriyas) for allergic disorders include Neti to cleanse the nasopharyngeal tracts, Dhouti to clean the stomach and Kapalabhaati to expel the phlegm from deeper airways (Vaid et al. 2021). They help in clearing the internal passages and developing voluntary mastery over hyper-reactive reflex responses such as sneezing, coughing, wheezing, etc., resulting in better tolerance to external allergens (Nagendra and Nagaratna 1986).

Jala Neti

It is nasal irrigation using warm saline water. Jala Neti is one of the widely practiced and popular kriyas in Yoga.

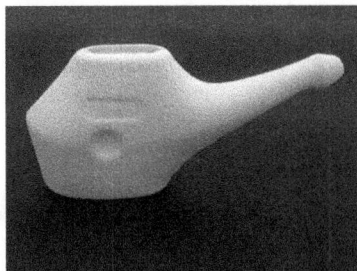

Figure 3. Neti Pot.

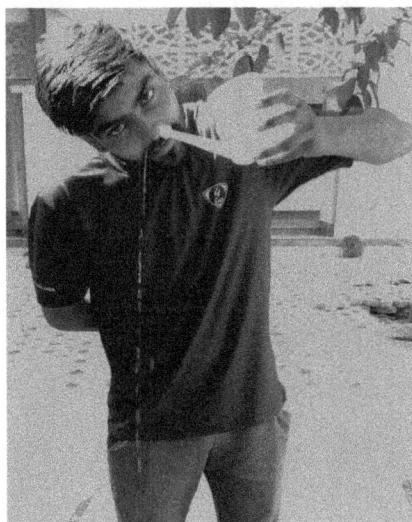

Figure 4. Demonstration of Jala Neti practice.

Procedure

Jala Neti should be practiced on an empty stomach early in the morning. Before the practice, Jala Neti one should ensure no nasal congestion (free air flow in both nostrils). Nasal congestion can be removed by performing Kapalabhati (forceful and dynamic exhalation by flapping the abdomen, i.e., 2 × 40 strokes/minute) (Malhotra et al. 2022).

Jala Neti is performed using lukewarm (39°C) saline water (2.5 grams NaCl/500 m water) (Georgitis 1994) using a Neti pot. As shown in the figure, one should stand straight, bend forward and tilt the neck to the right side. Nasal irrigation is done by inserting the Neti pot's nozzle into the right nostril. During nasal irrigation, one should breathe from the mouth. After the right nostril, repeat the procedure for the left nostril also. After completion, one should perform Kapalabhati to drain out the left saline water in the nostril (Satyananda 2014).

Advantages

Jala Neti cleanses the cranium and sinuses and alleviates the head and neck region (Muktanand 2014). It helps remove allergens and dust particles and improves blood circulation in the nasal mucosa. It is found to be effective in allergic rhinitis, asthma and insensitivity to smell. Jala Neti also improves attention and concentration (Meera et al. 2020).

Mechanism

Jala Neti reduces the inflammatory response to allergens in the nasal mucosa by reducing histamines and leukotriene (Georgitis 1994).

Contra-Indication

Jala Neti should be avoided in conditions like acute rhinitis, acute sinusitis and acute exacerbation of asthma, nasal polyps and severe form of the deviated nasal septum.

Asana (Yoga Postures)

Asana is the third step of the yoga discipline. Asana involves different yoga poses performed with mindfulness and slow breathing. According to Hatha Yoga Pradeepika, yoga postures bring stability, strength and lightness to the body (Satyananda 2014). In yoga, therapy-specific postures are recommended for a specific health condition, e.g., Bhujangāsana (cobras pose) is recommended for asthma. Studies have confirmed that asana practice is associated with enhanced autonomic balance, decreased sympathetic activity and increased vagal tone (Sarubin et al. 2014). Asana practice reduces inflammation and regulates immune function (Estevao 2022).

These yoga practices should be performed on an empty stomach or 2–2½ hours after a meal. Yoga postures should be done slowly with deep, slow and conscious breathing. Do not strain; try to attempt the pose at your ease (it is okay if a final/perfect posture is not possible). After reaching the final pose, one should hold the pose with their capacity with normal breathing.

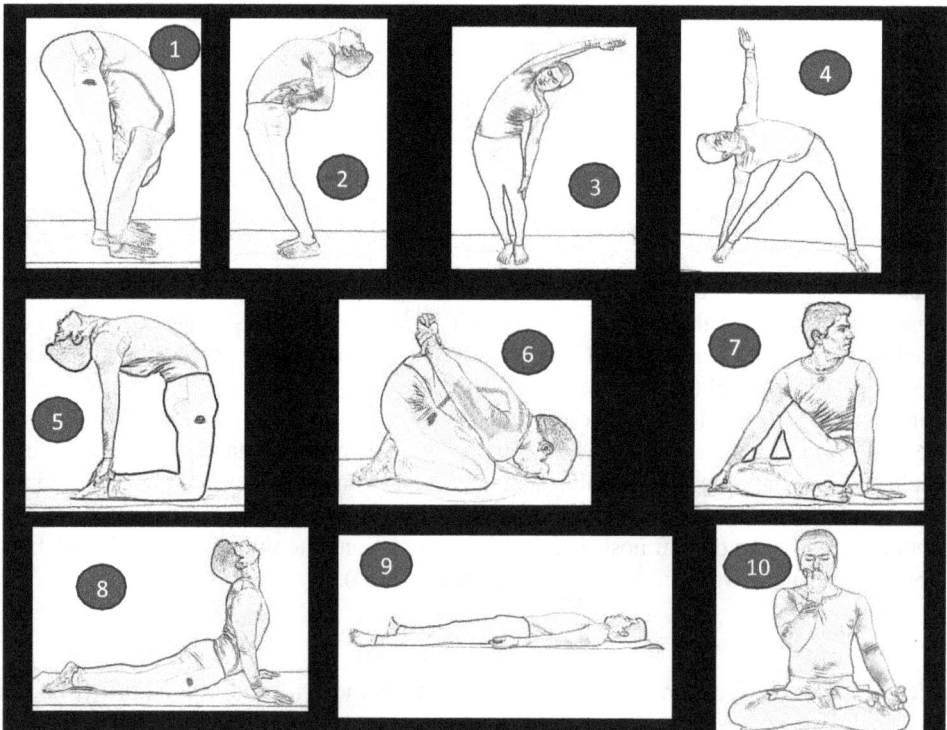

Figure 5. Yoga Postures Useful in Allergic Disorders. (1) PādaHastāsana (hand-to-foot pose), (2) Ardha Chakrāsana (half-wheel pose), (3) Ardhkati Chakrasana (half-waist bend), (4) Trikonasana (triangle pose), (5) Ustrāsana (camel pose), (6) Saśankasana (moon pose), (7) Vakrāsana (twisted spine pose), (8) Bhujangāsana (cobra pose), (9) Savāsana (corpse pose) and (10) Nādishuddhi Prāṇāyāma (alternate nostril breathing).

Pranayama (Yogic Breathing)

Prāṇāyāma is slow-paced mindful breathing. There are various types of breathing practices according to yoga, such as alternate nostril breathing (Nadishodhana Prāṇāyāma), left nostril breathing (Chandra Nadi Pranayama), right nostril breathing (Surya Nadi Pranayama), etc.

These breathing techniques have specific physiological benefits. Studies have reported the therapeutic benefits of Prāṇāyāma on the immune system and various chronic diseases, including allergic disorders (Arora et al. 2018; Das et al. 2021). Further, studies have reported that the practice of Prāṇāyāma helps to improve lung capacities, autonomic function, cardiac functions and cognitive abilities (Moventhan and Khode 2014). Prāṇāyāma improves vagal tone by promoting sino-respiratory arrhythmia and baroreflex (Bhavanani et al. 2012).

Meditation

Meditation is a yogic mental practice that involves the practice of mental focusing on a meditative object, thought, mantra, etc., followed by defocusing. There are various stages of meditation. In the initial phase, practitioners need to practice concentrating/chanting/visualising the object of meditation effortfully; this phase of meditation is called Dhāraṇa. The second phase is called Dhyāna, where the mind can be easily concentrated without/with minimum effort on the object of meditation; in this phase of meditation, mindfulness increases. Samādhi is the third phase of

Table 1. The list of yoga practices for allergic disorders.

Sl No	Practice	Duration – 60 Minutes
1	Loosening practices	10 Minutes
2	Quick Relaxation Technique (QRT)	
3	Breathing practices	15 Minutes
	Prasarita Hasta Swasah (Hands in and out breathing)	
	Utkashita Hasta Swasah (Hands stretch breathing)	
	Vyaghraswasah (Tiger breathing)	
	Ankle-stretch breathing	
	Straight-leg raising breathing	
	Sethubandhasana breathing (breathing in bridge pose)	
	Bhujangāsana breathing (Breathing in cobra pose)	
4	Asanas	20 Minutes
	Tadasana (straight pose)	
	Trikonasana (triangle pose)	
	Ardhachakrasana (half-wheel pose)	
	Padahasthasana (hand-feet pose)	
	Vajrayana (tree pose)	
	Ardhakaticharasana (half-waist pose)	
	Ustrāsana (camel Pose)	
	Shavasana (corpse pose)	
5	Deep relaxation technique (DRT)	10 Minutes
6	Prāṇāyāma (yogic breathing practices)	5 Minutes
	Bhastrika Pranayama (bellows breath)	
	Nadishodha Prāṇāyāma (alternate nostril breathing)	
	Brahmari Prāṇāyāma (humming)	

meditation, which is the state trance. In this phase, the mind is entirely free from all negative emotions, traumas and conflicts, and it becomes pure awareness of aloneness. In this phase, one attains purity, unconditional love, compassion, forgiveness and universal oneness; in the last few years lot of research on meditation (Kim et al. 2022). Their various tailor-made meditation techniques have evolved recently (Farias et al. 2020). Meditation is effective in allergic disorders (Lack et al. 2020). Mediations such as OM meditation, mindfulness meditation, Vipassana meditation and cyclic meditation are recommended for allergic diseases. Meditation is associated with decreased inflammatory cytokines, catecholamine, cortisol and sympathetic overactivity (Househam et al. 2017; Henneghan et al. 2021).

Scientific Evidence for Yoga

The therapeutic effects of yoga have attracted the attention of the medical and scientific community in the last three decades. The number of research publications on yoga for health benefits in healthy and clinical populations has increased (Alvarez et al. 2022).

Yoga and Immune Modulation

A large body of data confirmed the positive effects of yoga on the immune system. Yoga has immune-modulation properties. Yoga reduces inflammatory cytokines (Prinster 2014; Bower et al. 2014) and increases NK cell number and immune cell activity (Rao et al. 2008). Clinical trials have shown the positive role of yoga in immune-compromised conditions, such as HIV, tuberculosis and cancer (Dadang and Wahyu 2021; Visweswaraiah and Telles 2004; Sinclair 2020; Cramer et al. 2012; David et al. 2017; Jiang et al. 2021). Yoga intervention demonstrated an increase in NK-cell activity and T-lymphocytes, CD4, CD8 and NK-cell count and reduced inflammatory cytokines such as IL-1, IL-2, IL-6 and TNF alpha. Further, psychological factors such as anxiety, depression, stress and mood, which are known to affect immune function reduced after yoga intervention (Rao et al. 2008; Vempati and Telles 2002). Yoga brings the immune-modulation by reducing catecholamines, cortisol and inflammatory cytokines via down-regulating HPA axis hyperactivity and improving the vagal tone (Rajak et al. 2016; Ray et al. 2001).

Yoga in Allergic Rhinitis

Several RCT studies have demonstrated the benefits of yoga in allergic rhinitis. An RCT on an 8-week Hatha yoga intervention (3 times/week) among 27 allergic rhinitis patients has shown significant improvement in clinical symptoms of rhinitis and cytokine profiles (Chanta et al. 2019). Another study on 51 healthy volunteers and 51 allergic rhinitis patients who received 3 months of Hath yoga intervention showed a significant decrease in nasal airway resistance. It increased forced vital capacity and a non-significant increase in FEV1. Further, mental health measures and Sino-nasal outcome tests also improved significantly (Chellaa et al. 2019). Following yoga practice, the positive changes in allergic rhinitis may be attributed to immune modulation by reducing inflammatory cytokines, improved circulation to the nasal mucosa and decreased hypersensitivity of the nasal mucosa (Eda et al. 2018; Ye et al. 2020; Meera et al. 2020). Persons with allergic rhinitis are recommended regular yoga practices consisting of loosening practices, yoga postures and yoga breathing practices minimum (listed in Table 1) a minimum of three times a week, and Jala Neti practise a minimum of twice a week for a minimum of three months.

Yoga in Asthma

Several randomised controlled trials have been conducted to investigate the efficacy of yoga in asthma (Das et al. 2019; Cramer et al. 2014). These studies have reported a significant reduction in asthma symptoms, frequency of asthma episodes, inflammatory markers and need for bronchodilators. This study observed a significant improvement in lung function and quality of life (Cramer et al. 2014).

A systematic review of 11 clinical trials in adolescents 14–18 years with asthma reported the efficacy after 3–12 weeks of yoga. The study reported a positive impact of yoga on forced vital capacity, peak expiratory force, peak expiratory volume, reserve volume, respiratory rate, anxiety, stress, medication use and quality of life (Arora et al. 2017). A meta-analysis of 14 RCT studies on yoga in asthma found beneficial effects on various parameters of asthma, including symptoms, quality of life, asthma medication use and lung functions (Yang et al. 2016).

Yoga practice in asthma helps to improve lung capacities and reduce inflammatory cytokines (Papp et al. 2017; Swami et al. 2010; Venkatesh et al. 2020). It reduces hypersensitivity of the respiratory mucosa and improves breathing (Meera et al. 2020; Das et al. 2020).

Ayurveda

Ayurveda is an ancient life science, probably the first healthcare system on earth. The meaning of "Ayurveda" is "science of life." It is a science of a healthy lifestyle. The concept of "Tridosha" is unique to Ayurveda. It recognises three basic bio-energy principles in the body called Tridosha; Vāta, Pitta and Kapha are the Tridosha. These three bio-energy principles maintain normal functioning of the body such as vātagoverns all movements and transportation, pitta governs metabolism and temperature, Kapha governs growth and production, etc. Imbalance in the Tridosha results in disease. Each dosha disturbance leads to a specific disease when imbalanced (Padma 2005).

Prevention of the disease, according to Ayurveda, is through following a lifestyle that helps maintain balance in the Tridoshas, and treatment of the disease includes restoration of Tridosha balance. The Tridosha balance is affected by an unhealthy diet, inadequate or excessive physical activity, mental afflictions such as anxiety, depression, stress, hate, worry, etc. or seasonal variations. Ayurveda recommends a healthy lifestyle in Dinachary (daily regimes) and Rituchary (seasonal regimens) to maintain doshas in a balanced state (Mukherjee et al. 2017; Singh et al. 2007).

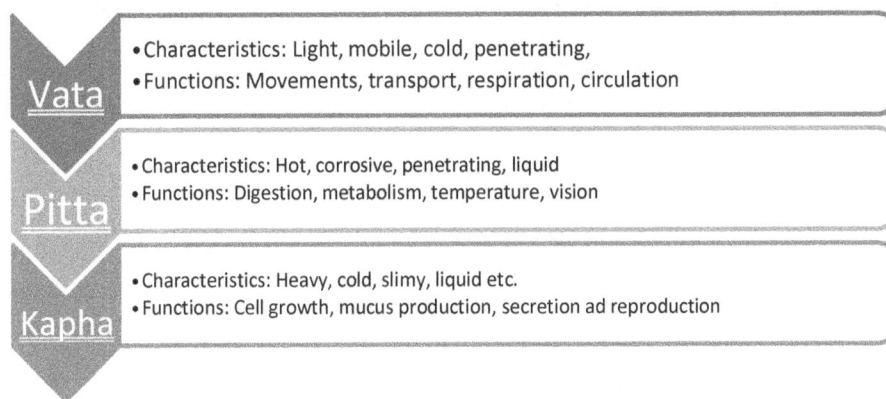

Vata
- Characteristics: Light, mobile, cold, penetrating,
- Functions: Movements, transport, respiration, circulation

Pitta
- Characteristics: Hot, corrosive, penetrating, liquid
- Functions: Digestion, metabolism, temperature, vision

Kapha
- Characteristics: Heavy, cold, slimy, liquid etc.
- Functions: Cell growth, mucus production, secretion ad reproduction

Figure 6. Characteristics of Tridosha: Vāta, Pitta and Kapha Have Distinctive characteristics.

Ayurveda Treatment Approach to Allergic Disorders

According to Ayurveda, allergic disorders such as skin allergies, food allergies, asthma, nasal allergy, etc., are due to an imbalance in the Tridosha.

Nidanaparivarjana (Avoidance of Causative Factors)

Ayurveda recommends Pathya (do's) and Apathya (dont's) for every disease. For allergic disorders, one should avoid the following things:

1. Exposure to cold weather, cold water bath, drinking cold water, milk and milk products.
2. Strongly Spiced foods, sweets, fried foods, heavy and cold food.

3. Excessive exercise or no exercise.

4. Avoid excess worry, stress and anxiety-provoking activities/situations.

Recommendations

- Eat food that is fresh, warm, free from preservatives and colouring agents and easy to digest, such as porridges, oats, etc.
- Keep yourself warm; drink warm water. Perform yoga, meditation, yoga Nidra and prayers to keep mental affliction away.
- One can use brown sugar and spices like ginger, turmeric, peppers, etc.
- Soups and warm drinks are beneficial.

Ayurveda recommends a specific daily regimen (Dinacharya) and season regimen (Ritucharya) for healthy living.

Dinacharya – Daily Regimens

In order to promote health and longevity, one has to wake up in Brahm muhurta (approximately 45 minutes before sunrise) in the morning. After completion of morning oblations, one should brush the teeth and perform Gandoosha (holding liquid/warm water or sesame oil for 1 minute). Following Gandoosha, Vyayama (exercise) should be performed at a moderate intensity. Have adequate relaxation after exercise. One may go for a whole-body massage followed by a bath. Warm water is advised for the bath for patients with allergic disorders. Clean, soft, cotton cloths that provide enough cool in the summer and warm in the winter should be used (Sharma and Bhagwan 2002).

Food should be light, wholesome and compatible. It should be consumed after feeling hungry (should not consume food when there is no proper hunger). Patients with asthma and respiratory diseases should consume light and small meals and drink warm water after meals. Patients with skin allergies should avoid the opposite food (Virudhanna), such as a combination of cold and hot food items, sweet and sour, milk, not consume curd at night and avoid sour fruits and pickles. Patients with nasal allergies should avoid taking head baths daily and eating milk products and sour fruits.

Ritucharya

Tridosha are subjected to changes to the change in season example; during winter Kapha Dosha increases and Pitta Dosha comes down; and during midsummer, Vātadosha increases and Kapha Dosha comes down. As disease results from an imbalance in the dosha and season can bring the imbalance in the dosha, one prevents this imbalance due to changes in the season by following certain seasonal norms called Ritucharya.

Ayurveda prescribes seasonal regimes for a healthy person to maintain health and prevent disease.

Hemant and Shishir (four months) are when Kapha gets aggravates and exacerbates respiratory-related allergic conditions. Hence, in these seasons, patients with respiratory-related allergies should avoid Kapha aggravating food and activities. Food items such as dairy products, black grams, sweets, deep-fried items, etc., should be avoided. Such patients should take warm soups, have a light diet, drink warm water, include ginger, pepper and turmeric in the diet, wear warm clothes, avoid exposure to cold and have a cold bath (Sharma and Bhagwat 2002). Similarly, the person with different dominant dosha should take care of their diet and lifestyle during different seasons.

Ayurveda Medications

A significant number of studies have shown the effects of Ayurveda in managing allergic disorders, including skin allergies, asthma, and nasal allergy. Ayurveda is an individualised system of practice based on individual assessments such as the basic and disturbed status of doshas (Prakriti and Vikriti), Agni, Dhatu and many other parameters. Hence, the clinician selects a combination of medications, such as Haridra Khanda, Chyavanaprash, Sitopaladichurna, Vasa Avaleha, etc., for allergic disorders after assessing each case. For chronic allergic conditions, Ayurveda recommends Panchakarma (systemic purificatory therapies), which is to be administered under the supervision of an Ayurveda physician (Patel et al. 2013).

Ayurveda Nasyachikitsa (nasal medication) is the administration of a few drops (3–10) of medicated oils or decoction in the nose. Clinical trials on Nasya therapy have shown positive effects on nasal allergy. Thirty-seven patients with nasal allergy received Anu tail Nasya therapy daily for two months in a study. Post-intervention, there was a significant decrease in nasal allergy symptoms, Total Leucocyte Count (TLC), Absolute Eosinophil Count (AEC), Neutrophils and Lymphocytes (Kumar et al. 2014).

Acknowledgement

Sujatha Reddy LPC. MSEd, BAMS, DCC Owner and CEO of Humanly Lakewood. Professional Counsellor and Ayurvedic Doctor.

Glossary of Abbreviations

HPA Axis – Hypothalamus-Pituitary-Adrenal Axis
NK Cells – Natural Killer Cells
IL – Interleukin
HIV – Human Immunodeficiency Virus
CD – Cluster of Differentiation
TNF Alpha – Tumour Necrosis Factor Alpha

References

Abishek, K., Bakshi, S. S. and Bhavanani, A. B. 2019. The efficacy of yogic breathing exercise Bhramari pranayama in relieving symptoms of chronic rhinosinusitis. International Journal of Yoga 12(2): 120.

Álvarez-Pérez, Y., Rivero-Santana, A., Perestelo-Pérez, L., Duarte-Díaz, A., Ramos-García, V., Toledo-Chávarri, A., Torres-Castaño, A., León-Salas, B., Infante-Ventura, D., González-Hernández, N., Rodríguez-Rodríguez, L. and Serrano-Aguilar, P. 2022. Effectiveness of mantra-based meditation on mental health: a systematic review and meta-analysis. International Journal of Environmental Research and Public Health 19(6): 3380. https://doi.org/10.3390/ijerph19063380.

Antonogeorgos, G., Priftis, K. N., Panagiotakos, D. B., Ellwood, P., García-Marcos, L., Liakou, E. et al. 2021. Exploring the relation between atopic diseases and lifestyle patterns among adolescents living in greece: evidence from the greek global asthma network (GAN) cross-sectional study. Children (Basel, Switzerland) 8(10): 932. https://doi.org/10.3390/children8100932.

Arora, P., Ansari, S. H., Anjum, V., Mathur, R. and Ahmad, S. 2017. Investigation of the anti-asthmatic potential of Kanakasava in ovalbumin-induced bronchial asthma and airway inflammation in rats. Journal of Ethnopharmacology 197: 242–249. https://doi.org/10.1016/j.jep.2016.07.082.

Arora, M., Ravindra, P., Ingole, S. G. and Gujarati, R. 2018. Efficacy of Jalaneti and Pranayama in managing Vataja Pratishyaya (allergic rhinitis). World Journal of Pharmaceutical Research 7(07): 925–935.

Arya, H., Bhandari, S. and Singh, S. K. 2021. Concept of allergic disorders in Ayurveda—a review. 10(12): 950–58.

Basavaraddi, I. V. 2015. Yoga: Its origin, history and development. Public Diplomacy, 1.

Banzal, A. and Rawat, V. 2021. Immediate effect of bhastrika pranayama on cognitive function of healthy adults. A PG Dissertation Report.

Bhagat, O. L. 2018. Yogic concepts of holistic health and wellness. J. Adv. Res. Ayur. Yoga UnaniSiddHomeo [serial online], 15–18.

Bhavanani, A. B. 2011. Yoga as therapy: A perspective. Yoga Mimamsa 42(4): 235–241.

Bhavanani, A. B., Madanmohan, Sanjay, Z. and Basavaraddi, I. V. 2012. Immediate cardiovascular effects of Pranava pranayama in hypertensive patients. Indian Journal of Physiology and Pharmacology 56(3): 273–278.

Bower, J. E., Greendale, G., Cross-well, A. D., Garet, D., Sternlieb, B., Ganz, P. A. et al. 2014. Yoga reduces inflammatory signaling in fatigued breast cancer survivors: a randomized controlled trial. Psychoneuroendocrinology 43: 20–29. https://doi.org/10.1016/j.psyneuen.2014.01.019.

Briançon-Marjollet, A., Weiszenstein, M., Henri, M., Thomas, A., Godin-Ribuot, D. and Polak, J. 2015. The impact of sleep disorders on glucose metabolism: endocrine and molecular mechanisms. Diabetology and Metabolic Syndrome 7: 25. https://doi.org/10.1186/s13098-015-0018-3.

Chanta, A., Klaewsongkram, J., Mickleborough, T. D. and Tongtako, W. 2019. Effect of Hatha yoga training on rhinitis symptoms and cytokines in allergic rhinitis patients. Asian Pacific Journal of Allergy and Immunology 10.12932/AP-260419-0547. Advance online publication. https://doi.org/10.12932/AP-260419-0547.

Chellaa, R., Soumya, M. S., Inbaraj, G., Nayar, R., Saidha, P. K., Menezes, V. H. et al. 2019. Impact of Hatha Yoga on the airway resistances in healthy individuals and allergic rhinitis patients. Indian Journal of Otolaryngology and Head and Neck Surgery: Official Publication of the Association of Otolaryngologists of India 71 (Suppl 3): 1748–1756. https://doi.org/10.1007/s12070-017-1098-1.

Cortelli, P. and Lombardi, C. 2005. Sleep and autonomic nervous system dysfunction. *In*: Handbook of Clinical Neurophysiology 6: 343–353. Elsevier.

Cramer, H., Lange, S., Klose, P., Paul, A. and Dobos, G. 2012. Yoga for breast cancer patients and survivors: a systematic review and meta-analysis. BMC Cancer 12: 412. https://doi.org/10.1186/1471-2407-12-412.

Cramer, H., Posadzki, P., Dobos, G. and Langhorst, J. 2014. Yoga for asthma: a systematic review and meta-analysis. Annals of Allergy, Asthma and Immunology: Official Publication of the American College of Allergy, Asthma, and Immunology 112(6): 503–510.e5. https://doi.org/10.1016/j.anai.2014.03.014.

Dadang, W. and Wahyu, H. 2021. Comparison of the effectiveness between defective cough and yoga breathing exercises in reducing breathlessness on tuberculosis patients at matahari room, Dr. M. Yunus Hospital, and Bengkulu. Indian Journal of Forensic Medicine and Toxicology 15(2).

Das, R. R., Sankar, J. and Kabra, S. K. 2019. Role of breathing exercises and yoga/pranayama in childhood asthma: a systematic review. Current Pediatric Reviews 15(3): 175–183. https://doi.org/10.2174/1573396315666190121122452.

Das, R. R., Sankar, J. and Kabra, S. K. 2021. Role of breathing exercises in asthma—Yoga and Pranayama. Indian Journal of Pediatrics, 1–7.

Das, R. R., Sankar, J. and Kabra, S. K. 2022. Role of breathing exercises in asthma—Yoga and Pranayama. Indian Journal of Pediatrics 89(2): 174–180. https://doi.org/10.1007/s12098-021-03998-w.

Dave, N. D., Xiang, L., Rehm, K. E. and Marshall, G. D., Jr. 2011. Stress and allergic diseases. Immunology and Allergy Clinics of North America 31(1): 55–68. https://doi.org/10.1016/j.iac.2010.09.009.

David, P. E., Luis-Benjamín, S. G., Luis-Antonio, I. A. and Delia, E. Á. E. A. 2017. Protective effect of Yoga against tuberculosis in people living with HIV. Indian Journal of Traditional Knowledge 16.

Dutta, A., Aruchunan, M., Mukherjee, A., Metri, K. G., Ghosh, K. and Basu-Ray, I. 2022. A comprehensive review of yoga research in 2020. Journal of Integrative and Complementary Medicine 28(2): 114–23.

Eda, N., Ito, H., Shimizu, K., Suzuki, S., Lee, E. and Akama, T. 2018. Yoga stretching for improving salivary immune function and mental stress in middle-aged and older adults. Journal of Women & Aging 30(3): 227–41.

Ellwood, P., Asher, M. I., García-Marcos, L., Williams, H., Keil, U., Robertson, C. et al. 2013. Do fast foods cause asthma, rhinoconjunctivitis and eczema? Global findings from the International Study of Asthma and Allergies in Childhood (ISAAC) phase three. Thorax 68(4): 351–360.

Estevao C. 2022. The role of Yoga in inflammatory markers. Brain, Behavior, and Immunity - Health 20: 100421. https://doi.org/10.1016/j.bbih.2022.100421.

Farias, M., Maraldi, E., Wallenkampf, K. C. and Lucchetti, G. 2020. Adverse events in meditation practices and meditation-based therapies: A systematic review. Acta Psychiatrica Scandinavica 142(5): 374–93.

Georgitis, J. W. 1994. Nasal hyperthermia and simple irrigation for perennial rhinitis: changes in inflammatory mediators. Chest 106(5): 1487–1492.

Guilliams, T. G. and Edwards, L. 2010. Chronic stress and the HPA axis. The Standard 9(2): 1–2.

Henneghan, A. M., Fico, B. G., Wright, M. L., Kesler, S. R. and Harrison, M. L. 2021. Effects of meditation compared to music listening on biomarkers in breast cancer survivors with cognitive complaints: secondary outcomes of a pilot randomized control trial. Explore (New York, N.Y.) S1550-8307(21)00230-5. Advance online publication. https://doi.org/10.1016/j.explore.2021.10.011.

Holgate S. T. 2000. Science, medicine, and the future. Allergic disorders. BMJ (Clinical Research ed.) 320(7229): 231–234. https://doi.org/10.1136/bmj.320.7229.231.

Househam, A. M., Peterson, C. T., Mills, P. J. and Chopra, D. 2017. The effects of stress and meditation on the immune system, human microbiota, and epigenetics. Advances in Mind-Body Medicine 31(4): 10–25.

Jiang, T., Hou, J., Sun, R., Dai, L., Wang, W., Wu, H. et al. 2021. Immunological and psychological efficacy of meditation/yoga intervention among people living with HIV (PLWH): A systematic review and meta-analyses of 19 randomized controlled trials. Annals of Behavioral Medicine: A Publication of the Society of Behavioral Medicine 55(6): 505–519. https://doi.org/10.1093/abm/kaaa084.

Johansson, S. G. O., Bieber, T., Dahl, R., Friedmann, P. S., Lanier, B. Q., Lockey, R. F. and Williams, H. C. 2004. Revised nomenclature for allergy for global use: Report of the Nomenclature Review Committee of the World Allergy Organization, October 2003. Journal of Allergy and Clinical Immunology 113(5): 832–836.

Khanna, P., Singh, K., Singla, S. and Verma, V. 2013. Relationship between Triguna theory and well-being indicators. International Journal of Yoga-Philosophy, Psychology and Parapsychology, 1(2): 69.

Kim, J., Yoon, D. W., Myoung, S., Lee, S. K. and Shin, C. 2022. Coexistence of moderate-to-severe obstructive sleep apnea and inflammation accelerates the risk of progression of arterial stiffness: a prospective 6-year study. Life 12(11): 1823.

Koinis-Mitchell, D., Craig, T., Esteban, C. A. and Klein, R. B. 2012. Sleep and allergic disease: a summary of the literature and future directions for research. The Journal of Allergy and Clinical Immunology 130(6): 1275–1281. https://doi.org/10.1016/j.jaci.2012.06.026.

Kuder, M. M., Clark, M., Cooley, C., Prieto-Centurion, V., Danley, A., Riley, I. et al. 2021. A systematic review of the effect of physical activity on asthma outcomes. The Journal of Allergy and Clinical Immunology. In Practice 9(9): 3407–3421.e8. https://doi.org/10.1016/j.jaip.2021.04.048.

Kumar, S., Debnath, P., Banerjee, S., Raj, A. and GR, R. P. 2014. Clinical investigations on the ayurvedic management of Allergic Rhinitis (Vatajapratishyaya) by Pratimarshanasyaas nasal drug delivery system. Explore Anim. Med. Res.) Exploratory Animal and Medical Research 4(2): 194–205.

Lack, S., Brown, R. and Kinser, P. A. 2020. An integrative review of yoga and mindfulness-based approaches for children and adolescents with asthma. Journal of Pediatric Nursing 52: 76–81. https://doi.org/10.1016/j.pedn.2020.03.006.

Liezmann, C., Klapp, B. and Peters, E. 2011. Stress, atopy and allergy: a re-evaluation from a psychoneuro-immunologic perspective. Dermato-endocrinology 3(1): 37–40.

Liezmann, C., Stock, D. and Peters, E. M. 2012. Stress-induced neuro-endocrine-immune plasticity: A role for the spleen in peripheral inflammatory disease and inflammation? Dermato-endocrinology 4(3): 271–279. https://doi.org/10.4161/derm.22023.

López-Varela, S., González-Gross, M. and Marcos, A. 2002. Functional foods and the immune system: a review. European Journal of Clinical Nutrition 56 Suppl 3: S29–S33. https://doi.org/10.1038/sj.ejcn.1601481.

Maeda, K., Caldez, M. J. and Akira, S. 2019. Innate immunity in allergy. Allergy 74(9): 1660–1674. https://doi.org/10.1111/all.13788.

Malhotra, V., Javed, D., Wakode, S., Bharshankar, R., Soni, N. and Porter, P. K. 2022. Study of immediate neurological and autonomic changes during kapalbhati pranayama in yoga practitioners. Journal of Family Medicine and Primary Care 11(2): 720.

Masatada Wachi, Masahiro Koyama, Masanori Utsuyama, Barry B. Bittman, Masanobu Kitagawa, Katsuiku Hirokawa Med. Sci. Monit, 2007; 13(2): CR57-70.

Meera, S., Vandana Rani, M., Sreedhar, C. and Robin, D. T. 2020. A review on the therapeutic effects of NetiKriya with special reference to JalaNeti. Journal of Ayurveda and Integrative Medicine 11(2): 185–189. https://doi.org/10.1016/j.jaim.2018.06.006.

Meera, S., Rani, M. V., Sreedhar, C. and Robin, D. T. 2020. A review on the therapeutic effects of Neti Kriya with special reference to Jala Neti. Journal of Ayurveda and Integrative Medicine 11(2): 185–189.

Misery, L., Chesnais, M., Merhand, S., Aubert, R., Bru, M. F., Legrand, C. et al. 2022. Perceived stress in four inflammatory skin diseases: an analysis of data taken from 7273 adult subjects with acne, atopic dermatitis, psoriasis or hidradenitis suppurativa. Journal of the European Academy of Dermatology and Venereology: JEADV, 10.1111/jdv.18016. Advance online publication. https://doi.org/10.1111/jdv.18016.

Moldofsky, H. 1995. Sleep and the immune system. International Journal of Immunopharmacology 17(8): 649–654.

Mooventhan, A. and Khode, V. 2014. Effect of Bhramari pranayama and OM chanting on pulmonary function in healthy individuals: A prospective randomized control trial. International Journal of Yoga 7(2): 104.

Mukherjee, P. K., Harwansh, R. K., Bahadur, S., Banerjee, S., Kar, A., Chanda, J. and Katiyar, C. K. 2017. Development of Ayurveda–tradition to trend. Journal of Ethnopharmacology 197: 10–24.

Myles, I. A. 2014. Fast food fever: reviewing the impacts of the Western diet on immunity. Nutrition Journal 13: 61. https://doi.org/10.1186/1475-2891-13-61.

Nagendra, H. R. and Nagarathna, R. 1986. An integrated approach of yoga therapy for bronchial asthma: A 3–54-month prospective study. Journal of Asthma 23(3): 123–37.

Nahhas, M., Bhopal, R., Anandan, C., Elton, R. and Sheikh, A. 2012. Prevalence of allergic disorders among primary school-aged children in Madinah, Saudi Arabia: two-stage cross-sectional survey. PloS One 7(5): e36848. https://doi.org/10.1371/journal.pone.0036848.

Nieman, D. C. and Wentz, L. M. 2019. The compelling link between physical activity and the body's defense system. Journal of Sport and Health Science 8(3): 201–217. https://doi.org/10.1016/j.jshs.2018.09.009.

Ozturk, L., Pelin, Z., Karadeniz, D., Kaynak, H., Cakar, L. and Gözükirmizi, E. 1999. Effects of 48 hours sleep deprivation on human immune profile. Sleep Research online: SRO 2(4): 107–111.

Papp, M. E., Wändell, P. E., Lindfors, P. and Nygren-Bonnier, M. 2017. Effects of yogic exercises on functional capacity, lung function and quality of life in participants with obstructive pulmonary disease: a randomized controlled study. European Journal of Physical and Rehabilitation Medicine 53(3): 447–461. https://doi.org/10.23736/S1973-9087.16.04374-4.

Padma, T. V. 2005. Ayurveda. Nature 436(7050): 486–486.

Patel, M., Desai, V. and Patel, V. 2013. Asthma therapy in Ayurveda: An ancient scientific approach. Pharmagene 1(1): 57–64.

Prinster, T. 2014. Yoga for Cancer: A Guide to Managing Side Effects, Boosting Immunity, and Improving Recovery for Cancer Survivors. Simon and Schuster.

Prossegger, J., Huber, D., Grafetstätter, C., Pichler, C., Braunschmid, H., Weisböck-Erdheim, R. et al. 2019. Winter exercise reduces allergic airway inflammation: a randomized controlled study. International Journal of Environmental Research and Public Health 16(11): 2040. https://doi.org/10.3390/ijerph16112040.

Rajak, C., Verma, R., Singh, P., Singh, A. and Shiralkar, M. 2016. Effect of Yoga on sérum adrenaline, serum cortisol levels and cardiovascular parameters in hyper-reactors to cold pressor test in young healthy volunteers. European Journal of Pharmaceutical and Medical Research 3(8): 496–502.

Rao, R. M., Nagendra, H. R., Raghuram, N., Vinay, C., Chandrashekara, S., Gopinath, K. S. et al. 2008. Influence of Yoga on mood states, distress, quality of life and immune outcomes in early stage breast cancer patients undergoing surgery. International Journal of Yoga 1(1): 11–20. https://doi.org/10.4103/0973-6131.36789.

Rao, R. M., Telles, S., Nagendra, H. R., Nagarathna, R., Gopinath, K., Srinath, S. and Chandrashekara, C. 2007. Effects of yoga on natural killer cell counts in early breast cancer patients undergoing conventional treatment. Comment to: recreational music-making modulates natural killer cell activity, cytokines, and mood states in corporate employees Masatada Wachi, Masahiro Koyama, Masanori Utsuyama, Barry B. Bittman, Masanobu Kitagawa, Katsuiku Hirokawa Med Sci Monit 13(2): CR57–70.

Ray, U. S., Mukhopadhyaya, S., Purkayastha, S. S., Asnani, V., Tomer, O. S., Prashad, R. et al. 2001. Effect of yogic exercises on physical and mental health of young fellowship course trainees. Indian Journal of Physiology and Pharmacology 45(1): 37–53.

Rico-Rosillo, M. G. and Vega-Robledo, G. B. 2018. Sueño y sistema immune [Sleep and immune system]. RevistaalergiaMexico (Tecamachalco, Puebla, Mexico: 1993) 65(2): 160–170. https://doi.org/10.29262/ram.v65i2.359.

Rohleder, N. and Kirschbaum, C. 2006, Mar. The hypothalamic–pituitary–adrenal (HPA) axis in habitual smokers. International Journal of Psychophysiology 59(3): 236–43.

Rosen, S. J. 2011. Food for the Soul: Vegetarianism and Yoga Traditions: Vegetarianism and Yoga Traditions. ABC-CLIO.

Rutkowski, K., Sowa, P., Rutkowska-Talipska, J., Sulkowski, S. and Rutkowski, R. 2014. Allergic diseases: the price of civilisational progress. Postepydermatologiiialergologii 31(2): 77–83. https://doi.org/10.5114/pdia.2014.40936.

Sarubin, N., Nothdurfter, C., Schüle, C., Lieb, M., Uhr, M., Born, C. et al. 2014. The influence of Hatha Yoga as an add-on treatment in major depression on hypothalamic-pituitary-adrenal-axis activity: a randomized trial. Journal of Psychiatric Research 53: 76–83. https://doi.org/10.1016/j.jpsychires.2014.02.022.

Sakiya, S. and Panda, S. K. 2011. Effect of Nadi Shodhan Pranayama on forced vital capacity*. Journal of Advances in Scholarly Researches and Allied Education 1: 309.

Satyananda, S. 2014. Shatkarma, Asana, Pranayama, Mudra, Bandha (4th Edition). Yoga Publications Trust, Bihar, p. 490.

Sharma, R. K. and Bhagwan Dash, V. Agniveśa's Caraka Saṃhitā (Text with English Translation and Critical Exposition Based on Cakrapāṇi Datta's Āyurveda Dīpikā) Chowkhamba Sanskrit Series Office, 1976–2002. Another good English translation of the whole text, with paraphrases of the commentary of Chakrapani Datta.

Shaw, A. and Kaytaz, E. S. 2021. Yoga bodies, yoga minds: contextualizing the health discourses and practices of modern postural Yoga. Anthropology and Medicine 28(3): 279–296.

Sicherer, S. H. and Burks, A. W. 2008. Maternal and infant diets for prevention of allergic diseases: understanding menu changes in 2008. Journal of Allergy and Clinical Immunology 122(1): 29–33.

Sinclair, K. L. 2020. Examining Psychological Symptoms as Moderators of the Effect of a Yoga Intervention on Sleep and Fatigue for Women With Breast Cancer Undergoing Chemotherapy (Doctoral dissertation, Sam Houston State University).

Singh, B. B., Khorsan, R., Vinjamury, S. P., Der-Martirosian, C., Kizhakkeveettil, A. and Anderson, T. M. 2007. Herbal treatments of asthma: a systematic review. Journal of Asthma 44(9): 685–698.

Stancak Jr, A., Kuna, M., Dostalek, C. and Vishnudevananda, S. 1991. Kapalabhati—yogic cleansing exercise. II. EEG topography analysis. Homeostasis in Health and Disease: International Journal Devoted to Integrative Brain Functions and Homeostatic Systems 33(4): 182–189.

Stevens, L. J., Kuczek, T., Burgess, J. R., Stochelski, M. A., Arnold, L. E. and Galland, L. 2013. Mechanisms of behavioral, atopic, and other reactions to artificial food colors in children. Nutrition Reviews 71(5): 268–281.

Swami, G., Singh, S., Singh, K. P. and Gupta, M. 2010. Effect of Yoga on pulmonary function tests of hypothyroid patients. Indian Journal of Physiology and Pharmacology 54(1): 51–56.

Vaid, M. and Verma, S. 2021. Kapalabhati: A physiological healer in human physiological system. Yoga Mimamsa 53(1): 69.

Valdez, C., Alvarez-Molina, K., Castro, L. A. and Tentori, M. 2023. Zens: Designing and evaluating a movement sonification interface to alter body and flexibility perception in Yoga. International Journal of Human-Computer Studies 7: 103084.

Vempati, R. P. and Telles, S. 2002. Yoga-based guided relaxation reduces sympathetic activity judged from baseline levels. Psychological Reports 90(2): 487–494. https://doi.org/10.2466/pr0.2002.90.2.487.

Venkatesh, H. N., Ravish, H., Wilma Delphine Silvia, C. R. and Srinivas, H. 2020. Molecular signature of the immune response to yoga therapy in stress-related chronic disease conditions: an insight. International Journal of Yoga 13(1): 9–17. https://doi.org/10.4103/ijoy.IJOY_82_18.

Visweswaraiah, N. K. and Telles, S. 2004. Randomized trial of Yoga as a complementary therapy for pulmonary tuberculosis. Respirology (Carlton, Vic.) 9(1): 96–101. https://doi.org/10.1111/j.1440-1843.2003.00528.x.

Von Ehrenstein, O. S., Aralis, H., Flores, M. E. and Ritz, B. 2015. Fast food consumption in pregnancy and subsequent asthma symptoms in young children. Pediatric Allergy and Immunology: Official Publication of the European Society of Pediatric Allergy and Immunology 26(6): 571–577. https://doi.org/10.1111/pai.12433.

White, D. G. 2019. Sinister Yogis. University of Chicago Press, 2019 Dec 31.

Woon, F. C., Chan, Y. S., Ismail, I. H., Chan, Y. M., Batterham, M., Latiff, A. H. A. et al. 2018. Contribution of early nutrition on the development of malnutrition and allergic diseases in the first year of life: a study protocol for the Mother and Infant Cohort Study (MICOS). BMC Pediatrics 18(1): 1–9.

Wu, D. and Yang, T. 2022. Late bedtime, uncertainty stress among Chinese college students: impact on academic performance and self-rated health. Psychology, Health and Medicine 1–12. Advance online publication. https://doi.org/10.1080/13548506.2022.2067337.

Yang, Z. Y., Zhong, H. B., Mao, C., Yuan, J. Q., Huang, Y. F., Wu, X. Y. et al. 2016. Yoga for asthma. The Cochrane Database of Systematic Reviews 4(4): CD010346. https://doi.org/10.1002/14651858.CD010346.pub2.

Ye, X., Chen, Z., Shen, Z., Chen, G. and Xu, X. 2020. Yoga for treating rheumatoid arthritis: a systematic review and meta-analysis. Frontiers in Medicine 7: 586665. https://doi.org/10.3389/fmed.2020.586665.

Zhang, Y. and Zhang, L. 2019. Increasing prevalence of allergic rhinitis in China. Allergy, Asthma and Immunology Research 11(2): 156–169. https://doi.org/10.4168/aair.2019.11.2.156.

Chapter 13B

Role of Acupuncture in Allergic Disorders

Parin Niranjan Parmar[1,]* and *Pudupakkam K. Vedanthan*[2]

Introduction

Acupuncture is one of the most important treatment methods in Traditional Chinese Medicine (TCM) - a system of healing that was developed in China. Similarly, in some of the Eastern countries, a vast number of herbs have been used tradtionally for treatment of allergic disorders for centuries. This chapter aims to discuss the role of acupuncture and herbal medicine in alllergy and various allergic disorders.

Basics of Acupuncture

Acupuncture plays an important role in healthcare in China Korea, Japan, Taiwan and Hong Kong. For the purpose of understanding acupuncture, it is important to know that Qi (pronounced as "chi") refers to the energy or vital force that keeps a living being alive. Meridians are the channels or pathways through which Qi flows, and acupuncture points are the points from where it is possible to influence the flow of Qi as well as the functioning of organs and tissues connected with the meridians. Until late in the second half of the twentieth century, meridians and acupuncture points were considered abstract and "non-existent" in the human body but recently several attempts have been made to identify and define them anatomically and physiologically (Maurer et al. 2019; Li et al. 2012). A recent systematic review has supported the existence of meridians and acupuncture points based on their electric, thermal, acoustic, optical, magnetic, isotopic and myoelectric characteristics (Li et al. 2012).

As per TCM, stimulation of acupuncture points can regulate the flow of Qi in the meridians and therefore it is possible to influence the functioning of internal organs by regulating the flow of Qi within the meridians connected with the corresponding organs. In addition to acupuncture, the points can also be stimulated by pressure, heat, cold, laser or other stimuli. Important steps of an acupuncture treatment are TCM diagnosis (i.e., diagnosis of imbalance within the person's body based on TCM principles), selection of acupuncture points based on TCM diagnosis, needling (insertion of acupuncture needles at the points) (Figure 1) and stimulation of the acupuncture points (manually or electrically). In a typical acupuncture session, the selected acupuncture points are

---

[1] Pediatric Allergy Consultant and Integrative Medicine Consultant, Rajkot, Gujarat, India.
[2] The University of Colorado at Anschutz Campus, Aurora, Colorado. USA.
* Corresponding author: parinmnparmar@gmail.com

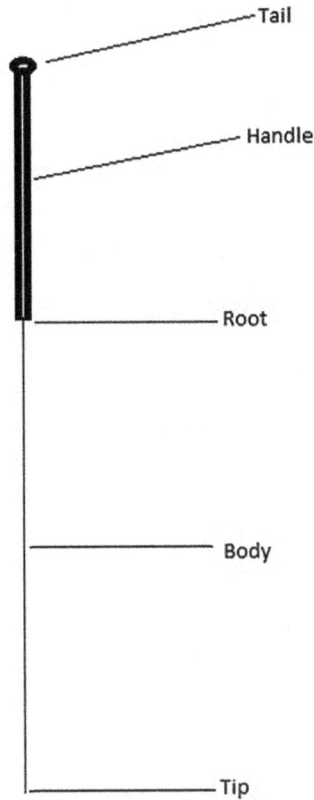

Figure 1. An acupuncture needle.

stimulated for 20 to 30 minutes. The frequency of the sessions usually ranges from once daily to twice weekly, and the duration of acupuncture treatment can range from a few weeks to a few months.

Based on various animal and human studies to date, beneficial effects of acupuncture in allergic disorders occur from a combination of multiple mechanisms such as complex neuro-endocrine-immunological interactions, anti-inflammatory effects mediated via hypothalamus-pituitary-adrenal axis and autonomic nervous system, altered cytokine responses, alterations in local blood flow, centrally mediated antipruritic effect and reduction in perceived and physiologic stress (McDonald et al. 2013; Yu et al. 2015).

Acupuncture in Allergic Disorders: Evidence

Allergic Rhinitis

Based on the evidence to date, acupuncture has shown beneficial effects significantly better in patients with allergic rhinitis as compared to other allergic disorders. Some of the clinical practice guidelines (Seidman et al. 2015; Cheng et al. 2018) also support the use of acupuncture as an important non-pharmacological intervention in the treatment of allergic rhinitis. A recent systematic review (Yin et al. 2020) and meta-analysis included 39 randomized controlled trials with 3,433 participants and showed that acupuncture was superior to sham acupuncture in improving total nasal symptoms score and quality of life in patients with allergic rhinitis. A recently published overview of systematic reviews and network meta-analysis (Zhang et al. 2020) compared the efficacy of different acupuncture therapies alone with that of conventional medicines and showed that manual acupuncture at the sphenopalatine ganglion point and San-Fu-Tie (a method of the herbal application over specific points on specific days during the year as per TCM) were more effective than conventional medicines for improving allergic rhinitis symptoms at 3, 6 and 12 months follow-up.

In addition to conventional acupuncture based on TCM diagnosis, acupuncture at the "sphenopalatine ganglion acupuncture point" requires special mention. The point is located between the zygomatic arch and coronoid of the mandible near the ST7 point and the needle is inserted through the point to reach the pterygopalatine fossa; both manual acupuncture and electroacupuncture have been used and both unilateral and bilateral sphenopalatine ganglion acupuncture have shown effectiveness. Possible mechanisms of this technique include stimulation of sympathetic nerve fibers in the local region causing vasoconstriction, reduced blood flow to the nasal mucosa and cavernous body, reduced glandular secretion and increased nasal ventilation (Zhang et al. 2020; Fu et al. 2019). A systematic review and meta-analysis involving ten studies and 943 participants concluded that acupuncture at only sphenopalatine ganglion acupuncture point is effective in relieving symptoms and improving quality of life in patients with allergic rhinitis as compared to acupuncture at other conventional points, sham acupuncture and Western medicine (Fu et al. 2019). However, the researchers felt the need for more studies because of the high heterogeneity of the studies included in the meta-analyses. No serious adverse effect has been reported to date, except for local hematoma and minor bleeding at the puncture points. This technique can be a good option for clinicians who are untrained in making TCM diagnoses and in acupuncture point selection.

Bronchial Asthma

There are many randomized controlled trials pointing to improved symptoms of asthma in children, adolescents as well as adults, the improvement reaching statistical significance. A recently published systematic review and meta-analysis included nine randomized controlled trials that compared acupuncture plus conventional treatment with conventional treatment alone in adolescents and adults with asthma (Jiang et al. 2019). Analysis of the pooled data from the nine trials showed statistically significant improvement in symptoms response rate and a statistically significant reduction in interleukin-6 levels in patients receiving combined acupuncture and conventional treatment than in patients receiving conventional treatment alone; however, the analysis did not suggest improvement in FEV_1 and FEV_1/FVC by addition of acupuncture in conventional treatment. In a systematic review including seven randomized controlled trials evaluating the efficacy of acupuncture in asthmatic children, beneficial effects on symptoms and lung function were reported by isolated trials, but no conclusion could be made because of methodologic variability in the trials (Liu and Chien 2015).

Chronic Urticaria

Although several studies have shown global symptom improvement with the use of acupuncture in patients with chronic urticaria, the overall quality of evidence for the effectiveness of acupuncture for chronic urticaria is low. Two recent systematic reviews concluded that a combination of acupuncture and antihistamines might be superior to antihistamines alone in the treatment of chronic urticaria, but the risk of bias was high in all the randomized controlled trials included in the study (Yao et al. 2016; Yan et al. 2015).

SP10, ST36, LI11 and SP6 were the most common acupuncture points stimulated in most of these trials. LI4, BL20, BL18 and GV11 were other common acupuncture points selected by the researchers for stimulation. A recently published systematic review and meta-analysis of seven randomized controlled trials evaluated auriculotherapy (auricular acupuncture, which uses only specific points on the auricle for stimulation) as a single intervention or in combination with other TCM interventions in the treatment of chronic spontaneous urticaria (Zhu et al. 2018). The results of the meta-analysis showed improved clinical features and safety of auriculotherapy, important limitations of the meta-analysis were small sample sizes and methodological flaws in the included studies.

Atopic Dermatitis

Acupuncture is widely used in itchy dermatological conditions including atopic dermatitis. Several case reports and small-sized studies suggest the beneficial effects of acupuncture in atopic dermatitis, but the number of quality randomized controlled trials is very low (Tan et al. 2015; Shi et al. 2017). In many of the studies, LI11 has been selected as an important "antipruritic acupuncture point" for stimulation, in addition to other acupuncture points (Akpinar et al. 2018). The anti-pruritic effect of acupuncture is known to occur due to a combination of both the peripheral and central mechanisms (Akpinar et al. 2018).

Food Allergies

Scientific literature evaluating the effects of acupuncture in patients with food allergies is very limited at present.

Adverse Effects of Acupuncture

One of the reasons why acupuncture is gaining popularity in patients with allergic disorders is its safety and lack of serious adverse effects or long-term complications. Results of a systematic review suggested that in patients with allergic rhinitis, acupuncture caused infrequent or negligible adverse effects as compared to adverse effects caused by drugs (Lee et al. 2009). Common adverse effects of acupuncture include pain at the site of needle insertion, minor local bleeding and local hematoma. Minor bleeding can be easily controlled by applying pressure over the bleeding point and hematoma usually subsides within one to three days. Because of the use of sterile, disposable acupuncture needles, infection is a rarity. Syncope is a known adverse effect and usually occurs immediately or several minutes after the first acupuncture treatment, especially when patients are in a sitting or semi-recumbent posture (Xu et al. 2013). Depending upon the location of the needling, injury to a local blood vessel, nerve or internal organ can occur; cases of pneumothorax and injury to structures of the peripheral and central nervous system as well as internal organs have been reported (Xu et al. 2013). However, avoidance of dangerous areas such as points in and around the orbit, side and back of the neck, intercostal spaces and points on prominent blood vessels could prevent such complications. Also, acupuncture is avoided on the nipple and breast, external genitalia, umbilicus and scalp (if the fontanelle is not closed) (Lohiya and Lohiya 2014).

In addition to acupuncture, other TCM treatments, such as moxibustion, cupping therapy, herbal application over acupuncture points, etc., are also used traditionally in the treatment of allergic disorders; however, their description is beyond the scope of this chapter. Important herbs and herbal formulations used in TCM for the treatment of allergic disorders are described under the heading of herbal medicine.

Explanation of the selection of acupuncture points for any disorder requires knowledge of the basics of TCM and is beyond the scope of this chapter. Acupuncture points that are commonly used in the treatment of allergic disorders are described in Table 1 (Figure 2).

Table 1. Commonly-used acupuncture points in the treatment of allergic disorders.

Acupuncture Point (Name in TCM Literature)	Location	Remarks (Relevant to Allergic Disorders Only, As Per TCM Literature)
BL13 (Feishu)	1.5 cun[a] lateral to the lower border of the spinous process of the third thoracic vertebra	Used for treatment of disorders related to the respiratory tract and skin
BL17 (Geshu)	1.5 cun lateral to the lower border of the spinous process of the seventh thoracic vertebra	Used in the treatment of cough and dyspnea Used in the treatment of urticaria
BL18 (Ganshu)	1.5 cun lateral to the lower border of the spinous process of the ninth thoracic vertebra	Used in the treatment of liver disorders and eye disorders Used in the treatment of muscle and tendon disorders
BL20 (Pishu)	1.5 cun lateral to the lower border of the spinous process of the eleventh thoracic vertebra	Used in the treatment of digestive disorders and allergic disorders
BL12 (Fengmen)	1.5 cun lateral to the lower border of the spinous process of the second thoracic vertebra	Used in the treatment of disorders related to the respiratory tract
ST36 (Zusanli)	3 cun below the kneecap and one finger breadth lateral to the lower end of the tibial tuberosity	An important point for improving immunity Used in several digestive disorders
SP6 (Sanyinjiao)	3 cun above the tip of the medial malleolus, posterior to the border of the tibia	Meeting point of three important meridians Used in the treatment of allergy Used in the treatment of digestive disorders
SP10 (Xuehai)	2 cun above the medial end of the upper border of the patella	Used in the treatment of urticaria, atopic dermatitis, allergic rhinitis and bronchial asthma
LI4 (Hegu)	In the web between the index finger and thumb on the dorsal aspect of the hand, at top of the first interosseous muscle when the thumb is adducted	Used in the treatment of allergic rhinitis and bronchial asthma
LI11 (Quchi)	At the outer end of the elbow crease when the elbow is semi-flexed	Used in the treatment urticaria and atopic dermatitis Used in the treatment of allergic rhinitis and bronchial asthma Used for improving immunity
LI20 (Yingxiang)	On the nasolabial grove, in the horizontal line drawn from the outermost point of the ala nasi	Used in the treatment of nasal congestion, allergic rhinitis and sinusitis
LU1 (Zhongfu)	In the infraclavicular fossa, 1.5 cun below the midpoint of the clavicle	Used in the treatment of cough, wheezing, bronchitis, bronchial asthma and other disorders of the lung Dangerous point for acupuncture; pneumothorax can be caused by deep insertion of the needle
DU11 (GV11, Shendao)	On the back, the midline between the dorsal spines of the fifth and sixth thoracic vertebrae	Used in the treatment of cough, shortness of breath, and shallow breathing
DU14 (GV14, Dazhui)	On the back, the midline between the dorsal spines of the seventh cervical and first thoracic vertebrae	Meeting point of several important meridians An important point for enhancing immunity Used in the treatment of frequent colds, coughs, bronchitis, and bronchial asthma Used in the treatment of atopic dermatitis and other skin disorders
RN4 (CV4, Guanyuan)	3 cun below the umbilicus in the midline	Used in the treatment of dry cough Used in the treatment of diarrhea and indigestion

Table 1 contd. ...

...Table 1 contd.

Acupuncture Point (Name in TCM Literature)	Location	Remarks (Relevant to Allergic Disorders Only, As Per TCM Literature)
RN8 (CV8, Shenjue)	In the center of the umbilicus	Used in the treatment of diarrhea, abdominal cramps, and borborygmi This point is not used for acupuncture but moxibustion and dry cupping can be done
Ex1 (Yintang)	Midway between the medial ends of the two eyebrows, on the ridge of the nose	Used in the treatment of allergic rhinitis and sinusitis
Ex17 (Dingchuan)	0.5 cun lateral to DU14 point	Used in the treatment of bronchial asthma
Bitong (Shangyingxiang)	Upper end of nasolabial groove, 0.5 cun superior and lateral to LI20 point	Used in the treatment of nasal congestion and allergic rhinitis

(aCun – a traditional Chinese unit of length; 1 cun = width of the patient's thumb at the interphalangeal joint).

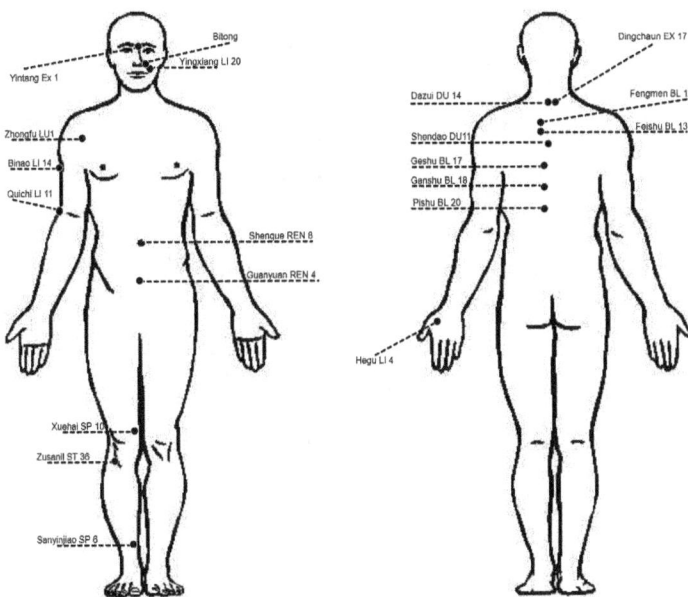

Figure 2. Commonly used acupuncture points in treatment of allergic disorders (see Table 1 for description).

Conclusion

In the treatment of allergic disorders, acupuncture offers a novel mode of treatment with mechanisms that are not addressed by conventional treatments. From the perspective of scientific research, it is desirable that studies evaluating the efficacy of acupuncture in allergic disorders are conducted by researchers who are trained in both modern medicine as well as in the basics of TCM. In experienced hands, acupuncture is safe.

Role of Herbal Medicine in Allergic Disorders

Over the last three decades, use of herbal medicine has progressively increased in Western countries as well. Out of many innumerable herbs traditionally used in the treatment of one or more allergic disorders in different countries, a relatively small number of herbs have undergone scientific evaluation and only a handful of them have shown conclusive evidence to support their use in patients with allergies. Hence, only some common and important herbs and herbal formulations are mentioned in Table 2.

Table 2. Commonly-used herbs and herbal formulations in allergic disorders.

Herb/Herbal Formulation	Mechanism of Action (Relevant to Allergic Disorders)	Remarks	References
Angelica sinensis (Angelica)	Possible immunomodulatory and anti-inflammatory actions	A common Chinese herb used in the treatment of asthma	Shergis et al. 2016; Amaral-Machado et al. 2020
Astragalus membranaceus (Astragali)	Modulation of Th1 and Th2 cytokines	A common Chinese herb used in the treatment of asthma	Shergis et al. 2016; Amaral-Machado et al. 2020
Berberine An alkaloid derived from herbs of the Berberis genus	Inhibition of IgE production by suppression of IgE isotype switching. Direct suppression of histamine release from mast cells	Used in the treatment of food allergy	Wang et al. 2021
Curcuma longa (Turmeric)	Contains the active compound curcumin, which has anti-inflammatory effects. Decreases Th2 cytokines and enhances Th1 cytokines	An add-on to conventional treatment in adults with asthma - improves lung function. Has shown beneficial effects in a murine model of food allergy	Amaral-Machado et al. 2020; Kohn and Paudyal 2017; Shin et al. 2015
Dianthus Superbus	Reduction of peanut-specific IgE level	Decreases anaphylaxis symptom scores in a murine model of peanut-induced anaphylaxis	Wang and Li 2012
Ginkgo biloba	Anti-inflammatory effects, inhibition of Th2 cytokines, inhibition of platelet-activating factor	Improves lung function in asthma patients. Increased risk of bleeding in patients taking anti-coagulant and anti-platelet drugs	Shergis et al. 2016 ; Chu et al. 2011
Glycyrrhiza uralensis (Licorice root)	Contains active compounds glycyrrhizinic acid (anti-inflammatory) and liquiritin apioside (anti-tussive). Inhibition of IgE production	A Chinese herb used in the treatment of asthma	Shergis et al. 2016, Amaral-Machado et al. 2020
Nigella sativa (black onion seed)	Anti-inflammatory, immunomodulatory, and antioxidant actions	Endonasal application of oil reduces symptoms of allergic rhinitis. Reduces IgE and eosinophil count in nasal discharge. Ingestion of oil in high dose can cause hepatic or renal toxicity	Kozlov et al. 2018

Table 2 contd. ...

...Table 2 contd.

Herb/Herbal Formulation	Mechanism of Action (Relevant to Allergic Disorders)	Remarks	References
Perilla frutescens	Contains luteolin that inhibits mucus overproduction	Extract enriched for rosmarinic acid has shown to improve nasal symptoms and quality of life as well as to decrease neutrophils and eosinophils in nasal lavage fluid in patients with allergic rhinitis	Guo et al. 2007 ; Kozlov et al. 2018
Petasites hybridus (Butterbur)	Inhibition of leukotriene synthesis	An effective and one of the most promising herbs for the treatment of seasonal and perennial allergic rhinitis Has been shown to decrease nasal resistance and reduce inflammatory mediator levels in nasal secretions	Guo et al. 2007; Kozlov et al. 2018 ; Hoang et al. 2021
Piper longum (long pepper) and Piper nigrum (black pepper)	Both contain the active compound piperine (inhibits eosinophil infiltration and reduces airway hyperresponsiveness) Piper longum also contains piperlongumine (inhibits the activity of multiple inflammatory mediators)	Used in the treatment of allergic rhinitis and asthma	Amaral-Machado et al. 2020; Guo et al. 2007
Radix Scutellariae	Contains the active compound wogonin Inhibits production of interleukin 5 and downregulation of expression of mediators of allergic inflammation	A traditional Chinese herb used in the treatment of atopic dermatitis	Wang et al. 2021
Rubia cordifolia	Reduction in peanut-specific IgE levels	Has been shown to decrease anaphylaxis symptom scores in the murine model of peanut-induced anaphylaxis	Wang and Li 2012, Wang et al. 2021
Sophora flavescens	Suppression of Th2 cells	A Chinese herb used in the treatment of asthma	Kohn and Paudyal 2016
Solanum xanthocarpum and Solanum trilobatum	Possible bronchodilator effects	Used in the treatment of asthma in the Siddha system of medicine	Kohn and Paudyal 2016; Amaral-Machado et al. 2020
Tinospora cordifolia	Anti-histamine and immunomodulatory effects	Extract from the herb has shown to improve symptoms of allergic rhinitis and to decrease eosinophils, neutrophils, and goblet cells in nasal smear	Guo et al. 2007; Kozlov et al. 2018
Tylophora indica	Anti-inflammatory, anti-histamine, antioxidant, and anxiolytic effects	A commonly used herb in India for the treatment of asthma	Rani et al. 2012

Zingiber officinale	Suppression of Th2-mediated immune responses	Used in the treatment of allergic rhinitis and asthma	Kohn and Paudyal 2016; Kawamoto et al. 2016
ASHMI (antiasthma simplified herbal medicine intervention)	Inhibition of the production of eotaxin and Th2 cytokines, inhibition of airway smooth muscle contraction, increased brain-derived neurotropic factor secretion	A TCM formula containing three herbs Has shown to improve lung function in adults with moderate-to-severe persistent asthma	Kohn and Paudyal 2016
FAHF-2 (Food Allergy Herbal Formula-2)	Inhibition of IgE production by human B cells Suppression of interleukin 5 and increased interferon γ Blockade of vascular leakage associated with anaphylaxis	A TCM formula containing nine herbs First USFDA botanical investigational new drug for food allergy Has shown safety and efficacy in murine models of peanut allergy and multiple food allergies Has shown safety in phase I and II clinical trials Butanol-purified (B-FAHF-2) and enhanced B-FAHF-2 have also shown efficacy in murine models	Wang et al 2021
Kakkonto	Modulation of Th1 cells, enhanced inhibition of Th2 cells, and enhancement of Treg cells	A traditional Japanese medicine (Kampo) formula containing seven herbs Used in the treatment of food allergy Has shown to suppress allergic diarrhea, decrease mast cells in the intestinal mucosa and have favorable immunological effects in the murine model	Wang and Li 2012, Wang et al. 2021
Pei Tu Qing Xin Tang	Anti-histamine and anti-inflammatory actions Possible reduction of IgE production	A TCM formula containing nine herbs Has shown efficacy superior to topical corticosteroids in the treatment of moderate-to-severe atopic dermatitis	Wang et al. 2021
Saiboku-to	Anti-histamine, anti-inflammatory and anxiolytic effects	A traditional Japanese medicine (Kampo) formula containing ten herbs Commonly used in the treatment of steroid-dependent asthma	Kohn and Paudyal 2016
Shi Zhen Tea	Inhibition of the production of IgE, eotaxin, and tumor necrosis factor α	A TCM formula containing 4 different herbs Used in the treatment of atopic dermatitis	Wang et al. 2021

Table 2 contd. ...

...Table 2 contd.

Herb/Herbal Formulation	Mechanism of Action (Relevant to Allergic Disorders)	Remarks	References
Sho-seiryu-to	Possible immunomodulation, inhibition of eosinophil infiltration, and reduction of IgE levels	A traditional Japanese medicine (Kampo) formula containing 8 different herbs Has shown to improve sneezing, running nose, and nasal congestion in allergic rhinitis	Guo et al. 2007
Yu ping feng san	Inhibits interleukin 1β, tumor necrosis factor α, and interferon γ	A TCM formulation containing three herbs Has shown beneficial therapeutic effects in adults with allergic rhinitis in more than 20 RCTs	Hoang et al. 2021

Evidence for Herbal Medicine in Allergic Disorders

A recent systematic review and meta-analysis conclude herbal medicine is safe and effective in improving symptoms and quality of life in adults as well as children with allergic rhinitis (Hoang et al. 2021; Zheng et al. 2018). However, it also suggests that the beneficial effects last only up to 12 weeks of the treatment and longer treatment is associated with tachyphylaxis. In patients with asthma, herbal medicine as an add-on therapy has been shown to improve lung function and asthma control and to reduce rescue medication use and acute asthma exacerbations in several recent studies (Shergis et al. 2016).

Similarly, a recent overview of multiple systematic reviews evaluating the effects of herbal medicine in atopic dermatitis concluded that herbal medicine might be effective for the treatment of atopic dermatitis, especially as an adjunctive therapy and that these therapeutic effects of herbal medicine were due to a combination of their anti-inflammatory and immunomodulatory effects (Kwon et al. 2020). Topical application of natural herbal oils such as olive oil, virgin coconut oil and mineral oil has also shown remarkable symptomatic improvement in patients with atopic dermatitis (Hussain et al. 2017). However, topical application of several other TCM herbal formulas has not been shown to be conclusively effective to date (Thandar et al. 2017; Gu et al. 2014).

Unlike non-pharmacological measures, such as yoga and acupuncture, herbal medicine has its own challenges. Based on available scientific literature to date, exact doses for all age groups and special populations are not clearly defined for many herbs. There is also a potential for drug interactions when herbal medicine is used in a patient taking conventional drugs. Some herbs can cause serious toxic effects, especially when consumed in large doses. In TCM, the selection of a specific formula is based on underlying TCM diagnosis and not on the conventional medical diagnosis and therefore an appropriate selection of TCM formulas for therapeutic purposes requires an understanding of the basic principles of TCM.

Conclusion

Herbal medicine is a wide subject, considering the fact that different herbs have been used in the treatment of allergic disorders in different traditional systems of medicine across the globe. Their safe integration into the conventional management of allergic disorders requires high-quality scientific research to know their mechanisms, efficacy, dose and safety before making evidence-based recommendations. At present, herbal medicine holds the potential to contribute to the relief of patients suffering from allergic disorders.

Acknowledgment

Sujatha Reddy LPC. MSEd, BAMS, DCC Owner and CEO of Humanly Lakewood. Professional Counselor and Ayurvedic Doctor.

Glossary of Abbreviations

ASHMI – Antiasthma Simplified Herbal Medicine Intervention
BL – Urinary Bladder Meridian
DU – Du Meridian (Governing Vessel)
Ex – Extra acupuncture point
FAHF-2 – Food Allergy Herbal Formula-2
FEV_1 – Forced Expiratory Volume in the first second
FVC – Forced Vital Capacity
IgE – Immunoglobulin E
LI – Large Intestine Meridian
LU – Lung Meridian

RN – Ren Meridian (Conception Vessel)
RCT – Randomized Controlled Trial
SP – Spleen Meridian
ST – Stomach Meridian
TCM – Traditional Chinese Medicine
Th1 – T Helper Cell Type 1
Th2 – T Helper Cell Type 2
Treg – Regulatory T Cell
USFDA – The United States Food and Drug Administration

References

Akpinar, R. and Karatay, S. 2018. Positive effects of acupuncture on atopic dermatitis. International Journal of Allergy Medications 4: 030.

Amaral-Machado, L., Oliveira, W. N., Moreira-Oliveira, S. S., Pereira, D. T., Alencar, E. N., Tsapis, N. et al. 2020. Use of natural products in asthma treatment. Evidence-Based Complementary and Alternative Medicine 2020: 1021258.

Cheng, L., Chen, J., Fu, Q., He, S., Li, H., Liu, Z. et al. 2018. Chinese society of allergy guidelines for diagnosis and treatment of allergic rhinitis. Allergy, Asthma & Immunology Research 10(4): 300–353.

Chu, X., Ci, X., He, J., Wei, M., Yang, X., Cao, Q. et al. 2011. A novel anti-inflammatory role for Ginkgolide B in asthma via inhibition of the ERK/MAPK signaling pathway. Molecules 16(9): 7634–7648.

Fu, Q., Zhang, L., Liu, Y., Li, X., Yang, Y., Dai, M. et al. 2019. Effectiveness of acupuncturing at the sphenopalatine ganglion acupoint alone for treatment of allergic rhinitis: a systematic review and meta-analysis. Evidence-Based Complementary and Alternative Medicine 2019: 6478102.

Gu, S., Yang, A. W., Li, C. G., Lu, C. and Xue, C. C. 2014. Topical application of Chinese herbal medicine for atopic eczema: a systematic review with a meta-analysis. Dermatology 228: 294–302.

Guo, R., Pittler, M. H. and Ernst, E. 2007. Herbal medicines for the treatment of allergic rhinitis: a systematic review. Annals of Allergy, Asthma & Immunology 99: 483–495.

Hoang, M. P., Chitsuthipakorn, W. and Snidvongs, K. 2021. Herbal medicines for allergic rhinitis: a systematic review and meta-analysis. Current Allergy and Asthma Reports 21: 25.

Hussain, Z., Thu, H. E., Shuid, A. N., Kesharwani, P., Khan, S. and Hussain, F. 2017. Phytotherapeutic potential of natural herbal medicines for the treatment of mild-to-severe atopic dermatitis: a review of human clinical studies. Biomedicine & Pharmacotherpy 93: 596–608.

Jiang, C., Jiang, L. and Qin, Q. 2019. Conventional treatments plus acupuncture for asthma in adults and adolescent: a systematic review and meta-analysis. Evidence-Based Complementary and Alternative Medicine 2019: 9580670.

Kawamoto, Y., Ueno, Y., Nakahashi, E., Obayashi, M., Sugihara, K., Qiao, S. et al. 2016. Prevention of allergic rhinitis by ginger and the molecular basis of immunosuppression by 6-gingerol through T cell inactivation. The Journal of Nutritional Biochemistry 27: 112–122.

Kohn, C. M. and Paudyal, P. 2017. A systematic review and meta-analysis of complementary and alternative medicine in asthma. European Respiratory Review 26: 160092.

Kozlov, V., Lavrenova, G., Savlevich, E. and Bazarkina, K. 2018. Evidence-based phytotherapy in allergic rhinitis. Clinical Phytoscience 4: 23.

Kwon, C.-Y., Lee, B., Kim, S., Lee, J., Park, M. and Kim, N. 2020. Effectiveness and safety of herbal medicine for atopic dermatitis: an overview of systematic reviews. Evidence-Based Complementary and Alternative Medicine 2020: 4140692.

Lee, M. S., Pittler, M. H., Shin, B.-C., Kim, J.-I. and Ernst, E. 2009. Acupuncture for allergic rhinitis: a systematic review. Annals of Allergy, Asthma, & Immunology 102: 269–279.

Li, J., Wang, Q., Liang, H., Dong, H., Li, Y., Ng, E. H. Y. et al. 2012. Biophysical characteristics of meridians and acupoints: A systematic review. Evidence-Based Complementary and Alternative Medicine 2012: 793841.

Liu, C. F. and Chien, L. W. 2015. Efficacy of acupuncture in children with asthma: a systematic review. Italian Journal of Pediatrics 41: 48.

Lohiya, P. B. and Lohiya, S. 2014. Acupuncture A Complete Textbook. Indian Academy of Acupuncture Science, Aurangabad.

Maurer, N., Nissel, H., Egerbacher, M., Gornik, E., Schuller, P. and Traxler, H. 2019. Anatomical evidence of acupuncture meridians in the human extracellular matrix: results from a macroscopic and microscopic interdisciplinary multicentre study on human corpses. Evidence-Based Complementary and Alternative Medicine 2019: 6976892.

McDonald, J. L., Cripps, A. W., Smith, P. K., Smith, C. A., Xue, C. C. and Golianu, B. 2013. The anti-inflammatory effects of acupuncture and their relevance to allergic rhinitis: a narrative review and proposed model. Evidence-Based Complementary and Alternative Medicine 2013: 591796.

Rani, A. S., Patnaik, S., Sulakshanaand, G. and Saidulu, B. 2012. Review of tylophora indica – an antiasthmatic plant. FS Journal of Pharmacy Research 1(2): 20–21.

Seidman, M. D., Gurgel, R. K., Lin, S. Y., Schwartz, S. R., Baroody, F. M., Bonner, J. R. et al. 2015. Clinical practice guideline: Allergic rhinitis. Otolaryngology-Head and Neck Surgery 152 (1 Suppl): S1–S43.

Shergis, J. L., Wu, L., Zhang, A. L., Guo, X., Lu, C. and Xue, C. C. 2016. Herbal medicine for adults with asthma: a systematic review. Journal of Asthma 0(0): 1–10.

Shi, Z., Song, T., Xie, J., Yan, Y. and Du, Y. 2017. The traditional chinese medicine and relevant treatment for the efficacy and safety of atopic dermatitis: a systematic review and meta-analysis of randomized controlled trials. Evidence-Based Complementary and Alternative Medicine 2017: 6026434.

Shin, H. S., See, H.-J., Jung, S. Y., Choi, D. W., Kwon, D.-A., Bae, M.-J. et al. 2015. Turmeric (Curcuma Longa) attenuates food allergy symptoms by regulating type 1/type 2 helper T cells (Th1/Th2) balance in a mouse model of food allergy. Journal of Ethnopharmacology 175: 21–29.

Tan, H. Y., Lenon, G. B., Zhang, A. L. and Xue, C. C. 2015. Efficacy of acupuncture in the management of atopic dermatitis: a systematic review. Clinical and Experimental Dermatology 40(7): 711–716.

Thandar, Y., Gray, A., Botha, J. and Mosam, A. 2017. Topical herbal medicines for atopic eczema: a systematic review of randomized controlled trials. British Journal of Dermatology 176(2): 330–343.

Wang, H. Liang, Dong, H., Li, Y., Ng, E. H. Y. et al. 2012. Biophysical characteristics of meridians and acupoints: a systematic review. Evidence-Based Complementary and Alternative Medicine 2012: 793841.

Wang, J. and Li, X.-M. 2012. Chinese herbal therapy for the treatment of food allergy. Current Allergy and Asthma Reports 12(4): 332–338.

Wang, Z., Zhen-Zhen, W., Geliebter, J., Tiwari, R. and Li, X.-M. 2021. Traditional Chinese medicine for food allergy and eczema. Annals of Allergy, Asthma, and Immunology 126(6): 639–654.

Xu, S., Wang, L., Cooper, E., Zhang, M., Manheimer, E., Berman, B. et al. 2013. Adverse events of acupuncture: a systematic review of case reports. Evidence-Based Complementary and Alternative Medicine 2013: 581203.

Yan, J., An, Y., Wang, L.-S. and Yang, S. 2015. Acupoint stimulation for chronic urticaria: a systematic review of randomized controlled trials. European Journal of Integrative Medicine 7: 586–592.

Yao, Q., Li, S., Liu, X., Qin, Z. and Liu, Z. 2016. The effectiveness and safety of acupuncture for patients with chronic urticaria: a systematic review. BioMed Research International 2016: 5191729.

Yin, Z., Geng, G., Xu, G., Zhao, L. and Liang, F. 2020. Acupuncture methods for allergic rhinitis: a systematic review and bayesian meta-analysis of randomized controlled trials. Chinese Medicine 15: 109.

Yu, C., Zhang, P., Lv, Z.-T., Li, J.-J., Li, H.-P., Wu, C.-H. et al. 2015. Efficacy of acupuncture in itch: a systematic review and meta-analysis of clinical randomized controlled trials. Evidence-Based Complementary and Alternative Medicine 2015: 208690.

Zhang, J., Zhang, Y., Huang, X., Lan, K., Hu, L., Chen, Y. et al. 2020. Different acupuncture therapies for allergic rhinitis: overview of systematic reviews and network meta-analysis. Evidence-Based Complementary and Alternative Medicine 2020: 8363027.

Zheng, Z., Sun, Z., Shou, X. and Zhou, Z. 2018. Efficacy of Chinese herbal medicine in treatment of allergic rhinitis in children: a meta-analysis of 19 randomized controlled trials. Journal of International Medical Research 46(10): 4006–4018.

Zhu, L., Kim, Y. and Yang, Z. 2018. The application of auriculotherapy to the treatment of chronic spontaneous urticaria: a systematic review and meta-analysis. Journal of Acupuncture and Meridian Studies 11(6): 343–354.

Chapter 14

Controversial Techniques in the Practice of Allergy

Hugo Van Bever[1],* and *Pudupakkam K. Vedanthan*[2]

Introduction

The prevalence of allergic diseases is still increasing worldwide in both developed and developing countries. Unfortunately, mainly in developing countries, there are not enough trained medical and paramedical personnel in this field of allergy. Due to this, and due to a large degree of ignorance about allergy in the general population—including wrong expectations on treatment—tests have been developed without any scientific background and only for financial benefits. These non-scientific diagnostic tests are very popular on social media, their spread seems unstoppable, and the list of tests is still growing (Ansotegui 2019).

Doctors, patients, and parents of allergic children should be aware of this. These tests have "no value" and most of them are very expensive. Moreover, the results of these tests lead to non-correct diagnoses and treatments, such as the prescription of extensive diets, which might be very troublesome (for the whole family) and harmful for the child, even leading to malnutrition. On the Internet, one can find many data and negative comments from many health authorities, and non-profit organizations on these tests (Wüthrich 2006). Not many reviews on non-diagnostic tests in allergy have been published. Hence, the readers are encouraged to refer to the articles in the attached bibliography for a detailed version of these procedures.

(The purpose of this text is to warn doctors, patients, and parents of allergic children about these tests, allowing/asking them to avoid the usage of these tests.)

The commonly used non-diagnostic tests can be divided into two groups: tests *in vivo* and tests *in vitro*.

In Vivo Tests

Applied Kinesiology: Muscle Testing for Allergies

The idea of this test is that every organ dysfunction is accompanied by a specific muscle weakness, which enables diseases to be diagnosed through muscle-testing procedures. The concepts of applied kinesiology (Figure 1) do not conform to scientific data about the causes or treatments of diseases,

---

[1] National University, Singapore.
[2] University of Colorado, Denver, Colorado USA.
* Corresponding author: paevbhps@nus.ed.sg

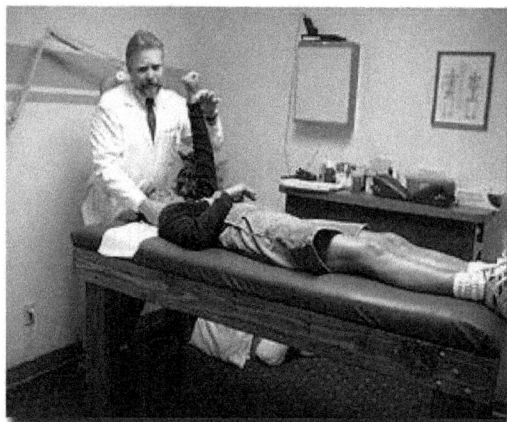

Figure 1. Applied kinesiology.

and controlled studies have found no difference between the results with test substances (usually food) and with a placebo.

Electrodermal Skin Testing, Bioresonance and Dubious Devices

Some physicians, neuropaths, dentists and chiropractors use "electrodiagnostic" devices (Figure 2) to help select the treatment they prescribe, which usually include homeopathic products. The devices they use are simply resistance-measuring instruments and the effectiveness or accuracy of these devices was never shown.

"Bioresonance" is based on the belief that human beings as well as any substances in the environment, such as allergens, emit electromagnetic waves, which may be either "good" or "bad." These waves can only be measured by specific bioresonance devices, but it was shown that the devices are not capable of measuring the electromagnetic wave presumed to be involved. Controlled studies failed to show any diagnostic or therapeutic value of bioresonance in adults suffering from allergic rhinitis and in children with eczema.

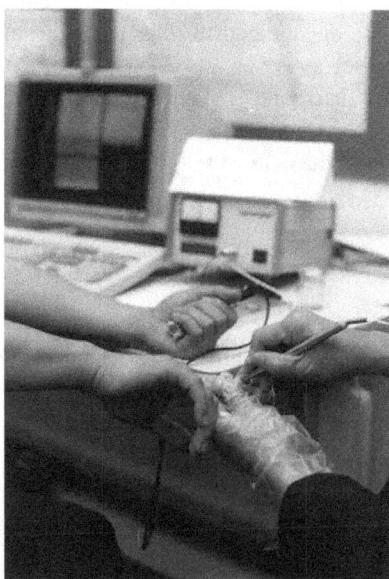

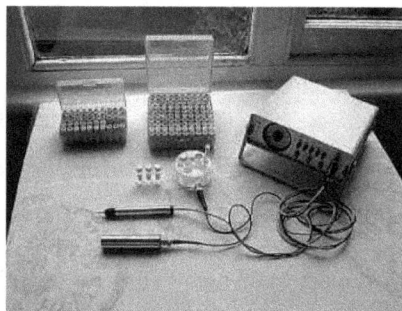

Figure 2. Electro-dermal tests have no value in diagnosing allergy.

Provocative and Neutralizing Testing (Subcutaneous)

This is a method used for both the diagnosis and treatment of allergic disorders. The allergen is injected subcutaneously in different concentrations and the patient is asked whether he/she is experiencing "any" symptoms. If the answer is affirmative, it is followed by an injection of either a "stronger" or "weaker" concentration to neutralize the symptoms. There has been no immunologic mechanism involved that has been demonstrated nor any clinical correlation has been established.

Provocative and Neutralizing Testing (Sublingual)

This was first described by Hansel in 1941 for the diagnosis and treatment of food allergy. Three drops of 1:100 dilution of the food antigen are placed under the patient's tongue, and the symptoms are assessed. The same procedure is repeated for the next suspected food antigen till the patient is fully assessed. Once the provocation is completed, the same antigen is diluted, and three drops are placed under the tongue for neutralization of symptoms. Several clinical trials have not been convincing. No immunological changes have been recorded.

Rinkel's Method of Skin Titration for Immunotherapy

Increasing concentrations of the antigen are placed by intradermal technique. The weakest dilution producing the positive wheal and flare reaction is considered the concentration for therapy. Dosage is started at 0.05 ml of that concentration with a maximum dose of 0.50 ml of the same weak dilution. This dose is claimed to relieve the symptoms within 4 hours. Controlled trials have proved that the Rinkel technique of allergen immunotherapy is equal to a placebo.

Urine Auto-Injection Therapy

The patient's urine is collected, sterilized by boiling and injected in varying doses between 0.25–5.00 ml intramuscular at different intervals. This method of treatment has no rationale and may have the risk of the development of autoimmunity.

Hair Analysis

This test assumes that food allergies cause nutritional deficiencies (e.g., zinc magnesium), which is untrue. In a study, the test could not distinguish allergic from nom-allergic subjects.

Iridology

Here, it is assumed that changes in the iris may suggest underlying systemic disease, including allergy. There's absolutely no scientific evidence for this.

In summary, the *in vivo* tests described above are used to diagnose non-existent health problems, select inappropriate treatments and defraud insurance companies. The practitioners who use them are either delusional, dishonest or both. These tests should be confiscated and the practitioners who use them should be prosecuted.

In Vitro Tests

Cytotoxic Testing: ALCAT TEST

The ALCAT test (test for cellular responses to foreign substances) has been launched in several countries for diagnosing so-called "non-IgE-mediated hypersensitivities." The promotion is mainly "for detecting adverse reactions to foods by advanced technology." The ALCAT test is a more sophisticated version of the previous "cytotoxic or leukocytotoxic testing," which was stopped in the USA by government actions of the FDA, after a negative statement of the American Academy of Allergy, Asthma and Immunology (AAAAI), concluding that cytotoxic testing is ineffective for diagnosing food or inhalant allergies.

The basic principle of the ALCAT test is measurement changes in white blood cell diameter after challenges with foods, molds, food additives, environmental chemicals, dyes and pharmaco-active agents in foods, antibiotics and other medications *in vitro*. The blood cells are passed through a narrow channel and are measured by an electronic instrument permitting to count instantaneously the number of cells, ranging from the smallest to the largest. The information brochure stated that the system has proven to be extremely reproducible and sensitive. On the company homepage, some references are listed, mainly from papers presented at congresses or articles in non-peer-reviewed journals. Therefore, it can be concluded that the ALCAT test system is relying on unproven statements that lack scientific and clinical proof of efficacy and is a test system that has no value in diagnosing allergic diseases in children.

Determination of Allergen-Specific IgG and IgG4

Specific IgG and IgG4 (which is a subclass of IgG) can be found in both adults and children in many different physiological (normal) and pathological (abnormal) conditions and their levels mainly

DIETARY ANTIGEN	ALLERGY					SENSITIVITY			
	IgE	IgE (µg/mL)	IMMUNE TOLERANCE TO IgE	IgG4	IgG4 (µg/mL)	IgG	IgG (µg/mL)	C3D	C3D (µg/mL)
Garlic		0.00		MODERATE	2.76	LOW	2.50	LOW	0.27
Ginger	LOW	0.12	YES	LOW	0.21		0.00	MODERATE	1.52
Gluten	HIGH	20.63	YES	HIGH	39.72	MODERATE	129.29	MODERATE	2.08
Goat's Milk	MODERATE	10.96	YES	MODERATE	12.84	LOW	43.84	LOW	0.46
Grapefruit		0.00		LOW	0.07		0.00		0.00
Grapes		0.00		LOW	0.11		0.32		0.00
Green Olive		0.00			0.00		0.00		0.04
Green Pea	HIGH	26.47	YES	HIGH	39.52	HIGH	80.97	MODERATE	2.25
Green Pepper		0.00		LOW	0.19		0.00	LOW	0.38
Halibut		0.00		MODERATE	2.59		0.18		0.00
Honeydew		0.00			0.00		0.00		0.00
Hops	LOW	0.16	YES	LOW	0.19		0.00	LOW	0.96
Kidney Bean	LOW	1.25	YES	LOW	3.90	LOW	8.18		0.04
Lemon		0.00			0.00		0.00		0.00
Lettuce		0.00		LOW	0.19		0.09	LOW	0.27
Lima Bean	HIGH	1.76	YES	HIGH	5.77	LOW	6.97		0.00
Lobster	LOW	0.16	YES	HIGH	0.67	HIGH	7.15	MODERATE	0.44
Mushroom		0.00		LOW	0.14		5.40		1.21
Mustard	HIGH	20.63		HIGH	7.67	HIGH	43.84	LOW	1.11
Navy Bean	HIGH	5.17	YES	MODERATE	9.49	LOW	19.56	LOW	0.73
Oat		0.00			0.02	MODERATE	5.78		0.00
Onion		0.00			0.00	LOW	0.74		0.00
Orange		0.00			0.00		0.00		0.00
Peach		0.00			0.00	LOW	0.88		0.00
Peanut	HIGH	17.07		HIGH	9.86	MODERATE	21.25	LOW	0.27
Pear		0.00			0.00		0.00		0.00
Pecan		0.00			0.00		0.00	MODERATE	0.71
Pineapple		0.00			0.00		0.00		0.00
Plum		0.00		LOW	0.09		0.00		0.00
Pork	MODERATE	0.67	YES	MODERATE	1.06	LOW	1.53	LOW	1.13
Rice		0.00			0.00		0.00	LOW	0.29
Rye		0.00		LOW	0.11		0.00		0.00
Salmon		0.00		MODERATE	4.58	LOW	0.93	LOW	0.19
Scallops		0.00			0.00		0.00		0.00
Sesame		0.00		MODERATE	0.26		0.00		0.00
Shrimp	MODERATE	0.43	YES	HIGH	0.70		0.00		0.00
Soybean	HIGH	4.27	YES	HIGH	36.97		0.00	LOW	0.27
Spinach	MODERATE	0.51		MODERATE	0.48		0.00	LOW	0.54
Strawberry		0.00			0.00		0.00		0.00
String Bean	MODERATE	0.35	YES	MODERATE	6.26	LOW	10.35	LOW	0.54
Sweet Potato	HIGH	1.14		HIGH	1.11	LOW	9.67		0.00
Tea		0.00			0.00		0.30		0.00
Tomato		0.00		LOW	0.04		0.00		0.00
Tuna		0.00		MODERATE	1.64	LOW	1.58	LOW	0.52
Turkey	MODERATE	0.31	YES	HIGH	3.01		0.00	MODERATE	0.52
Vanilla	HIGH	0.74			0.00		0.00	LOW	0.15
Watermelon	LOW	0.04	YES	LOW	0.09		0.00	LOW	0.17
White Potato		0.00		LOW	0.28	LOW	2.48	LOW	1.52
Whole Wheat		0.00		HIGH	7.23		0.00		0.00
Yellow Squash	HIGH	1.02		MODERATE	0.75	MODERATE	13.03	LOW	0.42

Summary Report of the Food Allergy Profile

Figure 3. IGG4 and IgE profile of food allergy.

"reflect contact with allergens (exposure to allergens)" and is in no way a measurement of the disease. Determination of allergen-specific IgG or IgG4 with different methods alone "does not prove the existence of an underlying allergy," as positive tests can also be found in healthy subjects. In most cases, the patient's serum is sent to a laboratory that performs tests to identify the specific IgE antibodies. The laboratory will automatically formulate the allergy vaccine based on these results and the vaccine is mailed back to the practitioner for initiation of an allergen immunotherapy program. Hence, there is a total lack of professionalism in this approach to patient needs.

The "Food Allergy Profile"

Now several alternative doctors use the so-called "food allergy profile IgE and IgG" against more than 100 types of food (Figure 3). The results are given in color with a scale of reactivity (0+ to 3+). The patient receives the information about results and therapy in the form of a "True Relief Guide" with instructions based on the first phase of an "Elimination Diet" of the IgG-positive foods and a second phase with a "Rotation Diet Schedule." In this second phase, foods that are not eliminated are allowed. The procedure lacks all scientific evidence and "can be dangerous" if a true IgE-mediated allergy is still present after the avoidance phase. Obviously, such a sophisticated guide is impressive for patients and parents, and together with the charisma of their healthcare providers using these mystic elimination, rotation and reintroduction diets, some placebo effects can be expected. However, no scientific evidence of any use of this method has been shown.

The Role of Food Additives and Hyperkinesis

Most studies done to evaluate the relationship between food additives, dyes and hyperactivity and learning disability syndromes have been inconclusive. This area continues to be controversial, and diets should not be used here.

Remote Practice of Allergy

The patient's serum is sent to a laboratory to identify the specific IgE antibodies. The laboratory will automatically formulate the allergy vaccine based on these results and the vaccine is mailed back to the practitioner for initiation of an allergen immunotherapy program. The sIgE may not have been validated; there are no steps taken to correlate patients' clinical picture with the sIgE profile. Hence, there is a complete lack of professionalism in this approach to patients' needs. Only a well-trained allergy specialist is capable of correlating a patient's clinical history and presentation with either an allergy skin test or *in vitro* sIgE data to formulate the proper management of the case (Shapiro and Anderson 1988).

Conclusion

Physicians need to be aware of these above-mentioned techniques that are still being practiced in the community. The public is unaware of the pitfalls associated with such unproven techniques of diagnosis and treatment. Proper advice and education will steer away such susceptible patients and families from undergoing unnecessary expenses and modalities of unproven methods of treatment.

Glossary of Abbreviations

ALCAT – Antigen Leukocyte Antibody Test

Further Suggested Reading

Allergy panel. 1987. Council on Scientific papers: *in vivo* diagnostic testing and immunotherapy for allergy. Report I Part I JAMA 258: 1363–1367.

Allergy panel. 1987. Council on Scientific Affairs: *in vivo* diagnostic testing and immunotherapy for allergy. Report I Part 2 JAMA 258: 1505–1508.

Allergy Panel. 1987. Council on Scientific Affairs: *In vitro* testing for allergy. Report 2. JAMA 258: 1639–1643.

American Academy of allergy. 1981. Position statements: controversial techniques. J. Allergy Clin. Immunol. 67: 333–338.

References

Ansotegui, I. J., Melioli, G., Canonica, G. W., Caraballo, L., Villa, E., Ebisawa, M. et al. 2020. IgE Allergy Diagnostics and Other Relevant Tests in Allergy, A World Allergy Organization Position Paper. WAO Jour.

Shapiro, G. and Anderson, J. 1988. Controversial techniques in allergy. Pediatrics Dec 1988 82(6): 935–937.

Wüthrich, B. 2005. Unproven techniques in allergy diagnosis. J. Invest. Allergol. Clin. Immunol. 15: 86–90.

Chapter 15

Aerobiology for Clinicians

Saibal Moitra[1],* and *Kavitha B.*[2]

◇◇◇

Introduction

The atmosphere around us contains a panoply of bio-particulate matter, which impacts our respiratory epithelium resulting in varied responses among different individuals. This consists of infectious particles, like bacteria, viruses and fungi, and non-infectious particles, like pollen grains, fungal spores, dust mite particles, animal dander, insect-derived particles, etc.

The collective term for the study of this airborne bio-particulate matter is called "aerobiology" and is used since 1930. The term was coined by American plant pathologist Fred Campbell Meier. Present-day aerobiology originated much earlier through the famous experiments of Spallanzani in 1776, but it is only in the last 50 years that it has emerged as a specialized multidisciplinary branch of science. With the inception of the International Biological Program (IBP) in 1954, the term has been extended to include all airborne materials of biological significance. Thus, it encompasses not only bio-particulates but also pollutants that exert specific biological effects. Edmonds and Benninghoof in 1973 described aerobiology as a scientific and multidisciplinary approach focused on the transport of organisms and biologically significant materials.

The majority of the aerobiological studies are carried out with reference to the "aerobiological triangle" (Figure 1). This is the path followed by an airborne particle, which is from source to release, dispersion, deposition and impact. The environmental factors affect each stage of this pathway and hence lead to geographical and temporal differences.

Aerobiological investigations are broadly classified into outdoor or extramural aerobiology and indoor or intramural aerobiology. Barometric pressure, the density of air and temperature decrease in the outdoor air with increasing height from the sea level. There is a microscopically thin layer of air known as a laminar boundary layer near the ground above, which is a variable turbulent boundary layer through which dispersion of most of the particles occurs and this extends up to the stratosphere. In addition, differential heating from Earth's surface on sunny days leads to pockets of air that are warmer than the surrounding air and which rise upwards as thermals lead to much wider and higher dispersal of various components of air spora. The indoor air or the microclimate inside the buildings is different and less variable than outdoor air leading to more homogeneous air spora compared to outdoors. The importance of these studies with respect to human health is paramount.

[1] Adjunct Professor and Senior Consultant, Division of Allergy and Immunology, Department of Respiratory Medicine, Apollo Multi Specialty Hospitals, Kolkata, India

[2] Associate Professor, Department of Microbiology, Government Science College (Autonomous), Nrupathnga Road, Bengaluru, Karnataka, India.

* Contributing author: saibal.moitra@icloud.com

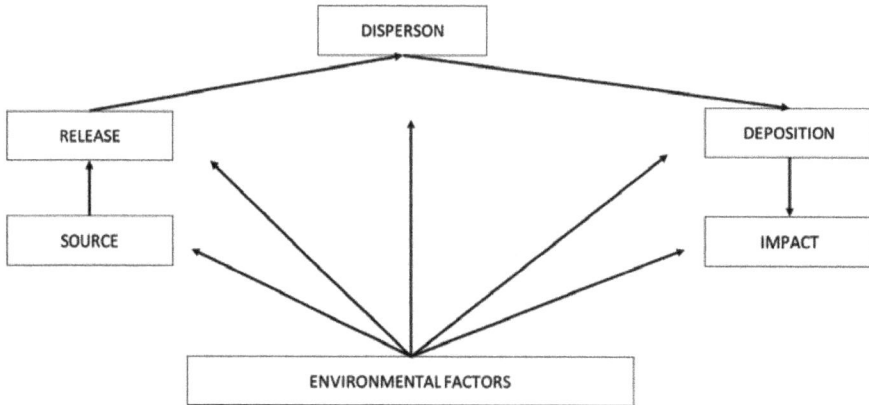

Figure 1. Aerobiological triangle.

The inhaled airborne pollen grains or mycospores impinge on the respiratory epithelium causing inflammation in predisposed individuals leading to symptoms of hay fever or asthma. Bostock (1819) was the first to suspect pollen grains as the causative agent of allergic rhinitis and Blackley (1873) established that grass pollens are an important cause of hay fever in the United Kingdom. The development of symptoms depends on the pollen load in the inhaled air. The majority of pollen grains in the air are liberated from wind-pollinated inconspicuous flowers of gymnosperms, grasses and some angiosperm trees. Insect-pollinated plants have large, colored flowers and the pollen grains are larger, heavier and often sticky so unlikely to be inhaled. Fungi, actinomycetes, lichens and non-spermatophyte plants reproduce by airborne spores, which are also dispersed by wind. The dispersion of pollens or spores in abundance is the goal of wind pollination, and this results in the health effects of these pollens. Pollen prevalence (grains per cubic meter) at any point is the composite effect of source strength from the plant, its location dynamics of the environment like climatic factors, wind direction, substrate precipitation, seasonal factors, air pollution and degree of exposure. This results in diurnal and seasonal variability of pollen grains and clinical symptoms commensurate to it.

Components of Air Spora

Air spora is a term associated with airborne particles of microbial, plant and animal origin. The gaseous suspension of these bioparticles referred to as bioaerosols can be introduced into the air through dust or water droplets. These remain suspended in the air for long periods and can be threatening to human health, which occurs through respiratory intake and deposition in nasal and bronchial airways. Airspora in the form of bioaerosols could be pollen from plants (10–100 µm); microorganisms like bacteria, fungi, viruses, parts of microorganisms/plants; microbial substances like endotoxin from G-ve bacteria and mycotoxin from fungi or even substances from animals like cat, dog, mite and cockroach. Individual bioaerosol particles can range in size from approximately 0.02 to 100 micrometers in diameter, depending on the type and source.

The atmosphere is, however, unsuitable for the growth of microorganisms due to extreme temperature variations, light, temperature and low amount of available water. Characteristics of the climate, vegetation and meteorology in a particular geographical setting determine the components and concentrations of these air spora. The distribution and amount of air spora in the outdoor environment fluctuate remarkably and is dependent upon the activities of the environment, such as speed of air current, size of bioaerosol and humidity of the environment.

The levels and dispersion of air spora in the indoor air is also determined by similar factors. The proliferation of indoor air spora is also affected by factors, such as building dampness, indoor temperature, relative humidity and hygiene conditions indoors and in the surrounding environment. Outdoor climate and weather conditions combined with occupant behavior can also affect indoor air quality. Both indoor and outdoor air spora contain allergens, which are responsible for many conditions of allergy including asthma, rhinitis and atopic dermatitis. Predominant among the aeroallergens in the air are pollen grains and fungal spores.

Pollen Grains

Pollen (Latin for flour or dust particle) is derived from Palynein (Gk.) meaning to spread and scatter around. The study of pollen is termed palynology and includes understanding its structural and applied aspects. Pollen grains are fine or coarse powder that functions as the male gametes found specifically in the anther of flower-bearing plants (angiosperms) or in the microsporangia of non-flowering/naked seeded plants (gymnosperms). Pollen grains can be round, ovule, triangular or disk-shaped with a smooth to spiky texture. The size of pollen grains generally varies with the species and ranges between 200–300 μm. The natural color of pollen grains is white, which may also vary depending on the plant species; some being yellow in color.

Pollen grains are minute and usually light and hence are able to be easily transported by water, wind or insect and animal pollinators. They are often structurally modified to assist in airborne transportation. For example, grass pollen is light, dry and released in large quantities. These airborne pollen grains, which come in contact with the mucosa of the eyes, nose, oral cavity or skin can produce immediate or delayed allergic symptoms. The presence of pollen and its concentration depends on climatic factors, such as temperature, humidity, wind direction, sunshine, substrate precipitation and other seasonal factors.

Based on the mode of pollen release from the anthers in the flower and pollination mechanism, plants are distinguished into Anemophilous or Entomophilous plants (Figure 2).

Pollen of Anemophilous plants is mostly allergenic since the pollen grains are dry, light and smooth-walled. The flowers of these plants are usually small in size, not brightly colored, odorless and do not produce any kind of nectar. These plants produce large quantities of pollen that are small in size and light in weight and hence are easily carried by wind to large distances. Examples include flowers of maize and grass.

Pollen of Entomophilous plants is non-allergenic since they are sticky and produced in fewer numbers. These flowers are pollinated by insects or animals and hence the pollen is usually heavy and large in size having a spiny or variously sculptured wall. The size of flowers is usually large, or flowers are present in large groups and brightly colored to attract pollinators. These flowers have an odor and produce nectar. Examples include hibiscus, jasmine and rose.

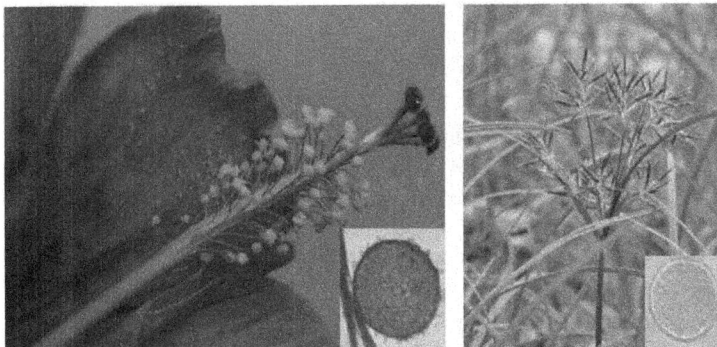

Figure 2. Entomophilous Plant (Hibiscus) and Anemophilous Plant (Grass) With their pollen grain as observed under light microscope.

The quantity of pollen production, which varies in individual species and the methods of dispersal are very important factors, which are directly or indirectly involved in manifestation of allergy.

Fungal Spores

Fungal aerosols are present in much higher concentrations than pollen grains in the air. Fungi or molds are ubiquitous in nature and the spores they produce can get airborne. The significance of airborne fungi in inciting allergies in human beings has been recognized, as has their role as important constituents of indoor bioaerosols. Numerous studies have shown that exposure to fungi may be associated with acute toxic effects, allergies and asthma (Bush and Portnoy 2001). Researchers believe that more than 80 genera of fungi are associated with symptoms of respiratory tract allergies (Black et al. 2000). Fungi implicated in allergic diseases are established to cause Type I hypersensitive diseases with IgE-mediated response. Many molecules of fungal origin can be potent sources of allergy like enzymes, fungal toxins (mycotoxins), cell wall components and phylogenetically highly conserved cross-reactive proteins. A triggering factor for respiratory allergy and asthma as well as atopic dermatitis can be exposure to indoor and outdoor fungal components mostly spores.

Fungi produce a huge amount of spores or conidia that are capable of long-range dispersal and our understanding of the seasonal diversity of these airborne fungal spores along with the spatial and temporal distribution becomes significant in the context of allergy. The fungal spores are between 2–20 μm in diameter and particles less than 5 μm in diameter are known to enter the lower respiratory airways leading to allergic symptoms.

Fungi are heterotrophic in nature due to the absence of chlorophyll. They have an absorptive mode of nutrition and can grow as a parasite, saprophytes or symbionts. Fungi produce a large number of spores and conidia and are resistant to the lack of water, hence can survive in a dry state for several years. Since they use different sources of energy they adapt to various environments. Additionally, they have the ability to synthesize a number of stress proteins that protect them against extreme environmental conditions.

Fungi are eukaryotic and multicellular and form the mycelium with the exception of yeast which is unicellular. The structure of the mycelium varies depending on the species, growing conditions and the presence of nutrients in the medium. Most fungi show both sexual and asexual states in their life cycle. Internally borne cells are termed spores and externally borne cells are called conidia. Generally, molds that have no sexual stage are known as Deuteromycota or imperfect fungi. For the most part, fungi that are known to cause human allergic diseases belong to this group.

Fungi are common in indoor and outdoor environments. Concentrations of fungal spores in the outdoor air vary depending on the weather and the climate. Airborne fungi found indoors originate both from outdoor air and various indoor sources and are present in the air space throughout the year. The number of spores in the air in some homes may exceed 250,000 per cubic meter. Their development is aggravated by poor access to light, windproof environment, limited ventilation and high humidity. These conditions occur mainly in basements, laundry rooms, bathrooms and kitchens and farm areas in the country, as well as in wooden cabins and summer houses. Significant invasion of mold can be identified by a characteristic musty smell, caused by volatile metabolites of fungi released into the air.

Both outdoor and indoor environments, especially in buildings frequented by a large number of people may be exposed to fungal aeroallergen, and studies indicate that the dominant fungi in the atmosphere and their concentration differed from place to place because of local environmental variables, fungal substrates and human activities.

Airborne fungi found indoors originate both from outdoor air and from various indoor sources. Significant correlations have been found between the airborne fungi of indoor and outdoor environments, but numerous fungi can also originate indoors. Fungal spores are found in all types of indoor settings, including homes, offices and other working environments and have the potential to affect occupants' health.

Sources of indoor air spora can occur through fresh air rushing through ventilators, coughing, sneezing, talking and mechanical disturbances, such as vacuum cleaning, sweeping, walking and making beds. Molds can grow on damp walls, wooden structures or furniture, can enter indoor areas either by means of passive ventilation or can be emitted by indoor sources, like animals, flowerpots and wastebaskets.

Fungi commonly considered allergenic include species of *Acremonium, Alternaria, Aspergillus, Curvularia, Cladosporium, Epicoccum, Fusarium, Rhizopus* and *Penicillium* (Figure 3). Most of these fungi are known to display a seasonal spore release pattern. Indoor fungi, very likely associated with water damage, include species of *Aspergillus* and *Penicillium*, Cladosporium and Alternaria are common outdoors; however, they grow well indoors in fiberglass insulation or on surfaces in high relative humidity conditions with occasional condensation. The outdoor concentration of fungal species from these genera has been associated with epidemics of asthma exacerbation. Species of *Alternaria* are found to be associated with carpets, textiles and window frames in building interiors, *Aspergillus* in water-damaged carpets, damp wood/wall or wallpaper glue, *Cladosporium* in supply ducts, *Penicillium* on damp walls, *Fusarium* in humidifiers and *Trichoderma* in the paper. Hidden Sources of mold may be on the backside of drywall/wallpaper, top of ceiling tiles (roof leaks), the underside of carpets, pipe chaises, utility tunnels, elevator shafts, drain pans in the HVAC system and insulation within the ductwork.

For a fungal spore to qualify as a potential aeroallergen, the spores must be produced in large quantities and be sufficiently buoyant to become airborne. The fungi must be widely and abundantly distributed and should contain an excitant of hay fever or asthma. Symptoms of allergy must occur when the spores are numerous in the air. Many fungal allergens are glycopeptides with enzymatic properties. They are found in spores, hyphae and fungal fragments but are released in greater amounts during germination and mycelial growth, which may occur inside the airways.

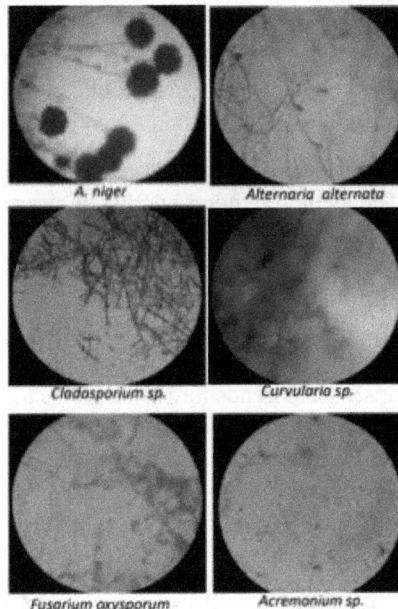

Figure 3. Fungi commonly considered allergenic as observed under light microscope.

Air Sampling Methods

Identification and monitoring of atmospheric pollen and spores is an important requirement in establishing allergy. The main objective is to detect and monitor the occurrence and relative abundance of pollen and spores in the atmosphere. This is greatly facilitated by the knowledge of local flora, especially the allergenic plants. Knowledge about diurnal, seasonal and annual fluctuations in airborne pollen and fungal spores in any area is essential for the effective diagnosis and treatment of allergies.

Aerobiological trapping and monitoring using a number of techniques can be carried out to determine the presence, sources and seasonal variations of air spora. Tracking both indoor and outdoor environments is also important for the evaluation of allergens. The aerobiological survey can be carried out in two phases—collection of material and sample analysis.

Collection of materials can be done using sampling devices that include gravimetric, impaction and suction samplers (Figure 4).

Gravimetric Sampler: It is based on the principle that bioparticles settle down on a surface due to gravitational force. Exposure to a horizontal surface on which particles settle down by gravity is the simple method of collecting airborne pollen and fungal spores. The sample that settles is retained by an adhesive on the sampling surface. The Durham sampler or the gravity slide sampler is one such sampling device consisting of two horizontal disks with a diameter of 22.1 cm and 8.1 cm. The upper disk protects the slide from rain and sun. The slides are exposed daily, at a fixed hour, coated with adhesive glycerine jelly. After exposure, the slides are mounted in a drop of molten glycerine jelly, for analysis.

Impaction Sampler: Wind impaction samplers are extensively used for pollen sampling. The vertical cylinder is most suitable due to its simple construction and efficiency. The spores are trapped on an adhesive-coated cellophane tape wrapped around a glass cylinder of 0.53 cm in diameter. This is suspended under a metallic shield. The sampler can be installed on the roof of high-rise buildings to facilitate the free flow of air around them. The pollen and spores get trapped irrespective of wind direction. The sellotape is mounted on slides with glycerin jelly, for analysis. Rotorod Sampler is a lightweight portable rotating impaction sampler that is electrically operated or battery-run. Rotorod Sampler has leucite rods of 1–3 mm coated with adhesive silicon grease which can collect airborne particles. The exposure time can be adjusted according to requirements.

Suction Samplers: These work on the principle that air to be sampled is drawn into an entrance by suction from a vacuum pump. The method requires suction of a certain volume of air according to a known velocity and for a chosen duration of trapping. The Hirst spore trap is one such device that allows bioparticles to adhere to slides coated with glycerin jelly. The slides can be replaced each day with fresh slides and provide quantitative data. It records the atmospheric concentration of pollen grains, fungal spores and other biological particles as a function of time through morphological identification. The Hirst trap was later modified to the Burkard trap which is one of the most widely used samplers to study diurnal or seasonal trends for pollen grains as well as fungal spores. Burkard portable slide sampler is a compact battery-operated sampler. It has a rectangular orifice at the top end and a slit on the slide to insert the microslide. The microslide is coated with glycerine jelly. The sampler sucks in 10 L of air per minute. The particles get impacted on the slide in the form of a streak. The slide can then be mounted in glycerine jelly and scanned for pollen grains/fungal spore count under the light microscope.

A Sampling of Airborne Fungi: In addition to using spore traps fungi can be cultured by the gravity or settling method. A common volumetric sampler is the Andersen sampler. In this sampler air after entering a circular orifice is drawn through a series of six circular perforated plates. The plates in the series have progressively smaller holes. The bioparticles are deposited on sterile media in Petri dishes which can then be cultured. The yield is lower in these cases simply because spores

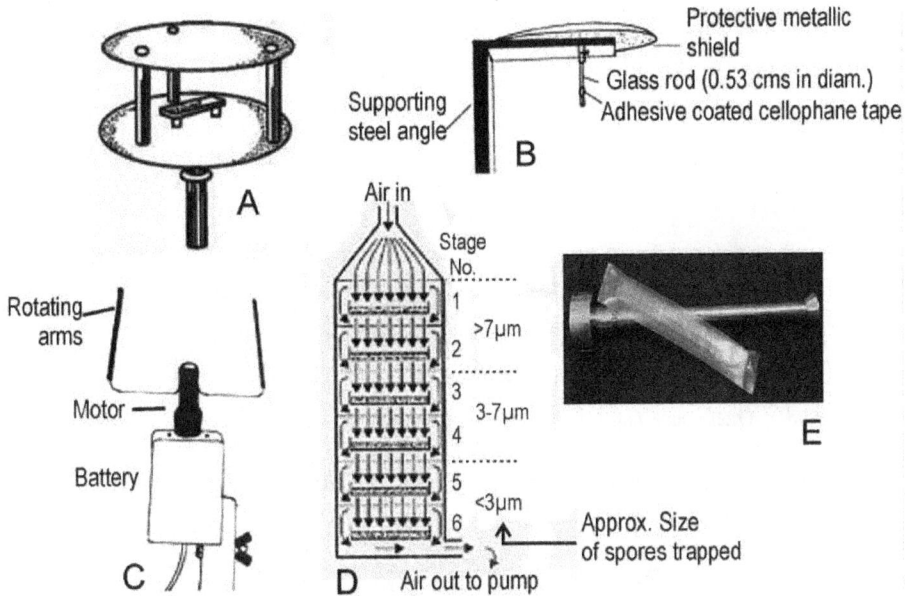

Figure 4. Examples of sampling devices. (A) Durham Sampler, (B) Vertical Cylinder trap, (C) Rotorod Sampler, (D) Andersons Sampler and (E) Handheld Sampler.

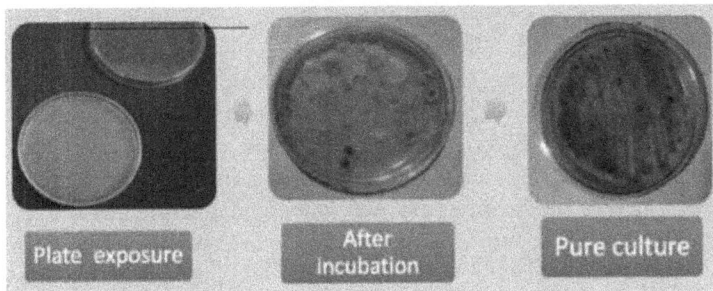

Figure 5. Plate exposure technique for culturing fungi.

may be non-viable, dormant or unable to grow on the media used. Fungi can also be sampled using portable handheld samplers.

One of the easiest techniques is the plate exposure technique (Figure 5), which follows the sedimentation method where plates with media are exposed to air for 10–15 minutes, and incubated at 25°C to 30°C for 3–5 days. Viable spores germinate and grow into colonies after incubation. Fungal colonies are then enumerated and identified. All fungal structures including spores, conidiophores and hyphal fragments are counted and presumptively identified by microscopy.

Analysis of Slides: Regardless of their method of collection, analysis can be performed by direct microscopic observation of the slides. Most of these bioparticles, including pollen grains, certain fungal spores like basidiospores, ascospores and spores of rust, smuts and downy mildew are identifiable by microscopic examination but fail to grow on most laboratory media. These bioparticles are identified microscopically based on shape, size and other morphological features of pollen and spores (Figure 6). Subsequent observation of morphological traits or cultural characteristics of colonies, such as their color and texture, conidial size and texture and conidiophore structure would help in the identification of the molds. The slides can be mounted in glycerine jelly if long-term storage is required. Glycerine jelly contains 2 parts gelatin, 12 parts water, 11 parts glycerine, 2% glycerine and 2% phenol. Mix gelatin and water; warm slightly dissolve, add water glycerine and

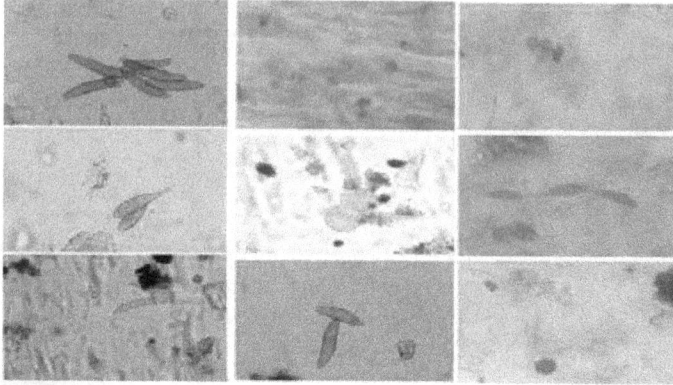

Figure 6. Slides of pollen and fungal spores collected from samplers and observed under a light microscope.

phenol. Let stand overnight and strain through cheesecloth. It can be warmed in a hot water bath until it flows from the dropper.

Pollens of Clinical Significance

Pollen grains of clinical significance are majorly classified into grass pollens, tree pollens and weed pollens. Grasses are ubiquitous worldwide and are the main contributors to seasonal inhalant allergies during spring as well as summer. The grass family (*Poaceae*) includes more than 600 genera with wide distribution. More than 95% of the clinically significant grass species belong to the three sub-families: *Pooideae, Chloridoideae* and *Panicoideae. Pooideae* dominate temperate climate zones, *Chloridoideae* are abundant in North American, African and Australian continents and *Panicoideae* is found mostly in the tropical and subtropical climates of Asia, Australia, Africa and South America. There are 10 designated groups of major and minor grass allergens. Grass allergen groups 1 and 5 are the immunodominant allergens in *Pooideae*. Pan-allergens profiling (Group 12) and polcalcin (group 7) cause cross-reactivity among grass, tree and weed pollens. The important genera of *Pooideae* consist of Orchard grass, Velvet grass, Timothy grass, Barley Wheat and rye. An important genus of *Chloridoideae* includes Bermuda grass, Rice and common reed. Those of *Panicoideae* include Bahia grass, Jonson grass, Corn and maize.

Weed pollen of clinical significance includes three main families. They are Amaranthaceae-Chenopodiaceae, Asteraceae and Urticaceae. Amaranthaceae contains pigweeds (*Amaranthus*), saltbushes (*Atriplex*) and tumbleweeds (*Salsola, Kochia* and *Bassia*) as well as other chenopod weeds (*Chenopodium*). The major tumbleweeds of North American plains are Russian thistle (*Salsola kali*) and burning bush (*Kochia scoparia*). Other species are common in the Middle East. Redroot pigweed (*Atriplex retroflexus*) is a common cosmopolitan weed of temperate regions. Asteraceae is the largest family of flowering plants. The genus *Ambrosia* contains all the ragweed, which are mainly North American natives but have been introduced in Europe. Pollination season is August and September. Another clinically important member of the genus *Artemesia* is sages of which the most prevalent is the mugwort. Cross-reactivity is very common among *Artemisia* species. Urticaceae includes two members of clinical relevance: pellitory (*Parietaria*) and nettle (*Urtica*). Pellitory is a common seasonal allergen of the Mediterranean region.

Tree pollens of allergic significance belong to three families: *Fagales, Oleaceae* and *Cupressaceae*. Fagale trees are widely distributed within the temperate climate of the Northern hemisphere and flower during spring. Oleaceae trees grow in the Mediterranean and other parts of the temperate zone. Their flowering season varies from January to June. Cupressaceae plants are widely distributed in Europe, Asia and North America with the flowering periods between January and April. Fagale allergies are mainly elicited by Bet v 1 like allergens that show cross-reactivity with homologous allergens of certain fruits and vegetables. Pan-allergens belonging to

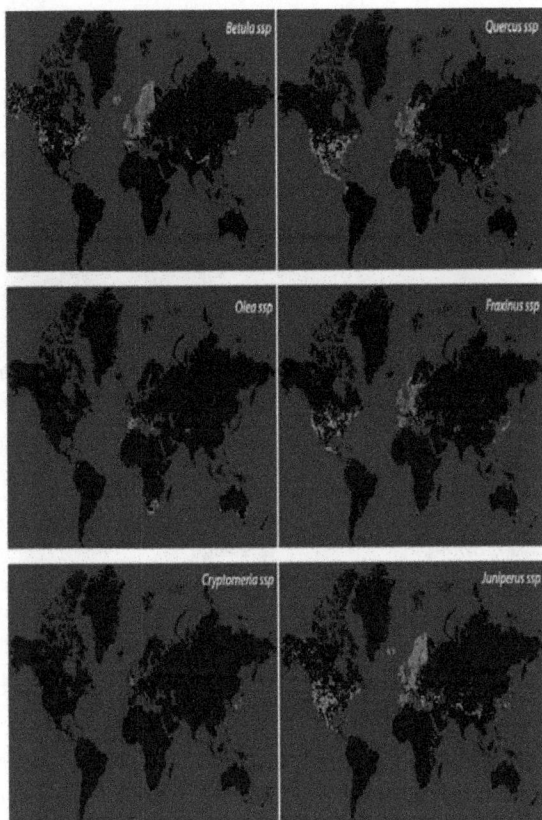

Figure 7. World maps showing the distribution of trees causing respiratory allergic reactions. Representative members of the Fagales family (Betula and Quercus), the Oleaceae family (Ole and Fraxinus) and the Cupressaceae family (Cryptomeria and Junipers) are depicted in the maps as the density of registered data (within the Global Biodiversity Information Facility (www.gbit.orgl), a free and open access data infrastructure funded by governments).

calcium-binding proteins and profilins also contribute to cross-reactive patterns among Fagale-sensitized persons.

Oleaceae trees like olive, ash, and privet contains the major allergen Ole e 1-like glycoproteins. Cupressaceae trees including cypress, mountain cedar and Japanese cedar show extensive cross-reactivity among themselves due to the presence of cross-reactive carbohydrate determinants. Their flowering season overlaps with the winter flu season (Figure 7).

An All India Coordinated Project on Aeroallergens and Human Health was conducted under the aegis of the Ministry of Environment and Forests, Government of India in 2000 to understand the allergenic pollens in India (Anonymous 2000). The dominant pollens of allergic significance as revealed in this project are listed in the table below (Singh 2003).

The dominant pollens from Northern India are *Holoptelea*, Poaceae, *Asteraceae, Artemisia, Eucalyptus, Casuarina, Morus* and *Putranjiva.* From Eastern India, the dominant types are *Trema orientalis*, Asteraceae, Chenopodiaceae, *Pongamia, Areca catechu, Xanthium* and *Cocos.* From Southern India, studies carried out revealed that *Casuarina, Parthenium, Spathodia*, Cheno/Amaranth, *Cocos, Eucalyptus*, Poaceae, *Peltophorum* and Cyperaceae are dominant pollen types. Pollens causing allergies are quite different in various ecozones which makes it important to identify them for proper clinical correlation.

Table 1. Clinically important Pollens in India.

	Spring (Feb–April)	Autumn (Sept–Oct)	Winter (Nov–Jan)
Grasses	*Cynodon dactylon*	*Bothriochloa pertusa*	*Cynodon dactylon*
	Dicanthium annulatum	*Cenchrus ciliaris*	*Eragrostis tenella*
	Imperata cylindrica	*Hetropogon contortus*	*Phalaris minor*
	Paspalum distichum	*Pennisetum typhoides*	*Poa annua*
	Poa annua	*Sorghum vulgare*	
	Polypogon monspeliensis		
Weeds	*Cannabis sativa*	*Amaranthus spinosus*	*Ageratum conyzoides*
	Chenopodium murale	*Artemisia scoparia*	*Argemone mexicana*
	Parthenium hysterophorous	*Cassia occidentalis*	*Chenopodium album*
	Suaeda fruiticosa	*Ricinus communis*	*Asphodelous tenuifolius*
	Plantago major	*Xanthium strumarium*	*Ricinus communis*
Trees	*Ailanthus excelsa*	*Anogeissus pendula*	*Cassia siamea*
	Holoptelea integrifolia	*Eucalyptus sp.*	*Salvadora persica*
	Prosopis juliflora	*Prosopis juliflora*	*Mallotus phillipensis*
	Putranjiva roxburghii	*Cedrus deodara*	*Cedrus deodara*

Pollen and Fungal Calendar

Pollen and fungal calendars can be used by allergologists and patients suffering from allergies for understanding seasonal pollen and spores that are present in a specific area. Aerobiologists compile pollen calendars of different regions and indicate types of pollen and their relative abundance in the air. This is the result of continuous surveys carried out by using samplers at specific locations, identification of pollen and spores and determination of their counts. The knowledge of the occurrence and concentration of allergenic pollen and spores can be inferred from pollen and spore calendars. This can also help in the immunological treatment of pollen allergies. Pollen calendars need to be compiled and updated every year to evaluate the change in trends of peak concentration over the years.

Pollen and Fungal Spore Allergy

Pollens are known to trigger symptoms in patients with allergic rhinitis, asthma and atopic dermatitis. A very old study investigating the relationship between pollen and spores and allergy was published by Hyde in Britain (1972). There has been increasing urban migration worldwide, which also results in increasing allergic symptoms due to aeroallergens. Allergy is a clinical condition characterized by Type 1 hypersensitivity reaction to environmental allergens. Aeroallergens being an important causative agent for nasobronchial allergy, the study of various air spora is important in clinical diagnosis and treatment. Pollen grains and fungal spores are constitutes the major part of this. Molecular biological techniques have enabled us to understand the structure of the antibody binding sites (or epitopes) of the allergens. Since certain protein structure has remained constant throughout evolution, they are shared among various members of the same family and in some cases in the entire plant kingdom. So, allergic patients showing sensitization to these proteins show cross-sensitizations among different genera of the same sub-family. This facilitates the allergy diagnosis by using a few cross-reactive allergens to know the sensitization pattern of an individual. Though at times it may create confusion by causing false sensitizations. For example, *Lolium perenne* is cross-reactive with *Acacia*, pineapple, *Oleaeuropaea*, *Dactylisglomerata*, *Ligustrum vulgare*, *Cynodon dactylon* and *Pinus radiata*. *Platanus acerifolia* has been found to cross-react with *Corylus avellana*, *Prunus persica*, *Malus domestica*, *Arachis hypogaea*, *Zea mays*, *Cicer arietinum*, *Lactuca virosa*, *Musa* spp., and *Apium* spp. *Ricinus communis*, commonly grown in India for its oil, cross-reacts with *Hevea brasiliensis*, *Mercurialis annua*, *Olea europaea*, *Betula*, *Zygophyllum fabago*, *Putranjiva roxburghii* and *Ricinus* (seed) *Areca catechu* cross-reacts with *Phoenix sylvestris*, *Cocos nucifera*, *Borassus flabelifer*. *Cynodon dactylons* (Bermuda grass) cross-reacts with *Pennisetum clandestinum*, *Stenotaphrum secundatum*, *Eragrostis*, *Brassica napus*, *Olea europaea*, *Ligustrum vulgare* and *Lolium perenne*. Cross-sensitizations also lead to a distinct clinical entity called pollen-fruit syndrome or oral allergy syndrome. In this condition, an individual showing cross-sensitizations to pollen and a particular edible fruit suffers from symptoms of burning and itching sensation of mouth and throat after consumption of that particular fruit or vegetable. Heiss (1996) showed that mugwort pollens are cross-reactive with celery, carrot, nuts, spices, mustard and Leguminoseae vegetables. Similarly, ragweed pollens are cross-reactive with Cucurbitaceae vegetables and fruits like melon, watermelon, banana and cucumber. Grass pollens are also cross-sensitized with tomato, potato, orange, apple, kiwi, orange, melon, watermelon and green peas. These cross-sensitizations are due to the presence of pan-allergens of plant kingdoms like lectins, cross-reactive carbohydrate determinants, profilins, major birch pollen allergen Bet v 1, etc. Wagner and Breiteneder (2002) have shown similar cross-sensitization between latex allergen (Hev b 6) and many fruits and vegetables like peach, tomato, bell pepper, potato, papaya, kiwi, avocado and chestnut due to structural homology between Hev b 6 and class I chitinases causing latex fruit syndrome.

Fungi are more numerous and are present worldwide. They occur indoors and outdoors. Fungal spores are small and light in weight and are easily dispersed in the air. Atmospheric fungal spore concentrations are 100–1,000 times more than pollen spore concentrations as shown by Burge (1989). Some fungi have specialized mechanisms for spore dispersal to rise above the stable laminar air column above the ground. These fungal spores cause immediate allergic reactions in the nose, sinuses, airways and skin among genetically predisposed individuals. Unlike pollen grains, fungal spores are not restricted to a particular region, though their concentration in the air may vary. They predominantly belong to Ascomycetes, Deuteromycetes and Basiodiomycetes. Common allergy-causing genera which belong to ascomycota are *Alternaria*, *Candida*, *Aspergillus*, *Bipolaris*, *Cladosporium*, *Epicoccum* and *Phoma*. The predominant basidiomycetes include *Calvatia*, *Ganoderma*, *Coprinus*, *Pleurotus* and *Psilocybe*. The average size of fungal spores is 2–10 micrometers, which is smaller than the size of pollen grains which allows fungal spores to reach deeper into the lungs and cause persistent airway inflammation.

There is also not much difference between the type of fungal spores in the indoor or outdoor air. Fungal spores can elicit both immediate and delayed-type hypersensitivity reactions and can also lead to life-threatening infections in susceptible individuals. Allergy to fungal allergens is a risk factor for asthma in patients suffering from allergic rhinitis. Though most allergenic fungi display seasonal spore release patterns, it is less well-defined than pollens. *Cladosporium*, *Alternaria*, *Epicoccum* and *Ganoderma* are the major outdoor fungal spores (Simon-Nobbe 2008). In India, the most important outdoor fungal spore is *Cladosporium* and common indoor fungi are *Aspergillus*, *Penicillium* and *Cladosporium*. Similar results were found in a Danish study (Gravesen 1999). Clinical manifestations of Type 1 fungal allergy include allergic rhinitis, allergic asthma and atopic dermatitis. Fungal allergy is associated with bronchial hyperreactivity in children and increased intensive care unit admissions and death among adults with severe asthma (Black 2000). *Malassezia furfur* belonging to Basidiomycota has been implicated in the pathogenesis of atopic dermatitis. Apart from this, fungal spores are known to cause type II, III and IV hypersensitivity reaction-related clinical conditions, like Allergic Bronchopulmonary Mycosis, Allergic Sinusitis and Hypersensitivity Pneumonitis.

Cross-reactivity is common among fungal allergens due to shared homologous B-cell epitopes. Fungal allergens show cross-reactivity not only among members of the same phylum but also among different phyla and among non-fungal phyla too. For example, Enolase is a common fungal allergen that is also found in *Cynodon dactylon* and *Hevea brasiliensis*. Apart from this fungal allergens have also been found to elicit auto-reactivity due to shared epitopes between fungal and human proteins leading to antigenic mimicry. Cross-reactivity between human and fungal proteins has been seen in manganese Superoxide Dismutase, thioredoxin, cyclophilin and acid ribosomal protein P2 (Appenzeller 1999).

The development of pollen allergy among different individuals depends upon diversified risk factors which may be related to the host or environment as allergy is the outcome of host-environment interaction. Host factors include atopy, gender (boys and adult females have more bronchial hyperreactivity), low lung function, smoking and viral infections of the respiratory tract (both upper and lower). Environmental factors include season, annual and diurnal variability, air pollution, environmental temperature, thunderstorms and wind speed. Exacerbation of asthma symptoms has been linked to high ambient pollen counts. Ghosh (2012) has demonstrated that asthma-related health admissions were more than 40% of the annual admission rates during the months of March and September when the pollen counts are higher. "September Epidemic" is also an increase in asthma admissions in countries like Australia and Canada, primarily affecting school children where the synergistic effect of rhinoviral infection and pollen exposure. Kitinoja (2020) estimated that for 10 grains/m^3 increase in pollen exposure, there is a 2% decrease in peak expiratory flow values.

But only exposure to high pollen may not cause hay fever symptoms, as rural areas show a lower prevalence of rhinitis and asthma though the people are exposed to more pollen. So, the dynamic interactions among various factors as stated before needs to be present in order to culminate into the manifestation of clinical allergic disease in a particular individual.

It has been also shown that exposure to various air pollutants increases the airway responsiveness to aeroallergens. The airway mucosal damage caused by air pollutants increases the penetration of aeroallergens into the mucosa and increases the interaction with the immune cells leading to their activation. The gaseous pollutants modify the morphology of the proteins and increase their allergenic potential. Diesel exhaust particles have been shown to cause enhanced IgE responses in atopic individuals. These all lead to increased allergic diseases in urban areas in conjunction with other factors.

Conclusion

Understanding aerobiology is an important aspect for allergists. This helps in choosing the right pollen and fungal allergens for testing in patients with allergic rhinitis or allergic asthma. The progress made in the field of aerobiology is impressive in the last two decades. This has enabled us to understand the prevalence of various allergenic pollens and fungal spores.

The continuing research on the molecular epitopes of the major allergens of pollens and spores is expanding our understanding of the pathologic mechanisms of pollinosis which will help in imparting more refined immunotherapy to patients with respiratory allergic diseases.

Glossary of Abbreviations

Air spora – The population of biological particles present in the air.

Allergen – A substance capable of causing an allergic reaction.

Allergy – A reaction of the body's immune system to the presence of a foreign substance

Bioaerosol – An aerosol of particles of biological origin or activity suspended in the air. Particle size may range from aerodynamic diameters of ca. 0.5 to 100 μm.

Burkard trap – Seven-day recording volumetric spore trap used by many for the daily spore count.

Daily counts – Daily counts of pollen or spores, often for allergy sufferers.
Daily (diurnal) periodicity – The cycle of high and low production of pollen and spores during the day.
Volumetric spore trap – The type of trap with which the volume of air sampled per unit of time is known.

References

Agashe, S. N. 2006. Palynology and its Applications. Oxford and IBH publication Co. Pvt Ltd.

Anand Bahadur Singh and Chandni Mathur. 2012. An aerobiological perspective in allergy and asthma. Asia Pac Allergy 2: 210–222.

Anonymous: All India Coordinated Project on Aeroallergens and Human Health. Report. Ministry of Environment and Forests, New Delhi 2000.

Appenzeller, U., Meyer, C., Menz, G., Blaser, K. and Crameri, R. 1999. IgE-mediated reactions to autoantigens in allergic diseases. Int. Arch. Allergy Immunol. 118: 193–196.

Black, P. N., Udy, A. A. and Brodie, S. M. 2000. Sensitivity to fungal allergens is a risk factor for life-threatening asthma. Allergy 55(5): 501–504.

Brooks, J. P., Gerba, C. P. and Pepper, I. L. 2004. Bioaerosol emission, fate, and transport from municipal and animal wastes. J. Residuals Sci. Technol. 1: 13–25.

Burge, H. A. 1989. Airborne allergenic fungi classification, nomenclature, and distribution. Immunol. Allergy Clin. North Am. 9: 307–319.

Bush, R. K. and Portnoy, J. M. 2001. The role and abatement of fungal allergens in allergic diseases. Journal of Allergy and Clinical Immunology 107(3): S430–S440.

Ghosh, D., Chakraborty, P., Gupta, J., Biswas, A., Roy, I., Das, S. et al. 2012. Associations between pollen counts, pollutants, and asthma related hospital admissions in a high-density Indian metropolis. J. Asthma 49: 792–9.

Gravesen, S., Nielsen, P. A., Iversen, R. and Nielsen, K. F. 1999. Microfungal contamination of damp buildings— examples of risk constructions and risk materials. Environ. Health Perspect. 107(suppl 3): 505–508.

Heiss, S., Fischer, S., Muller, W. D., Weber, B., Hirschwehr, R., Spitzauer, S., Kraft, D. and Valenta, R. 1996. Identification of a 60 kd cross-reactive allergen in pollen and plant-derived food. J. Allergy Clin. Immunol. 98: 938–947.

Hyde, H. A. 1972. Atmospheric pollen and spores in relation to allergy. Clin. Allergy 2: 153–179.

Kitinoja, M. A., Hugg, T. T., Siddika, N., Rodriguez Yanez, D., Jeakkola, M. S. and Jeakkola, J. J. K. 2020. Short-term exposure to pollen and the risk of allergic and asthmatic manifestations: a systematic review and meta-analysis. BMJ Open 10: e029069.

Magyar, D. 2007. Aeromycological aspects of mycotechnology. pp. 226–263. *In*: Rai, M. K. (ed.), Mycotechnology: Current Trends and Future Prospects. New Delhi: I.K. International Publishing House.

Simon-Nobbe, B., Denk, U., Pöll, V., Rid, R. and Breitenbach, M. 2008. The spectrum of fungal allergy. Int. Arch. Allergy Immunol. 145: 58–86.

Singh, A. B. and Kumar, P. 2003. Aeroallergens in clinical practice of allergy in India. An overview. Ann. Agric Environ. Med. 10: 131–136.

Tilak, S. T. and Pande, B. N. 2005. Current trends in aero mycological research. pp. 281–510. *In*: Rai, M. K. and Deshmukh, S. K. (eds.). Fungi: Diversity and Biotechnology. Jogpur: Scientific Publishers.

Wagner, S. and Breiteneder, H. 2002. The latex-fruit syndrome. Biochem. Soc. Trans. 30(Pt 6): 935–40.

Index

About the Editors

Pudupakkam K. Vedanthan

Pudupakkam K. Vedanthan (PK) is the lead editor of the Textbook of Diagnostic and Therapeutic Procedures in Allergy. He is a native of Mysuru, India and a graduate of Government Medical College, University of Mysore. He was awarded the 10th rank in the Pre University Course and distinctions in Physiology, Pharmacology and Pathology. He served as a lecturer in Pathology at his Almamater before moving to USA in 1971. He completed his residency in Pediatrics at Rhode Island Hospital at Brown University and Fellowship in allergy & Immunology at National Asthma Center, Denver, Colorado. He is board certified by the American Boards of Pediatrics and Allergy, Asthma and Immunology. He served for 35 years in Consultation practice in Colorado, as well as maintained academic affiliation with University of Colorado, Denver where he has been a Clinical Professor of Medicine for the past two decades. He has published in both national and international journals and has been active in the academic circle in various capacities. He was the lead editor for the Textbook of Allergy for the clinician published by the CRC Press in 2014 and 2019. He has contributed to Colorado Medical Society (CMS), Association of American Physicians of Indian origin (AAPI) in several capacities. His major contribution has been in Global medicine since he established a medical charity namely 'International Asthma Services (IAS)' (www.saahns.org) in 1992. IAS has been active in several developing countries like India, Sri Lanka, Mauritius, Kenya, Russia, Myanmar, Philippines, Argentina, Nepal conducting CMEs for health professionals and Asthma allergy Awareness camps for patients and their families and public in general. IAS has also partnered with major medical institutions in establishing formal PG diploma courses in allergy, asthma and immunology offered at Vellore Tamil Nadu, Delhi, Kolkata, and Bangalore INDIA and Barbados, West Indies. These courses have been sponsored/endorsed by the American Academy, Asthma & Immunology (AAAAI), and the Center for Global Health, College of Preventive Medicine, University of Colorado at Anschutz campus, Aurora, Colorado, USA. Nearly 1500 specialists have been trained under this program. Dr. PK has also been involved in providing voluntary medical care to the refugee population through Colorado Alliance for Health Education & Promotion (CAHEP), Denver, Colorado for the past three decades. He has also recently initiated the PRAANA Charitable Allergy Asthma clinics Initiative to serve the needy and sick in India, Nepal, Kenya and Barbados. In recognition of these activities, IAS was recognized in 2015 by the Centre for Global Health, School of Public Health, University of Colorado with the prestigious award of 'Excellence in Global health'. He has been the recipient of AAAAI Special recognition award for the year 2021, AMA Leadership award, UCD Distinguished Service award, Rotary 'Service Above Self Award', UCD International Faculty award, Special Innovator award from the department of Medicine, University of Colorado, Denver.

Harold S. Nelson

Dr. Nelson received an undergraduate degree in economics from Harvard College and later earned a doctor of medicine degree from Emory University. He then completed a residency in internal medicine at Letterman General Hospital and a fellowship in allergy/immunology at the University of Michigan. Dr. Nelson has published over 450 articles and book chapters. He has served on the Board of Regents of the American College of Allergy, Asthma, and Immunology (ACAAI), as well as on the Board of Directors of both the American Academy of Allergy, Asthma, and Immunology (AAAAI) and the American Board of Allergy and Immunology (ABAI). He was a member of the First, Second and Third Expert Panels of the NIH—NAEPP for developing the Guidelines for the Diagnosis and Management of Asthma. Dr. Nelson has been honored with the 'Fellow Distinguished Award' and 'Gold-Headed Cane Award' by the ACAAI; the 'Distinguished Clinician Award' 'Special Recognition Award' and 'Distinguished Service Award' by the AAAAI; the 'Outstanding Clinician Award' from the World Allergy Organization and the 'Lifetime Achievement Award' by National Jewish Health. He has also been honored with named 428 Textbook of Allergy for the Clinician lectureships at the annual meetings of the ACAAI 2008–2009, the AAAAI 2001–2013 and the Western Society of Allergy and Immunology 2018–2022.

Hugo P.S. Van Bever

Hugo P.S. Van Bever completed his medical studies at the State University of Ghent, Belgium (1971–1978) and did his training in pediatrics at Children's Hospital, State University of Ghent, Belgium from 1978–1983. Following that he became Resident in Paediatric Allergy and Pulmonology, University of Antwerp, Belgium from 1984–1993, Associate Professor in Paediatric Allergy and Pulmonology, University of Antwerp, Belgium from 1993–1997 and Professor in Paediatric Allergy and Pulmonology, University of Antwerp, Belgium from 1997. From 1997–2001 Hugo Van Bever was also the Head of the Department of Paediatrics, University of Antwerp, Belgium. He joined the National University Singapore as Professor, Senior Consultant, and Head of Paediatric Allergy and Immunology in the Department of Paediatrics in June 2002. Since 2002 he has been an active member of the Board of The Asian Pacific Academy of Paediatric Allergy, Respirology, and Immunology (APAPARI), in which he was responsible for research and education in pediatric allergy, organizing APAPARI workshops in different Asian countries. From 2019 till May 2021, he was the President of APAPARI. He is also a board member of APAAACI and committee member of the Immunotherapy Working Group of WAO. He has been Associate Editor of The European Respiratory Journal (1993–1998). Currently, he is reviewer for The European Journal of Paediatrics, Pediatrics, Paediatric Allergy and Immunology, Allergy, Paediatric Pulmonology, The European Respiratory Journal, Paediatric Research, British Medical Journal, The American Journal of Respiratory and Critical Care Medicine and Archives Diseases of Childhood. Hugo Van Bever defended his PhD thesis successfully in June 1993 at the University of Antwerp. The title of this thesis is: "Late asthmatic reactions in childhood asthma and Influence of specific immunotherapy upon the late asthmatic reaction". He has published more than 350 papers in national and international journals. His current research is focused on eczema, food allergy, allergic rhinitis, sublingual immunotherapy, and primary prevention of allergy. He runs clinics in NUH on pediatric allergy, especially on asthma, allergic rhinitis, eczema, and food allergy.

Mandakolathur R. Murali

Mandakolathur R. Murali M.D. received his undergraduate (MBBS) and postgraduate (MD) degrees in Internal Medicine at Stanley Medical College in Chennai, India. He was the recipient of the Government Gold medal, in both the MBBS and MD, as a recognition of being the best outgoing student of Madras University. He completed a residency in Internal Medicine and a fellowship in Allergy and Clinical Immunology as well as the Assistant training program Director in Allergy and Clinical Immunology at SUNY, Downstate Medical Center in Brooklyn, NY. He is boarded in Internal Medicine, Allergy and Clinical Immunology as well as Diagnostic and Laboratory Immunology. He was a full-time faculty in Allergy and Clinical Immunology at SUNY Brooklyn till 1992, and then served as the Director of Allergy Clinic as well as training program Director in Allergy and Immunology at SUNY Stony Brook in N.Y. Since 2002, he is the Director of Clinical Immunology laboratory at Massachusetts General Hospital, serving as full time faculty in departments of Medicine and Pathology, in the division of Rheumatology, Allergy and Clinical Immunology. He holds the rank of an Assistant Professor of Medicine at Harvard Medical School in Boston. Since 1979 he has been involved in teaching clinical and laboratory medicine to medical students, residents and fellows and has been recognized with several teaching awards at all 3 institutions he has served. He is a senior clinician with expertise in allergic and immunologic disorders and autoimmunity. His research interests and publications include immunopathology of autoimmune diseases, complement disorders, immunodeficiency diseases and evaluation of monoclonal gammopathies. He has been a member of the in-training exam committee of the AAAAI for over 25 years. He has contributed to chapters on immunodeficiency diseases, mechanisms of allergic diseases, complement disorders, cryoglobulins as well as evaluation of autoantibodies in systemic autoimmune diseases.

For Product Safety Concerns and Information please contact our EU
representative GPSR@taylorandfrancis.com
Taylor & Francis Verlag GmbH, Kaufingerstraße 24, 80331 München, Germany